Psychosocial Factors in Pain

Critical Perspectives

ROBERT J. GATCHEL
DENNIS C. TURK

Editors

THE GUILFORD PRESS

New York   London

© 1999 The Guilford Press
A Division of Guilford Publications, Inc.
72 Spring Street, New York, NY 10012
http://www.guilford.com

Printed in the United States of America

This book is printed on acid-free paper.

Last digit is print number: 9 8 7 6 5 4 3 2 1

Library of Congress Cataloging-in-Publication Data

Psychosocial factors in pain: critical perspectives / edited by
   Robert J. Gatchel, Dennis C. Turk.
       p.   cm.
     Includes bibliographical references and index.
     ISBN 1-57230-285-2 (hardcover)
     1. Pain—Psychological aspects. 2. Pain—Social aspects.
   I. Gatchel, Robert J., 1947-   . II. Turk, Dennis C.
     [DNLM: 1. Pain—psychology. 2. Pain—therapy. WL 704 P9748
   1999]
   RB127.P876   1999
   616'.0472—DC21
   DNLM/DLC
   for Library of Congress   98-50870
                                                                  CIP

To Mom, who, having the endless energy to raise five children, instilled in me by example a healthy work ethic and always reminded me of the Beverly Sills quote: "There are no shortcuts to any place worth going."

R. J. G.

In fondest memory of, and sincerest gratitude to, Kenneth S. Bowers, PhD, for nurturing my inquisitive nature, for helping me learn to think critically, and for modeling how to ask the "right" questions.

D. C. T.

About the Editors

Robert J. Gatchel, PhD, received his BA in psychology from the State University of New York at Stony Brook in 1969 and his PhD in clinical psychology from the University of Wisconsin in 1973. Dr. Gatchel is currently the Elizabeth H. Penn Distinguished Professor of Clinical Psychology and Professor in the Departments of Psychiatry and Rehabilitation Science at the University of Texas Southwestern Medical Center at Dallas, where he is the Director of Graduate Research, Division of Clinical Psychology. He is a Diplomate of the American Board of Professional Psychology and is on the Board of Directors of the American Board of Health Psychology. He has conducted extensive clinical research, much of it supported by grants from the National Institutes of Health, on the psychophysiology of stress and emotion, the comorbidity of psychological and physical health disorders, and the etiology, assessment, and treatment of chronic stress and pain behavior. He is also the recipient of a Research Scientist Development Award from the National Institute of Mental Health. He has published over 140 scientific articles and 45 book chapters, and has authored or edited 15 other books, including *Psychological Approaches to Pain Management: A Practitioner's Handbook* (with Dennis C. Turk). He is on the editorial board of numerous psychological and medical journals, and is also the editor of the Research Update section of the *Bulletin of the American Pain Society*.

Dennis C. Turk, PhD, is John and Emma Bonica Professor of Anesthesiology and Pain Research at the University of Washington. He is a founding member and currently serves on the Board of Directors of both the International Association for the Study of Pain (IASP) and the American Pain Society (APS). Dr. Turk was the recipient of the American Psychological Association, Division of Health Psychology, Outstanding Scientific Contribution Award in 1993 and the American Academy of Pain Medicine, Janet Travell Pain Management Award in 1998. Over 250 journal articles, invited papers, and chapters in edited books have been published by Dr. Turk in the areas of pain assessment, treatment, outcomes research, cost-effectiveness analyses, and clinical decision making. He has also written and edited 10 books and served as editor of the *Annals of Behavioral Medicine* from 1993 to 1997.

Contributors

Janet Abrams, PsyD, Division of Clinical Research, Fred Hutchinson Cancer Research Center, and Department of Psychiatry and Behavioral Sciences, University of Washington School of Medicine, Seattle, Washington

Sara M. Banks, MPH, PhD, Department of Anesthesiology, University of Rochester School of Medicine and Dentistry, Rochester, New York

Edward B. Blanchard, PhD, Center for Stress and Anxiety Disorders, University at Albany, SUNY, Albany, New York

Andrew R. Block, PhD, The WellBeing Group, Plano, Texas

Jennifer L. Boothby, MA, Department of Psychology, University of Alabama, Tuscaloosa, Alabama

William Breitbart, MD, Department of Psychiatry and Behavioral Sciences, Memorial Sloan-Kettering Cancer Center, New York, New York

C. Richard Chapman, PhD, Department of Anesthesiology, University of Washington, and Division of Clinical Research, Fred Hutchinson Cancer Research Center, Seattle, Washington

Robert H. Dworkin, PhD, Departments of Anesthesiology and Psychiatry, University of Rochester School of Medicine and Dentistry, Rochester, New York

Samuel F. Dworkin, DDS, PhD, Department of Oral Medicine, School of Dentistry, and Department of Psychiatry and Behavioral Sciences, School of Medicine, University of Washington, Seattle, Washington

Jake Epker, PhD, Division of Psychology, University of Texas Southwestern Medical Center at Dallas, Dallas, Texas

Michael Feuerstein, PhD, Departments of Medical and Clinical Psychology and Preventive Medicine and Biometrics, Uniformed Services University of the Health Sciences, Bethesda, Maryland; Department of Psychiatry, Georgetown University Medical Center, Washington, DC

Herta Flor, PhD, Institute of Psychology, Humboldt University of Berlin, Berlin, Germany

Leticia Y. Flores, PhD, Department of Anesthesiology, University of Washington, Seattle, Washington

Lucia Gagliese, PhD, Department of Psychology, The Toronto Hospital, Toronto, Ontario, Canada

Tara Galovski, MA, Center for Stress and Anxiety Disorders, University at Albany, SUNY, Albany, New York

John Paul Garofalo, PhD, Department of Behavioral Medicine and Oncology, Pittsburgh Cancer Institute, University of Pittsburgh Medical Center, Pittsburgh, Pennsylvania

Steven W. Harkins, PhD, Department of Gerontology, Virginia Commonwealth University, Richmond, Virginia

Kenneth A. Holroyd, PhD, Department of Psychology, Ohio University, Athens, Ohio

Grant D. Huang, BA, Department of Medical and Clinical Psychology, Uniformed Services University of the Health Sciences, Bethesda, Maryland

Mark P. Jensen, PhD, Department of Rehabilitation Medicine, University of Washington, Seattle, Washington

Joel Katz, PhD, Departments of Psychology and Anaesthesia, The Toronto Hospital; Department of Anaesthesia, Mount Sinai Hospital; and Department of Public Health Sciences and Anaesthesia, University of Toronto, Toronto, Ontario, Canada

Francis J. Keefe, PhD, Health Psychology Program, Department of Psychology, Ohio University, Athens, Ohio

Robert D. Kerns, PhD, Psychology Service, VA Connecticut Healthcare System, West Haven, Connecticut; Departments of Psychiatry, Neurology, and Psychology, Yale University, New Haven, Connecticut

Steven J. Linton, PhD, Department of Occupational and Environmental Medicine, Örebro Medical Center, Örebro, Sweden

Gay L. Lipchik, PhD, St. Vincent Health Center, Pain Management Center, Erie, Pennsylvania

Chris J. Main, PhD, Hope Hospital, Salford, United Kingdom; University of Manchester, Manchester, United Kingdom

Ronald Melzack, PhD, Department of Psychology, McGill University, Montreal, Quebec, Canada

Christine Miaskowski, PhD, RN, Department of Physiological Nursing, University of California, San Francisco, San Francisco, California

David B. Morris, PhD, Writer; Adjunct Professor, Department of Medicine, University of New Mexico, Albuquerque, New Mexico

Yoshio Nakamura, PhD, Department of Anesthesiology, University of Washington, and Talaria, Inc., Seattle, Washington

Akiko Okifuji, PhD, Department of Anesthesiology, University of Washington, Seattle, Washington

Peter Polatin, MD, PRIDE/Functional Restoration Associates, Dallas, Texas

Glenn Pransky, MD, MOccH, Department of Family and Community Medicine, Occupational and Environmental Health Program, University of Massachusetts Medical Center, Worcester, Massachusetts

Joseph L. Riley III, PhD, Claude Pepper Center for Research of Oral Health in Aging, College of Dentistry, and Department of Clinical Health Psychology, University of Florida, Gainesville, Florida

Michael E. Robinson PhD, Department of Clinical Health Psychology, University of Florida, Gainseville, Florida

Michael W. Stroud, PhD, Department of Rehabilitation Medicine, University of Washington, Seattle, Washington

Karen L. Syrjala, PhD, Division of Clinical Research, Fred Hutchinson Cancer Research Center, and Department of Psychiatry and Behavioral Sciences, University of Washington School of Medicine, Seattle, Washington

Raymond C. Tait, PhD, Department of Psychiatry, St. Louis University School of Medicine, St. Louis, Missouri

Beverly E. Thorn, PhD, Department of Psychology, University of Alabama, Tuscaloosa, Alabama

Michael Von Korff, ScD, Center for Health Studies, Group Health Co-operative of Puget Sound, Seattle, Washington

Gary A. Walco, PhD, Section of Pediatric Psychology, Hackensack University Medical Center, Hackensack, New Jersey; Department of Pediatrics, New Jersey Medical School, University of Medicine and Dentistry, Newark, New Jersey

James N. Weisberg, PhD, Pain Service, Department of Psychiatry and Behavioral Sciences, SUNY–Stony Brook, Stony Brook, New York

David A. Williams, PhD, Department of Psychiatry, Georgetown University Medical Center, Washington, DC

Preface

Pain has been a central concern to humans since earliest recorded history. The ancient Greeks noted the important role of psychological factors in understanding pain. For example, Aristotle conceptualized pain as an emotion similar to depression and anxiety. He specifically referred to pain as a "quality of the soul." Since that time, the importance of psychological factors in understanding pain has ebbed and flowed over the centuries. Developments in sensory physiology beginning in the 18th century and extending to the present tended to relegate psychological factors to secondary status as mere reactions to nociceptive stimulation. Beginning in the mid-1960s, however, a confluence of ideas and empirical research retrieved psychological factors from the periphery and moved them to a more central position.

Four main developments, each involving psychologists, served as the impetus for what must be viewed as a revolution in thinking about pain. In particular, Ronald Melzack and his colleagues' (Melzack & Casey, 1968; Melzack & Wall, 1965) formulation of the gate control hypothesis emphasized the role of the central nervous system in pain perception and, in particular, the importance of cognitive-evaluative and motivational-affective factors in the experience of pain. The work of John Basmajian, Neal Miller, and Edward Blanchard on voluntary control of the autonomic and somatic nervous systems also demonstrated that psychological factors were capable of influencing physiological activity of particular muscular and vascular factors that have been implicated in several pain syndromes (e.g., back pain, temporomandibular disorders, migraine and tension-type headaches). In addition, Wilbert Fordyce's seminal observations on the role of learning and conditioning factors in communication of pain highlighted the central role played by the environment and contingencies of reinforcement on the maintenance of overt communications of pain, distress, and suffering—"pain behaviors." Fordyce's classic work describing operant conditioning and the treatment of chronic pain was published in 1976. Finally, Dennis Turk, Donald Meichenbaum, and Myles Genest (1983) integrated the insights of Melzack, Miller, and Fordyce into a comprehensive clinical model and approach to treatment that they labeled a "cognitive-behavioral perspective."

The revolution initiated by these four trends has stimulated an explosion of research and subsequent evolution in all aspects of the understanding of pain, as well as serving as the basis for new interventions that are often complementary to traditional biomedical interventions. The evolution of thinking and treatment of pain beginning in the 1960s was quite robust and continues at the present time.

What we have attempted to do in this volume is to provide a status report addressing the question, What is the current state of knowledge regarding the role of psychological factors in pain? We have brought together the major contributors to this revolution and evolution. We asked them to describe their major insights about pain in general and how these are related to specific disorders on the basis of their own research, as well as that of others. We have also asked the authors to project their ideas into the future; that is to say, In what directions do they see the field moving? What are the central questions that remain? and What are the most promising directions for research?

We have divided this volume into three major sections. Part I includes contributions that focus on contextual factors, not only providing a perspective on the contributions of individual factors such as predispositional variables, mood, thought, and consciousness in the experience of pain but also expanding beyond the individual to the sociocultural and religious influences. The dynamic interaction among the individual pain sufferer, his or her sociocultural context, and principles of learning are emphasized in attempts to better understand pain, suffering, and responses to treatment.

Part II includes chapters that address many of the most prevalent pain syndromes. Each contributor provides background on a particular pain syndrome and then describes the role that psychological factors play in the maintenance, exacerbation, or experience of the pain associated with the syndrome. Although there are unique features of each syndrome or disorder, as one reads through these chapters it becomes apparent that there are sufficient commonalties that transcend each one. Health care professionals who target their research or treatment to only one of these syndromes or disorders would do well to review the other chapters for valuable insights that may be applied to particular disorders and syndromes of greatest interest to them.

The final section, Part III, addresses issues relating to prevention and management, including the potentially important role of pain management in primary care settings. The role of psychosocial factors in prediction of response to pain and response to treatment is also covered, as well as the influence of gender. Discussions of evaluation methods on an individual basis, as well as on a program level, are provided. The section ends with our attempt to integrate the material presented throughout the volume with speculations about the future (always a hazardous endeavor).

We believe that the material included in the present volume provides not only a status report but also a guide for the continuing evolution of the field. We trust that the insights of the contributors will serve as a stimulus to researchers and clinical investigators to address many of the pressing needs that still exist in this evolving field. Moreover, we hope that these insights will stimulate clinicians to broaden their perspective and to think more comprehensively about their patients. Finally, this volume should be of considerable interest to specialists in applied pain management and clinical researchers—physicians, dentists, nurses, physical therapists, and chiropractors, as well as psychologists. It should also be of use not only to health care professionals but also to those who are receiving advanced training in undergraduate courses, graduate courses, postdoctoral programs, internships, and residencies.

ROBERT J. GATCHEL
DENNIS C. TURK

REFERENCES

Melzack, R., & Casey, K. L. (1968). Sensory, motivational, and central control determinants of pain: A new conceptual model. In D. Kerschal (Ed.), *The skin senses* (pp.423–443). Springfield, IL: Charles C Thomas.

Melzak, R., & Wall, P. D. (1965). Pain mechanisms: A new theory. *Science, 50,* 971–979.

Turk, D. C., Meichenbaum, D., & Genest, M. (1983). *Pain and behavioral medicine: A cognitive-behavioral perspective.* New York: Guilford Press.

Contents

Part I

BIOPSYCHOSOCIAL CONTEXT

Chapter 1

Perspectives on Pain: A Historical Overview

ROBERT J. GATCHEL

As I have noted elsewhere, the quest to understand and control pain has been a significant human pursuit since earliest recorded history (Gatchel & Turk, 1996). For example, the mention of pain treatment has been found in Egyptian papyri dating back to 4000 BC. Acupuncture therapy, which was used for pain reduction, originated in ancient China almost 2,000 years ago. Temporomandibular joint disorder was recognized in the fifth century BC by Hippocrates, who speculated about its origins and possible treatment (Ruffer, cited in Speculand, Goss, Hughes, Spence, & Pilowsky, 1983). Indeed, as Turk, Meichenbaum, and Genest (1983) have noted, the alleviation of pain is not a recent concern. For example, they provide a cogent illustration of the treatment for pain that Charles II of England was administered:

> Consider the treatment that Charles II of England endured at the hands of the best physicians of his day. A pint of blood was extracted from his right arm, and a half-pint from his left shoulder. This was followed by an emetic, two physics, and an enema comprising 15 substances. Next, his head was shaved and a blister raised. Following in rapid succession were more emetics, sneezing powder, bleedings, soothing potions, a plaster of pitch, and pigeon dung was smeared on his feet. Potions containing ten different substances, chiefly herbs, as well as 40 drops of extract of human skull, were swallowed. Finally, application of bezoar stones (gallstones from sheep and goats) was prescribed. Following this extensive treat-

ment, the king died (Haggard, 1929). Whether death was attributable to a medical condition or iatrogenic complications is unclear. (pp. 75–76)

Turk et al. (1983) also note that in centuries past, peasants in Western cultures often treated pain by impaling the affected area of the body with a "vigorous" twig of a tree, with the assumption that this twig would absorb the pain from the body. Next, in order to prevent other people from getting the pain from that twig, they buried the twig deeply in the ground. Some other early practices for controlling pain were not so "exotic." However, they were frequently crudely applied, even by physicians. In 19th-century America, for example, alcoholic beverages and "medicines" that contained opium were readily available for individuals to use to alleviate pain. In the early 1840s, diethyl ether and chloroform began to be used by surgeons in order to render patients insensate to pain during surgical procedures. Thus, as can be seen, attempts to treat pain have a long history. It was not until the 19th century, however, that there was a concurrent attempt to better understand pain in order to more effectively treat it. In the present chapter, I present a historical overview of these more recent attempts to better understand pain. As is clearly emphasized, the more recent transition from a strict *biomedical reductionist* theory to an integrated *biopsychosocial* approach to understanding pain has led to more effective treatment of this phenomenon that accounts for more than 70 million office visits to physicians each year.

HISTORICAL OVERVIEW OF THE MIND–BODY RELATIONSHIP

The history of understanding the etiology and treatment of pain parallels the historical changes that have occurred in medicine in general (Figure 1.1 presents the sequence of the historical changes that will be discussed). As I have reviewed elsewhere (Gatchel, 1993), the association between the mind and the body has long been controversial among philosophers, physiologists, and psychologists. The perspective that there can be intricate interrelationships between the mind and the body can be found in very ancient literary writings from Babylonia and Greece. Moreover, the ancient Greek physician Hippocrates (400–300 BC) proposed one of the earliest temperamental theories of personality when he hypothesized that four bodily fluids (or what he called "humors") were responsible for specific personality or temperament types, as well as for various physical or mental illnesses. The four proposed humors he hypothesized were blood, black bile, yellow bile, and phlegm. Galen (AD 130–200) subsequently elaborated on Hippocrates' four-humor

theory by proposing that a preponderance of yellow bile was associated with a choleric temperament; an excess of black bile was associated with a melancholic personality type; a preponderance of blood was associated with a sanguine personality type; and an excess of phlegm was associated with the phlegmatic personality type. This four-humor theory remained quite popular until only a few centuries ago. It is a good illustration of how physical and biological factors were viewed through the ages as significantly interacting with and/or directly affecting the personality or psychological status of an individual. It was believed that psychological factors might be significantly associated with bodily diseases and processes.

This historical view of the interaction between mind and body, though, began to lose favor in the 17th century with the advent of physical medicine during the Renaissance. In the Renaissance period, the perspective that the mind (or the soul) influenced the body began to be regarded as unscientific. The goal of understanding the mind and soul was viewed as the purview of religion and philosophy; the understanding of the body was viewed as a separate realm of the growing attraction of physical medicine. This was due to the new wave or approach in the investigation of physical phenomena that emerged during this period. Work based

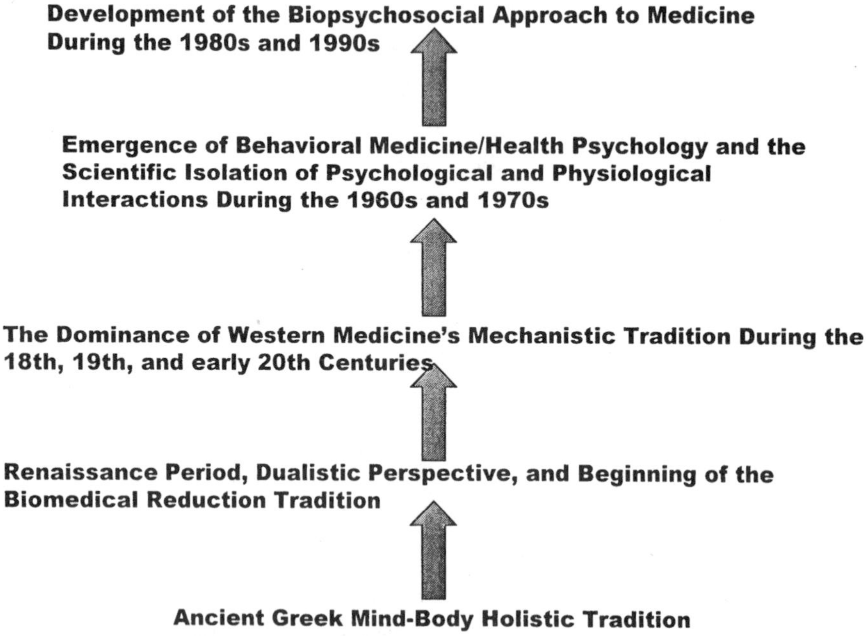

Development of the Biopsychosocial Approach to Medicine During the 1980s and 1990s

⬆

Emergence of Behavioral Medicine/Health Psychology and the Scientific Isolation of Psychological and Physiological Interactions During the 1960s and 1970s

⬆

The Dominance of Western Medicine's Mechanistic Tradition During the 18th, 19th, and early 20th Centuries

⬆

Renaissance Period, Dualistic Perspective, and Beginning of the Biomedical Reduction Tradition

⬆

Ancient Greek Mind-Body Holistic Tradition

FIGURE 1.1. Sequence of the historical changes that have occurred in medicine.

on the dissection of the human body and associated experimentation stimulated a revolution in method toward gaining more knowledge through careful observation, experimentation, and objective quantification rather than relying on common sense, mythology, or outdated dogma. A number of revolutionary works appeared, such as the seminal textbook on anatomy, *De Humani Corporis Fabrica*, which was published in 1543 by the Dutch physician and teacher Andreas Vesalius, and in 1628, the English physician William Harvey discovered that blood circulates in the body and is propelled by the heart.

These influential works marked the advancement of the view that the body can be explained by its own mechanisms. This viewpoint initiated the trend toward a *biomedical reductionism* approach, which argued that concepts such as the mind or soul were not needed to explain physical functioning or behavior. It also stimulated a great revolution in knowledge, with sciences such as anatomy, biology, physiology, and physics evolving simultaneously, all of which were based on the principles of scientific investigation.

Unfortunately, this new mechanistic approach to the study of human anatomy and physiology also fostered a "dualistic" viewpoint that mind and body functioned separately and independently. Before the Renaissance period, physicians had approached the understanding of mind–body interactions in a more holistic way. They also served the multiple roles of philosopher, teacher, priest, and healer. The individual who is usually viewed as popularizing and solidifying this dualistic viewpoint was the 17th-century French philosopher René Descartes (1596–1650). He argued that the mind or soul was a separate entity parallel to, and incapable of affecting, physical matter or somatic processes in any significant or direct way. This dualistic viewpoint gained additional acceptance during the 19th century with the discovery that microorganisms caused certain diseases. This new biomedical reductionism philosophy of medicine became the only acceptable basis for explaining disease through understanding mechanical laws and physiological principles.

Early Theories of Pain

The same medical mechanistic approach to pain was also dominant during the Renaissance period. For example, in 1644, Descartes conceptualized pain as some specific type of activity in the sensory nervous system. He conceived that the pain system was a "straight-through" channel from the skin directly to the brain. He provided the analogy that the system was similar to the bell-ringing mechanism in a church. If an individual pulls the rope at the bottom of the tower, the bell rings in the belfry. Similarly, as he proposed, a flame applied to the foot sets particles in the foot into activity, and that motion is transmitted up the leg and back into the head, where it activates something like an alarm system. The person thus feels the pain and begins to respond to it. As Melzack and Wall (1965) noted, a more formal model of pain was proposed by Von Frey in 1894, which was labeled the *specificity theory of pain*. This theory hypothesized that there were specific sensory receptors responsible for the transmission of sensations such as pain, warmth, touch, and pressure. It was assumed that various sensory receptors had different structures and that these differences made them sensitive to different kinds of stimulation. Pain was perceived as having specific central, as well as peripheral, mechanisms similar to those of other bodily senses.

Melzack and Wall (1965) also point out that at about the same time that Von Frey was proposing his specificity theory of pain, Goldschneider proposed an alternative conceptualization of pain that he labeled the *pattern theory of pain*. Goldschneider contended that pain sensations were the result of the transmission of nerve impulse *patterns* that were produced and coded at the peripheral stimulation site. He proposed that the differences in the patterning and quantity of these peripheral nerve fiber discharges caused the differences in the quality of sensation. For example, a minimal tactile stimulus to an area might cause a feeling of touch, whereas a stronger pattern of tactile stimuli could cause pain. He further argued that if the same nerve fibers were stimulated and discharged, then the difference in sensation had to be due to an increased discharge. This pattern of stimulation that was produced by a specific stimulus then had to be coded by the central nervous system. Thus, the experience of pain resulted from central nervous system coding of nerve impulse patterns and was not simply the result of a specific connection between pain receptors and pain sites.

As has been noted elsewhere (Baum, Gatchel, & Krantz, 1997), subsequent research has demonstrated that the aforementioned two theories were not sufficient to explain pain, even though there has been some level of support reported for each. More important, a number of reported findings cannot be accounted for by either theory. Many of these findings have indicated that psychological factors such as anxiety can significantly affect the pain experienced from a noxious stimulus. Bonica (1953) had earlier documented the shortcomings of both of these purely mechanistic theories of pain.

By this time, the strict mechanistic, dualistic approach of medicine began to mellow because of the influential initial work of Sigmund Freud (1856–1939) in Europe. Freud emphasized the potential interaction of psychological and physical factors in various disorders. In the United States, Benjamin Rush (1745–1813) wrote the first textbook on psychiatry in 1812, which highlighted the fact that "actions of the mind" were possible causes of many diseases and that treatment of such "actions of the mind" might be medically beneficial. Although the major emphasis in medicine was still on the role that the body, microorganisms, and physiological factors had in determining disease, medicine gradually became aware of other significant influences, such as the psychological state of the patient. The concept of "psychogenesis," or the belief that psychological factors could affect bodily processes in some way, gradually began to be resurrected.

Subsequently, the 20th century further evidenced a great deal of growth in the acceptance of an integrated, holistic approach to health and illness, especially because of the advent of modern psychiatry and psychology. The principal area for this integration was in a new field of medicine that came to be known as *psychosomatic medicine*. As I have noted elsewhere (Gatchel, 1993), this field of psychosomatic medicine underwent a great deal of change during the 1950s because of disenchantment with the psychoanalytic principles that were the major theoretical driving force in the field. Dissatisfaction with the psychodynamic formulations used to explain how psychological processes interacted with bodily functioning to produce disease led to the emergence of a more objective and scientifically based behavioral-cognitive approach to the field in the 1970s. This change was stimulated by the formation of, and rapid growth in, the area of health psychology/behavioral medicine. This specialty, which was responsible for developing a scientifically acceptable bridge between psychology and medicine, produced some of the most systematic and scientifically rigorous research yet done to demonstrate the importance of understanding the interaction of psychological and physiological processes that could result in disease and illness behavior (see Baum, Gatchel, & Krantz, 1997). A more comprehensive *biopsychosocial* model of ill-

ness was proposed that emphasized the unique interactions of biological, psychological, and social factors that need to be taken into account for a better understanding of health and illness.

This trend toward a more comprehensive biopsychosocial approach to illness that was occurring in medicine in general was paralleled by a similar approach to the understanding of pain. This synergy in developing a more comprehensive understanding of pain first began to emerge with some preliminary work that demonstrated the importance of the psychological status of a person in determining his or her response to pain. For example, Beecher (1956) reported a classic investigation in which he studied wounded soldiers returning from battle during World War II. Beecher evaluated requests for painkilling medications by soldiers taken to combat hospitals following wounds received in combat at the Battle of Anzio. The soldiers' requests were compared with those made by civilians with comparable surgical wounds. Beecher found that only 25% of the combat-wounded soldiers actively requested medication and that the majority of the soldiers either denied having pain from their extensive wounds or reported that they had so little pain that they did not think medication was necessary. In striking contrast, the civilians with similar wounds from surgery experienced much more pain, with greater than 80% requesting pain medication. These reports were interpreted by Beecher as suggesting that psychological factors, such as a person's emotional state and secondary gain, could significantly affect pain. "Secondary gain" refers to a benefit of being sick or in pain, such as receiving more attention or not having to go back to an uncomfortable situation or environment. In the case of Beecher's investigation, the secondary gain was most likely experienced by soldiers who were allowed to leave the aversive, life-threatening combat zone environment because of their wounds, which would probably allow them to eventually be sent home.

The Gate Control Theory of Pain

Since this pioneering study by Beecher (1956), numerous studies have demonstrated the importance of how the psychological state of an individual can affect the perception of pain (see Baum, Gatchel, & Krantz, 1997). The major theory that had the greatest influence on the subsequent acceptance of the fact that there was a close interaction between psychological and physiological processes and pain was that of Melzack and Wall (1965). They introduced the *gate control theory* of pain to take into account the many diverse factors involved in pain perception. Although their initial theory had limitations, its major contribution was introducing the scientific community to the importance of central and psychological factors in the pain-perception process. It also highlighted the potentially significant role that psychological factors played in the perception of pain (Melzack, 1993).

Melzack and Wall's theory assumed that there were a number of structures within the central nervous system that significantly contributed to pain. They theorized that the interplay among these structures was critical in determining whether and to what extent specific stimuli lead to pain. They argued that pain was not a result of a "straight-through" transmission of impulses from the skin surface to the brain. Rather, this pathway was much more complex, involving considerable opportunity for the alteration of incoming pain signals by other sensations, even by descending inhibiting impulses from higher brain centers. This theory represented a major advance in our conceptualization of pain because it was comprehensive enough to take into account the evidence that suggested specific types of pain receptors, as well as allowing for the possibility that pain stimulation and transmission might occur in patterns of sensations. Moreover, it provided for the potentially significant role that "downward" central nervous system mediation could play in pain perception. Thus, the door was opened to the possibility of such downward mediation being psychological in nature. It also partially took into account different types of pain, as well as the different effects of time on the pain process (Fordyce & Steger, 1979). It viewed pain as a complex set of phenomena rather than as a simple specific or discrete entity and converged nicely with the biopsychosocial approach to medicine that began to emerge during the 1970s and 1980s. Of course, clinical researchers do not view the original gate control theory proposed by Melzack and Wall (1965) as comprehensively accounting for the etiology, evaluation, and treatment of pain. As new understanding of pain neurophysiology, neurotransmission, and endogenous opioids increases, a more refined model will naturally evolve over time.

The Biopsychosocial Model of Pain

The major contribution of this biopsychosocial model of pain has been a movement away from the traditional descriptions of pain in purely physiological terms. In the past, there was a tendency to view organic pain as a different type of pain from psychogenic pain. The term "psychogenic" was used to suggest that the pain was due to psychological causes only, that it was "all in the patient's head," and that it was not "real" pain because a specific organic basis for it could not be found. This was an unfortunate perspective, and its perpetuation by a purely mechanistic approach in medicine as a myth hindered the development of good pain management strategies. Today, fortunately, it is now accepted that psychogenic pain is not experienced any differently than pain that arises from clearly delineated injury or tissue damage. Psychogenic and organic pain both hurt equally! Moreover, the assessment or diagnosis of organically caused pain does not rule out the important role that psychological factors can play for any particular patient. Indeed, as is clear from the discussion of the gate control theory of pain, the experience of pain may be produced by psychological factors through a hypothesized central control trigger mechanism that descends to the periphery.

This acceptance of a biopsychosocial perspective on pain occurred gradually, as did its acceptance in medicine as a whole. Indeed, conventional medicine has always been slow to change. For example, the Scottish physician James Linn (1716–1794) developed a method for preventing scurvy (caused by a prolonged deficiency of vitamin C, or ascorbic acid, in the diet) in sailors. However, his prevention method (introducing citrus fruits such as lime juice into the diet) was not accepted as a standard medical prevention method by the British navy for more than 40 years. Similarly, the work of the Hungarian obstetrician Igraz Semmelweis (1818–1865), which introduced the concept of antiseptic prophylaxis, was not accepted by medicine for more than 30 years. Semmelweis, who worked in a maternity ward of the Vienna General Hospital, observed that pregnant women, examined in a particular ward by student doctors (who had not washed their hands after performing cadaver autopsy dissections), demonstrated much greater infection and subsequent mortality rates from bacterial infections relative to women who were examined by midwives in another ward. In fact, there was almost a 400% difference in infection rates between the two wards. Semmelweis subsequently ordered all the doctors to wash their hands with chlorinated lime before examining patients; this measure resulted in maternal mortalities falling from about 12% to 1%. Nevertheless, he encountered major opposition from hospital officials because of his "unorthodox" antiseptic practices. He was subsequently released from his duties at that hospital and was discharged from three other hospitals. It was not until much later that his "washing hands of germs" before treating patients became an accepted medical practice. This "germ theory" of disease was later advocated by Louis Pasteur.

Finally, as another example of how medicine can be slow in accepting a new theory or approach, even if it is proposed by a distinguished scientist, is the case of rabies vaccine treatment. The world-renowned French chemist and biologist Louis Pasteur (1822–1895) spent the last years of his life conducting research on rabies. His theory about the cause of rabies, as well as the treatment, was not accepted by medicine for more than 30 years. Thus, this serves as another example of how slow conventional medicine changes in response to any new "unconventional" idea or concept.

The Recent Advent of Chaos Theory

It should also be noted that Kossman and Bullrich (1997) review the development of a new scientific discipline called "General Systems Theory," initially proposed by von Bertalanffy (1969). This theory proposed that the study of systems requires the understanding of the dynamics of the "whole" rather than a traditional reductionistic analysis of its parts. Before this time, the biomedical reductionistic approach, using logical empiricism, was unquestionably embraced because the dominant scientific perspective was that there was an objectively verifiable set of principles that can be delineated in order to understand all human functioning, as well as the universe as a whole. However, as Perna and Masterpasqua (1997) have pointed out, with the advent of quantum physics at the beginning of the century and its acceptance of "uncertainty" as an important component of the scientific discovery process, a new scientific paradigm has been stimulated. Philosophers of science such as Kellert (1993), theoretical biologists (e.g., Goodwin, 1994), and mathematicians (e.g., Stewart, 1989) have emphasized that unpredictability and "chaos" are important aspects in understanding how dynamic systems evolve and are often nonlinear in nature. *Chaos theory* in science is a revolutionary new way of conceptualizing the world. It is helping to explain many, until now, unexplainable phenomena in biology, chemistry, and phys-

ics that could not be easily accounted for by a simple reductionistic linear model or approach to science and medicine. In nonlinear systems, even minor external changes (or differences in inputs) can lead to major differences in reactivity and temporary "chaos" in the system (or differences in output). Such chaotic system states are not predictable, but they are stable in their irregular patterns over time. Thus, acceptable scientific method will continue to evolve in medicine, including the area of pain, as new phenomena are unveiled.

THE SIGNIFICANT CLINICAL CONTRIBUTIONS OF WILBERT FORDYCE

Wilbert Fordyce has been one of the leading investigators in the field involving the psychosocial variables that influence the experience of chronic pain (see Fordyce, Roberts, & Sternbach, 1985). Fordyce was especially influential in the field by pointing out the importance of the behavioral assessment and treatment of chronic pain. He cogently argued that it is not enough to simply evaluate and attempt to modify an individual's subjective experience of pain. Rather, one must comprehensively evaluate pain *behavior*, which involves not only what the patient is verbalizing but also the patient's actual observable functioning. This led to the development of the prototypic pain clinic during the 1960s. As Fordyce et al. (1985) have emphasized:

> Behavioral methods for treating pain problems (chronic pain behaviors) are not intended to "treat pain" in the traditional sense in which this implies directing attention to sources and mechanisms of noxious stimuli generating injury signals which lead to "pain." Behavioral pain methods do *not* have as their principal objective the modification of nociception, nor the direct modification of the experience of pain, although it very frequently happens that both are influenced by these methods. Rather, *behavioral methods* in pain-treatment programs are *intended to treat excess disability and expressions of suffering.* . . . The goal is to render chronic pain patients functional again and as normal in behavior as possible. (p. 115)

Fordyce noted that one of the major problems with traditional medical treatment and theoretical approaches to chronic pain was too great a focus on the mere subjective experience of pain. A distinction had to be made between "pain" (i.e., the subjective experience) and *pain behavior*, or behavioral functioning. The emphasis was placed on focusing on observable and objectively evaluated functioning or behavior, along with self-report, in order to comprehensively assess chronic pain behavior. Thus, pain, similar to any other form of complex behavior, must be thought of as having multiple behavioral components.

There have been many self-report instruments developed for measuring the subjective component of pain. For example, the McGill Pain Questionnaire (Melzack, 1975) was devised to evaluate chronic pain. This scale allowed for the evaluation of both self-reported quantitative, as well as qualitative, aspects of pain. There have been numerous other self-report tests and measures of pain. Williams (1988) and Jensen and Karoly (1992) have provided comprehensive reviews of many of these other self-report tests and measures. However, taking the lead from Fordyce and colleagues, many pain clinicians became wary of relying solely on self-report measures because of potential reporting biases in these measures. They, therefore, developed additional ways of evaluating pain behaviors that could be observed and objectively measured by independent raters. Such alternative ways of measuring pain include the use of observation of various pain behaviors, such as bracing, grimacing, lying down, and so forth. The need for standardizing such "objective" indices of pain has led to the development of various taxonomies of pain behavior such as the one developed by Follick, Ahern, and Aberger (1985). They delineated operational definitions for 16 common pain behaviors: asymmetry, slow response time, guarded movement, limping, bracing, personal contact, position shifts, partial movement, absence of movement, eye movement, grimacing, quality of speech, pain statements, limitation statements, sounds, and pain-relief devices. Keefe and Williams (1992) have provided a review of the process involved in the assessment of such pain behaviors.

The above development and use of pain behavior measures helped to reinforce the biopsychosocial approach to pain that Turk comprehensively reviews in Chapter 2 of this volume. Indeed, the focus on behavioral or physiological measures rather than on simple self-report indices does not necessarily yield a more valid or reliable measure of a person's pain than does a simple self-report (Fernandez & Turk, 1992). Pain is a complex behavior and not purely a sensory event. One needs to consider its multiple components—self-report, observable behavior, and physiological indices—in the comprehensive assessment and treatment of

this behavior. Thus, as noted by Fordyce (1988), pain is different from suffering (the former causing the latter), and although it is caused by real or imagined injury or tissue damage, it is separable from that injury and not simply the sum of all damage to bodily tissues. Psychosocial factors can significantly affect the sensation of pain and the subsequent display of pain behaviors.

THE DEVELOPMENT OF BIOPSYCHOSOCIAL PAIN TREATMENT METHODS

Comprehensive Operant Conditioning: The Initial Establishment of the Pain Clinic

Fordyce and Steger (1979) differentiated between two basic types of inpatient strategies generally employed in pain clinics: (1) a "pure" operant or behavioral treatment program in which reinforcement methods for "well behavior" are the major components in the treatment program; and (2) "mixed" behavioral and other treatment programs in which treatment involves strategies other than simple reinforcement for "well behavior." Other strategies might include support group discussion with other patients, relaxation and placebo methods, and family therapy approaches that are not related to direct pain behavior management. The prototype of the "pure" operant conditioning pain treatment program was initially developed by Fordyce and colleagues at the University of Washington's Department of Rehabilitation Medicine (Fordyce, Fowler, Lehman, & De Lateur, 1968). This program, which involved a 4- to 8-week inpatient period designed to gradually increase the general activities of daily living and socialization of the patient, as well as a decrease in medication usage, was based on the assumption that although pain may initially result from some underlying organic pathology, environmental consequences (such as attention of the patient's family and the rehabilitation staff) can significantly modify and further maintain various aspects of pain behavior. As discussed above, such pain behaviors may consist of complaining, grimacing, bracing, requesting pain medication, and so forth. In viewing pain as an operant behavior, Fordyce and colleagues assumed that the consequences, such as concern and attention from others, rest, medication, and avoidance of unpleasant responsibilities and duties, would frequently reinforce the maladaptive pain behaviors and, therefore, hinder a patient's progress in treatment.

In their operant treatment program, Fordyce and coworkers systematically controlled environmental events such as attention, rest, and medication and made these events contingent on adaptive behaviors such as increased activity, socialization, and so forth. The major goal of the program was to increase such behaviors as participation in therapy and activity level while simultaneously decreasing or eliminating pain behaviors. Members of the patients' families were actively involved in the treatment program and worked closely with the rehabilitation staff. They were taught to react to the patient's behavior in a manner that would reduce pain and maximize the patient's compliance with the rehabilitation program. Throughout this operant program approach, the patient was taught to reinterpret the sensation of pain and to tolerate it while performing more adaptive behaviors that would gain the attention and approval of others. Such a program was initially conducted in the hospital and later continued on an outpatient basis.

A major feature of this program was the reduction in the amount of pain medication used by these chronic pain patients. This was seen as important for reducing the possibility of addiction and habituation of the analgesic medication, thereby reducing the patient's general dependence on drugs. Often, medication was provided on a p.r.n., or as-needed, basis. Unfortunately, the medication would then be contingent on the very pain behavior that the rehabilitation staff wanted to decrease (e.g., complaints of pain, requests for medication, etc.). Such a reinforcement system would therefore inadvertently increase various pain behaviors. In order to avoid such a problem, the delivery of medication was made contingent on the passage of time rather than on patients' pain behavior. Fordyce developed intervals between pain medication delivery that gradually increased during the treatment program. Moreover, the medication itself was presented to the patient in the form of a liquid that masked the color and taste of the medication (such as cherry syrup or Robitussin). It was found that, over a period of approximately 2 months, the dosage level of the medication in this "pain cocktail" was gradually decreased until the patient was given only the masking liquid without an active ingredient. The patient and the patient's family were informed of this medication-reduction procedure either before or after the medication had been eliminated.

This type of comprehensive operant conditioning program was shown to produce significant decreases in the patients' complaints of pain and in the use of analgesic medication (Fordyce & Steger, 1979). Subsequently, many pain clinics were developed throughout the country using the operant conditioning procedures that were first introduced by Fordyce and colleagues. Sanders (1996) has provided an excellent review of the current use of operant conditioning procedures in the management of chronic pain.

Cognitive-Behavioral Treatment Approaches

During the 1960s and 1970s, while Fordyce's prototypic pain clinic was being widely adopted, the field of clinical psychology was simultaneously developing a number of effective cognitive-behavioral treatment procedures that were employed with a host of problem behaviors such as anxiety, depression, inappropriate social behaviors, and so forth. Subsequently, the application of these approaches, modified to adapt their use to medical settings and to provide new ways of reducing distress and enhancing psychological adjustment in medical patients, became a hallmark of the growing field of health psychology. An important attribute of these cognitive-behavioral interventions was the fact that they were empirically based and tested, and emphasized the patients' ability to help themselves rather than depending on the therapist to "take care" of them. As Baum, Gatchel, and Krantz (1997) have highlighted, in the area of disease management alone, various cognitive-behavioral interventions have demonstrated efficacy in the reduction of pain, the control of essential hypertension, the management of depression and other emotional disturbances, and the management of various symptoms and medical-procedure-related distress, as well as in increasing compliance and quality of life. We have also pointed out that "even though contemporary therapeutic approaches have been divided into those that primarily emphasize 'behavior' and those that emphasize 'cognitions,' they are quite similar. Moreover, there is empirical support for the treatment efficacy of both approaches. The real problem confronting the practitioner at this point in time is selecting from among the wide range of these very promising and effective cognitive and behavioral approaches" (Baum, Gatchel, & Krantz, 1997, p. 294). These cognitive-behavioral therapy techniques include the following: systematic desensitization, progressive muscle relaxation, modeling, behavior rehearsal, contingency management, stimulus-control techniques, cognitive restructuring, self-control techniques, and comprehensive stress-management programs.

Lazarus (1971) initially coined the term "broad-spectrum behavior therapy" to highlight the fact that most therapists utilize several different treatment procedures for a specific disorder in order to deal effectively with all the important controlling or causal variables. The term "broad-spectrum cognitive-behavioral therapy" is now used to emphasize again that therapists use several different cognitive-behavioral treatment methods for a specific disorder in order to deal with all of the potentially multiple factors that are contributing to the disorder. There are a number of excellent books that comprehensively review these cognitive-behavioral techniques (e.g., Dattilio & Freeman, 1994). Indeed, the availability of a host of different treatment methods gives broad-spectrum cognitive-behavioral therapy a major advantage over traditional forms of treatment for a disorder.

In the area of pain management, broad-spectrum cognitive-behavioral therapy has also been applied. As Bradley (1996) cogently notes, all of these interventions share a common set of theoretical assumptions pertaining to the interactions among environmental events, cognitions, and behaviors that interact to determine a patient's subjective pain perceptions and overt displays of pain. This particular broad-spectrum approach directly evolved from the development of this approach to psychiatric disorders and to addressing health psychology issues. Table 1.1 delineates the goals of

TABLE 1.1. The Four Major Objectives of Cognitive-Behavioral Therapy

1. Help patients alter their beliefs that their problems are unmanageable; that is, help them to become resourceful problem solvers instead of individuals with little hope of coping effectively with their pain, emotional distress, and other psychosocial difficulties.

2. Help patients to learn to monitor their thoughts, emotions, and behaviors to identify relationships among these factors and environmental events, pain, emotional distress, and psychosocial difficulties.

3. Help patients learn to perform behaviors at appropriate times to cope effectively with pain, emotional distress, and psychosocial difficulties.

4. Help patients develop and maintain increasingly effective and adaptive ways of thinking, feeling, and responding that can be used to cope with problems that may be experienced after treatment termination.

Note. From Bradley (1996, p. 134). Copyright 1996 by The Guilford Press. Reprinted by permission.

broad-spectrum cognitive-behavioral therapy that Bradley (1996) described in effectively dealing with chronic pain patients.

The efficacy of these approaches has been demonstrated for patients with a variety of pain-related disorders (cf. Bradley, 1996), as well as a wide range of psychophysiological disorders (cf. Gatchel & Blanchard, 1993). As Bradley (1996) notes, research efforts are now being devoted toward providing patients with relapse-prevention training throughout the administration of cognitive-behavioral therapy in the hopes of showing that such interventions can produce long-term reductions in pain perceptions and behaviors. Finally, Gatchel and Turk (1996) have provided a comprehensive review of the various psychological approaches to pain management that are now being employed.

Multidisciplinary/Interdisciplinary Approaches to Pain Management

Springing from the tradition of the prototypic pain clinic developed by Fordyce in the 1960s, as well as from the growing acceptance of a biopsychosocial perspective on chronic pain, multidisciplinary treatment programs started to develop a reputation as the most effective method of comprehensively treating chronic pain patients. These multidisciplinary programs represent what Fordyce referred to as "mixed" programs, in contrast to the "pure" operant or behavioral treatment program he initially developed. These programs employ a host of the various cognitive-behavioral approaches reviewed earlier, as well as approaches from other disciplines such as physical therapy and occupational therapy. At the outset, it should be clearly noted that the term "multidisciplinary pain clinic" refers to those clinics in which multiple disciplines are utilized for assessment and treatment. However, many of the disciplines are not necessarily housed "under one roof" but are used on a consultant basis. In contrast, an "interdisciplinary treatment program" signifies that all of the specialties are housed under one roof, which maximizes clear and immediate communication among the various disciplines. With that slight, but sometimes significant, difference in mind, it should be noted that Gatchel and Turk (see Chapter 27, this volume) have provided a comprehensive review of these specialty pain treatment facilities. The philosophy of such clinics is that complex pain behaviors can be more effectively managed by a multidisciplinary team, with each team member contributing his or her specialized knowledge and skills to the common goals of making a correct diagnosis and of developing the most effective therapeutic strategy tailored for a particular patient. The philosophy is that patients with complex pain conditions can be best served by a team of specialists with different health care backgrounds. Moreover, it is accepted that the complaint of pain is not just the result of some bodily damage but also has an array of cognitive, affective, and environmental origins as well. A major aim is to improve the patient's physical performance and coping skills, thereby allowing a transfer of control of pain and the management of its related problems from the therapist back to the individual patient. Treatments are designed to increase functional ability so that the patient can make appropriate changes in quality of life, environmental stressors, and various psychosocial factors such as self-esteem and mood, all of which will assist in pain control and management.

The multidisciplinary treatment team, as noted by Gatchel and Turk (in Chapter 27, this volume), consists of a core group of professionals. This core group and their roles are delineated in Table 1.2. The general body of scientific literature available

TABLE 1.2. Core Group of Professionals and Their Roles in a Multidisciplinary Treatment Program

Physician: Deals with the medical issues involved in the diagnosis and management of anatomical, pathological, and physiological processes related to pain complaints.

Nurse: Obtains patient histories, evaluates lifestyle issues that may affect patients, and assists in the monitoring and/ or the tapering of medications.

Physical therapist: Conducts comprehensive musculoskeletal evaluations involving the assessment of range of motion and strength, the examination of gait and postural abnormalities, the examination of sensation and reflexes, and the performance of neurological tests; coordinates a physical rehabilitation program.

Occupational therapist: Performs physical capacity evaluations and job assessments; provides evaluations prior to treatment and at termination that focus on body mechanics and energy conservation in activities of daily living, work, and leisure.

Psychologist: Evaluates current psychosocial functioning, personality, social and relationship functioning, mental status, and so forth that help to determine whether there are any significant "barriers" to rehabilitation; provides treatment to help patients progress through the program.

has provided evidence that such multidisciplinary pain clinics can significantly improve the overall functioning of chronic pain sufferers (see Chapter 27, this volume). These improvements have been shown on various outcome criteria—such as return to work, change in medication use, subsequent utilization of the health care system, and resolution of litigation cases—not simply on changes in self-report of pain and disability (see Chapter 27, this volume). In striking contrast, patients who have to rely on conventional medical support appear to languish and even show deterioration. The cost savings of multidisciplinary treatment programs have also been found to be quite significant. Thus, the close integration of professionals composing a multidisciplinary team that has a comprehensive biopsychosocial perspective on pain has been shown to be the most likely treatment of choice for chronic pain. This again demonstrates the significant improvement in medical, as well as pain, treatment outcomes when one moves away from the traditional reductionistic biomedical view of disease and health.

Functional Restoration Treatment

During the last decade, an even more effective and comprehensive interdisciplinary approach to chronic musculoskeletal pain, *functional restoration*, has been developed. The term "functional restoration" refers not only to the basic treatment methodology for chronic musculoskeletal pain patients but also to a broader conceptualization of the entire pain problem, its diagnosis, and its management. This approach does not simply accept current limits in history taking based solely on patients' self-reports of pain and on diagnoses through skeletal imaging technology but involves more objective quantification of functioning. Structured interviews and quantified self-report measures, as well as objective assessment of physical capacity and effort, has added a new dimension to diagnosis. This approach is modeled after a sports medicine approach, which permits the development of treatment programs of varied intensity and duration aimed primarily at restoring physical functional capacity and social performance. Besides the simple alteration of pain complaints, the objectives of this approach are more far-reaching, including decreasing medication, improvement in quality of life, increasing physical capacity, and decreasing social problems associated with chronic pain. A focus on realistic goals, such as returning patients back to work and reducing the use of the medical care system, has already helped to change the focus of traditional treatment programs, as well as the criteria for evaluation of effectiveness. This orientation emphasizes function. This is in keeping with the tradition of Fordyce in emphasizing that it is not enough to simply evaluate and modify an individual's subjective experience of pain. Rather, one must comprehensively evaluate pain behavior that involves not only what the patient is verbalizing but also his or her actual functioning. There has been a great deal of research demonstrating the clinical efficacy of functional restoration in managing chronic musculoskeletal pain disability (e.g., Hazard, 1995; Mayer & Gatchel, 1988).

Alternative/Complementary Medicine Approaches

In a seminal survey study conducted by Eisenberg, Kessler, Foster, Norlock, Calkins, and Delbanco (1993) on the use of alternative medicine approaches in the United States, published in *The New England Journal of Medicine*, there were some striking data reported on the prevalence, cost, and patterns of use of such "unconventional" medicine in the United States. Findings from this national survey revealed that an estimated 60 million Americans used alternative medical therapies in 1990 at an estimated cost of $13.7 billion. Moreover, the estimated number of annual visits to providers of alternative medicine amounted to 425 million visits, which far exceeded the number of visits to all primary care physicians in the United States (388 million visits). In addition, it was found that 70% of patients who acknowledged using alternative therapy never mentioned it to their physicians. These data stimulated a great deal of attention and debate concerning this "invisible mainstream" that exists within the U.S. health care system. More recently, there has been a national trend for third-party payers to authorize alternative therapies in the form of "expanded benefits." Eisenberg (1997) has further elaborated on this trend.

The term "alternative medicine" often seems to have an antagonistic or oppositional quality when it is encountered by those who embrace conventional medicine. However, it should *not* be viewed in this light. This is why the term "behavioral medicine," which is widely embraced in the field today, has not developed a threatening connotation. Alternative medicine is also a nonoppositional new area *within* medicine. In fact, some prefer to use the terms "complementary medicine"

or "integrative medicine." All three terms simply imply a new area within medicine that is gaining a groundswell of support in the general population, as well as developing a scientific basis that is starting to grow and to demonstrate significant contributions to medicine. Indeed, the National Institutes of Health now has an Office of Alternative Medicine to help stimulate new research in this area. However, as noted earlier in discussing the work of Pasteur, Linn, and Semmelweis, conventional medicine has been historically slow in embracing new concepts and treatment approaches.

There are many misconceptions about alternative medicine. Often it is viewed as some type of voodoo or "fringe medicine." In fact, however, this is far from the truth. Also, as indicated above, it is viewed as a threat to traditional medicine; that is, individuals erroneously think that they need to choose between conventional/traditional medicine and alternative medicine. Again, this is not the case. Alternative or complementary medicine is an important area within medicine. It is simply a continuation of the tradition of medicine to incorporate new approaches that have been demonstrated to be efficacious based on scientific research. For example, therapies based on herbs have been used to treat pain for hundreds of years. Ingesting an extract from poppy seeds (opiates) or from willow bark (aspirin), as well as applying a local anesthetic such as the extract of coca leaves (cocaine), have a long tradition in pain management. The Chinese practice of acupuncture also has a long history. Moreover, a committee of medical experts selected by the National Institutes of Health has recently concluded that there is now clear evidence that acupuncture can be effectively used to treat pain after surgery or dental procedures, as well as to control nausea and vomiting caused by chemotherapy or pregnancy. We must always remember the symbol of medicine, the caduceus of Hermes (Figure 1.2). As we develop new knowledge of a

CADUCEUS OF HERMES

KNOWLEDGE AND WISDOM

FIGURE 1.2. Caduceus of Hermes.

particular area, we also have to concurrently develop the wisdom to apply this knowledge appropriately. We are now on the brink of developing a new knowledge base within medicine, and, therefore, we also need to start to develop the wisdom to incorporate it appropriately within our clinical practice and research endeavors.

Various alternative medicine approaches are starting to be used for the treatment of pain. Berman and Swyers (1998) have recently reviewed research on the efficacy of alternative medicine therapies, such as acupuncture, chiropractic, and various mind–body techniques for treating various chronic pain syndromes. One of the traditional approaches has been biofeedback. It should be noted that many times these approaches cannot be used as the sole treatment modality. Rather, they can be effectively used as "complementary" approaches to be used with other conventional approaches. Other alternative or complementary approaches that are being used in the area of pain management include herbalism, hypnosis, and massage therapy. For those readers who are interested in further reviews of alternative or complementary medicine, there is a growing list of publications, including Rosenfeld (1996), Micozzi (1996), and Lewith, Kenyon, and Lewis (1996). For the specific area of pain treatment, Davis (1997) has presented a number of alternative/complementary modalities that can be employed by physical therapists and other health care professionals in the management of chronic pain patients.

PHYSIOLOGICAL UNDERPINNINGS OF PAIN

The development of more effective psychological approaches to pain management (c.f. Gatchel & Turk, 1996) has not dampened the efforts to better understand the neurophysiological and neurogenic factors of basic nociception processes. Indeed, there has been much recent research demonstrating a number of different structures within the nervous system that appear to be involved in pain. The term "nociceptor" has replaced the much older term "pain receptor" in order to emphasize the fact that these sensory units contribute to, rather than create, the pain experience. Nociceptors, which are nerve endings that transmit pain, are specialized transducer-like units that terminate in the skin, muscle, deep tissues, and viscera. Various groups of peripheral nerve fibers involved in nociception

have been delineated, such as A-delta and C fibers. There has also been a great deal of work on neurochemical bases of pain during this decade. For example, there has been an expanding interest in endogenous opiate-like substances that compose a neurochemically based internal pain-regulation system, such as *beta-endorphins*, *proenkaphalins*, and *prodynorphins*. These chemicals are similar to morphine and other opiates in their pain-reducing characteristics, but they are produced inside the body in many parts of the brain and glands and are assumed to play a significant role in pain reduction. Thus, there is a continuation of scientific work aimed at delineating the underlying physiological bases of pain. However, this is not being done in ignorance of the fact that psychosocial processes can interact in a significant way in the physiological underpinnings of pain. As discussed earlier, the gate control theory of Melzack and Wall stimulated interest in the importance of taking into account a more comprehensive psychophysiological approach to the etiology of pain. The chapter by Melzack (Chapter 6) in this book presents an interesting insight into the importance of evaluating the role of strss in the pain process. He suggests that the hypothalamic pituitary adrenal (HPA) axis and the sympathetic adrenal medullary system form major homeostatic mechanisms for the regulation of pain and stress. Thus, neuroendocrine modulation of the pain mechanism is now beginning to receive more research attention.

Finally, as noted by Hopkin (1997), research on pain mechanisms and pathways has greatly expanded in scope during the past few years (after failing to produce many new important findings over the last decade). A wide array of techniques, including anatomical, electrophysiological, genetic, molecular biological, and pharmacological, are being used in this research. Hopkin (1997) provides a concise review of this new research, which is beginning to reveal the following:

1. Especially for chronic or inflammatory pain, the nervous system can be sensitized, leading to the stimulation of chemical, functional, and structural changes that "prime the pain-processing pump."
2. Inflammation can trigger the lowering of the threshold of pain-sensing neurons and concomitantly stimulate the release of growth factors that act to reinforce the pain message.
3. Pain can also shape the central nervous system by using neurotransmitters such as gluta-

mate and substance P to further reinforce and strengthen its message.

4. We are beginning to understand how descending pathways passing from the cerebral cortex to the spinal cord allow the brain to mediate the sensation of pain.

5. New imaging technology is helping to identify which areas in the brain are responsible for the processing of pain.

6. Genetic research is being conducted to assess potential differences in a person's predisposition to pain.

Such research as the preceding will obviously have great clinical implications for developing the most effective way to manage pain, because it will help us understand how the nervous system senses, interprets, and responds to pain.

SUMMARY AND CONCLUSIONS

In this chapter, I have provided a historical overview of how pain has been conceptualized and treated. The quest to understand and control pain has been a major human pursuit since earliest recorded history, starting with the ancient Egyptians and Chinese. As was pointed out, the history of understanding the etiology and treatment of pain parallels the historical changes that have occurred in medicine in general. These changes have been quite significant, starting with the perspective of an intricate interrelationship between the mind and body proposed by the early Greek physician Hippocrates. This historical perspective of the interaction between mind and body began to lose favor in the 17th century with the advent of physical medicine during the Renaissance and its emphasis on a biomedical reductionism approach that contended that concepts such as the mind or soul were not needed to explain physical functioning or behavior. This new mechanistic approach to the study of medicine also fostered a "dualistic" viewpoint that mind and body functioned separately and independently. The reductionism philosophy of medicine was viewed as the only acceptable basis for explaining disease through understanding mechanical laws and physiological principles. This same medical mechanistic approach to pain was also dominant during the Renaissance period. Pain theories proposed by Descartes, Von Frey, and Goldschneider were all in keeping with the biomedical reductionistic philosophy.

This strict mechanistic, dualistic approach to medicine and pain began to subside in influence during the 19th and 20th centuries. Influential writings began to appear that emphasized the importance of taking an integrated, holistic approach to health and illness. A more comprehensive biopsychosocial model of illness was proposed that emphasized the unique interactions of biological, psychological, and social factors that need to be taken into account for better understanding of health and illness. The gate control theory of pain proposed by Melzack and Wall (1965) was a major contribution that highlighted the potentially significant role that psychosocial factors played in the perception of pain. Since that time, a number of significant clinical contributions occurred in the field of pain research, starting with the work of Wilbert Fordyce, who developed the initial prototypic pain clinic based on a comprehensive operant conditioning approach to the treatment of pain behavior. Subsequently, a number of cognitive-behavioral approaches were simultaneously being developed in the field of health psychology for dealing with a host of problems such as anxiety, depression, and so forth. These approaches were then applied to pain patients during the 1960s and 1970s. This work ultimately led to the development of multidisciplinary/interdisciplinary approaches to the comprehensive management of pain. These programs are now the major effective treatment programs for pain. Their philosophy is that complex pain behaviors can be more effectively managed by a multidisciplinary team, including a medical director, nurse, physical therapist, occupational therapist, and psychologist, with each team member contributing his or her specialized knowledge and skills to the common goal of making a correct diagnosis and then developing the most effective therapeutic strategy tailored for a particular patient. The general body of scientific literature has provided evidence that such multidisciplinary/interdisciplinary pain clinics can sigificantly improve the overall functioning of chronic pain sufferers. Newer alternative medicine approaches are also now being introduced to these multidisciplinary/interdisciplinary clinics.

Finally, as I have discussed, the development of these more effective comprehensive multidisciplinary approaches to pain management has not dampened efforts to better understand the neurophysiological and neurogenic factors underlying basic nociception processes. Indeed, in recent years there has been an increase in research on pain mechanisms and pathways highlighted by a greatly expanded scope of investigation. A wide array of techniques, including anatomical, electrophysiological, genetic, molecular biological, and pharmacological, are being used in such investigations. This exciting new research, which will aid in better understanding of how the nervous system senses, interprets, and responds to pain, will have great clinical implications for developing even more effective ways of managing pain.

ACKNOWLEDGMENT

The writing of this chapter was supported in part by Grant Nos. R01 DE10713 and K02 MH01107 from the National Institutes of Health.

REFERENCES

Baum, A., Gatchel, R. J., & Krantz, D. (1997). *An introduction to health psychology* (3rd ed.). New York: McGraw-Hill.

Beecher, H. K. (1956). Relationship of significance of wound to the pain experienced. *Journal of the American Medical Association, 161,* 1609-1613.

Berman, B. M., & Swyers, J. P. (1998). Applying complementary/alternative medicine approaches to managing chronic pain syndromes: If not now, when? *American Pain Society Bulletin, 8,* 4-6.

Bertalanffy, L. von (1969). *General systems theories: Foundations, development, and applications.* New York: Braziller.

Bonica, J. J. (1953). *The management of pain.* New York: Lea & Febiger.

Bradley, L. A. (1996). Cognitive-behavioral therapy for chronic pain. In R. J. Gatchel & D. C. Turk (Eds.), *Psychological approaches to pain management: A practitioner's handbook.* New York: Guilford Press.

Dattilio, F. M., & Freeman, A. (Eds.). (1994). *Cognitive-behavioral strategies in crisis intervention.* New York: Guilford Press.

Davis, C. M. (Ed.). (1997). *Complementary therapies and rehabilitation.* Thorofare, NJ: Slack.

Eisenberg, D., Kessler, R. C., Foster, C., Norlock, F. E., Calkins, D. R., & Delbanco, T. L. (1993). "Unconventional" medicine in the United States: Prevalence, cost, and patterns of use. *New England Journal of Medicine, 328,* 246-252.

Eisenberg, D. M. (1997). Advising patients who seek alternative medical therapies. *Annals of Internal Medicine, 127,* 61-69.

Fernandez, E., & Turk, D. C. (1992). Sensory and affective components of pain: Separation and synthesis. *Psychological Bulletin, 112,* 205-217.

Follick, M. J., Ahern, D. K., & Aberger, E. W. (1985). Development of an audiovisual taxonomy of pain behavior: Reliability and discriminant validity. *Health Psychology, 4,* 555-568.

Fordyce, W. E. (1988). Pain and suffering: A reappraisal. *American Psychologist, 43,* 276-283.

Fordyce, W. E., Fowler, R., Lehmann, J., & De Lateur, B. (1968). Some implications of learning in problems of chronic pain. *Journal of Chronic Disabilities, 21,* 179-190.

Fordyce, W. E., Roberts, A. H., & Sternbach, R. A. (1985). The behavioral management of chronic pain: A response to critics. *Pain, 22,* 112-125.

Fordyce, W. E., & Steger, J. C. (1979). Chronic pain. In O. F. Pomerleau & J. P. Brady (Eds.), *Behavioral medicine: Theory and practice.* Baltimore: Williams & Wilkins.

Gatchel, R. J. (1993). Psychophysiological disorders: Past and present perspectives. In R. J. Gatchel & E. B. Blanchard (Eds.), *Psychophysiological disorders: Research and clinical applications.* Washington, DC: American Psychological Association.

Gatchel, R. J., & Blanchard, E. B. (Eds.). (1993). *Psychophysiological disorders: Research and clinical applications.* Washington, DC: American Psychological Association.

Gatchel, R. J., & Turk, D. C. (Eds.). (1996). *Psychological approaches to pain management: A practitioner's handbook.* New York: Guilford Press.

Goodwin, B. (1994). *How the leopard changed its spots: The evolution of complexity.* New York: Scribner.

Hazard, R. G. (1995). Spine update: Functional restoration. *Spine, 20,* 2345-2348.

Hopkin, K. (1997). Show me where it hurts: Tracing the pathways of pain. *Journal of NIH Research, 9,* 37-43.

Jensen, M. P., & Karoly, P. (1992). Self-report scales and procedures for assessing pain in adults. In D. C. Turk & R. Melzack (Eds.), *Handbook of pain assessment.* New York: Guilford Press.

Keefe, F. J., & Williams, D. A. (1992). Assessment of pain behaviors. In D. C. Turk & R. Melzack (Eds.), *Handbook of pain assessment.* New York: Guilford Press.

Kellert, S. H. (1993). *In the wake of chaos.* Chicago: University of Chicago Press.

Kossman, M. R., & Bullrich, S. (1997). Systematic chaos: Self-organizing systems and the process of change. In F. Masterpasqua & P. A. Perna (Eds.), *The psychological meaning of chaos: Translating theory into practice.* Washington, DC: American Psychological Association.

Lazarus, A. A. (1971). *Behavior therapy and beyond.* New York: McGraw-Hill.

Lewith, G., Kenyon, J., & Lewis, P. (1996). *Complementary medicine: An integrated approach.* Oxford: Oxford University Press.

Mayer, T. G., & Gatchel, R. J. (1988). *Functional restoration for spinal disorders: The sports medicine approach.* Philadelphia: Lea & Febiger.

Melzack, R. (1975). The McGill Pain Questionnaire: Major properties and scoring methods. *Pain, 1,* 277-299.

Melzack, R. (1993). Pain: Past, present, and future. *Canadian Journal of Experimental Psychology, 47,* 615-629.

Melzack, R., & Wall, P. (1965). Pain mechanisms: A new theory. *Science, 50,* 971-979.

Micozzi, M. S. (Ed.). (1996). *Fundamentals of complementary and alternative medicine.* New York: Churchill Livingstone.

Perna, P. A., & Masterpasqua, F. (1997). Introduction: The history, meaning, and implications of chaos and complexity. In F. Masterpasqua & P. A. Perna (Eds.), *The psychological meaning of chaos: Translating theory into practice*. Washington, DC: American Psychological Association.

Rosenfeld, I. (1996). *Dr. Rosenfeld's guide to alternative medicine*. New York: Random House.

Sanders, S. H. (1996). Operant conditioning with chronic pain: Back to basics. In R. J. Gatchel & D. C. Turk (Eds.), *Psychological approaches to pain management: A practitioner's handbook*. New York: Guilford Press.

Speculand, B., Goss, A. N., Hughes, A., Spence, N. D., & Pilowsky, I. (1983). Temporomandibular joint dysfunction: Pain and illness behavior. *Pain, 17,* 139–150.

Stewart, I. (1989). *Does God play dice?: The mathematics of chaos*. New York: Blackwell.

Turk, D. C., Meichenbaum, D., & Genest, M. (1983). *Pain and behavioral medicine: A cognitive-behavioral perspective*. New York: Guilford Press.

Williams, R. C. (1988). Toward a set of reliable and valid measures for chronic pain assessment and outcome research. *Pain, 35,* 239–251.

Chapter 2

Chronic Pain:
A Biobehavioral Perspective

DENNIS C. TURK
HERTA FLOR

The question, What is pain? has perplexed philosophers, healers, and lay persons since the earliest recorded history. A model based primarily if not exclusively on anatomy and physiology gained ascendancy in the 19th century with the advances in knowledge of anatomy and sensory physiology. This model—the biomedical model—has directed attention primarily to the role of sensory input from the periphery that impinges on specific receptors and to the modulation and transmission of this information from the periphery to the central nervous system, the endpoints being different locations within the brain at which the sensory input sets off a signal that is realized as pain.

A tremendous amount of effort has been expended in an attempt to understand the neurological and biochemical bases of pain. Most recently, a number of investigators have used sophisticated procedures such as positron emission tomograpy (PET) and functional magnetic resonance imaging (fMRI) to image structures and information processing within the brain. In addition to attempting to understand pain, these efforts have as their ultimate goal to relieve pain and suffering. With the increased knowledge, innovative surgical and pharmacological interventions have developed, with many more on the horizon. Despite these efforts and the advances made, there continue to be a significant number of individuals for whom no identifiable

objective pathology is observed and for whom pain persists despite extensive efforts to ameliorate the symptoms and accompanying suffering.

It is well to recall John Bonica's comment in the preface to the first edition (1954) of his volume *The Management of Pain*, repeated in the second edition some 36 years later (1990):

> The crucial role of psychological and environmental factors in causing pain in a significant number of patients only recently received attention. As a consequence, there has emerged a sketch plan of pain apparatus with its receptors, conducting fibers, and its standard function which is to be applicable to all circumstances. But . . . in so doing, medicine has overlooked the fact that the activity of this apparatus is subject to a constantly changing influence of the *mind*. (p. 12)

Bonica's observation is particularly relevant for chronic pain syndromes, although it is applicable for acute pain as well. The advances referred to here have brought relief and improved quality of life to many patients with acute pain and some chronic pain syndromes; however, conventional efforts have failed to successfully alleviate pain for many of those who are diagnosed with chronic pain syndromes and symptoms such as chronic back pain, irritable bowel syndrome, osteoarthritis and rheumatoid arthritis, temporomandibular disorders, complex regional pain syndromes, headaches, and pain associated with neoplasms.

In addition to the failure of even the most advanced pharmacological and surgical armamentarium to alleviate pain and suffering consistently and permanently for many individuals, several observations also pose challenges to the biomedical model. If there were a direct transmission line from the periphery to the spinal cord and eventually the brain, then it is difficult to explain how different individuals with the same objective pathology or diagnosis, treated with the same treatment, can have variable responses. Procedures designed to cut or block the "pain pathways" should eliminate the report of pain, yet in many instances they do not. Studies have also shown that asymptomatic individuals may show significant pathology on computerized tomography scans (CT scans; Wiesel, Tsourmas, & Feffer, 1984) and MRI scans (M. C. Jensen, Brant-Zawadski, Obuchowski, Modic, & Malkasian Ross, 1994). From the biomedical model, it would be predicted that there would be a highly significant if not isomorphic relationship between objective pathology and the resulting disability, yet this is patently not the case.

Pain in the absence of pathology, pathology in the absence of pain, individual differences in response to identical treatments, failure of neurosurgical procedures and potent analgesic agents to consistently eliminate pain, and the low association between impairment and disability fail to conform to a model of pain that presumes a direct transmission from the periphery to central nervous system structures. Two responses to the set of challenges posed have been frequently invoked. Reports of pain in the absence of physical pathology, the variability in treatment response, and the less-than-perfect association between impairment and disability have been attributed to a lack of knowledge. The argument claims that these problems will be resolved with improved imaging or other diagnostic procedures. In short, the variability noted is assumed to be simply due to our ignorance. This argument has some difficulty explaining why up to 35% of asymptomatic individuals reveal significant pathology on MRI and CT scans.

An alternative response is that different psychological factors are involved in some of the problems noted. For example, one view holds that in the absence of physical explanations to account for reports of symptoms, the variability in response to symptoms and treatments and the modest association between objective pathology and subjective response are explained by psychological factors. Simply put, the symptoms are psychogenic—caused by a range of psychological factors.

There are at least two etiological variants of the psychogenic perspective. One suggests that reports of pain in the absence of objective pathology are caused by conscious efforts of the individual (motivation) to achieve some secondary gain (e.g., attention, financial compensation). Alternatively, principles of reinforcement may maintain reports of pain even in the absence of pathology. This latter view, based on operant conditioning, does not make specific assumptions about the individual's motivation. Rather, contingencies of reinforcement may serve to maintain behaviors (so-called "pain behaviors"; i.e., expressions of pain, distress, and suffering) that originally responded to nociception even after the cause of the noxious stimulation has been resolved. As was the case with the biomedical model, these psychogenic views do not have a ready explanation for the presence of pathology in the absence of reported symptoms.

Although the perspectives briefly discussed provide valuable insights into understanding reports of pain, they are inadequate. Viewing reports of pain and variations in responding to treatment in a dichotomous fashion—that the pain is either physically based (somatogenic) or psychologically based (psychogenic)—therefore creates an artificial distinction between *mind* and body that can be traced back to the philosopher René Descartes in the 18th century. We might do better if we heeded the words of Bonica, cited previously, and acknowledged the role of physical, psychological, and sociobehavioral factors if we truly wish to understand pain and to treat people who report pain more effectively.

A model that integrates this range of factors might be labeled "biopsychosocial" or "biobehavioral." In the latter case, the "behavioral" portion of the model broadly subsumes psychological and social factors. In contrast to the biomedical model's emphasis on disease, the biopsychosocial or biobehavioral model focuses on illness, the result of a complex interaction of biological, psychological, and social variables. From this perspective, the diversity in illness expression (which includes its severity, duration, and consequences for the individual) is accounted for by the complex interrelationships among predispositional, biological, and psychological characteristics (e.g., genetic or prior learning history), biological changes, psychological status, and the social and cultural contexts that shape the patient's perceptions and response to illness. For example, the biological substrate of disease is known to affect psychological factors (e.g., mood) and sociological factors (e.g., interpersonal relationships). Similarly, the psychological and sociological aspects of disease are known to reciprocally affect biomedical outcomes. Specifically, the impact of stress on biological systems is well documented (see Melzack, Chapter 6, this volume), and the influence of sociocultural variables on health care access is widely recognized (see Morris, Chapter 8, this volume). The biopsychosocial model stands in sharp contrast to the traditional biomedical perspective, which conceptualizes illness in terms of more narrowly defined physiochemical dimensions.

The biopsychosocial way of thinking about the differing responses of patients to symptoms and the presence of chronic conditions is based on an understanding of the dynamic nature of these conditions. That is, by definition, chronic syndromes extend over time. Therefore, these conditions need to be viewed longitudinally as ongoing, multifactorial processes in which there is a dynamic and reciprocal interplay among biological, psychological, and sociocultural factors that shapes the experience and responses of patients (Dworkin, Von Korff, & LeResche, 1992). Predispositional factors and current biological factors may initiate, maintain, and modulate physical perturbations; predispositional and current psychological factors influence the appraisal and perception of internal physiological signs; and social factors shape the behavioral responses of patients to the perceptions of their physical perturbations. Thus the observation of pain in the absence of pathology, pathology in the absence of pain, individual variability in treatment response, and the modest association between impairment and disability are explicable by positing the complex interactions among predispositional, biomedical, psychosocial, and behavioral factors.

We can now consider current understanding of physical, cognitive, affective, and behavioral factors related to pain. We begin by reviewing Melzack and Wall's (1965) seminal gate control theory and the extension proposed by Melzack and Casey (1968) that was the first attempt to develop an integrative model designed to address the inconsistencies created by unidimensional models and to integrate physiological and psychological factors. We then describe recent advances in the understanding of the roles of both psychological and physiological factors in states of chronic pain. Finally, we describe an integrative model that attempts to integrate biomedical and psychosocial factors within a biobehavioral model.

GATE CONTROL THEORY

Perhaps the most important contribution of the gate control theory is the way it changed thinking about pain perception. Melzack and Casey (1968) differentiate three systems related to the processing of nociceptive stimulation—sensory-discriminative, motivational-affective, and cognitive-evaluative—that are all thought to contribute to the subjective experience of pain. Thus the gate control theory specifically includes psychological factors as an integral aspect of the pain experience. It emphasizes the central nervous system (CNS) mechanisms and provides a physiological basis for the role of psychological factors in chronic pain.

The gate control theory proposes that a mechanism in the dorsal horn substantia gelatinosa of the spinal cord acts as a spinal gating mechanism that inhibits or facilitates transmission of nerve impulses from the body to the brain on the basis of the diameters of the active peripheral fibers, as well as of the dynamic action of brain processes. It was postulated that the spinal gating mechanism was influenced by the relative amount of excitatory activity in afferent large-diameter (myelinated) and small-diameter fibers (unmyelinated nociceptor) converging in the dorsal horns. It was further proposed that activity in A-beta (large-diameter) fibers tends to inhibit transmission of nociceptive signals (closes the gate) whereas A-delta and C (small-diameter) fibers primary afferent activity tends to facilitate transmission (open the gate). The hypothetical gate is proposed to be located in the dorsal horn, and it is at this point that sensory input is modulated by the balance of activity of small-diameter (A-delta and C) and large-diameter (A-beta) fibers.

Melzack and Wall (1965) postulated further that this spinal gating mechanism is influenced not only by peripheral afferent activity but also by efferent neural impulses that descend from the brain. They proposed that a specialized system of large-diameter, rapidly conducting fibers (the central control trigger) activate selective cognitive processes that then influence, by way of descending fibers, the modulating properties of the spinal gating mechanism. They suggested that the brainstem reticular formation functions as a central biasing mechanism inhibiting the transmission of pain signals at multiple synaptic levels of the somatosensory system.

The gate control theory maintains that the large-diameter fibers play an important role in pain by inhibiting synaptic transmission in dorsal horn cells. When large fiber input is decreased, mild stimuli that are not typically painful trigger severe pain. Loss of sensory input to this complex neural system, such as occurs in neuropathies, causalgia, and phantom limb pain, tend to weaken inhibition and lead to persistent pain. Herniated disc material, tumors, and other factors that exert pressure on these neural structures may operate through this mechanism. Emotional stress and medication that affect the reticular formation may also alter the biasing mechanisms and thus the intensity of pain.

From the gate control perspective, the experience of pain is an ongoing sequence of activities, largely reflexive in nature at the outset but modifiable even in the earliest stages by a variety of excitatory and inhibitory influences, as well as the integration of ascending and descending nervous system activity. The process results in overt expressions communicating pain and strategies by the individual to terminate the pain. In addition, considerable potential for shaping of the pain experience is implied, because the gate control theory invokes continuous interaction of multiple systems (sensory-physiological, affect, cognition, and ultimately, behavior).

The gate control model describes the integration of peripheral stimuli with cortical variables, such as mood and anxiety, in the perception of pain. This model contradicts the notion that pain is either somatic or psychogenic and instead postulates that both factors have either potentiating or moderating effects on pain perception. In this model, for example, pain is not understood to be the result of depression or vice versa, but rather the two are seen as evolving simultaneously. Any significant change in mood or pain will necessarily alter the others.

The theory's emphasis on the modulation of inputs in the dorsal horns and the dynamic role of the brain in pain processes and perception has resulted in psychological variables, such as past experience, attention, and other cognitive activities, being integrated into current research on and therapy for pain. Prior to this formulation, psychological processes were largely dismissed as reactions to pain. This new model suggested that cutting nerves and pathways was inadequate because a host of other factors modulated the input. Perhaps the major contribution of the gate control theory was that it highlighted the central nervous system as an essential component in pain processes and perception.

The physiological details of the gate control model have been challenged, and it has been suggested that the model is incomplete (Nathan, 1976; Price, 1987; R. F. Schmidt, 1972). As additional knowledge has been gathered since the original formulation in 1965, specific points of posited mechanisms have been disputed and have required revision and reformulation (Nathan, 1976; Wall, 1989). For example, large-diameter fibers may under certain conditions (e.g., inflammation) increase rather than inhibit pain perception (cf. Treede & Magerl, 1995; Siddal & Cousins, 1997; Woolf, 1995) and can cause hyperalgesia and allodynia at the site of the injury. In addition, plastic alterations in the properties of spinal cord neurons may be the consequence of acute pain states and may lead to secondary hyperalgesia (cf. Woolf, 1995). Overall, however, the gate control theory has proved remarkably resilient and flexible in the face of accumulating scientific data and challenges to it and still provides a "powerful summary of the phenomena observed in the spinal cord and brain, and has the capacity to explain many of the most mysterious and puzzling problems encountered in the clinic" (Melzack & Wall, 1982, p. 261). This theory has had enormous heuristic value in stimulating further research in the basic science of pain mechanisms.

The gate control theory can be credited as a source of inspiration for diverse clinical applications to control or manage pain, including neurophysiologically based procedures (e.g., neural stimulation techniques from peripheral nerves and collateral processes in the dorsal columns of the spinal cord; North, 1989), pharmacological advances (Abram, 1993), behavioral treatments (Fordyce, Roberts, & Sternbach, 1985), and those interventions that target modification of attentional and perceptual processes involved in the pain experience (Turk, Meichenbaum, & Genest, 1983). After the gate control theory was proposed in 1965, no one could try to explain pain exclusively in terms of peripheral factors.

Although the gate control theory provides a physical basis for the role of psychological factors in pain, it does not address the nature of the psychological factors in depth. That is, it does not incorporate a number of the specific psychological variables. We review some of these in the next section of this chapter.

BEHAVIORAL FACTORS

Operant Learning Mechanisms

A new era in thinking about pain began with Fordyce's (1976) description of the role of operant factors in chronic pain. The operant approach stands in marked contrast to the biomedical model of pain described above.

In the operant formulation, behavioral manifestations of pain rather than pain per se are central. It is suggested that when an individual is exposed to a stimulus that causes tissue damage, the immediate response is withdrawal and attempts to escape from noxious sensations. This may be accomplished by avoidance of activity believed to cause or exacerbate pain, seeking help to reduce symptoms, and so forth. These behaviors are observable and, consequently, subject to the principles of operant conditioning.

The operant view proposes that acute "pain behaviors" such as limping to protect a wounded limb from producing additional nociceptive input may come under the control of external contingencies of reinforcement and thus develop into a chronic pain problem. Pain behaviors (e.g., complaining, inactivity) may be positively reinforced directly, for example, by attention from a spouse or health care providers. Pain behaviors may also be maintained by escaping from noxious stimulation through the use of drugs or rest or the avoidance of undesirable activities such as work. In addition "well behaviors" (e.g., activity, working) may not be sufficiently reinforcing, and the pain behaviors reinforced may, therefore, be maintained. The pain behavior originally elicited by organic factors may come to occur, totally or in part, in response to reinforcing environmental events. Because of the consequences of specific behavioral responses, it is proposed that pain behaviors may persist long after the initial cause of the pain is resolved or greatly reduced.

The operant conditioning model does not concern itself with the initial cause of pain. Rather it considers pain an internal subjective experience that may be maintained even after an initial physical basis of pain has been resolved. The operant conditioning model focuses on overt manifestations of pain and suffering expressed as pain behaviors such as limping, moaning, and avoiding activity. Emphasis is placed on the communicative function of these behaviors. Thus, in one sense, the operant conditioning model can be viewed as analogous to the psychogenic models described above. That is, psychological factors are treated as secondary, as reactions to sensory stimulation, rather than as being directly involved in the perception of pain per se.

Although operant factors undoubtedly play a role in the maintenance of disability, exclusive reliance on the operant conditioning model to explain the experience of pain has, however, been criticized for its exclusive focus on motor pain behaviors, its failure to consider the emotional and cognitive aspects of pain (A. J. M. Schmidt, 1985a, 1985b; A. J. M. Schmidt, Gierlings, & Peters, 1989; Turk & Flor, 1987), and its failure to treat the subjective experience of pain (Kotarba, 1983). The applicability of this model is somewhat problematic for pain associated with cancer, as the initiation of such pain behaviors as talking about pain and requesting medication are encouraged and even essential to inform health care providers regarding disease progress (Wilkie, Keefe, Dodd, & Copp, 1992).

In recent years evidence has accumulated that suggests that not only observable pain behaviors but also verbal-subjective and physiological responses to pain are subject to operant learning, for example, the mere presence of a pain (Flor, Breitenstein, Birbaumer, & Fürst, 1995). It was also shown that increases in muscle tension reduce the impact of aversive stimulation selectively in chronic pain patients (Knost, Flor, Schugens, & Birbaumer, in press). It appears that this negative reinforcement mechanism is also acting on the cortical processing of pain. It concurrently reduces the pain-evoked potential of the electroencephalogram (EEG). It is thus likely that operant learning mechanisms have a pervasive yet largely still unrecognized effect on all levels of pain processing.

Respondent Learning (Classically Conditioned) Mechanisms

Factors contributing to chronicity that have previously been conceptualized in terms of operant learning may also be initiated and maintained by respondent conditioning (Gentry & Bernal, 1977). Fordyce, Shelton, and Dundore (1982) hypothesized that avoidance behavior does not necessarily require intermittent sensory stimulation from the site of bodily damage, environmental reinforcement, or successful avoidance of aversive social activity to account for the maintenance of protective movements. Avoidance of activities has been shown to be related more to anxiety about pain than to actual reinforcement (Linton, 1985).

Lethem, Slade, Troup, and Bentley (1983) and Linton, Melin, and Götestam (1985) have suggested that once an acute pain problem exists, fear of motor activities that the patient *expects* to result in pain may develop and motivate avoidance of activity. Nonoccurrence of pain is a powerful reinforcer for reduction of activity, and thus the original respondent conditioning may be followed by an operant learning process whereby the nociceptive stimuli and the associated responses need no longer be present for the avoidance behavior to occur. In acute pain states, it may be useful to reduce movement and consequently avoid pain to accelerate the healing process. Over time, however, anticipatory anxiety related to activity may develop and act as a conditioned stimulus (CS) for sympathetic activation (conditioned response, CR) that may be maintained after the original unconditioned stimulus (US; e.g., injury) and unconditioned response (UR; pain and sympathetic activation) have subsided (Lethem et al., 1983; Linton et al., 1985; Philips, 1987).

Pain related to sustained muscle contractions might, however, also be conceptualized as an unconditioned stimulus in the case where no acute injury was present, and sympathetic activation and tension increases might be viewed as unconditioned responses that may elicit more pain; conditioning might thus proceed in the fashion outlined here. Thus, although the original association between pain and pain-Drelated stimuli results in anxiety regarding these stimuli, with time the expectation of pain related to activity may lead to avoidance of adaptive behaviors even if the nociceptive stimuli and the related sympathetic activation are no longer present. (See Seligman & Johnston, 1973, on the role of expectation in learning processes.)

In acute pain, many activities that are neutral or pleasurable may elicit or exacerbate pain and are thus experienced as aversive and are avoided. Over time, more and more activities may be seen as eliciting or exacerbating pain and will be avoided (stimulus generalization). Fear of pain may become conditioned to an expanding number of situations. Avoided activities may involve simple motor behaviors, as well as work, leisure, and sexual activity (Philips, 1987). In addition to the avoidance learning, pain may be exacerbated and maintained in these encounters with potentially pain-increasing situations due to the anxiety-related sympathetic activation and muscle tension increases that may occur in anticipation of pain and also as a consequence of pain (Flor, Birbaumer, & Turk, 1990). Thus psychological factors may directly affect nociceptive stimulation and need not be viewed as merely reactions to pain. We will return to this point later.

The persistent avoidance of specific activities will reduce disconfirmations that are followed by corrected predictions (Rachman & Arntz, 1991).

The prediction of pain promotes pain-avoidance behavior, and overpredictions of pain promote excessive avoidance behavior, as demonstrated in A. Schmidt's (1985a, 1985b) studies. Insofar as pain avoidance succeeds in preserving the overpredictions from repeated disconfirmation, they will continue unchanged (Rachman & Lopatka, 1988). By contrast, repeatedly engaging in behavior that produces significantly less pain than was predicted will be followed by adjustments in subsequent predictions, which also become more accurate. These increasingly accurate predictions will be followed by increasingly appropriate avoidance behavior, even to elimination of all avoidance if that is appropriate. These observations add support to the importance of physical therapy, with patients progressively increasing their activity levels despite fear of injury and discomfort associated with renewed use of deconditioned muscles.

Thus, from a conditioning perspective, the patient may have learned to associate increases in pain with all kinds of stimuli that were originally associated with nociceptive stimulation (stimulus generalization). Sitting, walking, engaging in cognitively demanding work or social interaction, sexual activity, or even thoughts about these activities may increase anticipatory anxiety and concomitant physiological and biochemical changes (Philips, 1987). Subsequently, patients may display maladaptive responses to many stimuli and reduce the frequency of performance of many activities other than those that initially induced pain. The physical abnormalities often observed in chronic pain patients (such as distorted gait, decreased range of motion, muscular fatigue) may thus actually be secondary to changes initiated in behavior through learning. As the pain symptoms persist, more and more situations may elicit anxiety and anticipatory pain and depression because of the low rate of reinforcement obtained when behavior is greatly reduced (cf. Lethem et al., 1983). With chronic pain, the anticipation of suffering or prevention of suffering may be sufficient for the long-term maintenance of avoidance behaviors.

Social Learning Mechanisms

Social learning mechanisms have received some attention in the development and maintenance of chronic pain states. From this perspective, the acquisition of pain behaviors may occur by means of observational learning and modeling processes. That is, individuals can acquire responses that were not previously in their behavioral repertoire by observing others performing these activities. Bandura (1969) has described and documented the important role of observational learning in many areas of human functioning. Children acquire attitudes about health and health care, the perception and interpretation of symptoms, and physiological processes, as well as appropriate responses to injury and disease, from their parents and social environment and thus may be more or less likely to either ignore or overrespond to symptoms they experience (Pennebaker, 1982). The culturally acquired perception and interpretation of symptoms determines how people deal with illness (Nerenz & Leventhal, 1983). The observation of others in pain is an event that captivates attention. This attention may have survival value, may help an individual to avoid experiencing more pain and to learn what to do about acute pain.

Expectancies and actual behavioral responses to nociceptive stimulation are based, at least partially, on prior learning history. This fact may contribute to the marked variability in response to objectively similar degrees of physical pathology noted by health care providers.

AFFECTIVE FACTORS

Pain is ultimately a subjective, private experience, but it is invariably described in terms of sensory and affective properties. As defined by the International Association for the Study of Pain: "[Pain] is unquestionably a sensation in a part or parts of the body but it is also always unpleasant and therefore also an emotional experience" (Merskey, 1986, p. S217). The central and interactive roles of sensory information and affective state are supported by an overwhelming amount of evidence (Fernandez & Turk, 1992).

The affective components of pain include many different emotions, but they are all primarily negative in quality. Anxiety and depression have received the greatest amount of attention in chronic pain patients. The importance of anxiety in the maintenance of chronic pain has been described above. Research suggests that from 40% to 50% of chronic pain patients suffer from depression. In the majority of cases, depression appears to be patients' reaction to their plight. Some have suggested that chronic pain is a form of masked depression; although this may be true in a small number of cases, the research on this topic does

not suggest that depression precedes the development of chronic pain (Turk & Salovey, 1984).

Given what has been discussed above, it is not surprising that a large number of chronic pain patients are depressed. It is interesting to ponder the other side of the coin: Given the nature of the symptom and the problems created by chronic pain, how is it that all such patients are *not* depressed? Turk and colleagues (Rudy, Kerns, & Turk, 1988; Turk, Okifuji, & Scharff, 1994, 1995) examined this question and determined that patients' appraisals of the impact of the pain on their lives and of their ability to exert any control over the pain and their lives mediated the pain–depression relationship. That is, those patients who felt that they could continue to function and to maintain some control despite their pain did not become depressed.

Anger has been widely observed in individuals with chronic pain (e.g., Kinder & Curtiss, 1988; L. Schwartz, Slater, Birchler, & Atkinson, 1991). Pilowsky and Spence (1975) found an incidence of "bottled-up anger" in 53% of chronic pain patients. Kerns, Rosenberg, and Jacob (1994) noted that the internalization of angry feelings accounted for a significant proportion of variance in measures of pain intensity, perceived interference, and reported frequency of pain behaviors. Corbishley, Hendrickson, and Beutler (1990) reported that even though chronic pain patients in psychotherapy might present an image of themselves as even-tempered, 88% of the patients treated acknowledged their feelings of anger when such acknowledgment was explicitly sought. Summers, Rapoff, Varghese, Porter, and Palmer (1992) examined patients with spinal cord injuries and found that anger and hostility explained 33% of the variance in pain severity.

Frustrations related to persistence of symptoms, limited information on etiology, and repeated treatment failures, along with anger toward employers, the insurance and health care systems, family members, and themselves, all contribute to the general dysphoric mood of these patients. The impact of anger and frustration on exacerbation of pain and treatment acceptance has not received much attention, but it would not be unreasonable to expect that the presence of anger may serve as a complicating factor, increasing autonomic arousal and blocking motivation and acceptance of treatments oriented toward rehabilitation and disability management rather than cure, which are often the only treatments available for chronic pain (Fernandez & Turk, 1995).

COGNITIVE FACTORS

People with pain often have negative expectations about their own ability to control certain motor skills without pain. Moreover, pain patients tend to believe they have limited ability to exert any control over their pain. Such negative, maladaptive appraisals about the situation and personal efficacy may reinforce the experience of demoralization, inactivity, and overreaction to nociceptive stimulation (Biedermann, McGhie, Monga, Shanks, 1987; Brown & Nicassio, 1987). These cognitive appraisals and expectations are postulated to have an effect on behavior that leads to reduced efforts and activity and that may contribute to increased psychological distress (helplessness) and subsequent physical limitations.

If one accepts that pain is a complex, subjective phenomenon that is uniquely experienced by each individual, then knowledge about idiosyncratic beliefs, appraisals, and coping repertoires become critical for optimal treatment planning and for accurately evaluating treatment outcome. This was demonstrated in a study reported by Reesor and Craig (1988). They showed that the primary difference between chronic low back pain patients who were referred because of the presence of many "medically incongruent" signs and those who did not display these signs was *maladaptive thoughts.* Interestingly, there were no significant differences between these groups on the number of surgeries, compensation, litigation status, or employment status. These maladaptive cognitive processes may amplify or distort patients' experiences of pain and suffering. Thus the cognitive activity of chronic pain patients may contribute to the exacerbation, attenuation, or maintenance of pain, pain behavior, affective distress, and dysfunctional adjustment to chronic pain (Turk & Rudy, 1986, 1992).

Biomedical factors that may have initiated the original report of pain play less and less of a role in disability over time, although secondary problems associated with deconditioning may exacerbate and serve to maintain the problem. Inactivity leads to increased focus on and preoccupation with the body and pain, and these cognitive-attentional changes increase the likelihood of misinterpreting symptoms, of overemphasizing symptoms, and of perceiving oneself as disabled. Reduction of activity, fear of reinjury, pain, loss of compensation, and an environment that, perhaps unwittingly, supports the "pain patient role" can impede alleviation of pain, successful rehabilitation, reduction of disabil-

ity, and improvement in adjustment. As has been noted, cognitive factors may not only affect the patient's behavior and, indirectly, his or her pain but may also actually have a direct effect on physiological factors believed to be associated with the experience of pain.

Individuals respond to medical conditions in part based on their subjective representations of illness and symptoms (schemata). When confronted with new stimuli, the individual engages in a "meaning analysis" that is guided by the schemata that best match the attributes of the stimulus (Cioffi, 1991). It is on the basis of the patients' idiosyncratic schema that incoming stimuli are interpreted, labelled, and acted on. People build fairly elaborate representations of their physical state, and these representations provide the basis for action plans and coping (Nerenz & Leventhal, 1983; Turk, Rudy, & Salovey, 1986).

Beliefs about the meaning of pain and one's ability to function despite discomfort are important aspects of the cognitive schemata about pain (Slater, Hall, Atkinson, & Garfin, 1991). These representations are used to construct causal, covariational, and consequential information from their symptoms. For example, a cognitive schemata that one has a very serious debilitating condition, that disability is a necessary aspect of pain, that activity is dangerous, and that pain is an acceptable excuse for neglecting responsibilities will likely result in maladaptive responses (M. P. Jensen, Turner, Romano, & Lawler, 1994; D. P. Schwartz, DeGood, & Shutty, 1985; Williams & Thorn, 1989). Similarly, if patients believe they have a serious condition that is quite fragile and a high risk for reinjury, they may fear engaging in physical activities (Philips, 1987). Through a process of stimulus generalization, patients may avoid more and more activities and become more physically deconditioned and more disabled.

Patients' beliefs, appraisals, and expectations about their pain, their ability to cope, their social supports, their disorder, the medicolegal system, the health care system, and their employers are all important, as they may facilitate or disrupt the patient's sense of control and ability to manage pain. These factors also influence patients' investment in treatment, acceptance of responsibility, perceptions of disability, adherence to treatment recommendations, support from significant others, expectancies for treatment, and acceptance of the treatment rationale (Slater et al., 1991; Turk & Rudy, 1991).

Cognitive interpretations also will affect how patients present symptoms to significant others, including health care providers and employers. Overt communications of pain, suffering, and distress will enlist responses that may reinforce the pain behaviors (overt communications of pain such as limping, moaning, ambulating in a guarded or distorted fashion) and impressions about the seriousness, severity, and uncontrollability of the pain. That is, complaints of pain may lead physicians to prescribe more potent medications, order additional diagnostic tests, and, in some cases, perform surgery. Family members may express sympathy, excuse the patient from usual responsibilities, and encourage passivity, thereby fostering further physical deconditioning. It should be obvious that the cognitive-behavioral perspective integrates the operant conditioning emphasis on external reinforcement and respondent view of learned avoidance within the framework of information processing.

From our perspective, people with chronic pain, as is true for all individuals, are viewed as active processors of information. They have negative expectations about their own ability and responsibility to exert any control over their pain. Moreover, they often view themselves as helpless. Such negative, maladaptive appraisals about their condition, their situation, and their personal efficacy in controlling their pain and problems associated with pain serve to reinforce their experience of demoralization, inactivity, and overreaction to nociceptive stimulation. These cognitive appraisals are posed as having an effect on behavior, leading to reduced effort, reduced perseverance in the face of difficulty and activity, increased psychological distress, and physiological arousal.

The specific thoughts and feelings that patients experience prior to exacerbations of pain, during an exacerbation or intense episode of pain, and following a pain episode can greatly influence physiological arousal, the experience of pain, and subsequent pain episodes (Newton & Barbaree, 1987). Moreover, the methods patients use to control their emotional arousal and symptoms have been shown to be important predictors of both cognitive and behavioral responses (Flor & Turk, 1988; Reesor & Craig, 1988). As described previously, interrelated sets of cognitive variables, including thoughts about the controllability of pain, attributions about one's own ability to use specific pain coping responses, expectations concerning the possible outcomes of various coping efforts, and common erroneous beliefs about pain and disability influence the experience of pain.

To this point our focus has been on the role of psychological factors in chronic pain. We now need to incorporate the current understanding of the physical mechanisms of pain.

ANATOMICAL, PHYSIOLOGICAL, AND CHEMICAL BASES OF PAIN

Between the stimulus of tissue injury and the subjective experience of pain is a series of complex electrical and chemical events. In considering pain, it is important to have a conceptual understanding of the physiological processes involved, as well as the anatomical structures that are believed to be important. It is equally important to be aware that the understanding of pain is far from complete, and thus what is described in this section must be viewed as a puzzle with many pieces missing and some that may be incorrectly placed.

Four distinct physiological processes have been identified in pain: transduction, transmission, modulation, and perception (Fields, 1987). Consideration of these processes will help guide a review of anatomical, physiological, and chemical bases subserving the experience of pain.

Transduction

Embedded in the various tissues are nerve endings that respond best to noxious stimuli. Transduction or receptor activation is the process by which one form of energy (chemical, mechanical, or thermal) is converted into another—in this case, the electrochemical nerve impulse in the primary afferents. By this process, information about a stimulus is converted to a form that is accessible to the brain. Information is coded by the frequency of impulses in the primary afferents activated by the stimulus. Noxious stimuli lead to electrical activity in the appropriate sensory nerve endings.

Transmission

Transmission refers to the process by which coded information is relayed to those structures of the central nervous system (CNS) whose activity produces the sensation of pain. The first stage of transmission is the conduction of impulses in primary afferents to the spinal cord. At the spinal cord, activity in the primary afferents activates spinal neurons that relay the nociceptive message to the brain. This message elicits a variety of responses ranging from withdrawal reflexes to the subjective perceptual events ("It hurts!"). Once the noxious stimulus has been coded by the impulses in the peripheral nerve, the sensations that result are determined by the neurons of the nociceptive transmission system.

There are three major neural components of the nociceptive transmission system: the peripheral sensory nerves, which transmit impulses from the site of transduction to their terminals in the spinal cord; a network of relay neurons that ascend the spinal cord to brainstem and thalamus; and reciprocal connections between the thalamus and cortex. CNS neurons receive convergent input from numerous primary afferents, often of different types, including both nociceptive and non-nociceptive neurons that have spatially extensive receptive fields that in some cases include the entire body surface. In addition, the responses of CNS neurons to noxious stimuli are variable because they are subject to inhibitory influences elicited by peripheral stimulation or originating within the brain itself.

The neurons activated by noxious stimuli and their pattern of activity is thus a complex function of the primary afferent barrage that arrives at the spinal cord and the inhibitory influences that are active at the time. The primary afferent nociceptors terminate in the dorsal horn of the spinal cord. The axons of spinal neurons activated by these afferent nociceptors cross primarily to the anterolateral quadrant on the side opposite to the activated nociceptors. The message then ascends to the brainstem and via the thalamus to the cortex.

Melzack and Casey (1968) proposed that the paramedian pathway, with its diffuse projection to the limbic system and to the frontal lobe, primarily subserves the affective-motivational aspects of pain. Consistent with this idea is the well-established role of the brainstem reticular formation in behavioral arousal and in cortical arousal produced by a variety of sensory stimuli. In addition to producing arousal, the paramedian reticular formation plays an important role in escape behavior.

Noxious stimuli activate peripheral endings of the primary afferent nociceptor by the process of transduction. The message is then transmitted over the peripheral nerve to the spinal cord, where it synapses with cells of origin of the two major ascending nociceptive pathways, the spinothalamic and spinoreticulothalamic. The message is relayed in the thalamus to both the frontal and the somatosensory cortices. By tracing the pain message

along neural pathways from peripheral receptors to the cortex, it would appear that the relationships among stimulus intensity, activity in nociceptive transmission cells, and the perceived intensity of pain are simple and reproducible. This has an appealing simplicity; however, clinical observations indicate that the correlation between stimulus intensity and reported pain is actually unusual. In fact, the severity of reported pain may range from *minimal to unbearable in different individuals with apparently similar injuries, and* it is obvious that the subjectively experienced intensity of pain depends not only on the stimulus intensity but also to a very large extent on psychological factors, as described previously.

Recent imaging studies suggest that the primary somatosensory cortex plays an important role in coding sensory-discriminative aspects of the pain experience, whereas limbic structures subserve the affective evaluation of nociception (Coghill et al., 1994; Talbot et al., 1991). For example, in a study reported by Rainville, Duncan, Price, Carrier, and Bushnell (1997), hypnotic induction was used to reduce the affective processing of painful stimuli; this was accompanied by concomitant reduced activity in the anterior cingulate, whereas activity in primary somatosensory cortex remained unaltered.

Modulation

Modulation refers to the neural activity that leads to control of the nociceptive transmission pathway. Input from the frontal cortex and hypothalamus activate cells in the midbrain, which control spinal nociceptive transmission cells by means of cells in the medulla. The activity of this modulatory system is one reason why people with apparently severe injuries may deny significant levels of pain (Beecher, 1959; Wall, 1979).

Although we are far from understanding all the complexities of the human mind and consciousness, we know that there are specific pathways in the CNS that control pain transmission, and there is evidence that these pathways can be activated by the psychological factors described above. The midbrain, periaqueductal gray matter, and adjacent reticular formation that project to the spinal cord via the rostroventral medulla are all involved in the modulation of nociceptive signals (Fields, 1987). This pathway inhibits spinal neurons that respond to noxious stimuli. There is also a pain-modulating pathway from the dorsolateral pons to the cord. The pathway from the rostral medulla to the cord is partly serotonergic, whereas that from the dorsolateral pons is at least noradrenergic.

In addition to the biogenic-amine-containing neurons, endogenous opioid peptides are present in all the regions implicated in pain modulation. The opioid-mediated analgesia system can be activated by electrical stimulation or by opiate drugs such as morphine. It can also be activated by nociception, stress, and suggestion. Opioids produce analgesia by direct action on the CNS and activate the nociceptive modulating system. Opioid receptors have two distinct functions: chemical recognition and biological action. Researchers reasoned that the brain itself ought to synthesize molecules that would act at these highly specific receptor sites. Endogenous opioid peptides—namely, leucine-enkephalin, methionine-enkephalin, beta-endorphin, dynorphin, and alpha-neoendorphin—that are pharmacologically similar to morphine and reversed by opioid antagonists such as naloxone have all been identified.

The action of the endogenous opioids is also modifiable by learning processes. For example, Maier (1989) has shown that stress-induced analgesia can be conditioned and that this conditioned analgesia is also opioid-mediated. We (Flor, Birbaumer, Schulz, Mucha, & Grüsser, 1997) have recently shown that stress-induced analgesia can also be classically (respondent) conditioned in humans and have suggested that these learning processes can be used to enhance the efficacy of treatments for acute and chronic pain. Wiertelak et al. (1994) have also reported that illness-related hyperalgesia can be classically conditioned. The implications of this finding for the development of chronic pain in humans have not yet been sufficiently explored but deserve attention.

Perception

The final physiological process involved with pain is perception. Somehow, the neural activity of the nociceptive transmission neurons produces a subjective experience. How this comes about is obscure, and it is not even clear in which brain structures the activity occurs that produces the perceptual event. The question remains, How do objectively observable neural events produce subjective experience? Because pain is fundamentally a subjective experience, there are inherent limitations to understanding it (see, however, Chapman, Nakamura, & Flores, Chapter 3, this volume, for an attempt to clarify this process).

Pain responses cannot be predicted with certainty because there is great subjective variability. In some individuals, innocuous stimuli produce excruciating pain. In other situations, patients with severe injuries deny any significant pain. This variability presents a conundrum to health care providers and patients alike.

To understand the variability in individual experiences, it is useful to distinguish between *pain detection threshold* and *pain tolerance*. Pain threshold is a property of the sensory system that depends on the stimulus. It is highly reproducible in different individuals and in the same individual at different times. In contrast to this reproducibility, pain tolerance is highly variable. No two individuals react to nociception and pain in quite the same way. This distinction helps to understand the variability of pain. Pain tolerance is a manifestation of a person's reaction to noxious stimuli and is highly dependent on psychological variables, as described earlier. Not only does it vary between different individuals in the same situation, but also the same individual may react differently in different situations.

There are several reasons for the variability. There may be an injury to the nociceptive transmission system or to the activity of the modulatory system that lowers pain intensity. There may be abnormal neural activity, producing hypersensitivity that can result from self-sustaining processes set in motion by an injury but that may persist beyond the time it takes for the original injury to heal. This self-sustaining process may even create a situation in which pain is experienced without the noxious stimulus produced by an active tissue-damaging process (neuropathic pain, complex regional pain syndrome, type 2, phantom limb pain). Finally, the psychological processes and factors described herein may affect normal pain intensity, creating unpredictable responses.

If pain were simply a sensation, these neural pain mechanisms would probably be sufficient to explain most of the clinically observed variability. However, pain is more than a sensation. The close association of the nociceptive sensory system with the function of protection of the body from damage is unique among sensory systems. It is essential for understanding pain patients that the desire to escape from or terminate the sensation be considered. If it is not unpleasant, it is not pain.

As noted in the discussions of our biobehavioral model earlier, the meaning of pain is one important factor in determining pain tolerance. Different individuals have learned different ways of coping with pain; some minimize it and some overreact. Thus for many patients it may be as important to know what they think their pain means as to know what its cause is. Because of the importance of the patient's interpretation, it is imperative, especially for persistent or recurrent pain, to make some inquiry about this issue for treatment.

Pathophysiology of Pain

Now that we have considered the four general physiological processes of transduction, transmission, modulation, and perception, we can examine some of the specific physical factors involved in pain. When a stimulus of sufficient intensity to be tissue-damaging (i.e., noxious) is applied to a sensitive part of the body such as the skin or the somatic (musculoskeletal) and visceral structures, a chain of events is set in motion that eventually results in a sensation labeled as painful. The capacity of tissues to elicit pain when noxious stimuli are applied to them depends on their innervation of nociceptors. Nociceptors are primary afferent nerves with peripheral terminals that can respond specifically and differentially to noxious stimuli. The peripheral terminals of the nociceptive afferents (pain receptors or nociceptors) are directly sensitive to brief intense thermal, mechanical, and chemical stimuli. Some of the chemicals that excite the nociceptors include kinins, histamine, and K^+ and H^+ ions that usually result from inflammation.

By the complex cascade of events described previously, nociceptor activity produces several results. On the peripheral side there is prolongation of noxious sensations long after the termination of the stimulus and the development of hyperalgesia (stimuli above normal pain threshold perceived as more intense than in uninjured areas). In the peripheral tissues, the activity in nociceptors acts synergistically with the other processes initiated by tissue damage to produce increased blood flow and edema.

In addition to transient responses to these brief stimuli, nociceptors show relatively long-lasting increases in sensitivity when noxious stimuli are repeatedly applied. Long-lasting enhancement of nociceptor activity can be produced by a variety of diffusible substances that activate (potassium, serotonin, bradykinin, histamine) or sensitize (prostaglandins, leukotrienes, substance P) the primary afferent. Schaible and Schmidt (1988) have discovered so-called silent nociceptors that only become active

when they are sensitized (e.g., by an inflammatory process).

Of the afferent sensory fibers, A-delta and C fibers, readily found in skin, muscle, and fascia, are slow-conducting small-diameter fibers that carry nociception, whereas A-beta fibers are activated by touch and pressure. The nociceptive fibers, which utilize substance P as a neurotransmitter, synapse at the dorsal horn, cross to the other side, and ascend via the spinothalamic tract. The spinal neurons are also subject to sensitization and may thus contribute to the development of chronic states of pain (Woolf, 1995). On the spinal level, the nociceptive afferents connect with sympathetic efferents, as well as the efferents of the motor system, and may thus lead to secondary muscular reflexes and enhance sympathetic activation (Mense, 1993). The spinothalamic tract transmits connecting fibers to the reticular formation of the brainstem and thalamic nuclei before ending in the somatosensory cortex. Contrary to previous belief, the cortex plays an essential role in pain perception, and it integrates the cognitive and behavioral aspects of pain (Kenshalo & Douglass, 1995). Changes in representational size of pain-affected body areas and the size of receptive fields have been reported for both the thalamus (Guilbaud, Bernard, & Besson, 1994) and the cortex (Flor, Braun, Elbert, & Birbaumer, 1997).

The important endogenous pain inhibitory system involves (1) descending analgesic pathways from the periaqueductal grey areas of midbrain to spinal dorsal horn via raphe magnus nucleus of the pons; (2) local enkephalinergic interneurons in the spinal cord; and (3) peripheral A-beta sensory fibers that presynaptically inhibit A-delta and C-fibers at the dorsal horn. The inhibitory system utilizes several neurotransmitters, including serotonin, enkephalin, norepinephrine, gamma-aminobutyric acid (GABA), and somatostatin. The periaqueductal grey receives neuronal fibers from cortex, hypothalamus, and the limbic system, probably explaining the interaction of cognitive and emotional elements with pain perception and inhibition. Given the same noxious stimuli, pain perception between two individuals may vary according to the phenomenon of attention or inhibition, both of which are probably modulated by various descending neurons. Emotion, attention, and motivation may all influence pain perception, probably through a complex network of reticular, limbic, and cortical fibers.

We will now describe our biobehavioral model. Our model attempts to integrate some of the behavioral and psychosocial, as well as physiological aspects of pain perception discussed previously.

BIOBEHAVIORAL MODEL

We proposed that preconditions for chronic pain, including predisposing factors, precipitating stimuli, precipitating responses, and maintaining processes were all required to explain the processes involved (Flor et al., 1990; see also Okifuji & Turk, Chapter 15, in this volume). The existence of a physiological predisposition or diathesis involving a specific body system is the first component of this model. This predisposition consists of a reduced threshold for nociceptive activation that may be related to genetic variables, previous trauma, or social learning experiences and results in a physiological response stereotypy of the specific body system. The existence of persistent aversive external or internal stimuli (pain-related or other stressors) with negative meaning (e.g., various aversive emotional stimuli such as familial conflicts or pressures related to employment) activate the sympathetic nervous system and muscular processes as unconditioned and conditioned stimuli and motivate avoidance responses. Aversive stimuli may be characterized by "excessive" intensity, duration, or frequency of an external or internal stimulus. A behavioral, cognitive, or physiological repertoire that is inadequate or maladaptive to reduce the impact of these aversive environmental or internal stimuli on the individual are among the precipitating responses. Operant and respondent learning of behavioral, verbal-subjective, and physiological pain responses may maintain the pain experiences.

We (Flor et al., 1990) suggested that an important role is played by the cognitive processing of external or internal stimuli related to the experience of stress and pain: for example, increased perception, preoccupation with and overinterpretation of physical symptoms, or inadequate perception of internal stimuli such as muscle tension levels. Moreover, we believe that the nature of the coping response—active avoidance, passive tolerance, or depressive withdrawal—may determine the type of problem that develops, as well as the course of the illness.

We propose further that subsequent maladaptive physiological responding, such as increased and persistent sympathetic arousal and increased and persistent muscular reactivity, as well as sensitization of central structures including the cortex,

may induce or exacerbate pain episodes. Thus we suggest that learning processes in the form of respondent conditioning of fear of activity (including social, motor, and cognitive activities), social learning, and operant learning of pain behaviors—but also operant conditioning of pain-related covert and physiological responses, as described previously—make a contribution to the chronicity of pain.

It is important to note that these learning processes lead to both implicit and explicit memories for pain that subsequently guide the patient's behavior and determine his or her pain perception. For example, it has been shown that chronic pain leads to the formation of somatosensory pain memories that are specific for the site of pain and manifest themselves in an enlarged representation of the pain-affected body part in the primary somatosensory cortex (Flor, Braun, et al., 1997). This type of implicit pain memory is completely outside of the patient's conscious awareness but will lead to enhanced responsivity to stimuli that originate in the affected body region. It has also been shown that the explicit recall of a pain-related episode leads to the activation of a large cortical network subserving pain, as shown by the enhanced dimensional complexity of the EEG in chronic pain patients (Lutzenberger, Flor, & Birbaumer, 1997). Thus learned pain memories (i.e., psychological processes) influence directly the physiological processing of pain (cf. Birbaumer, Flor, Lutzenberger, & Elbert, 1995).

An even more dramatic example of a learned memory for pain has been described for phantom limb pain patients (cf. Flor, Elbert, et al., 1995). In traumatic upper limb amputees, the magnitude of phantom limb pain is proportional to the amount of reorganization in the primary somatosensory cortex, namely, the magnitude of the shift of the cortical mouth representation into the area that was formerly occupied by the now-absent hand representation. The amount of this shift is positively related to preamputation pain, and this shift does not occur in congenital amputees who never learned to associate the affected body part with a specific cortical representational zone.

The primary focus of our biobehavioral model is thus on the patient, rather than on symptoms and pathophysiology. In this model, we emphasize the patient's explicit thoughts and feelings in addition to implicit conditioning factors, as these will all influence behavior and physiology. From this perspective, assessment and treatment of the patient with persistent pain requires a broader strategy than those based on the previous dichotomous models described that examine and address the entire range of psychosocial and behavioral factors in addition to biomedical ones (Turk & Rudy, 1989; 1991).

In short, our biobehavioral model places greatest emphasis on the role of learning factors in the onset, exacerbation, and maintenance of pain for those patients with persistent pain problems. We (Flor et al., 1990) suggested that a range of factors predisposes individuals to develop chronic or recurrent acute pain; however, the predisposition is necessary but not sufficient. In addition to anticipation, avoidance, and contingencies of reinforcement, cognitive factors, particularly expectations, are also of central importance in our model of chronic pain. Conditioned reactions are viewed as self-activated on the basis of learned expectations as well as being automatically evoked. The critical factor in our model, therefore, is not that events occur together in time but that people learn to predict them and to summon appropriate reactions (Turk et al., 1983). It is the individual patient's processing of information that results in anticipatory anxiety and avoidance behaviors.

Our biobehavioral perspective on pain management focuses on providing the patient with techniques to gain a sense of control over the effects of pain on his or her life, as well as actually modifying the affective, behavioral, cognitive, and sensory facets of the experience (Flor & Turk, in press). Behavioral experiences help to show patients that they are capable of more than they assumed, thereby increasing their sense of personal competence. Cognitive techniques help to place affective, behavioral, cognitive, and sensory responses under the patient's control.

Our assumption is that long-term maintenance of behavioral changes will occur only if the patient has learned to attribute success to his or her own efforts. There are suggestions that these treatments can result in changes in beliefs about pain, coping style, and reported pain severity, as well as direct behavior changes (Dolce, Crocker, Moletteire, & Doleys, 1986; Turner & Clancy, 1986, 1988). Furthermore, treatment that results in increases in perceived control over pain and decreased catastrophizing also are associated with decreases in pain severity ratings and functional disability (M. P. Jensen, Turner, Romano, & Karoly 1991; M. P. Jensen, Turner, & Romano, 1991) and changes in physiological activity (Flor, Turk, & Birbaumer, 1985).

CONCLUDING COMMENTS

The emotional distress that is prevalent in a majority of pain patients may be attributed to a variety of factors, including fear, inadequate or maladaptive support systems and other coping resources, iatrogenic complications, overuse of tranquilizers and narcotic medication, inability to work, financial difficulties, prolonged litigation, disruption of usual activities, and sleep disturbance. Moreover, the experience of "medical limbo"—the presence of a painful condition that eludes diagnosis and that carries the implication of either psychiatric causation and malingering on the one hand or an undiagnosed life-threatening disease on the other—is itself a source of stress and can initiate psychological distress or aggravate a premorbid psychiatric condition. In the case of cancer, the stress of pain is superimposed on the general fear of living and possibly dying from a potentially lethal disease.

Individuals with persistent pain complaints become enmeshed in the medical community as they proceed from doctor to doctor, diagnostic test to diagnostic test, and treatment to treatment in a continuing, often futile, quest to have their pain eradicated. For many patients, the pain becomes the central focus of their lives. As patients withdraw from society, they lose their jobs, alienate family and friends, and become isolated. In this ongoing search for relief, it is hardly surprising that patients experience feelings of demoralization, helplessness, hopelessness, and outright depression.

In sum, persistent pain creates a demoralizing situation that confronts the individual not only with the stress created by pain but also with a cascade of ongoing stressors that compromises all aspects of their lives. Living with persistent pain conditions requires considerable emotional resilience, tends to deplete one's emotional reserve, and taxes not only the individual but also the capacity of family, friends, coworkers, and employers to provide support.

From the patient's point of view, the pain complaint connotes distress and is a plea for assistance. The subjective experience includes an urge to escape from the cause or, if that is not possible, to obtain relief. It is the overwhelming desire to terminate it that gives pain its power. It can produce fear and, if it persists, depression and erosion of the will to live.

It has become abundantly clear that no isomorphic relationship exists among tissue damage, nociception, and pain report. The more recent conceptualizations discussed view pain as a perceptual process that results from the nociceptive input and is modulation on a number of different levels in the CNS.

Pain is a subjective perceptual experience; one characteristic that differentiates it from pure sensation is its affective quality. Thus pain appears to have two defining properties: (1) bodily sensation and (2) an aversive affect (Fernandez & Turk, 1992; Melzack & Casey, 1968). Quintessentially, pain is experienced at both a sensory level and an affective level, as underscored by the definition of pain presented by the International Association for the Study of Pain (Merskey, 1986).

In this chapter, conceptual models were presented to explain the subjective experience of pain. As was noted, the current state of knowledge suggests that pain must be viewed as a complex phenomenon that incorporates physical, psychosocial, and behavioral factors. Failure to incorporate each of these factors will lead to an incomplete understanding. The range of psychological variables that have been identified as being of central importance in pain, along with the current understanding of the physiological basis of pain, were reviewed. We outlined a biopsychosocial model that integrates the current understanding of pain. Pain has become a vigorous research area, and the virtual explosion of information will surely lead to refinements in our biopsychosocial model and advances in clinical management.

ACKNOWLEDGMENTS

Preparation of this chapter was facilitated by grants from the National Institutes of Health to D. C. T. (Nos. P01 HD33989 and R01 AR44724) and from the Deutsche Forschungsgemeinschaft to H. F. (Nos. Fl 156/16 and Bi 195/24).

REFERENCES

Abram, S. E. (1993). Advances in chronic pain management since gate control. *Regional Anesthesia, 18,* 66–81.

Bandura, A. (1969). *Principles of behavior modification.* New York: Holt, Rinehart & Winston.

Beecher, H. K. (1959). *Measurement of subjective responses: Quantitative effects of drugs.* New York: Oxford University Press.

Biedermann, H. J., McGhie, A., Monga, T. N., & Shanks, G. L. (1987). Perceived and actual control in EMG treatment of back pain. *Behaviour Research and Therapy, 25,* 137–147.

Birbaumer, N., Flor, H., Lutzenberger, W., & Elbert, T. (1995). The corticalization of chronic pain. In B. Bromm & J. Desmedt (Eds.), *Pain and the brain: From nociception to cognition* (pp. 331–344). New York: Raven Press.

Bonica, J. J. (1954). *The management of pain.* Philadelphia: Lea & Febiger.

Bonica, J. J. (1990). *The management of pain* (2nd ed.). Philadelphia: Lea & Febiger.

Brown, G. K., & Nicassio, P. M. (1987). Development of a questionnaire for the assessment of active and passive coping strategies in chronic pain patients. *Pain, 31,* 53–62.

Cioffi, D. (1991). Beyond attentional strategies: A cognitive-perceptual model of somatic interpretation. *Psychological Bulletin, 109,* 25–41.

Coghill, R. C., Talbot, J. D., Evans, A. C., Meyer, E., Gjedde, A., Bushnell, M. C., & Duncan, G. H. (1994). Distributed processing of pain and vibration by the human brain. *Journal of Neuroscience, 14,* 4095–4108.

Corbishley, M., Hendrickson, R., & Beutler, L. (1990). Behavior, affect, and cognition among psychogenic pain patients in group expressive psychotherapy. *Journal of Pain and Symptom Management, 5,* 241–248.

Dolce, J. J., Crocker, M. F., Moletteire, C., & Doleys, D. M. (1986). Exercise quotas, anticipatory concern and self-efficacy expectancies in chronic pain: A preliminary report. *Pain, 24,* 365–372.

Dworkin, S. F., Von Korff, M., & LeResche, L. (1992). Epidemiologic studies of chronic pain: A dynamic-ecologic perspective. *Annals of Behavioral Medicine, 14,* 3–11.

Fernandez, E., & Turk, D. C. (1992). Sensory and affective components of pain: Separation and synthesis. *Psychological Bulletin, 112,* 205–217.

Fernandez, E., & Turk, D. C. (1995). The scope and significance of anger in the experience of chronic pain. *Pain, 61,* 165–175.

Fields, H. L. (1987). *Pain.* New York: McGraw-Hill.

Flor, H., Birbaumer, N., Schulz, R., Mucha, R. F. & Grüsser, S. M. (1997). *Opioid mediation of conditioned stress analgesia in humans.* Manuscript submitted for publication.

Flor, H., Birbaumer, N., & Turk, D. C. (1990). The psychobiology of chronic pain. *Advances in Behavior Research and Therapy, 12,* 47–84.

Flor, H., Braun, C., Elbert, T., & Birbaumer, N. (1997). Extensive reorganization of primary somatosensory cortex in chronic back pain patients. *Neuroscience Letters, 224,* 5–8.

Flor, H., Breitenstein, C., Birbaumer, N., & Fürst, M. (1995). A psychophysiological analysis of spouse solicitousness toward pain behaviors, spouse interaction, and pain perception. *Behavior Therapy, 26,* 255–272.

Flor, H., Elbert, T., Wienbruch, C., Pantev, C., Knecht, S., Birbaumer, N., Larbig, W., & Taub, E. (1995). Phantom limb pain as a perceptual correlate of cortical reorganization. *Nature, 357,* 482–484.

Flor, H., & Turk, D. C. (1988). Chronic back pain and rheumatoid arthritis: Predicting pain and disability from cognitive variables. *Journal of Behavioral Medicine, 11,* 251–265.

Flor, H., & Turk, D. C. (in press). *A biobehavioral perspective on chronic pain. A comprehensive assessment and treatment guide.* New York: Plenum.

Flor, H., Turk, D. C., & Birbaumer, N. (1985). Assessment of stress-related psychophysiological reactions in chronic back pain patients. *Journal of Consulting and Clinical Psychology, 53,* 354–364.

Fordyce, W. E. (1976). *Behavioral methods for chronic pain and illness.* St. Louis, MO: Mosby.

Fordyce, W. E., Roberts, A. H., & Sternbach, R. A. (1985). The behavioral management of chronic pain: A response to critics. *Pain, 22,* 113–125.

Fordyce, W. E., Shelton, J., & Dundore, D. (1982). The modification of avoidance learning pain behaviors. *Journal of Behavioral Medicine, 4,* 405–414.

Gentry, W. D., & Bernal, G. A. A. (1977). Chronic pain. In R. Williams & W. D. Gentry (Eds.), *Behavioral approaches to medical treatment* (pp. 171–182). Cambridge, MA: Ballinger.

Guilbaud, G., Bernard, J. F., & Besson, J. M. (1994). Brain areas involved in nociception and pain. In P. D. Wall & R. Melzack (Eds.), *Textbook of pain* (3rd ed., pp. 113–124). Edinburgh: Churchill Livingstone.

Jensen, M. C., Brant-Zawadski, M. N., Obuchowski, N., Modic, M. T., & Malkasian Ross, J. S. (1994). Magnetic resonance imaging of the lumbar spine in people without back pain. *New England Journal of Medicine, 331,* 69–73.

Jensen, M. P., Turner, J. A., & Romano, J. M. (1991). Self-efficacy and outcome expectancies: Relationship to chronic pain coping strategies and adjustment. *Pain, 44,* 263–269.

Jensen, M. P., Turner, J. A., Romano, J. M., & Karoly, P. (1991). Coping with chronic pain: A critical review of the literature. *Pain, 47,* 249–283.

Jensen, M. P., Turner, J. A., Romano, J. M., & Lawler, B. K. (1994). Relationship of pain-specific beliefs to chronic pain adjustment. *Pain, 57,* 301–309.

Kenshalo, D. R., & Douglass, D. K. (1995). The role of the cerebral cortex in the experience of pain. In B. Bromm & J. E. Desmedt (Eds.), *Pain and the brain: From nociception to cognition* (pp. 21–34). New York: Raven Press.

Kerns, R. D., Rosenberg, R., & Jacob, M. C. (1994). Anger expression and chronic pain. *Journal of Behavioral Medicine, 17,* 57–68.

Kinder, B. N., & Curtiss, G. (1988). Assessment of anxiety, depression, and anger in chronic pain patients: Conceptual and methodological issues. In C. D. Spielberger & J. N. Butcher (Eds.), *Advances in personality assessment* (pp. 651–661). Hillsdale, NJ: Erlbaum.

Knost, B., Flor, H., Schugens, M., & Birbaumer, N. (in press). The learned maintenance of pain: Muscle tension reduces central nervous system processing of painful stimulation in chronic pain patients. *Psychophysiology.*

Kotarba, J. A. (1983). *Chronic pain: Its social dimensions.* Beverly Hills, CA: Sage.

Lethem, J., Slade, P. O., Troup, J. P. G., & Bentley, G. (1983). Outline of a fear-avoidance model of exaggerated pain perception. *Behaviour Research and Therapy, 21,* 401–408.

Linton, S. (1985). The relationship between activity and chronic back pain. *Pain, 21,* 289–294.

Linton, S. J., Melin, L., & Götestam, K. G. (1985). Behavioral analysis of chronic pain and its management. In M. Hersen, R. Eisler, & P. Miller (Eds.), *Progress in behavior modification* (Vol. 7, pp. 1–38). New York: Academic Press.

Lutzenberger, W., Flor, H., & Birbaumer, N. (1997). Enhanced dimensional complexity of the EEG during memory for personal pain in chronic pain patients. *Neuroscience Letters, 266,* 167–170.

Maier, S. F. (1989). Determinants of the nature of environmentally induced hypoalgesia. *Behavioral Neuroscience, 103,* 131–143.

Melzack, R., & Casey, K. L. (1968). Sensory, motivational and central control determinants of pain: A new conceptual model. In D. Kenshalo (Ed.), *The skin senses* (pp. 423–443). Springfield, IL: Thomas.

Melzack, R., & Wall, P. D. (1965). Pain mechanisms: A new theory. *Science, 50,* 971–979.

Melzack, R., & Wall, P. D. (1982). *The challenge of pain.* New York: Basic Books.

Mense, S. (1993). Nociception from skeletal muscle in relation to clinical muscle pain. *Pain, 54,* 241–289.

Merskey, H. (1986). Classification of chronic pain: Descriptions of chronic pain syndromes and definitions of pain terms. *Pain* (Suppl. 3), S1–S225.

Nathan, P. W. (1976). The gate control theory of pain: A critical review. *Brain, 99,* 123–158.

Nerenz, D. R., & Leventhal, H. (1983). Self regulation theory in chronic illness. In T. Burish & L. A. Bradley (Eds.), *Coping with chronic illness* (pp. 13–37). Orlando, FL: Academic Press.

Newton, C. R., & Barbaree, H. E. (1987). Cognitive changes accompanying headache treatment: The use of a thought-sampling procedure. *Cognitive Therapy and Research, 11,* 635–652.

North, R. B. (1989). Neural stimulation techniques. In C. D. Tollison (Ed.), *Handbook of chronic pain management* (pp. 136–146). Baltimore, MD: Williams & Wilkins.

Pennebaker, J. W. (1982). *The psychology of physical symptoms.* New York: Springer.

Philips, H. C. (1987). Avoidance behaviour and its role in sustaining chronic pain. *Behaviour Research and Therapy, 25,* 273–279.

Pilowsky, I., & Spence, N. D. (1975). Patterns of illness behaviour in patient with intractable pain. *Journal of Psychosomatic Research, 19,* 279–287.

Price, D. D. (1987). *Psychological and neural mechanisms of pain.* New York: Raven Press.

Rachman, S., & Arntz, A. (1991). The overprediction and underprediction of pain. *Clinical Psychology Review, 11,* 339–356.

Rachman, S., & Lopatka, C. (1988). Accurate and inaccurate predictions of pain. *Behaviour Research and Therapy, 26,* 291–296.

Rainville, P., Duncan, G. H., Price, D. D., Carrier, B., & Bushnell, M. C. (1997). Pain affect encoded in human anterior cingulate but not somatosensory cortex. *Science, 277,* 968–971.

Reesor, K. A., & Craig, K. (1988). Medically incongruent chronic pain: Physical limitations, suffering and ineffective coping. *Pain, 32,* 35–45.

Rudy, T. E., Kerns, R. J., & Turk, D. C. (1988). Chronic pain and depression: Toward a cognitive behavioral mediation model. *Pain, 35,* 179–183.

Schaible, H. G., & Schmidt, R. F. (1988). Direct observation of the sensitization of articular afferents during experimental arthritis. In R. Dubner, G. F. Gebhart, & M. R. Bond (Eds.), *Proceedings of the Fifth World Congress on Pain: Vol. 3. Pain research and clinical management* (pp. 44–50). Amsterdam: Elsevier.

Schmidt, A. J. M. (1985a). Cognitive factors in the performance of chronic low back pain patients. *Journal of Psychosomatic Research, 29,* 183–189.

Schmidt, A. J. M. (1985b). Performance level of chronic low back pain patients in different treadmill test conditions. *Journal of Psychosomatic Research, 29,* 639–646.

Schmidt, A. J. M., Gierlings, R. E. H., & Peters, M. L. (1989). Environment and interoceptive influences on chronic low back pain behavior. *Pain, 38,* 137–143.

Schmidt, R. F. (1972). The gate control theory of pain: An unlikely hypothesis. In R. Jansen, W. D. Keidel, A. Herz, C. Streichele, J. P. Payne, & R. A. P. Burt (Eds.), *Pain: Basic principles, pharmacology, therapy* (pp. 57–71). Stuttgart: Thieme.

Schwartz, D. P., DeGood, D. E., & Shutty, M. S. (1985). Direct assessment of beliefs and attitudes of chronic pain patients. *Archives of Physical Medicine and Rehabilitation, 66,* 806–809.

Schwartz, L., Slater, M., Birchler, G., & Atkinson, J. H. (1991). Depression in spouses of chronic pain patients: The role of pain and anger, and marital satisfaction. *Pain, 44,* 61–67.

Seligman, M. E. P., & Johnston, J. C. (1973). A cognitive theory of avoidance learning. In F. J. McGuigan & D. B. Lumsden (Eds.), *Contemporary approaches to conditioning and learning* (pp. 69–110). Washington, DC: Winston.

Siddal, P. J., & Cousins, M. J. (1997). Spinal pain mechanisms. *Spine, 22,* 98–104.

Slater, M. A., Hall, H. F., Atkinson, J. H., & Garfin, S. R. (1991). Pain and impairment beliefs in chronic low back pain: Validation of the Pain and Impairment Relationship Scale (PAIRS). *Pain, 44,* 51–56.

Summers. J. D., Rapoff, M. A., Varghese, G., Porter, K., & Palmer, K. (1992). Psychological factors in chronic spinal cord injury pain. *Pain, 47,* 183–189.

Talbot, J. D., Merrett, S., Evans, A. C., Meyer, E., Bushnell, M. C., & Duncan, G. H. (1991). Multiple representations of pain in human cerebral cortex. *Science, 251,* 1355–1359.

Treede, R.-D., & Magerl, W. (1995). Modern concepts of pain and hyperalgesia: Beyond the polymodal C-nociceptor. *News in the Physiological Sciences, 10,* 216–228.

Turk, D. C., & Flor, H. (1987). Pain > pain behaviors: The utility and limitations of the pain behavior construct. *Pain, 31,* 277–295.

Turk, D. C., Meichenbaum, D., & Genest, M. (1983). *Pain and behavioral medicine: A cognitive-behavioral perspective.* New York: Guilford Press.

Turk, D. C., Okifuji, A., & Scharff, L. (1994). Assessment of older women with chronic pain. *Journal of Women and Aging, 6,* 25–42.

Turk, D. C., Okifuji, A., & Scharff, L. (1995). Chronic pain and depression: Role of perceived impact and perceived control in different age cohorts. *Pain, 61,* 93–102.

Turk, D. C., & Rudy, T. E. (1986). Assessment of cognitive factors in chronic pain: A worthwhile enterprise? *Journal of Consulting and Clinical Psychology, 54,* 760–768.

Turk, D. C., & Rudy, T. E. (1989). A cognitive-behavioral perspective on chronic pain: Beyond the scalpel and syringe. In C. D. Tollison (Ed.), *Handbook of chronic pain management* (pp. 222–236). Baltimore: Williams & Wilkins.

Turk, D. C., & Rudy, T. E. (1991). Persistent pain and the injured worker: Integrating biomedical, psychosocial, and behavioral factors. *Journal of Occupational Rehabilitation, 1,* 159–179.

Turk, D. C., & Rudy, T. E. (1992). Cognitive factors and persistent pain: A glimpse into Pandora's box. *Cognitive Therapy and Research, 16,* 99–112.

Turk, D. C., Rudy, T. E., & Salovey, P. (1986). Implicit models of illness: Description and validation. *Journal of Behavioral Medicine, 9,* 453–474.

Turk, D. C., & Salovey, P. (1984). "Chronic pain as a variant of depressive disease": A critical reappraisal. *Journal of Nervous and Mental Disease, 172,* 398–404.

Turner, J. A., & Clancy, S. (1986). Strategies for coping with chronic low back pain: Relationship to pain and disability. *Pain, 24,* 355–363.

Turner, J. A., & Clancy, S. (1988). Comparison of operant behavioral and cognitive-behavioral group treatment for chronic low back pain. *Journal of Consulting and Clinical Psychology, 56,* 261–266.

Wall, P. D. (1979). On the relationship of injury to pain. *Pain, 6,* 63–64.

Wall, P. D. (1989). The dorsal horn. In P. D. Wall & R. Melzack (Eds.), *Textbook of pain* (2nd ed., pp. 102–111). New York: Churchill Livingstone.

Wiertelak, E. P., Smith, K. P., Furness, L., Mooney-Heiberger, K., Mayr, T., Maier, S. F., & Watkins, L. R. (1994). Acute and conditioned hyperalgeric responses to illness. *Pain, 56,* 227–234.

Wiesel, S. W., Tsourmas, N., & Feffer, H. (1984). A study of computer assisted tomography: I. The incidence of positive CAT scans in an asymptomatic group of patients. *Spine, 9,* 549–551.

Wilkie, D. J., Keefe, F. J., Dodd, M. J., & Copp, L. A. (1992). Behavior of patients with lung cancer: Description and associations with oncologic and pain variables. *Pain, 51,* 231–240.

Williams, D. A., & Thorn, B. E. (1989). An empirical assessment of pain beliefs. *Pain, 36,* 251–258.

Woolf, C. (1995). Somatic pain: Pathogenesis and prevention. *British Journal of Anesthesiology, 75,* 169–176.

Chapter 3

Chronic Pain and Consciousness: A Constructivist Perspective

C. RICHARD CHAPMAN
YOSHIO NAKAMURA
LETICIA Y. FLORES

Pain is a normal part of life. As awareness of tissue trauma, it serves an important protective function. However, pain can persist beyond the healing time needed for recovery from injury, and it can also accompany progressive degenerative disease. When pain exists indefinitely under these conditions, physicians call it *chronic* pain. Chapman and Stillman (1996) described chronic pain as severe persisting pain of moderate or long duration that disrupts sleep and normal living, ceases to serve a protective function, and instead degrades health and functional capability. It typically becomes a source of suffering and disability for patients and a vexing frustration for physicians.

The biomedical model of chronic pain, anchored in classical neurophysiology, assumes that pain is a time-limited sensory experience signaling tissue damage or pathology. Nonetheless, pain persists indefinitely in many people who lack definable injury or disease. The inability of conventional medical intervention to relieve chronic pain has spawned substantial psychological thinking about the problem. This approach—commonly termed the biopsychosocial model—emphasizes that persisting pain can become a habit pattern, a weltanschauung, and, in some cases, a lifestyle for the person who lives with it. Moreover, it raises the possibility that chronic pain is not only something one feels but also a social role that one assumes. Rather than competing with the biomedical model, the biopsychosocial model extends and enhances it, attempting to explain the development and maintenance of chronic pain and disability. Although this approach represents an important advance in understanding, it does not integrate smoothly with the knowledge base on pain in medicine. Nor can it explain how social and psychological factors engender or produce chronicity and disability.

We are developing a third perspective from the new and rapidly growing field of consciousness research. Consciousness is an emergent property of a self-organizing nervous system, and pain is an aspect of consciousness. Fundamentally, consciousness is a necessary precondition of pain: The conventional wisdom holds that pain does not occur in unconscious persons. The consciousness viewpoint builds on the rich information base of classical neurophysiology and also on the broader position of biopsychosocial thinking, which recognizes that many factors besides tissue pathology determine chronic pain. We propose that the consciousness framework approach can help clarify the nature of chronic pain and also provide a context for more completely integrating biomedical and biopsychosocial standpoints.

This chapter briefly reviews the three perspectives on chronic pain: the biomedical, the biopsychosocial, and a third one, emerging from consciousness research. We suggest ways of integrating biomedical and psychological approaches within a broader, overarching consciousness framework.

THE BIOMEDICAL MODEL

The biomedical concept of pain holds that pain is a sensory experience that signals tissue damage. The transmission of tissue trauma information from the periphery to the cerebral cortex causes the experience of pain. In a nutshell, pain involves (1) transduction of tissue trauma into neural signals, (2) transmission of such signals to the dorsal horn of the spinal cord and from there to the thalamus, and (3) central registration of the sensory information in somatosensory cortex. The modulation of the signals along the way is an important feature of pain and a mechanism for pain relief. The biomedical model also recognizes pain states that originate with injury to neurological pathways (neuropathic pain). A chronic pain state is neuropathic when the brain interprets signals originating from the abnormal firing of damaged nerves as true sensory experience.

Basic Assumptions about Pain

The classical biomedical perspective holds that pain is a mechanistic sensory experience that signals tissue damage. It takes place in a passive nervous system: Pain happens to people when either immediate tissue trauma or neuropathy is present; people do not make pain. Pain control options include (1) alleviating the cause of tissue trauma or tissue sensitization in the periphery, (2) blocking or interrupting pathways carrying noxious signals, and (3) activating endogenous modulation mechanisms by pharmacological or neurosurgical means.

Duthie (1994) provides a succinct statement of the biomedical view of pain:

> The appreciation of pain requires that the energy of a painful stimulus be transformed by peripheral receptors into impulses which are conducted along sensory neurones to the CNS. Onward transmission to higher centers triggers the appreciation of pain. Pain may be alleviated either by impeding the transmission of impulses or by enhancing the mechanisms which modulate onward transmission. (p. 120)

Duthie further notes (p. 125) that "pain appreciation has never been localized to a particular region of the brain. The postcentral gyrus and parietal operculum are both possibilities." These statements reveal some important assumptions: A neural message signals pain from the moment trauma activates the sensory end organ (indeed, this particular statement suggests that pain is a property of the stimulus), and the awareness of pain depends on the activation of specific regions in the brain. Duthie's words and many other statements like it suggest that the 19th-century doctrine of specific nerve energies still influences current thinking.

The biomedical model holds that pain is a sensory message of peripheral tissue trauma, specifically and accurately coded in peripheral nerves as well as in pathways of central neural transmission and in the brain. Figure 3.1 illustrates the biomedical concept, indicating that pain is predomi-

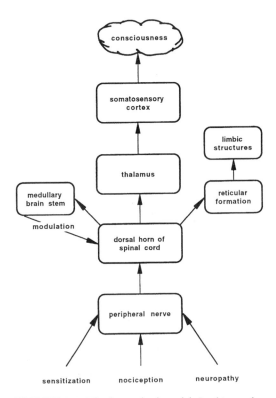

FIGURE 3.1. The biomedical model. In this mechanistic perspective, pain is a modality-specific sensory message of tissue trauma. Awareness of pain, a sensory experience, corresponds to the arrival of the message at the somatosensory cortex. Along the way, the message undergoes modulation. Patients become aware of pain (or appreciate pain); they do not produce pain in response to injury.

nantly a product of rigid, unidirectional, straight-through (albeit modulated) information transmission. It is not at all clear who or what interprets the signals that complete their journey from periphery to cortex. The model tacitly assumes that a conscious self receives and interprets pain alarm signals, like a person attending to shouts of "Fire!" while watching a film in a motion picture theater. Where did this idea originate?

Contemporary understanding of pain reflects the strong influence of Descartes, who in the 17th century construed bodily processes as clockwork mechanics (Damasio, 1994). Descartes held that body and mind were separate entities. For Descartes, pain was a specific modality—a straight-through sensory projection system that moved injury signals from damaged tissue to the brain, where the mind could appreciate them. This perspective went unchallenged for two centuries, and it still exerts considerable subtle influence. Scientists and physicians alike assumed, until the 1960s, that tissue trauma activates specific receptors and that signals of tissue trauma follow specific pain pathways through the spinal cord to a pain center in the brain. In biomedical thinking, pain is the sensory end product of an essentially passive information transmission process that operates as a biologically adaptive mechanism.

Basic Mechanisms

Transduction

The transduction of tissue trauma into neural signals depends on sensory end organs known as nociceptors (Besson & Chaouch, 1987; Heppelmann, Messlinger, Schaible, & Schmidt, 1991; Willis & Westlund, 1997). The free nerve endings of thinly myelinated A-delta fibers function as thermal and/or mechanical nociceptors, conducting impulses at 4–44 meters per second. In addition, certain unmyelinated C fibers that conduct slowly (roughly 0.5–1 meters per second) act as polymodal nociceptors, responding to various high-intensity mechanical, chemical, and thermal stimuli. Both types of fibers distribute widely in skin and in deep tissue. Repetitive stimulation of these receptors produces pain. In addition, some primary afferents act as "silent nociceptors." Normally, these end organs will not respond to harmless sensory stimuli, but noxious events or chemical changes can sensitize them so that they function thereafter as nociceptors (McMahon & Koltzenburg, 1990; Willis, 1993).

Nociceptors innervate skin, muscle, fascia, joints, tendons, blood vessels, and visceral organs. From a sensory perspective, these tissues group into cutaneous, deep, and visceral types. Nociception appears to serve somewhat different functions in the three types of tissues, and the quality of the pain that ensues from their activation varies across types. Most cutaneous pain is well localized, sharp, pricking, or burning. A-delta fibers produce sharp, pricking pain sensations of short duration whereas C fibers typically generate burning sensations. Deep-tissue pain usually seems diffuse and dull or aching in quality, although deep tissues can produce bright, sharp pains under certain conditions (e.g., muscle rupture). Visceral pain is very diffuse, often referred to the body surface, perseverating, and frequently associated with a queasy quality that patients describe as "sickening." Severe visceral pain typically produces an accompaniment of profuse sweating, nausea, and vomiting.

The adequate stimuli for nociception differ across tissue types. Cutaneous receptors detect injurious stimuli from the surrounding environment, and so they respond to severe mechanical and thermal events such as cutting, burning, or freezing. Nociceptors in deep tissue such as muscle detect overuse strain, deep mechanical injury such as tearing and contusion, spasm or cramping, and ischemia. Their function resembles that of nociceptors in cutaneous tissue, but their responses may link more intimately to flexor reflexes than do those of their counterparts in skin. Muscle pain tends to foster muscle stiffness and splinting, which serves a protective function by bracing or supporting injured muscle. Visceral nociceptors do not respond to cutting or burning injury as do their counterparts in cutaneous tissue but instead fire in response to pathological change. A hollow viscus needs to identify and transduce distention, stretch, and isometric contraction. A solid organ needs to signal distention of the capsule that contains it and inflammation. Gebhart and Ness (1991) listed the following as naturally occurring visceral stimuli: distention of hollow organs, ischemia, inflammation, muscle spasm, and traction. The peripheral origins of pain vary markedly, depending on whether the nociceptors involved lie in superficial or deep tissues.

Sensitization of Nociceptors

Sensitization of nociceptors plays a major role in clinical pain states (Alexander & Black, 1992). As nociceptors become sensitized, pain thresholds diminish (allodynia), and the painful qualities of subsequent noxious stimuli increase (hyperalgesia). Such alterations may reflect changes in the transduction process, central changes that facilitate the transmission of noxious messages, or both. Sensitization of nociceptors can result from either inflammation or repetitive stimulation of nociceptors. Enhanced sensitivity is usually adaptive because it promotes recuperation and repair, minimizing further injury by discouraging all contact rather than just contact with noxious stimuli.

Once traumatized, tissue normally becomes inflamed. It is now clear that the process of inflammation sensitizes nociceptors and thereby increases their signal-generating capability (Woolf, 1989). Chemical by-products of inflammation, such as the prostaglandins, alter the chemical environment of nociceptors, lowering their thresholds for firing and in some cases recruiting other fibers to function as nociceptors. Thus injured peripheral tissues can become extraordinarily sensitive because of local chemical changes.

A key feature of sensitization is that it can awaken nociceptors that are otherwise silent—so-called sleeping nociceptors (McMahon & Koltzenburg, 1990). Furthermore, it can recruit sensory endings that are normally not nociceptive to function, like volunteer firemen, as nociceptors. Sensitization drastically alters the process of transduction.

Neuropathophysiology That Masquerades as Transduction

Some painful conditions, collectively termed neuropathic pain, arise from dysfunction of the peripheral or central nervous system. When pain originates in disturbed neural function, it is neurogenic in origin. Patients with neurogenic pain may experience ongoing or episodic electrical sensations or paresthesias, painful paroxysms, or a general hypersensitivity that makes harmless stimuli exquisitely painful (Bowsher, 1991; Davar & Maciewicz, 1989; Elliott, 1994; Galer, 1995). Injury to a peripheral nerve can produce pathophysiological changes in electrical excitability that generate abnormal ongoing and evoked discharge (Devor, 1991). Changes in the afferent impulse barrage can induce long-term shifts of central synaptic excitability, as well as changes in spinal cord cell excitability (Wall, 1991).

Chronic nerve root compression, for example, a herniated disc, can generate pain by causing severe demyelination and fibrosis (Boulu & Benoist, 1996). Certain mono- and polyneuropathies associated with diabetes (Boulton, 1992) or alcoholism

(Galer & Portenoy, 1991) sometimes produce persisting pain. In addition, pain can arise from iatrogenic or adventitious injury to peripheral nerves or neural plexuses (Vecht, Van de Brand, & Wajer, 1989) or to central structures such as the spinal cord (Siddall, Taylor, & Cousins, 1995). Severed nerves occasionally form neuromas that generate abnormal impulse discharge (Fried, Govrin, Rosenthal, Ellisman, & Devor, 1991). Bowsher (1991) estimated that such cases make up about one-fourth of the patient population of most pain clinics; however, neuropathic pain is rare and afflicts at most about 1% of the general population. Not all neuropathy is painful; why some lesions produce pain and others do not is still an enigma.

Vecht and colleagues (Vecht et al., 1989) described a classical iatrogenic neuropathic pain syndrome. Breast cancer patients who have undergone radical breast amputation with an axillary lymph node dissection sometimes develop electric-shock-like pain in the axilla, the inner side of the upper arm and/or shoulder. This syndrome occurs when the surgical procedure produces a lesion of the intercostobrachial nerve. This is a difficult pain to control.

Damage to neural tissue may disturb a central regulating mechanism and thereby produce a condition in which the sympathetic nervous system plays a role in nociception (Roberts, 1986). Terms for this include Sympathetically Maintained Pain (SMP) and Complex Regional Pain Syndrome (CRPS) (Stanton-Hicks et al., 1995). Such conditions are rare, but excruciatingly painful, conditions in which altered function of the sympathetic nervous system contributes to a painful hypersensitivity in an affected area of the body. Abnormal skin color, temperature change, abnormal sudomotor activity, and edema accompany this type of pain. There are two types of SMP. The first occurs without a definable nerve injury, and the second, commonly called causalgia, occurs in response to a definable nerve lesion. Causalgia illustrates the complexity of this type of pain state.

Causalgia typically appears after a high-velocity wound (a bullet, shrapnel, or knife injury) that has damaged a major nerve in a limb (Bonica, 1990). Most patients experience surface pain of a burning quality immediately in the periphery of the injured extremity, and they develop shiny skin and edema in the affected area. The pain worsens and evolves into a constant hyperesthesia and allodynia (everything touching the area causes pain). With time, the pain spreads and eventually involves the entire limb. Temperature changes, light touch, friction from clothing, blowing air, movement of the limb, and any stimulus that affects the patient's emotional state can exacerbate the pain. Minor events like the cry of a child, the rattling of a newspaper, or watching a television program can provoke intense pain. Any stimulus that activates the sympathetic nervous system, even social stimuli that are emotion-eliciting, can provoke severe pain. Consequently, patients suffer greatly, become reclusive and withdrawn, and become tragically incapacitated by the pain.

Transmission

The centripetal transmission of noxious signals takes place in the spinal cord. Nociceptive afferents enter the spinal cord primarily through the dorsal route, terminating principally in lamina I (the marginal zone) but also in laminae II (the substantia gelatinosa) and V of the dorsal horn (Craig, 1991). The spinal and medullary dorsal horns are much more than simple relay stations; these complex structures participate directly in sensory processing, performing local abstraction, integration, selection, and appropriate dispersion of sensory impulses (Bonica, 1990; Dubner, 1991; Jänig, 1987; Perl, 1984; Willis, 1988). Upon entry, nociceptive afferents synapse with projection neurons that convey information to higher centers, facilitory interneurons that relay input to projection neurons, and inhibitory interneurons that modulate the flow of nociceptive signals to higher centers (Jessell & Kelly, 1991). Similar neural processing occurs in the spinal cord and the medullary dorsal horn.

The spinal cord contains a complex network of interneurons. These networks not only relay signals to higher levels of the central nervous system but also modulate signal transmission and initiate motor reflexes. Peripheral trauma can sensitize dorsal horn nociceptive neurons, making them sensitive to normal inputs and also excessively responsive to those inputs (Willis & Westlund, 1997; Woolf & King, 1990). The exaggerated response of transmission cells in the spinal cord is central sensitization. Enduring central sensitization could cause persisting pain.

There are two principal types of projection neurons in the spinal cord: nociceptive specific and multireceptive or wide dynamic range (WDR) neurons (Jänig, 1987). The former convey only tissue trauma signals; the latter respond to stimuli of increasing intensity. Ascending tracts include spinothalamic, spinoreticular, spinomesencephalic, spino-

cervical, and postsynaptic dorsal cord tracts. Willis and Westlund (1997) and Besson and Chaouch (1987) provide useful reviews of nociceptive transmission mechanisms. In biomedical thinking, the spinothalamic tract is clearly the most important. Lesions of the anterolateral quadrant of the spinal cord result in a loss of pain sensation below the segmental level of the lesion on the contralateral side of the body (Bonica, 1990).

Central Registration

The thalamus is a gateway and relay center for afferent input coming to the brain; therefore, it is the key structure in central registration. It consists of several functionally distinct nuclei that are reciprocally connected to many parts of the limbic system and the cortex (Willis & Westlund, 1997). Medial and ventrobasal thalamic nuclei relay noxious signals to the primary and secondary somatosensory cortices (SI, SII) where refined localization and discrimination occur. In biomedical thinking, the appreciation of pain occurs in these cortical areas.

Recent work acknowledges the existence of spinoreticular, spinomesencephalic, and spinolimbic pathways as nociceptive pathways (Willis & Westlund, 1997), but to date neurophysiologists do not link them to appreciation of pain sensation. Chapman and Stillman (1996) suggested that spinolimbic and spinoreticular pathways play a major role in the emotional component of pain and that this determines the aversive quality of the pain experience.

Modulation

Pain is the end product of modulated transmission. The concept of modulation revolutionized biomedical thinking about pain. Historically, gate control theory (Melzack & Wall, 1965) brought modulation to the forefront in pain research. What had been a rigid, bottom-up information transmission system incorporated a top-down influence when the gate control concept came onto the scene. Gate control theory postulated a gating mechanism at the dorsal horn of the spinal cord that could modulate the transmission of noxious signaling. The signal dampening action of the gate depends on the relative amount of activity in large- versus small-diameter fibers in the periphery. It also suggested descending inhibitory influences from higher centers.

Numerous, and more elegant, models of modulation have emerged over the past three decades, and they have displaced the original gate control concepts many times over. Currently, the dominant model is the Diffuse Noxious Inhibitory Control (DNIC) concept that focuses on counterirritation—the phenomenon by which an additional noxious stimulus reduces the pain caused by the initial noxious stimulus (DeBroucker, Cesaro, Willer, & LeBars, 1990; Talbot, Duncan, & Bushnell, 1989). In humans, counterirritation induces parallel decreases in the sensation of pain and the RIII nociceptive spinal flexion reflex simultaneously evoked by electrical stimulation of the sural nerve (Willer, DeBroucker, & LeBars, 1989). The mechanism of DNIC is at issue and apparently involves, but may not be limited to, inhibition of the activity of WDR neurons in the dorsal horn.

Before moving on, we return to our movie viewer analogy in light of the modulation concept. We see that the person in the movie theater, hearing shouts of "Fire!," now finds that the shouting varies in clarity as a function of the sound and activity level of the ongoing movie. Furthermore, the clarity of the shouted message may increase or diminish as a function of how much interest the viewer has in receiving alarming news messages.

Pain and the Mind

The mechanistic assumptions of classical neurology, which hold that pain is a purely sensory phenomenon, have survived over the centuries because they have proven useful as simple working models of pain and symptom perception. However, this viewpoint becomes ever more tenuous as consciousness research and philosophy progress. It is not so much the clockwork mechanics of Cartesian thinking that creates the problem for contemporary biomedical thinking as the assumption of duality. Descartes held that the awareness of pain, like awareness of other bodily sensations, must occur in a special location from which the mind observes the mechanistic body. Dennett (1991) and others concerned with consciousness characterize this concept as the Cartesian Theater. The mind observes and interprets the array of multimodality signals that the body produces. Contemporary neurophysiology, of course, rejects out of hand the existence of such a theater (Damasio, 1994), but the notion is endemic in Western culture and intransigent.

One of the intriguing limitations of implicit Cartesian dualism is the double transduction dilemma (Dennett, 1996). The biomedical thinker first postulates a transduction of stimulus energy into neural impulses (see the earlier quote from

Duthie). In order to account for the entry of a sensory message into awareness, he or she must postulate a second transduction from neural messaging into the mind stuff of awareness. Although Dennett did not address pain specifically, his challenge applies directly to pain concepts in medicine. Postulating a second transduction reifies the concept of a mind separate from the body and is pure dualism.

Summary of the Biomedical Position

The biomedical sensory neurophysiological model of pain holds that nociception, transmission of noxious signaling, modulation, and sensory registration of pain are biologically predetermined processes. This is a predominantly bottom-up, unidirectional, sequential information processing model, rooted in Cartesian dualist assumptions. Although mechanisms of modulation exist, pain is something that happens in the awareness of an injured or sick person, like a written message that arrives. No straightforward explanation exists for chronicity, although neuropathy and sensitization are potential factors. Why patients with little or no definable pathology sometimes suffer debilitating, chronic pain remains an enigma. This position also has major problems in explaining how a sensory experience can contribute so powerfully to suffering; why pain hurts is still unclear.

This model to date has not addressed the knotty problem that challenges consciousness researchers: How do signals of tissue trauma make their way into consciousness? Thus far, the biomedical model has equated consciousness with activity in the cerebral cortex, with no reflection on how or why this might be. Mind-body dualism, although implicit, still dominates biomedical thinking about pain.

THE BIOPSYCHOSOCIAL PERSPECTIVE

Cognitive-behavioral psychologists offer a different perspective on pain. For them pain is not a simple alarm message arriving at the cerebral cortex like a radio signal exciting a beeper. Rather, sensory messaging binds inextricably to complex associations that embed it in personal and social context and imbue it with meaning. The perception of a chronic pain patient involves a constellation of unpleasant bodily awareness sensations, beliefs about one's health and physical status, fears and uncertainties, and interpretation of the vocational, family, and other social implications of possible disease.

Historically, biopsychosocial thinking began about 1970. Melzack and Casey (1968), in an attempt to expand gate control theory, had speculated about the nature and the location of higher order processes in the brain. They postulated that the neospinothalamic projection system mediates pain sensation, whereas reticular and limbic structures determine the motivation and negative affect necessary to initiate action. Unspecified neocortical processes match input with prior experience and with the neospinothamalmic, reticular, and limbic systems. This elaboration represented and encouraged a growing openness for discussion of the brain's complex influence on the body.

Other psychological professionals were independently developing other theories on the brain/body relationship with implications for pain research. For example, Engel (1977) argued for an alternative to the biomedical model that would bring psychological and social factors to the table. Moreover, pain clinicians, including Bonica (1953) and others, had become increasingly frustrated with the often inadequate care available to chronic pain patients and were seeking new ways of managing pain more effectively. Many realized that pain affected the entire person and suspected that psychological history and context influenced the experience of pain.

Behavioral models based on operant conditioning made important inroads for psychology into medicine. Fordyce (1976) pointed to the influence of operant learning mechanisms on the pain behaviors of patients. His approach directly addressed the discrepancy between tissue damage and pain behavior, and this captured the attention of some medical clinicians. Fordyce contended that chronic pain is not simply something that patients feel; it is what they do. It is reasonable to look at pain as a learned behavior and to treat inappropriate pain behavior. In this perspective, hurt does not equal harm if medical evaluation shows no link between the pain and immediate tissue trauma. Because this is the case, rest only promotes deconditioning and disability. The Fordyce approach, which emphasized rehabilitation and restoration of function, competed successfully with classical psychiatric practice that, at the time, tended to simply label chronic pain patients lacking detectable pathology as either hysterical or depressed and offered little or no intervention.

During the same era, Sternbach (1966) addressed psychophysiological pain syndromes, frequently called "stress-induced pain disorders." This effort engendered greater consideration of environmental, as well as psychological, factors in illness. Mason, Brady, and Tolson (1966), Engel (1968), and Frankenhaeuser (1972) lent further support to these ideas by emphasizing the importance of psychological determinants in the stress response and in illness. Gradually, it became clear that pain was not only a complex experience but also a social role. Causal factors included life stress, as well as tissue trauma.

Brody's (1973) early system model and later Levi's (1974) diathesis-stress model attempted to further integrate environmental factors into the etiology of illness. Levi's model was the first to reference explicitly a biopsychosocial framework of illness, a framework that extends to the present day. His model attempted to incorporate a patient's biological and psychophysiological vulnerabilities with environmental (social) circumstances in describing the patient's disease. Like basic gate control theory, the biopsychosocial model of illness has undergone numerous refinements, but it continues to serve as a useful tool in our quest to understand chronic pain.

The current biopsychosocial model of chronic illness comprises three major factors: (1) integrated action, (2) reciprocal determinism, and (3) evolution (Turk, 1996). The idea of integrated action emphasizes that chronic pain does not occur in a vacuum; biological, psychological, and social elements are integrated to color the chronic pain patient's experience. For example, a male patient's site of injury (back), emotional state (anger at his supervisors for making him work overtime), and manner of expressing his pain to others based on social and/or cultural beliefs ("men don't cry" stoicism) all affect how he will make meaning of his pain. The concept of reciprocal determinism states that biological, psychological, and social factors can influence each other. For example, the man's physiological changes, stemming from pain (increased sympathetic arousal), can affect emotional aspects of the pain experience (increased anger); and these consequently influence his response to the environment (hostility to others), which can further alter his physiological state. Finally, the concept of evolution states that the patient's pain experience is not a static condition but is instead constantly changing over time to adapt to the biological, psychological, and social circumstances. Therefore, when we observe the man in pain at any point in time, we are receiving only a snapshot of his experience; his condition will likely change in some manner after he receives comfort from social contacts, again after he speaks with work supervisors, and yet again when he experiences some pain relief through analgesic medications.

In this model, biological factors are most important in initiating, continuing, and modulating pain in the acute stage. Psychological factors come into play by shaping the individual's understanding of resulting physiological cues and determining the patient's consequent behavior. Such factors include beliefs about the cause and effect of pain, as well as beliefs about self-efficacy. A patient who believes that an increase in pain indicates a worsening physical condition will interpret cues more negatively than a patient who holds more benign beliefs about an increase in pain (Spiegel & Bloom, 1983). Additionally, patients who, based on past experiences of pain, anticipate pain and believe that they will be unable to function if they engage in certain activities will perform poorly on exercise tasks (Council, Ahern, Follick, & Kline, 1988; Schmidt, 1985a, 1985b). Thus actions are often determined more by memories of past pain than by actual pain experienced in the present. The social and cultural context further influences how a patient acts based on this understanding (Sternbach & Tursky, 1965; Zborowski, 1952; Zola, 1966). For instance, children of chronic pain patients visit the school nurse more often and complain more frequently about their pain than children of healthy subjects (Richard, 1988). Figure 3.2 illustrates the biopsychosocial perspective.

The biopsychosocial framework of chronic pain has spawned numerous studies that seek to expand on older concepts, as well as validate new concepts that have formed since Fordyce's behavioral model (Costa & Vandenbas, 1990; Craig & Weiss, 1990; Fernandez & Turk, 1989; Flor, Turk, & Rudy, 1989; Fordyce, 1988; Fordyce, Fowler, & DeLateur, 1968; Fordyce, Fowler, Lehmann, & DeLateur, 1968; Fordyce, Roberts, & Sternbach, 1985; Gatchel & Blanchard, 1993; Kabat-Zinn, Lipworth & Burney, 1985; Keefe, 1994; Keefe, Dunsmore, & Burnett, 1992; Linton, 1986; Linton, Melin, & Gotestam, 1984; McCauley, Thelen, Frank, Willard, & Callen, 1983; Romano et al., 1992; Sanders, 1979, 1985, 1989, 1996; Shumaker, Schron, & Ockene, 1990; Spiegel & Bloom, 1983; Syrjala, Cummings, & Donaldson, 1992; Syrjala, Donaldson, Davis, Kippes, & Carr,

1995; Turner & Jensen, 1993). Cognitive aspects of behavior change have assumed greater importance as time has passed, and the current treatment regimens of multidisciplinary pain clinics usually include cognitive-behavioral techniques. Typical techniques include cognitive reframing of certain painful stimuli into more benign sensory information rather than interpreting the stimuli as signals of progressing disease (e.g., attributing soreness to exercise). Identifying, challenging, and altering automatic thoughts about pain (e.g., "my pain will prevent me from enjoying anything") is another common technique. Patients often find monitoring their behavior useful because it allows them to determine whether any patterns of behavior or particular situations increase their pain and to take steps to change. These interventions illustrate the power of altering beliefs in order to sustain behavioral change over time.

The two major goals of cognitive-behavioral treatment for chronic pain are: (1) to develop and bolster patients' beliefs that they can function adaptively in everyday living and manage pain, and (2) to teach patients skills for effectively handling future pain-related challenges (Bradley, 1996). Often patients believe that their ability to enjoy life is destroyed by their pain; they may think that they can no longer enjoy their favorite habits and pastimes or that their ability to perform everyday tasks is forever lost. Few patients realize that their thoughts, emotions, and behaviors constantly influence their pain and disability. By becoming more aware of and experiencing their ability to positively (and negatively) alter their pain experience through thinking and action, patients can then feel more in control over their lives, and they see alternatives to complete disability. Consequently, they can more realistically evaluate how their lifestyles will and will not change as a result of their pain. Moreover, the new skills they learn to manage their pain (reframing, relaxation, monitoring, etc.) can generalize to future challenges that may contribute to pain (e.g., job stress and interpersonal problems).

In contrast to the biomedical model, the biopsychosocial model does not emphasize curing the patient of pain. The pursuit of cure often leads to disappointment for the patient and the physician alike. Instead, the biopsychosocial approach aims to enable patients to cope more effectively with their pain and improve daily functional capability. Essentially, this framework encourages patients to adopt a more adaptive life perspective that may frequently entail pain rather than letting pain be-

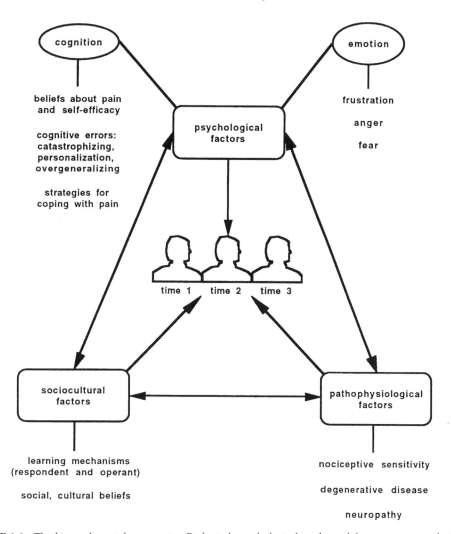

FIGURE 3.2. The biopsychosocial perspective. Biological, psychological, and social factors continuously interact with each other and exert varying influence on the pain patient across time. Each view of the patient is a snapshot of a continuously evolving chronicity process.

come a barrier to normal living. Although these treatments have provided relief to and increased coping skills in many chronic pain patients, they have not succeeded uniformly. Clearly, there is more to learn about optimizing biopsychosocial interventions.

Where does this leave us in our understanding of chronic pain and disability? Although the current biopsychosocial framework has enabled providers to identify more factors that contribute to chronic pain, it deals in broad generalities and offers no explanation of how psychosocial factors affect the brain and the body. Because current

understanding of psychological and sociocultural influences stems solely from observation of overt patient behaviors, one can only make assumptions and inferences about the mental processes that evoke these behaviors. Without a solid theoretical basis for explaining the mechanisms under which these factors drive pain chronicity, the model will prove interesting but useless for those in the medical community who are attempting to treat chronic pain. Although psychologists have broken free of the biomedical model of pain, they have not been able to replace it with a better theory.

CONSCIOUSNESS AND THE CONSTRUCTIVIST FRAMEWORK

Consciousness

We contend that, in consciousness, pain represents tissue trauma. Scientifically, what is consciousness? As a field of research, consciousness is inchoate, multidisciplinary, and multilevel in focus. Its scientific community comprises quantum mechanical physicists, neurophysiologists, neural network computationalists, psychologists, ethologists, sociologists, and anthropologists, among others (see Hameroff, Kaszniak, & Scott, 1996, for an overview). We cannot, therefore, characterize it comprehensively in this limited space, but a few relevant generalizations hold for much of the work in progress.

First, much consciousness research makes use of the concepts of decentralized, dynamical, nonlinear self-organization processes and complexity (Resnick, 1995). Biology offers thousands of examples of how organisms, ranging from colonies of bacteria to herds of caribou, organize themselves as a leaderless collective in the course of adapting to an environment. The behavior of a flock of birds is a common example. One can argue that crowd behavior, traffic jams, and culture itself are human aspects of this process. Nonlinear systems dynamics, as a field, lends itself nicely as a descriptive framework for this process (Bar-Yam, 1997; Freeman, 1995). One can characterize seemingly chaotic phenomena as complex systems. The amount of information one needs to describe the behavior of such a system is a measure of the system's complexity.

Second, the concept of emergence (and emergent property) is a major building block for many workers in the consciousness field (Baas, 1996; Scott, 1996). Emergence simply means that combining certain elements produces a complex system that possesses properties lacking in the individual elements and unpredictable from knowledge of the individual elements. Expressed as a familiar cliché, the whole is greater than the sum of the parts. Atoms of hydrogen and atoms of oxygen at room temperature are gases, but when one combines them, the curious property of liquidity emerges. Emergent properties are just this—the spontaneous emergence of hitherto nonexistent features. The apparent intelligence of an anthill is an emergent property of the collective. No individual ant is intelligent, and nothing we know about individual ants allows us to predict the astonishing intelligence that the colony displays. The concept of emergent property helps one escape the constrained thinking of Cartesian clockwork mechanics.

Inherent in the concept of emergence is the importance of hierarchy in scientific endeavor (Scott, 1995). Interesting, unprecedented properties emerge as one goes from lower to higher levels of scientific inquiry. Emergent properties often define domains of study by specifying the boundaries of a given paradigm. The researcher who attempts to explain subjective reality from the activity of neurons and circuits in the brain simply comes to the edge of the territory. To work with subjective reality, one needs the paradigms of psychology. Curiously, workers engaged at one level of scientific inquiry tend to ignore the efforts of colleagues working at higher or lower levels and sometimes consider them to be misguided. The ultimate goal of science, of course, is to build knowledge bases at each level and then achieve explanatory bridges across levels. Consciousness research recognizes the importance of building knowledge and bridges at all levels.

In light of these considerations, we construe consciousness as an emergent property of the brain: a dynamical self-organizing process operating in a distributed neural network. The legacy of evolution, it increases the repertoire of behaviors and the functional capability of the individual. Viewed neurologically, consciousness has certain on–off features (coma, sleep, anesthesia), but it is useful for psychological purposes to think of it as a gradation, varying in degree of arousal. This gradation is like the degree of illumination of a theater stage on which various characters appear. Specific subjects emerge into the spotlight of consciousness and then fade into the background. Consciousness involves constant ebb and flow in focus. Many important functions are preconscious. That is, they occur outside of awareness, require faster computation than conscious thought can muster, are nonlinear, and are often nonverbal. Examples include the use of overlearned skills such as riding a bicycle or using the rules of grammar, intuition, and creativity.

Currently, the field of consciousness research lacks a single definition for consciousness that suits all applications. We agree broadly with Greenfield's (1995) admittedly complex description of consciousness as

spatially multiple yet effectively single at any one time. It is an emergent property of non-specialized, divergent groups of neurons (Gestalt) that is continuously variable with respect to, and always entailing, a stimulus epicenter. The size of the Gestalt, and hence the depth of prevailing consciousness, is a product of the interaction between the recurring strength of the epicenter and the degree of arousal. (p. 104)

Like an electron that has at a given instant both a position and velocity, consciousness has a stimulus-defined focus and a degree of arousal.

Constructivism and Pain

Constructivism is only one niche in the complex field of consciousness research, but it can deal directly with the question of pain. It assumes that the brain deals not with reality itself but with an internal representation of reality that it constructs from moment to moment, using sensory information, networks of association, and memory stores. Subjective reality undergoes constant revision (self-organization), includes sensory information, emotion, ratiocination, and other aspects of cognition, and always has a point of view. The point of view is the sense of self, which is closely tied to the sense of body–self (Damasio, 1994).

For the constructivist, pain is a complex, emotionally negative awareness characterized by sensory qualities and normally consequent to tissue trauma (Chapman, 1995; Chapman & Nakamura, 1998). It is a threat to the biological integrity of the self. The transduction, transmission, and modulation aspects of biomedical thinking are basic mechanisms for the constructivist framework. However, whereas the biomedical model focuses on the transmission of nociceptive impulses as specific sensory signals, the constructivist perspective emphasizes the central processing of such signals and the construction of the contents of consciousness. Our model does not include a simple sensory registration of pain as a message. We suggest instead that pain emerges from complex patterns of massive parallel distributed processing in the perceiver's model of the self and world.

Features of Human Consciousness

Consciousness develops from birth through differentiation. In the newborn, awareness is largely incoherent, but over time a unity emerges and creates the sense of self. Learning, memory, expectation, and beliefs become parts of the self and, partly through the self's executive functions, shape consciousness. The following features characterize consciousness.

Coherence

In the mature individual, consciousness tends toward coherence. That is, consciousness is self-organizing and continually works toward meta-stability. At its root, awareness is inherently fragmented, a cacophony of inner voices and visions. Such fragments may well arise from multiple origins. However, consciousness tends to form meaningful wholes from elements of awareness and to create a working model of both the external world and the body. It also organizes experience across time. We perceive a connectedness in moving from one thing to another. Moreover, our model of reality is situated: Mental events have a time and place reference.

Sense of Self

What organizes awareness and ensures coherence across place and time? How does a brain engaged in massive parallel processing achieve a singular point of view? One could describe the sense of self as an epiphenomenon of the brain's tendency to achieve coherence. The concept of self is particularly important for pain research for two reasons. First, individuals have a strong sense of the body self. A mental map of the body that Melzack calls the body matrix (Melzack, 1990) exists in human consciousness. When a person loses a limb or other body part, the persistence of the mental image of the body creates the experience of a phantom. That is, the sense of whole remains even when a part is lost. A twisted or distorted phantom limb represents an injury to the body self within the realm of consciousness and can be a cause of great distress to the patient.

Second, at a higher level of self-organization, namely society, people have social selves. Names and roles in family and society define individuals. Chronic pain syndromes, in particular, demonstrate the ways in which the persistence of pain can become a part of the social self. The representation of self is complex and multidimensional.

Purposiveness

Adaptation and survival, along with the goals and purposes of an individual, direct activity and also consciousness. Because we use limited mental resources, consciousness requires resource allocation. It seems, therefore, to involve a searchlight of attention. This searchlight ensures that consciousness has a center and a periphery. In addition consciousness involves intentionality. That is, it is always about something. Our biological, psychological, and social motivations drive the focus of attention. Except perhaps in certain meditation states, we are never simply aware in a vacuum.

Personal Nature and Affect

The personal nature of consciousness is so obvious that we risk overlooking it. We cannot share our thinking or feelings with one another other than by verbal or gestural communication. My back pain is something that is mine alone; you cannot share it or even know quite what it is like for me. This feature sets the phenomena of consciousness apart from those phenomena that neuroscience addresses. The objective features of a neuroscience phenomenon are the same for all observers, but the things in my awareness at this moment are mine alone and cannot be yours.

Finally, consciousness often involves an affective tone: Emotion colors everything we experience. Things seem good or bad to us to varying degrees, and this serves an important biological function in protecting us from harm and helping to ensure that we sustain those resources that we need for survival. The emotional quality of pain represents in consciousness the meaning or importance of a tissue trauma event, whereas the sensory aspect of pain provides information about what has happened and where (Chapman, 1995).

A Constructivist Model for Pain

Figure 3.3 offers an overview of our model. Like biomedical thinking, this approach has a strong bottom-up element, and the mechanisms of neural transmission are the same as those in the biomedical framework. Biomedical models, however, like that described by Duthie (1994), limit pain mechanisms to the transmission of signals to the thalamus and from there to the somatosensory cortex, as Figure 3.1 indicates. In contrast, we build on the observations of several studies of regional cerebral blood flow associated with pain—observations that indicate massive parallel distributed processing. We ascribe such processing to self-organization. It integrates, produces coherence, and sets the stage for the individual's construction of immediate experience and meaning.

A number of recent positron emission tomography (PET) studies of brain metabolic activity during pain indicate that central processing is far more complex than a sensory registration model allows (Casey et al., 1994; Casey, Minoshima, Morrow, & Koeppe, 1996; Coghill et al., 1994; Jones, Brown, Friston, Qi, & Frackowiak, 1991; Jones et al., 1994; Talbot et al., 1991; Vogt, Derbyshire, & Jones, 1996). Although the time resolution of PET studies does not permit investigators to specify strictly which aspects of distributed processing are serial and which are parallel, these studies demonstrate unequivocally that extensive distributed processing occurs in many different areas of the brain.

The complexity of central processing of painful events is striking. In people who are experiencing pain, distributed processing involves the internal capsule (lenticular nucleus), anterior cingulate, insular cortex, frontal areas, thalamus, somatosensory cortices, superior and inferior frontal cortex, straight gyrus, and cerebellar vermis (Casey et al., 1994; Casey et al., 1996; Coghill et al., 1994; Derbyshire et al., 1994; Jones et al., 1991; Jones et al., 1994; Talbot et al., 1991; Vogt et al., 1996). These studies reveal that the limbic brain, the seat of emotion, undertakes a major part of the processing that builds the experience of pain. The emotional aspects of pain are invariably negative, and the noradrenergic pathways may play a central role in building the disturbing emotional quality of pain (Chapman, 1995).

As the PET studies cited here show, the brain displays multifocal, parallel, and complex central processing (Mesulam, 1990; Mesulam, 1994). Therefore, we propose that dynamically distributed processing in large-scale networks, operating in parallel, integrates and synthesizes noxious signaling and other products of central processing to construct the contents of consciousness. Pain is but one aspect of this complex, constantly self-organizing process, and yet it is a prominent aspect because of its strong emotional component.

How parallel distributed processing in various brain regions constructs the awareness of pain and the associated suffering is still uncertain. We suggest that parallel distributed processing initiated by tissue trauma involves self-organized response patterns and that dynamically emerging response patterns, rather than fixed anatomical pathways, are the proper focus for interpreting PET observations of people experiencing pain.

The following processes characterize central processing: (1) multiple central response patterns compete for dominance (this is an evolutionary theory concept of cell assemblies, well articulated by Calvin, 1987; see Taylor, 1996, for similar ideas

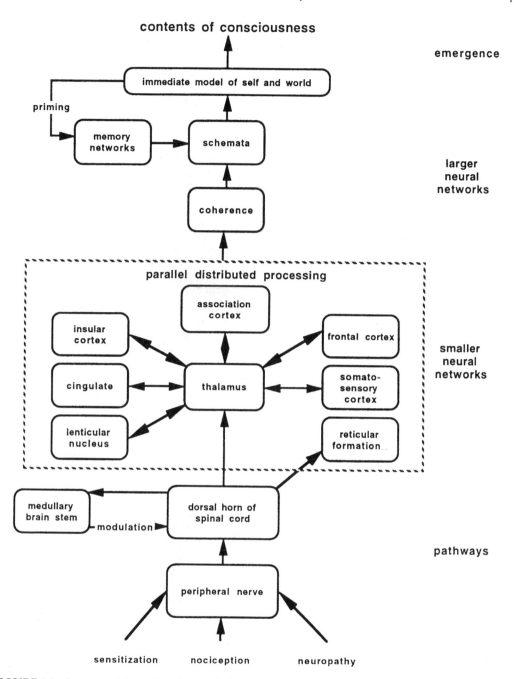

FIGURE 3.3. A constructivist model of pain. The lower part of this figure corresponds to the biomedical mechanisms: transduction, transmission, and modulation. The box with the dashed line indicates that, at higher levels of the central nervous system, massive parallel distributed processing takes place. In the interest of simplicity, we characterize these processes as loops from the thalamus to various other structures. This processing integrates multimodal neural information and produces a coherent set of sensory and emotional associations. Schemata emerge from parallel distributed processing and memory networks and compete with one another for entry into the contents of consciousness. To qualify for emergence, a schema must fit memory associations and the individual's immediate model of the self and the world to incoming noxious signaling. This figure represents a snapshot of a complex dynamical system evolving over time. In this framework, patients construct pain from immediate sensory information, memory networks, and the immediate model of the world and self.

about neural networks); (2) sensory signaling integrates with expectation and other components of memory networks, various associations and motives appropriate to the immediate situation, and the long-range goals of the person; and (3) self-organization forms a coherent whole from the sum of the many parts of the distributed processing. This coherent whole is dynamical by nature: The contents of consciousness evolve constantly, but (with the exception of dreaming) they maintain coherence.

As the cognitive-behaviorists recognize, pain never exists in sensory isolation. It is embedded in contextual experience, and the brain constantly works toward reconciling the disharmony that it causes. The experience of pain, ordinarily a signal of injury or disease, typically triggers various high-level responses directed at escaping from or stopping the threat to biological integrity.

Pain, Schemata, and Consciousness

How can something like low back pain intrude into consciousness, amidst a mingled and ever-varying composite of other experiences? Let us assume that this type of pain originates with a compression lesion of a nerve root, due perhaps to a herniated disc. A complex barrage of multisensory afferent signals arrives at the brain constantly, and this array changes over time. The signals from the injured nerve are but minor features of the stream of neural signals that reach the brain. We propose that the brain constantly forms and reforms short-lived perceptual wholes from the constantly changing arrays of information. Immediately after a noxious stimulus (in this case, provocation of a neuropathic condition), nonconscious and parallel distributed processing integrates the signals from nociceptors with other representations in the brain and various memories and associations. Such processing forms a stable pattern of primary activations and associations, which we call a schema.[1]

The general notion of a schema as a pattern of activation and association is familiar in cognitive psychology, clinical psychology, artificial intelligence, and neural network modeling (Rumelhart, Smolensky, McClelland, & Hinton, 1986; Williams, Watts, MacLeod, and Mathews, 1988). Although applications and specific definitions of the word schema vary markedly, the term refers to a normally nonconscious pattern of concepts or affects and associations that reflects a person's past experience and influences, as well as expectations for the present and future.

We construe schemata as fuzzy, preconscious, and dynamical, roughly related to neural network patterns. Rumelhart and colleagues (1986) usefully described schemata in this way:

> Schemata are not single things. There is no representational object which is a schema. Rather schemata emerge at the moment they are needed from the interaction of large numbers of much simpler elements, all working in concert with one another. Schemata are not explicit entities, but rather are implicit in our knowledge and are created by the very environment that they are trying to interpret as it is interpreting them. (p. 20)

A schema may emerge as a new network of associations, or it may be a partially preformed pattern of imagery that emerges from memory (e.g., a visual image or a tune). It is not a simple memory trace. Alternatively, a schema could be a pattern of motor skills formed from learning processes that involved extensive practice (e.g., riding a bicycle). Presumably the brain stores certain images and motor patterns associated with somatosensory and visceral sensory awareness. As it periodically retrieves, uses, and restores this information, it alters it. In other words, retrieving and using memory contents (which are more akin to networks of association than stored computer records) alters those contents to some degree.

The process of constructing consciousness is dynamical and complex. The available construction materials include schemata associated with immediate sources of physiological stimulation (sensory experience), immediate cognitive and affective schemata, schemata produced in imagination, and schemata stored in memory. Most schemata are short-lived because the constant changes of perception overwrite the neural circuitry before they have a chance to consolidate. However, some are learned; that is, they survive indefinitely in memory. Learned schemata are readily available for recall, and certain sensory events or other schemata can act as triggers for a particular schema.

The schema construct helps explain a painful, trigger-sensitive condition known as phantom limb pain that exists across individuals and cultures. Phantom body parts tend to appear in consciousness after a person has lost a limb. They are kinesthetically vivid realizations of a body part that is physically absent. Sometimes a phantom limb will hurt, and no treatment directed at the

---

[1]The word comes from the Greek, and its plural is schemata.

stump or administered systemically can relieve it (Melzack, 1990).

In a study of 68 patients with phantom limb pain, Katz and Melzack (1990) found that patients had experienced various postamputation pains, all localized to the missing limbs. The patients described these pains as immediate and real, quite unlike recollection of a past pain state. In constructivist terms, the patients were reproducing or reconstructing pain and not simply recalling a past event. Interestingly, some of the phantom experiences involved painless experience (e.g., feeling a shoe on a missing foot), and some had multimodal sensory qualities. Katz and Melzack speculated that "a higher order somatosensory memory component, once formed, can be activated when only some of its elements are present in the sensory input" (p. 333).

For the constructivist, this means that simple somatosensory stimuli can serve as triggers, activating preformed schemata that become part of the contents of consciousness. This leads to the principle that one schema can trigger another. Triggers for phantom limb pain are not invariably sensory. Sometimes they are cognitive or emotional in nature (Hill, Niven, & Knussen, 1996). This suggests that cognitive and affective schemata may function as triggers for chronic pain states, when tissue trauma is no longer the predominant cause of noxious signaling.

Our model also assumes that some schemata dominate others for a place in the content of consciousness at a given moment. Why some emerge and others recede begs explanation. Marcel (1983), as Williams et al. (1988) interpret, proposes that multiple schemata (in Marcel's terms, "perceptual hypotheses") become activated simultaneously, and each is tested automatically against the records of nonconscious processing for goodness of fit. The prevailing schema is the one that best accounts for the most data in the records (i.e., noxious signaling from tissue trauma). Pain researchers often refer to the multidimensional nature of pain as a complex theoretical construct (Chapman, 1995). In our view, the multidimensionality of schemata and consciousness is the underlying system-level mechanism that gives rise to pain.

Evidence for Schemata

The neurophysiologist may be tempted to dismiss the notion of schema as a fanciful construct of psychologists, unrelated to demonstrable neurophysiological function. However, organized patterns of neural action resembling schemata must exist. Neurosurgical studies of patients with epilepsy indicate that complex and highly coherent patterns of multisensory experience reside in the brain, as do rather complicated patterns of motor experience. Focal electrical stimulation of the brain of an awake patient during surgery can cause chronologically distant memory fragments to suddenly emerge into consciousness. Penfield (1975) described a single case in which he repeatedly stimulated the interpretive cortex. On one trial, the patient said, "I had a little memory, a scene in a play, they were talking and I could see it. I was just seeing it in my memory . . ." (p. 27). This and other examples indicate that the activated memory patterns are multimodal and dynamic (that is, they are more like multimedia movie clips of events than simple snapshots). On another trial, the same patient said, "Just a tiny flash of feeling, of familiarity, and a feeling that I knew everything that was going to happen in the near future . . ." (p. 25). This example indicates that (1) some patterns are emotional rather than sensory in quality and that (2) the emotional schemata seem to be present and real as compared to the memory quality of predominantly visual or auditory events. Penfield also described eliciting involuntary motor movements from patients by stimulating motor cortex regions. These observations suggest that the brain not only forms multimodal sensory, motor, emotional, and cognitive schemata, but it also stores them in memory. It is reasonable to suppose that the brain may form schemata on its own, drawing upon intrinsic memories, associations, and ratiocination.

How many schemata can the contents of consciousness sustain at a given moment? In principle, consciousness can reflect several schemata simultaneously, but the consciousness is a limited resource. Normally, there is only a single focus of consciousness at a given moment in time. That exceptions can occur is quite clear. During neurosurgical brain electrical stimulation, patients appear to be fully aware of the surgical setting and of an elicited experience simultaneously (Penfield, 1975), and persons with agenesis or surgical transsection of the corpus callosum appear to have two simultaneous arenas of consciousness under certain experimental conditions (Gazzaniga & LeDoux, 1978).

Self-Organization

Unlike the classical theorist, the constructivist does not need to assume that the brain is a passive arena through which information passes. Clearly, the human brain can generate its own patterns of awareness and imagery in the absence of extrinsic signaling. Moreover, it can store these patterns in memory, retrieve them selectively, modify them, and put them back into storage. Perception is more an act of constantly building and remodeling one's view of the world than it is of receiving and registering information.

How does consciousness handle changes in information across time? Dennett and Kinsbourne (1992) assert that mental representation of reality changes constantly in a nonlinear way, relatively independent of time. That is, instead of generating conscious representation of stimulus events in a chronologically serial fashion, the brain constantly produces revised drafts of awareness, mixing old and newer sensory, affective, and cognitive representations without particular regard for time. Put another way, elements of memory and expectation compete and eventually integrate with recent sensory messages from the environment for a place in the representation of reality. If this is the case, then schemata emerging from nonconscious processing into the contents of consciousness need not carry the most recent information that the brain has processed. A part of our immediate representation of reality comes from memory.

The "multiple drafts" concept of consciousness suggests that the most remarkable feature of consciousness formation is its extraordinary plasticity. The brain creates a representation of immediate reality by interweaving records of the past with sensory input from the immediate present, and it forecasts images of the future. Far from being a passive entity that merely registers information that comes in from various sensory channels, the brain is an active, adaptive system that constantly simulates the world and the body in which it dwells. Nociceptive signals may trigger complex responses and schemata, leading to elaborate experiences of pain with sensory, affective, cognitive, and motor dimensions.

The Role of Evolution

Constructivist thinking about pain has deep roots in the theory of evolution. Pain is not an accident of human development but rather a protective mechanism that fosters adaptation and survival in a primitive world. From a Darwinian perspective, one must ask why we would evolve the capability for complex pain schemata when a simple sensory warning signal might suffice. We hold that high plasticity in modeling the world increases survival value by increasing the adaptation of an individual to a changing environment.

In normal life, a pain schema merits high priority in the contents of consciousness because it represents a violation of biological tissue integrity. However, under conditions of emergency such as combat, pain can prove catastrophically maladaptive by interfering with the very functions on which survival depends. During combat, observers often note that wounded combatants do not experience pain despite visually startling tissue trauma. For the soldier under fire, victory or escape are more important goals than recognizing and tending to injury. Therefore, we suggest that those schemata that serve the individual's goals for the immediate situation are the most likely ones to prevail in competition for a place in consciousness. Protection and survival are high on the list of goals in most situations, and pain is normally relevant to these goals.

Advantages of the Constructivist Approach

This position, unlike the biomedical framework, can account for emerging observations of widespread parallel distributed processing in the brain during the pain experience. Such processes are the preconscious workings of the construction process. In addition, constructivism offers several advantages for understanding pain and its treatment. For one, this position can help explain the vast differences in response to painful events that one sees in clinical settings. People differ because they create and live with unique subjective realities. Two persons with identical lesions do not have identical subjective realities.

For another, we can account for the effects of various psychological interventions such as hypnosis on pain (Chapman & Nakamura, 1998). These are interventions that recognize and address the uniqueness of the individual. Hypnotic suggestion alters the construction of the pain experience. This suggests that the processes of competition and integration are as much targets for pain intervention as the neural structures and synapses that transmit nociception. Biopsychosocial interventions directed at altering maladaptive beliefs are attempts to reconstruct patient subjective reality.

In preventing or relieving pain, it is important to fit the intervention to the person. The assumptions behind biomedical thinking do not permit this type of accommodation. One assumes that human sensory mechanisms are basically all alike. In the constructivist model, everyone is unique in experiencing pain, and it is necessary to understand something of each person's model of reality in order to alter it. Because of this feature, constructivist thinking may ultimately provide a rationale for the development and refinement of biopsychosocial interventions for pain.

Finally, the link of pain to suffering, which forever eludes the biomedical theorist, is readily evident in this framework. We suffer with pain because we bundle awareness of tissue trauma with complex schemata that have negative cognitive and affective features.

CONCLUSION

We have described three approaches to understanding pain. The first two, biomedical and biopsychosocial, are bastions of parochialism: Neither camp shows any interest in the scientific efforts and issues of the other. Indeed, biomedical researchers reading this chapter have probably skipped or skimmed over the section on biopsychosocial models, and biopsychosocial readers have probably skipped the section on biomedical mechanisms. This situation represents a failure in communication across levels of inquiry. We propose the consciousness framework because it offers some hope for relating, if not integrating, these two fields.

The biomedical approach, despite the severe historical constraints of Cartesian thinking, has served medicine well. A clear need exists for more basic fact-gathering on nociceptive transmission and its modulation within this framework, but biomedical thinking has locked itself, quite unnecessarily, into a bottom-up focus. Commitment to reductionism does not imply that one must work from the bottom up. It is equally legitimate to start with a higher level process and decompose it by working downward (Churchland, 1994).

Biomedical pain researchers may lack the necessary incentive for top-down research because the field suffers from a limited vision of the brain processes associated with pain. It now must confront challenging brain imaging data obtained from persons in pain. Neurophysiologists cannot interpret the findings emerging from PET studies of brain metabolism during pain, and future development in the neuroimaging field is likely to widen the gap between biomedical assumptions and brain imaging observations. The pain field will soon need

to acknowledge and address the issues that consciousness researchers are currently approaching in vision and other areas: What is the nature of massive parallel distributed processing? What, if any, role does binding play in consciousness? How do complex patterns of electrical and metabolic activity in the brain produce the phenomenon of awareness? Ultimately, pain research must confront these and other difficult questions.

The biopsychosocial field has done well in building a conceptual framework that can account for chronic pain at the psychological level, and definitive work at this level is absolutely essential for the advance of the pain field overall. Unfortunately, biopsychosocial research has never extended a hand to biomedical research. Many biopsychosocial researchers have a thin understanding of the physiological basis of pain and make no effort to develop a knowledge base in this fundamental area. Most biomedical researchers are barely aware that the biopsychosocial field exists. It is hard to imagine how pain research can function effectively as a multidisciplinary field if researchers at different levels will not learn one another's language.

As a scientific discipline, the biopsychosocial field is somewhat aberrant. One might ask whether it is science at all. On the one hand, biopsychosocial researchers employ standard scientific method and hypothesis testing. They measure their constructs and replicate one another's findings. In keeping with the principle of parsimony, they attempt to produce the simplest possible explanation to account for their observations. In conducting research, biopsychosocial researchers have kept the rules and colored inside the lines.

On the other hand, the biopsychosocial field lacks some of the essential features of a science. First, science is, above all, about the process of discovery. Just what biopsychosocial researchers have discovered, in the classical sense of the term, or what they envision one could discover within this framework is quite unclear. The second feature of a solid science is strong heuristics. An area should generate new research and thinking, not only within its own ranks but also in related areas. It is difficult thus far to discern how biopsychosocial research has influenced biomedical research and thinking. Finally, because of its parochial tendencies, the field lacks solid consilience (interconnection of concepts and findings with other areas). These limitations are largely deficiencies of parochialism.

Biopsychosocial pain investigators exist in a multidisciplinary field dominated by the biomedical model, but their constructs and explanations do not connect with, nor are they formally complementary to, biomedical research and theory. Although the scientific survival of biopsychosocial thinking surely depends on its interaction with, and links to, biomedical research, there is no ongoing effort to forge such linkage at the level of basic science.

Entering the scientific arena in the full light of the day will prove to be challenging for the biopsychosocial field. Currently, eliminative materialism is a formidable force. This position holds that scientific explanation of mental activity and behavior will ultimately reduce to neurophysiology (materialism). Moreover, it assumes that the inexorable march of science will eventually prove many of the contemporary accepted constructs accounting for human behavior inadequate (eliminative). The history of science is littered with constructs that could not withstand the test of time. Biopsychosocial researchers are well aware of the demise of the pure behaviorist approach. Will their constructs survive? Is the construct of belief, for example, really defensible in an open multidisciplinary science? Only time will tell.

We suggest that the consciousness research framework, in particular the constructivist approach, offers an environment for integrating pain research across levels. Viewing pain as a phenomenon of consciousness and embedding the issues of pain research in the broader framework of consciousness issues will help establish bridges across levels of inquiry that are now quite separate. Hopefully, it will also call attention to the phenomena of emergence, which demand investigation in their own right. Understanding pain means the elucidation of coherent, integrated explanations from the whole brain through neural systems, neural networks, pathways, synapses, and neurons.

Our goal in suggesting a constructivist approach is to offer a framework, constrained by existing findings at many levels of the neuraxis but with sufficient heuristic value to generate multiple hypotheses at those same levels. Our framework encompasses a range of processes involved in consciousness. Ultimately, this perspective, which is still incipient, will have to generate models that are open to falsification. Ideally, constructivist research on pain will involve phenomena that are well defined in psychological research and theory, reliably quantifiable, clearly related to brain regions in brain imaging studies, and well linked to activity in other brain regions. The brain activity of a person feeling pain must differ in multiple ways from that of a person who is equally awake and attentive but not in pain. Pain research needs to determine sys-

tematically what those differences are. Constructivism contends that the field needs to understand these differences as process differences in the construction of subjective reality.

There is much in the consciousness field that can assist and empower biopsychosocial research. For example, Nelson's (1996) work on consciousness and metacognition fits well with biopsychosocial notions of cognitive errors. The metacognition concept presumes that introspection is not infallible; instead, the individual is "an imperfect measuring device of his or her cognitions" (p. 106). People commit cognitive illusions, which misrepresent the real world. This work, along with many other papers on consciousness, could provide a fruitful entry for biopsychosocial researchers into the field of consciousness study.

The consciousness framework suggests that biomedical and biopsychosocial researchers could work together in a complementary fashion, each camp presenting challenges and questions to the others. Coordinated, parallel lines of pain research at different levels of inquiry, guided by an overarching theory of consciousness, could produce noteworthy and rapid advances in our understanding of pain.

REFERENCES

Alexander, J., & Black, A. (1992). Pain mechanisms and the management of neuropathic pain. *Current Opinion in Neurology and Neurosurgery, 5*(2), 228–234.

Baas, N. A. (1996). A framework for higher order cognition and consciousness. In S. R. Hameroff, A. W. Kaszniak, & A. W. Scott (Eds.), *Toward a science of consciousness* (pp. 633–648). Cambridge, MA: MIT Press.

Bar-Yam, Y. (1997). *Dynamics of complex systems.* Reading, MA: Addison-Wesley.

Besson, J. M., & Chaouch, A. (1987). Peripheral and spinal mechanisms of nociception. *Psychological Review, 67*(1), 67–186.

Bonica, J. J. (1953). *The management of pain.* Philadelphia: Lea & Febiger.

Bonica, J. J. (1990). *The management of pain* (2nd ed.). Philadelphia: Lea & Febiger.

Boulton, A. (1992). What causes neuropathic pain? *Journal of Diabetes and Its Complications, 6*(1), 58–63.

Boulu, P., & Benoist, M. (1996). Recent data on the pathophysiology of nerve root compression and pain. *Revue du Rhumatisme. English Edition, 63*(5), 358–363.

Bowsher, D. (1991). Neurogenic pain syndromes and their management. *British Medical Bulletin, 47*(3), 644–666.

Bradley, L. A. (1996). Cognitive-behavioral therapy for chronic pain. In R. J. Gatchel & D. C. Turk (Eds.), *Psychological approaches to pain management: A practi-*

tioner's handbook (pp. 131–147). New York: Guilford Press.

Brody, H. (1973). The systems view of man: Implications of medicine, science, and ethics. *Perspectives in Biology and Medicine, 17,* 71–91.

Calvin, W. H. (1987). The brain as a Darwin machine. *Nature, 330,* 33–34.

Casey, K. L., Minoshima, S., Berger, K. L., Koeppe, R. A., Morrow, T. J., & Frey, K. A. (1994). Positron emission tomographic analysis of cerebral structures activated specifically by repetitive noxious heat stimuli. *Journal of Neurophysiology, 71*(2), 802–807.

Casey, K. L., Minoshima, S., Morrow, T. J., & Koeppe, R. A. (1996). Comparison of human cerebral activation pattern during cutaneous warmth, heat pain, and deep cold pain. *Journal of Neurophysiology, 76*(1), 571–581.

Chapman, C. R. (1995). Affective dimension of pain: A model. In B. B. Bromm & J. E. Desmedt (Eds.), *Pain and the brain: From nociception to cognition* (pp. 283–302). New York: Raven Press.

Chapman, C. R., & Nakamura, Y. (1998). Hypnotic analgesia: A constructivist framework. *International Journal of Clinical and Experimental Hypnosis, 46*(1), 6–27.

Chapman, C. R., & Stillman, M. (1996). Pathological pain. In L. Kruger (Ed.), *Pain and touch* (2nd ed., pp. 315–342). New York: Academic Press.

Churchland, P. S. (1994). Can neurobiology teach us anything about consciousness? In American Philosophical Association, *Proceedings and addresses of the American Philosophical Association* (Vol. 67, pp. 23–40). Lancaster, PA: Lancaster Press.

Coghill, R. C., Talbot, J. D., Evans, A. C., Meyer, E., Gjedde, A., Bushnell, M. C., & Duncan, G. H. (1994). Distributed processing of pain and vibration by the human brain. *Journal of Neuroscience, 14*(7), 4095–4108.

Costa, P. T., & Vandenbas, G. R. (1990). *Psychological aspects of serious illness: Chronic conditions, fatal diseases, and clinical care.* Washington, DC: American Psychological Association.

Council, J. R., Ahern, D. K., Follick, M. J., & Kline, C. L. (1988). Expectancies and functional impairment in chronic low back pain. *Pain, 33,* 323–331.

Craig, A. D. (1991). Supraspinal pathways and mechanisms relevant to central pain. In K. L. Casey (Ed.), *Pain and central nervous system disease: The central pain syndromes* (pp. 157–170). New York: Raven Press.

Craig, K. D., & Weiss, S. M. (1990). *Health enhancement, disease prevention, and early intervention: Biobehavioral strategies.* New York: Springer.

Damasio, A. R. (1994). *Descartes' error: Emotion and reason in the human brain.* New York: Grosset/Putnam.

Davar, G., & Maciewicz, R. J. (1989). Deafferentation pain syndromes. *Neurologic Clinics, 7*(2), 289–304.

DeBroucker, T., Cesaro, P., Willer, J. C., & LeBars, D. (1990). Diffuse noxious inhibitory controls in man. Involvement of the spinoreticular tract. *Brain, 113,* 1223–1234.

Dennett, D. (1991). *Consciousness explained.* Boston: Little, Brown.

Dennett, D. C. (1996). The myth of double transduction. Paper presented at the meeting *Toward a Science of Consciousness 1996,* Tucson, Arizona.

Dennett, D. C., & Kinsbourne, M. (1992). Time and the observer: The where and when of consciousness in the brain. *Behavioral and Brain Sciences, 15*(2), 183–247.

Derbyshire, S. W., Jones, A. K., Devani, P., Friston, K. J., Feinmann, C., Harris, M., Pearce, S., Watson, J. D., & Frackowiak, R. S. (1994). Cerebral responses to pain in patients with atypical facial pain measured by positron emission tomography. *Journal of Neurology, Neurosurgery and Psychiatry, 57*(10), 1166–1172.

Devor, M. (1991). Neuropathic pain and injured nerve: Peripheral mechanisms. *British Medical Bulletin, 47*(3), 619–630.

Dubner, R. (1991). Neuronal plasticity and pain following peripheral tissue inflammation of nerve injury. In M. R. Bond, C. J. Woolf, & J. E. Charlton (Eds.), *Proceedings of the Sixth World Congress on Pain* (pp. 263–276). Amsterdam: Elsevier.

Duthie, D. J. R. (1994). The physiology and pharmacology of pain. In W. S. Nimmo, D. J. Rowbotham, & G. Smith (Eds.), *Anaesthesia* (Vol. 1, pp. 119–131). Oxford: Blackwell.

Elliott, K. J. (1994). Taxonomy and mechanisms of neuropathic pain. *Seminars in Neurology, 14*(3), 195–205.

Engel, G. L. (1968). A life setting conducive to illness: The giving up–given up complex. *Bulletin of the Menninger Clinic, 32,* 355–365.

Engel, G. L. (1977). The need for a new medical model: A challenge for biomedicine. *Science, 196,* 129–136.

Fernandez, E., & Turk, D. C. (1989). The utility of cognitive coping strategies for altering pain perception: A meta-analysis. *Pain, 38,* 123–135.

Flor, H., Turk, D. C., & Rudy, T. E. (1989). Relationship of pain impact and significant other reinforcement of pain behaviors: The mediating role of gender, marital status, and marital satisfaction. *Pain, 38,* 45–50.

Fordyce, W. E. (1976). *Behavioral methods for chronic pain and illness.* St. Louis, MO: Mosby.

Fordyce, W. E. (1988). Pain and suffering: A reappraisal. *American Psychologist, 43,* 276–283.

Fordyce, W. E., Fowler, R., & DeLateur, B. (1968). An application of behavior modification technique to a problem of chronic pain. *Behaviour Research and Therapy, 6,* 105–107.

Fordyce, W. E., Fowler, R., Lehmann, J., & DeLateur, B. (1968). Some implications of learning in problems of chronic pain. *Journal of Chronic Disease, 21,* 179–190.

Fordyce, W. E., Roberts, A. H., & Sternbach, R. A. (1985). The behavioral management of chronic pain: Response to critics. *Pain, 22,* 113–125.

Frankenhaeuser, M. (1972). *Biochemical events, stress, and adjustment* (Rep. No. 368). Stockholm, Sweden: University of Stockholm, Psychological Laboratories.

Freeman, W. J. (1995). *Societies of brains.* Hillsdale, NJ: Erlbaum.

Fried, K., Govrin, L. R., Rosenthal, F., Ellisman, M. H., & Devor, M. (1991). Ultrastructure of afferent axon endings in a neuroma. *Journal of Neurocytology, 20*(8), 682–701.

Galer, B. S. (1995). Neuropathic pain of peripheral origin: Advances in pharmacologic treatment. *Neurology, 45*(12, Suppl. 9), S17–S25, S35–S36.

Galer, B. S., & Portenoy, R. K. (1991). Acute herpetic and postherpetic neuralgia: Clinical features and management. *Mount Sinai Journal of Medicine, 58*(3), 257–266.

Gatchel, R. J., & Blanchard, E. B. (1993). *Psychophysiological disorders: Research and clinical applications*. Washington, DC: American Psychological Association.

Gazzaniga, M. S., & LeDoux, J. E. (1978). *The integrated mind*. New York: Plenum Press.

Gebhart, G. F., & Ness, T. J. (1991). Central mechanisms of visceral pain. *Canadian Journal of Physiology and Pharmacology, 69*(5), 627–634.

Greenfield, S. A. (1995). *Journey to the centers of the mind: Toward a science of consciousness*. New York: Freeman.

Hameroff, S. R., Kaszniak, A. W., & Scott, A. W. (Eds.). (1996). *Toward a science of consciousness*. Cambridge, MA: MIT Press.

Heppelmann, B., Messlinger, K., Schaible, H. G., & Schmidt, R. F. (1991). Nociception and pain. *Current Opinion in Neurobiology, 1*(2), 192–197.

Hill, A., Niven, C. A., & Knussen, C. (1996). Pain memories in phantom limbs: A case study. *Pain, 66*(2,3), 381–384.

Jänig, W. (1987). Neuronal mechanisms of pain with special emphasis on visceral and deep somatic pain. *Acta Neurochirurgica Supplementum (Wien), 38*, 16–32.

Jessell, T. M., & Kelly, D. D. (1991). Pain and analgesia. In E. R. Kandel, J. H. Schwartz, & T. M. Jessell (Eds.), *Principles of neural science* (3rd ed., pp. 385–398). New York: Elsevier.

Jones, A. K., Brown, W. D., Friston, K. J., Qi, L. Y., & Frackowiak, R. S. (1991). Cortical and subcortical localization of response to pain in man using positron emission tomography. *Proceedings of the Royal Society of London. Series B: Biological Sciences, 244*(1309), 39–44.

Jones, A. K., Cunningham, V. J., Hakawa, S., Fujiwara, T., Luthra, S. K., Silva, S., Derbyshire, S., & Jones, T. (1994). Changes in central opioid receptor binding in relation to inflammation and pain in patients with rheumatoid arthritis. *British Journal of Rheumatology, 33*(10), 909–916.

Kabat-Zinn, J., Lipworth, L., & Burney, R. (1985). The clinical use of mindfulness meditation for the self-regulation of chronic pain. *Journal of Behavioral Medicine, 8*, 163–190.

Katz, J., & Melzack, R. (1990). Pain "memories" in phantom limbs: Review and clinical observations. *Pain, 43*(3), 319–336.

Keefe, F. J. (1994). Behavior therapy. In P. D. Wall & R. Melzack (Eds.), *Textbook of pain* (pp. 392–406). Edinburgh: Churchill Livingstone.

Keefe, F. J., Dunsmore, J., & Burnett, R. (1992). Behavioral and cognitive-behavioral approaches to chronic pain: Recent advances and future directions. *Journal of Consulting and Clinical Psychology, 60*, 528–536.

Levi, L. (1974). Psychosocial stress and disease: A conceptual model. In E. K. Gunderson & R. H. Rahe (Eds.), *Life stress and illness* (pp. 8–33). Springfield, IL: Thomas.

Linton, S. J. (1986). Behavioral remediation of chronic pain: A status report. *Pain, 24*, 125–141.

Linton, S. J., Melin, L., & Gotestam, K. G. (1984). Behavioral analysis of chronic pain and its management. In R. Hersen, M. Eisler, & P. M. Miller (Eds.), *Progress in behavior modification* (Vol. 18, pp. 1–42). New York: Academic Press.

Marcel, A. (1983). Conscious and unconscious perception: Experiments on visual masking and word recognition. *Cognitive Psychology, 15*, 197–237.

Mason, J. W., Brady, J. V., & Tolson, W. W. (1966). Behavioral adaptations and endocrine activity. In R. Levine (Ed.), *Endocrines and the central nervous system* (pp. 227–250). Baltimore: Williams & Wilkins.

McCauley, J. D., Thelen, M. H., Frank, R., Willard, R., & Callen, K. (1983). Hypnosis compared to relaxation in the outpatient management of chronic low back pain. *Archives of Physical Medicine and Rehabilitation, 64*, 548–552.

McMahon, S., & Koltzenburg, M. (1990). The changing role of primary afferent neurones in pain. *Pain, 43*(3), 269–272.

Melzack, R. (1990). Phantom limbs and the concept of a neuromatrix. *Trends in Neurosciences, 13*, 88–92.

Melzack, R., & Casey, K. L. (1968). Sensory, motivational, and central control determinants of pain: A new conceptual model. In D. Kenshalo (Ed.), *The skin senses* (pp. 423–443). Springfield, IL: Thomas.

Melzack, R., & Wall, P. D. (1965). Pain mechanisms: A new theory. *Science, 150*, 971–979.

Mesulam, M. M. (1990). Large-scale neurocognitive networks and distributed processing for attention, language, and memory. *Annals of Neurology, 28*(5), 597–613.

Mesulam, M. M. (1994). Neurocognitive networks and selectively distributed processing. *Revue Neurologique (Paris), 150*(8–9), 564–569.

Nelson, T. O. (1996). Consciousness and metacognition. *American Psychologist, 51*(2), 102–116.

Penfield, W. (1975). *The mystery of the mind*. Princeton, NJ: Princeton University Press.

Perl, E. R. (1984). Characterization of nociception and their activation of neurons in the superficial dorsal horn: First steps for the sensation of pain. In L. Kruger & J. C. Liebeskind (Eds.), *Advances in pain research and therapy* (Vol. 6, pp. 23–52). New York: Raven Press.

Resnick, M. (1995). Beyond the centralized mindset. *Journal of the Learning Sciences, 5*(1), 1–22.

Richard, K. (1988). The occurrence of maladaptive health-related behaviors and teacher-related conduct problems in children of low back pain patients. *Journal of Behavioral Medicine, 11*, 107–116.

Roberts, W. J. (1986). A hypothesis on the physiological basis for causalgia and related pains. *Pain, 24*(3), 297–311.

Romano, J. M., Turner, J. A., Friedman, L. S., Bulcroft, R. A., Jensen, M. P., Hops, H., & Wright, S. F. (1992). Sequential analysis of chronic pain behaviors and spouse responses. *Journal of Consulting and Clinical Psychology, 60*, 777–782.

Rumelhart, D. E., Smolensky, P., McClelland, J. L., & Hinton, G. E. (1986). Schemata and sequential thought processes in PDP models. In J. L. McClelland & D. E. Rumelhart (Eds.), *Parallel distributed processing: Explorations in the microstructure of cognition: Vol. 2. Psychological and biological models* (pp. 7–57). Cambridge, MA: MIT Press.

Sanders, S. H. (1979). Behavioral assessment and treatment of clinical pain: Appraisal and current status. In M. Hersen, R. Eisler, & P. Miller (Eds.), *Progress in behavior modification* (Vol. 8, pp. 249–291). New York: Academic Press.

Sanders, S. H. (1985). The role of learning in chronic pain states. In S. F. Brena & S. Chapman (Eds.), *Clinics in anesthesiology: Pain control* (pp. 57–73). Philadelphia: Saunders.

Sanders, S. H. (1989). Contingency management and the reduction of overt pain behavior. In D. Tollison (Ed.), *Handbook of chronic pain management* (pp. 210–221). Baltimore: Williams & Wilkins.

Sanders, S. H. (1996). Operant conditioning with chronic pain: Back to basics. In R. J. Gatchel & D. C. Turk (Eds.), *Psychological approaches to pain management: A practitioner's handbook* (pp. 112–130). New York: Guilford Press.

Schmidt, A. J. M. (1985a). Cognitive factors in the performance level of chronic low back pain patients. *Journal of Psychomatic Research, 29*(2), 183–189.

Schmidt, A. J. M. (1985b). Performance level of chronic low back pain patients in different treadmill test conditions. *Journal of Psychomatic Research, 29*(6), 639–646.

Scott, A. C. (1995). *Stairway to the mind.* New York: Springer.

Scott, A. C. (1996). The hierarchical emergence of consciousness. In S. R. Hameroff, A. W. Kaszniak, & A. C. Scott (Eds.), *Toward a science of consciousness* (pp. 659–671). Cambridge, MA: MIT Press.

Shumaker, S. A., Schron, E. B., & Ockene, J. K. (1990). *The handbook of health behavior change.* New York: Springer.

Siddall, P. J., Taylor, D., & Cousins, M. J. (1995). Pain associated with spinal cord injury. *Current Opinion in Neurology, 8*(6), 447–450.

Spiegel, D., & Bloom, J. R. (1983). Pain in metastatic breast cancer. *Cancer, 52,* 341–345.

Stanton-Hicks, M., Janig, W., Hassenbusch, S., Haddox, J. D., Boas, R., & Wilson, P. (1995). Reflex sympathetic dystrophy: Changing concepts and taxonomy. *Pain, 63*(1), 127–133.

Sternbach, R. A. (1966). *Principles of psychophysiology.* New York: Academic Press.

Sternbach, R. A., & Tursky, B. (1965). Ethnic differences among housewives in psychophysical and skin potential responses to electric shock. *Psychophysiology, 1,* 241–246.

Syrjala, K. L., Cummings, C., & Donaldson, G. (1992). Hypnosis or cognitive-behavioral training for the reduction of pain and nausea during cancer treatment: A controlled clinical trial. *Pain, 48,* 137–146.

Syrjala, K. L., Donaldson, G. W., Davis, M. W., Kippes, M. E., & Carr, J. E. (1995). Relaxation and imagery and cognitive-behavioral training reduce pain during cancer treatment: A controlled clinical trial. *Pain, 63*(2), 189–198.

Talbot, J. D., Duncan, G. H., & Bushnell, M. C. (1989). Effects of diffuse noxious inhibitory controls (DNICs) on the sensory-discriminative dimension of pain perception. *Pain, 36*(2), 231–238.

Talbot, J. D., Marrett, S., Evans, A. C., Meyer, E., Bushnell, M. C., & Duncan, G. H. (1991). Multiple representations of pain in human cerebral cortex. *Science, 251*(4999), 1355–1358.

Taylor, J. G. (1996). A competition for consciousness. *Neurocomputing, 11*(2–4), 271–296.

Turk, D. C. (1996). Biopsychosocial perspective on chronic pain. In R. J. Gatchel & D. C. Turk (Eds.), *Psychological approaches to pain management: A practitioner's handbook* (pp. 3–32). New York: Guilford Press.

Turner, J. A., & Jensen, M. P. (1993). Efficacy of cognitive therapy for chronic low back pain. *Pain, 52,* 169–177.

Vecht, C. J., Van de Brand, H. J., & Wajer, O. J. (1989). Post-axillary dissection pain in breast cancer due to a lesion of the intercostobrachial nerve. *Pain, 38*(2), 171–176.

Vogt, B. A., Derbyshire, S., & Jones, A. K. (1996). Pain processing in four regions of human cingulate cortex localized with co-registered PET and MR imaging. *European Journal of Neuroscience, 8*(7), 1461–1473.

Wall, P. D. (1991). Neuropathic pain and injured nerve: Central mechanisms. *British Medical Bulletin, 47*(3), 631–643.

Willer, J. C., DeBroucker, T., & LeBars, D. (1989). Encoding of nociceptive thermal stimuli by diffuse noxious inhibitory controls in humans. *Journal of Neurophysiology, 62*(5), 1028–1038.

Williams, J. M. G., Watts, F. N., MacLeod, C., & Mathews, A. (1988). *Cognitive psychology and emotional disorders.* Chichester, England: Wiley.

Willis, W. D. J. (1988). Dorsal horn neurophysiology of pain. *Annals of the New York Academy of Sciences, 531,* 76–89.

Willis, W. D. J. (1993). Mechanisms of somatic pain. In C. R. Chapman & K. M. Foley (Eds.), *Current and emerging issues in cancer pain* (pp. 67–81). New York: Raven Press.

Willis, W. D. J., & Westlund, K. N. (1997). Neuroanatomy of the pain system and of the pathways that modulate pain. *Journal of Clinical Neurophysiology, 14,* 2–31.

Woolf, C. J. (1989). Recent advances in the pathophysiology of acute pain. *British Journal of Anaesthesia, 63*(2), 139–146.

Woolf, C. J., & King, A. E. (1990). Dynamic alterations in the cutaneous mechanoreceptive fields of dorsal horn neurons in the rat spinal cord. *Journal of Neuroscience, 10*(8), 2717–2726.

Zborowski, M. (1952). Cultural components in responses to pain. *Journal of Social Issues, 8,* 16–30.

Zola, I. K. (1966). Culture and symptoms—an analysis of patients presenting complaints. *American Sociological Review, 31*(5), 615–630.

Chapter 4

Personality, Individual Differences, and Psychopathology in Chronic Pain

JAMES N. WEISBERG
FRANCIS J. KEEFE

One of the most challenging tasks for pain clinicians is dealing with personality factors in the patients they treat. Patients with neurotic tendencies may continue to worry about minor painful physical complaints long after the tissue pathology has been resolved. Patients having long-standing depressive personality features may seem hopeless about the future course of their pain and helpless when it comes to taking an active role in their own treatment. Patients with clear-cut personality disorders (e.g., borderline personality) may demand immediate attention or request unnecessary medications or referrals for specialized care and may respond in a threatening and angry fashion when their demands are not met. To deal with such challenges, pain specialists have developed and refined a number of approaches to better understand and assess personality factors in chronic pain. The purpose of this chapter is to provide an overview of these approaches. The chapter is divided into three sections. The first section provides a conceptual background for the assessment of personality factors in chronic pain. In this section, we trace the evolution of theories of personality and pain, highlighting the development of psychodynamic, trait, and biopsychosocial theories. The second section describes and critically evaluates empirical studies on personality and chronic pain. Two groups of studies are reviewed in detail: those examining personality traits and those examining personality disorders in chronic pain patients. The third section of this chapter highlights a number of important clinical and research issues in this area.

CONCEPTUAL BACKGROUND

Over the past 100 years, a number of theories have addressed the relationship of personality to the pain experience. These theories can be grouped into three basic categories: (1) psychodynamic theories, (2) trait theories, and (3) biopsychosocial theories.

Psychodynamic Theories

Psychodynamic theorists maintain that deep-rooted unresolved personality conflicts can either serve as the basis for persistent pain or complicate the management of chronic pain. Freud (Breuer & Freud, 1893–1895/1957) was one of the first to recognize the connection between pain and underlying emotional conflicts. Freud viewed persistent pain as an affective, or emotional, response to an actual loss or injury. Because he viewed perceived loss as critical to the development of persistent pain, Freud likened the experience of chronic pain to that of mourning. A key component of Freud's model of pain was the notion of "conversion," that is, the idea that emotional pain can be expressed through physical mechanisms. In *Studies on Hysteria* (Breuer & Freud, 1893–1895/1957), Freud postulated that individuals with personality attributes that disallowed the expression of emotional pain through emotional symptoms are likely to "convert" their emotional pain to somatic pain symptoms. The specific pain symptoms that would occur in such cases were considered to be symbolic of the underlying emotional issues. Thus pain located in the pelvic area may well be an expression of an unresolved conflict regarding unacceptable sexual urges. In sum, the hallmarks of the Freudian perspective on persistent pain were (1) that underlying, often unconscious, emotional conflicts are important in understanding pain; (2) that these emotional conflicts can, through psychodynamic mechanisms, be converted to physical pain symptoms; and (3) that the particular pain symptoms that occur are symbolic of underlying emotional conflicts. These basic tenets of psychodynamic theory are important because they have had a strong influence on subsequent psychodynamic theories of chronic pain.

In his book *Pain and Pleasure*, Szasz (1957) took a psychodynamically based object-relations approach to understanding the development and maintenance of chronic pain. According to Szasz, persistent pain was the end product of a threat to the integrity of the individual as a whole. Szasz argued that whether the threat was real or imagined was unimportant; rather, it was the individual's interpretation that mattered. An important feature of Szasz's formulation of pain was the notion that persistent pain can serve numerous functions. At the most basic level, persistent pain provided subjective symptoms that the individual can focus on. At a secondary level, pain can affect interaction with others by providing a reason to ask for help or assistance. Finally, at the deepest level, pain has a symbolic function in that it serves as a symbol for unexpressed emotional pain, giving the individual a way to cope with that emotional pain. Like Freud (Breuer & Freud, 1893–1895/1957), Szasz (1957) maintained that pain could serve as a substitute for past emotional hurt and anguish that the individual was not able to express or experience appropriately. Descriptions of the severity, location, and character of physical pain, therefore, can provide the individual with an "acceptable" means of expressing emotional hurt and serve as a further defense against the earlier emotional suffering.

George Engel (1959), in his classic article "'Psychogenic' Pain and the Pain-Prone Patient," further discussed the various meanings that persistent pain may have. Engel argued that, although persistent pain can have a pathophysiological basis, the individual's interpretation of that pain is a "psychological phenomenon." Engel believed that pain, whether related to disease processes or of unclear etiology, may serve several important psychological functions. First, pain may provide a means of absolving one of guilty feelings by turning the suffering inward. Second, a focus on pain may enable an individual to displace attention from aggressive or hostile feelings that he or she is unable to express directly. Finally, persistent pain may be related to a lifelong history of suffering and defeat and serve as a protagonist that enables an individual to continue in the role of being victimized. Engel (1959) also noted that certain psychiatric diagnoses were quite common in persons having chronic pain. These diagnoses, from the *Diagnostic and Statistical Manual of Mental Disorders*, first edition (DSM-I; American Psychiatric Association, 1952), included hysteria, depression, hypochondriasis, and paranoid schizophrenia. Engel's formulations of pain were important for two reasons. First, they underscored the notion that pain is a complex phenomenon. Second, they maintained that psychodynamic formulations are important not only in understanding pain due to hysteria or psychiatric disorders but also in understanding how people adjust to pain due to injuries or disease.

Trait Theories

Trait theorists argue that long-standing personality traits or dispositions can have a strong influence on how one responds to the onset, persistence, and treatment of pain. Sternbach (1974) was one of the first to highlight the role that personality traits can play in adjustment to chronic pain. Sternbach cited research conducted by Bond (1971) and Bond and Pearson (1969) showing that personality factors such as neuroticism predisposed individuals to chronic pain. Sternbach also suggested the reverse may be true. The experience and expression of pain may predispose people to neuroticism and hypochondriacal worries (Sternbach, 1974). Finally, he noted that, although most people understand acute pain as a warning sign of danger, many struggle with their inability to understand chronic pain. Chronic pain is an ambiguous phenomenon that has no obvious meaning and does not serve a protective function to the organism. Sternbach (1974) argued that, in response to such an ambiguous situation, the meaning that the person ascribes to his or her pain becomes very important. This meaning often reflects the individual's personality and history. Sternbach found that chronic pain patients often felt punished, hopeless, and helpless in relation to their pain. More recently, Blumer and Heilbronn (1982) have argued that certain personality factors place people at risk for chronic pain disorders. They reported anecdotal evidence that patients often referred to themselves as "solid citizens" prior to pain onset and had idealized views of their interpersonal relationships and their own independence. They went on to use the term "egomania" to describe such patients (Blumer & Heilbronn, 1982) and argued that these traits predispose individuals to chronic pain and disability. Blumer and Heilbronn (1982) felt that such "pain prone" individuals are suffering from a variant of depressive disorder and are best treated with a conservative approach once physical pathology is ruled out.

Biopsychosocial Models

The biopsychosocial model maintains that personality traits and dispositions interact with biological factors to determine how one responds to pain. The biopsychosocial model was first conceived by Engel (1977). Engel maintained that illness represented a complex interaction of biological, psychological, and social influences. The interaction may be linear or nonlinear, with each component affected by and affecting each other. For example, an individual sprains his or her ankle. This biological event may initiate and maintain a psychological reaction, such as anger or frustration. The psychological response may, in turn, be affected by the person's social environment; that is, family and friends may be overly solicitous and provide excessive attention or sympathy when pain is reported. These social responses may lead the individual to avoid use of his or her ankle and become overly sedentary, which can result in muscle weakness and deconditioning—biological factors that can perpetuate the ankle pain. Thus a seemingly simple event (sprained ankle), when viewed from a biopsychosocial perspective, can precipitate a cascade of biological, psychological, and social responses that can interact to exacerbate and maintain pain. The biopsychosocial perspective is especially relevant to

understanding chronic pain, because, in the case of persistent pain, many opportunities exist for biological, psychological, and social factors to influence pain. The biopsychosocial model of pain has served as the basis for multidisciplinary treatment programs for chronic pain. These programs incorporate a variety of medical, psychological, and social interventions to teach patients to control their pain and resume a functionally effective lifestyle and to promote more adaptive social interactions with family, friends, and employers. Another model that has been applied to the understanding of pain is the diathesis–stress model. According to the diathesis–stress model, illness develops as an interaction between an underlying biological or genetic substrate (diathesis) and the expression of that substrate under certain situations (stress). The model has been successfully applied to medical illnesses such as diabetes, ulcerative disease, and heart disease, as well as to psychiatric conditions that include schizophrenia, depressive disorders, and substance abuse. The diathesis–stress model has been proposed as an explanation for why some individuals develop chronic pain disorders while others do not (Flor & Turk, 1984; Turk & Flor, 1984). According to the diathesis–stress model, chronic pain disorders are a function of the interaction between the individual's premorbid biological and psychological predispositions (diathesis) and the challenges or stressors (stress) that he or she faces as a result of the physical impairment and tissue damage (Banks & Kerns, 1996). The diathesis includes the individual's personality strengths and vulnerabilities, and the stress includes the biochemical and nociceptive changes that occur at the outset of the pain disorder. The diathesis–stress model has been used to account for muscular hyperreactivity that occurs in certain low back pain patients. Flor, Turk, & Birbaumer (1985) have argued, for example, that poor coping resources for managing stressful situations, coupled with depressed mood, place individuals at risk for developing excessive muscle-tension responses to pain. Indeed, research studies of patients with low back pain have shown that only those people who are depressed, worried, and emotionally affected by their pain are likely to show high levels of low back muscle tension in response to stress (e.g., Flor et al., 1985). In another study of chronic pain patients, we found that depression mediated the degree to which a novel mental stressor (problem solving) precipitated excessive trapezius muscle reactivity (Weisberg, Gorin, Drozd, & Gallagher, 1996). When depressed patients were exposed to the stressor, they showed very high levels of bilateral trapezius muscle tension. Nondepressed patients exposed to the same stressor, however, showed relatively little muscle tension response.

EMPIRICAL STUDIES OF PERSONALITY AND CHRONIC PAIN

Empirical studies on personality and chronic pain can be divided into two basic categories: (1) those that examine personality traits and (2) those that examine personality disorders.

Personality Traits and Chronic Pain

Numerous research studies have examined personality traits in patients who have chronic pain. In this section, we consider (1) psychometric instruments used to assess personality traits, (2) descriptive studies identifying common personality traits, and (3) predictive studies examining the relationship of personality traits to treatment outcome and the development of chronic pain.

Instruments Used to Assess Personality Traits

Over the past 50 years, psychologists have developed a number of standardized psychological test instruments for assessing personality traits. These instruments have several basic features. First, they are self-administered paper-and-pencil tests that can be easily used in clinical settings. Second, their scoring is standardized. Third, they have been administered to normative populations, thereby enabling one to compare a given patient to relevant comparison groups. Finally, they are psychometrically strong; that is, they show good evidence of reliability and validity.

Much of the research on personality traits in chronic pain patients has used the Minnesota Multiphasic Personality Inventory (MMPI; Hathaway & McKinley, 1943). The MMPI was originally developed by using psychiatric inpatients who represented a broad range of disorders as the criterion group; it was normed on 724 friends and relatives (representative of the Minnesota population) of hospital inpatients. The MMPI contains 566 items and consists of three validity scales and 10 clinical scales. The validity scales aim to assess the individual's test-taking attitude. They include (1) the Lie scale (*L*), which attempts to uncover a

person's attempts to present him- or herself in the most favorable manner; (2) the Frequency scale (*F*), which was developed to detect deviant ways of responding to the test; and (3) the Correction scale (*K*), a more sensitive version of the *L* scale, aimed at ascertaining whether an individual is attempting to present him- or herself in a more or less psychologically healthy light. High scores on the *K* scale are indicative of a defensive test-taking manner. In addition to the three validity scales, the "cannot say" scale consists of simply tallying the number of items to which the individual did not respond. When scoring the MMPI, the interpreter looks at the pattern of the *L*, *F*, and *K* scales to determine the validity and manner in which the examinee approached the test. There are 10 clinical scales, including (1) Hypochondriasis (*Hs*), preoccupation with one's body and somatic symptoms; (2) Depression (*D*), general dissatisfaction with one's life; (3) Hysteria (*Hy*), tendency to convert emotional symptoms into physical complaints, often characteristic of psychological immaturity; (4) Psychopathic Deviate (*Pd*), tendency to be amoral and engage in delinquent acts; (5) Masculinity–Femininity (*Mf*), the extent to which an individual is engaged in traditional gender roles (originally intended to detect homosexual tendencies); (6) Paranoia (*Pa*), feelings of grandiosity, ideas of reference, or persecution; (7) Psychasthenia (*Pt*), the propensity to doubt oneself, act compulsively, and ruminate (closest to obsessive–compulsive disorder); (8) Schizophrenia (*Sc*), aberrant thoughts and behavior often considered psychotic; (9) Hypomania (*Ma*), elevated mood, behavior, and irritability; and (10) Social Introversion (*Si*), the proclivity toward being withdrawn and avoid social contact and responsibilities. There are standardized norms, and both high and low scores (defined as two or more standard deviations from the norm) are interpreted. A more recent revision of the MMPI has been developed (MMPI-2; Butcher, Dahlstrom, Graham, Tellegen, & Kaemmer, 1989). The MMPI-2 has 567 items and was normed on 2,600 individuals drawn from a much more diverse population that was chosen to be representative of the 1980 population census data. Additional advantages of the MMPI-2 over the first version include stronger evidence of reliability and validity and the updating of questions. Despite the potential advantages of the MMPI-2 in assessing personality traits in chronic pain patients, this instrument has not been widely used by pain researchers or clinicians (Deardorff, Chino, & Scott, 1993). This may be due to the fact that the instrument is relatively new or that users may prefer the original MMPI, which has been shown to have utility in the assessment of chronic pain patients.

Another standardized personality test that has been used in pain assessment is the NEO-PI (Neuroticism, Extroversion, Openness Personality Inventory). The NEO-PI is a broad-based self-report inventory originally developed in the 1980s (Costa & McCrae, 1985) to assess a variety of interpersonal and intrapsychic functions in healthy individuals. The NEO-PI is a 181-item self-report measure that taps five domains of personality: Neuroticism, the tendency to worry excessively; Extroversion, an individual's inclination to remain either relatively reserved and serious or outgoing and "high-spirited"; Openness, the ability to view situations from other standpoints; Agreeableness, the capacity to demonstrate warmth interpersonally, to avoid conflict, and to trust others; and Conscientiousness, having high standards for oneself and others. These domains were empirically derived through factor analytic studies and demonstrate good reliability and validity across a variety of populations. Within each domain, there are six subcategories that tap a variety of interpersonal, intrapsychic, and defensive structures. The NEO-PI has been the focus of numerous reliability and validity studies (McCrae, 1991; McCrae & Costa, 1987).

Descriptive Studies

Descriptive studies have attempted to identify personality traits that are common in patients having chronic pain. One of the first descriptive studies of chronic pain patients was conducted by Hanvik (1951). Hanvik used the MMPI to differentiate between low back pain patients whose pain was either functional (i.e., of psychological origin) or organic (i.e., of physical origin). Hanvik demonstrated that individuals without physical findings were clearly distinguishable on the MMPI from those patients with organic findings. Those individuals without a physical basis for pain had significantly elevated scores on scales measuring impulsivity (Pd), anxiety (Pt), and odd thinking (Sc), in addition to elevations on scales assessing somatic concern (Hs), hysteria (Hy), and depression (D). From these findings, Hanvik constructed the Low Back Pain (Lb) scale to distinguish between low back pain patients with physical causes (organic) from those without physical findings (functional). This scale attracted considerable attention, since it purported to provide a simple means of discriminating functional from organic pain and led to

increased use of the MMPI in low back pain assessment. However, subsequent studies provided somewhat mixed support for Hanvik's claims regarding the utility of the MMPI in differentiating functional from organic pain (Armentrout, Moore, Parker, Hewitt, & Felts, 1982; Bradley, Prokop, Margolis, & Gentry, 1978; Gentry, Shows, & Thomas, 1974; McCreary, Turner, & Dawson, 1977; Sternbach, Wolf, Murphy, & Akeson, 1973a, 1973b). Hanvik (1951) also described the "conversion-V" originally described by Gough (1946). The conversion-V consists of clinically significant elevations ($T > 70$) on scale 1 (Hypochondriasis) and scale 3 (Hysteria), with a lower score on scale 2 (Depression), resulting in a "V" pattern on the first three scales of the MMPI. This profile was believed to represent conversion hysteria, whereby the individual "converts" his or her unacceptable depressive feelings into somatic complaints. Studies showed that when MMPI data from a large number of pain patients were averaged and graphed, the conversion-V pattern was often observed. This observation raised questions about whether or not the conversion-V was normative for chronic pain patients or whether there were subpopulations within diverse chronic pain populations that showed a variety of MMPI profiles. Sternbach et al. (1973a) noted that, in addition to elevation on the Hypochondriasis and Hysteria scales, chronic pain patients also often had a significant elevation on the Depression scale of the MMPI. Therefore, many of these individuals were clearly depressed, and it was hypothesized that they were unable to fully convert their affect into psychophysiological symptoms. Based on their findings, Sternbach et al. (1973a) concluded that depression and neurotic disturbances in the form of preoccupation with physical symptoms are common in patients having chronic pain. They also discuss invalidism, or a pattern of behavior characterized by what he later referred to as a "professional pain patient" (Sternbach, 1974). Sternbach et al. (1973b) also used the MMPI to study personality traits in acute (less than 6 months' duration) and chronic (more than 6 months' duration) low back pain patients with and without physical findings. They found that the profiles of the chronic patients were significantly higher than those of the acute patients on the Hysteria, Depression, and Hypochondriasis scales. When they compared the MMPI profiles of patients with physical findings (defined by a variety of clinical and x-ray findings) from those without physical findings, there were relatively few differences between these two groups.

In his classic text *Pain Patients: Traits and Treatment*, Sternbach (1974) summarizes four commonly observed patterns on the MMPI. The first pattern, hypochondriasis, reflects excessive somatic concerns and consists of T scores above 70 on Hypochondriasis (Hy) and Hysteria (Hs) scales. The second subtype, named "reactive depression" by Sternbach, had significant elevations on scales Hy, D, and Hs, with depression higher than either of the other elevations. In this subtype, individuals are often depressed and anxious, perhaps in response to their somatic pain, and tend to benefit the most from treatment. The third subgroup is the classic conversion-V previously described. The final profile Sternbach (1974) identified was the manipulative reaction, which consisted of elevations on scale 4 (Psychopathic Deviate), as well as on scales 1–3. The patients were believed to be angry and manipulative and often acted out, using their physical symptoms to get needs met.

Gentry et al. (1974) attempted to combine the MMPI and other psychological tests with biographical and historical data to derive a "psychological profile" of patients with chronic low back pain. Patients in the study completed the MMPI, a sentence completion test, and the Draw-A-Person test. They were also given an interview to assess their familial history of chronic pain. The MMPI profile obtained from this group of patients conformed to the conversion-V pattern characteristics of individuals who are excessively somatic-focused, use defense mechanisms of denial and repression, and tend to be outwardly sociable, dependent, and self-centered. Gentry et al. (1974) also noted that, as a group, these patients often had familial role models for pain and received a significant amount of support and attention at the onset of their symptoms.

McCreary et al. (1977) conducted a study comparing personality differences of individuals having functional as opposed to organic pain. They found that individuals with functional pain had significantly higher elevations on scales measuring hypochondriasis (Hs), hysteria (Hy), mania (Ma), schizophrenia (Sc), aberrant behavior (Pd), and extroversion (Si). In addition, patients without organic findings scored significantly lower on the defensiveness scale (K). The authors concluded that their findings are consistent with those of Hanvik (1951). However, they cautioned the reader to avoid using these findings to diagnose functional versus organic pain, since the differences on MMPI scale between these two groups of patients, although present, were relatively small (less than 1 standard deviation difference between groups).

Bradley et al. (1978) argued that one reason for the divergent findings regarding the MMPI and chronic pain was that data from diverse groups of patients were being averaged to form composite profiles. They conducted a study designed to reveal whether one could identify homogeneous, replicable MMPI subgroups within a diverse low back pain population. Using multivariate cluster analytic methods, they identified four distinct MMPI profile subgroups for females and three for males. One subgroup, present in both genders, had MMPI elevations on scales Hs, D, and Hy similar to the "reactive depressed" subtype previously identified by Sternbach (1974). These patients may be somatically focused and concerned about a variety of physical symptoms that may be related to the pain. The second subgroup common to both genders had elevations on scales K, Hs, and Hy, but none of these elevations exceeded a T score of 70, or 2 standard deviations from the mean. Bradley et al. (1978) suggested that individuals in this subgroup might be dependent and might be achieving unmet dependency issues through their symptoms. The third MMPI subgroup identified in both males and females had greater psychopathology and had elevations on multiple MMPI scales (i.e., Hs, D, Hy, and Sc). Bradley et al. (1978) maintained that the patients in this subgroup were very depressed, preoccupied with their physical concerns, and isolated and that the pain may serve their unmet emotional needs through socially acceptable means. The final subgroup identified by Bradley et al. (1978) had clinically significant elevations on scales Hs and Hy but not on the D scale. This subgroup, present in females only, showed a pattern similar to that of Sternbach's conversion-V (1973a, 1974). Bradley et al. (1978) noted Sternbach's (1974) observation that these patients tended to enjoy the sick role. Bradley et al. concluded that low back pain patients were not a homogeneous group, as previously believed, and that distinct, replicable MMPI subgroups could be identified.

Armentrout et al. (1982) also used multivariate cluster analysis methods to identify MMPI subgroups. Their results yielded three clusters that were similar to those found by Bradley et al. (1978). The three clusters included a subgroup showing a virtually normal profile, a subgroup having elevations on scales measuring hypochondriacal concerns, and a subgroup that had elevations on numerous MMPI scales (a "psychopathological" profile). Patients in the psychopathological profile subgroup reported the highest levels of pain, those in the hypochondriasis subgroup the next highest level of pain, and those in the normal group the lowest level of pain. Armentrout et al. (1982) argued that clinicians working with chronic pain patients need to be aware of these subgroups because patients in each subgroup may require somewhat different approaches to assessment and treatment.

As noted earlier, relatively few studies have used the MMPI-2 to assess personality traits in chronic pain patients. One example of such studies is a relatively recent report by Deardorff, Chino, & Scott (1993). This study factor analyzed MMPI-2 data collected from 114 chronic pain patients recruited from an outpatient pain treatment facility. The factor analysis revealed five factors, four of which were interpretable. Factor 1 was characterized by elevations on scales F, PD, Pa, Pt, and Sc and was interpreted to reflect general psychological distress. Factor 2 was characterized by very low scores on scales K and Si and subscales of Hy and was interpreted to reflect social isolation and introversion. Factor 3 was characterized by low scores on Ma and on subscales of D and Hy and was interpreted to reflect psychomotor retardation. The final factor was characterized by elevations on scales Hs, Hy, and subscales on Hy and was interpreted to represent physical dysfunction. Although theirs is not a temporal mode, the authors believe each of their factors may represent one aspect in the development of chronic pain, from the subacute to chronic phases (Deardorff et al., 1993).

Wade, Dougherty, Hart, and Cook (1992) used the NEO-PI profile to differentiate between subgroups previously found on the MMPI (Sternbach, 1974). Fifty-nine subjects were placed into one of the four MMPI subgroups based on their MMPI profiles, and NEO-PI scores were generated for each of the five domains. Following statistical analysis, only the Neuroticism domain score on the NEO-PI differentiated any of the MMPI subgroups—the emotionally overwhelmed subgroup (Sternbach, 1974)—from those in the other three MMPI subgroups. Interestingly, the NEO-PI responses of patients who fell in the hypochondriasis, somaticizing, and adaptive coping MMPI subgroups were similar to those of normal controls. On the basis of these NEO-PI results, the authors conclude that "chronic pain patients typically present with unremarkable adult personality structure" (Wade et al., 1992). The authors conclude that the NEO-PI is sensitive enough to identify chronic pain patients scoring high on Neuroticism, but that it does not appear to discriminate between a number of MMPI subtypes identified in the research literature. In general, the NEO-PI responses of chronic pain patients are similar to those of normal, well-adjusted adults.

Comment. There does not appear to be any consistent evidence that chronic pain patients fit into one profile, as previously believed, although some traits may be common between individuals.

Predictive Studies

A number of studies have examined the degree to which personality traits measured by standard psychological tests can predict the outcome of treatments for chronic pain. The basic design of these studies involves administering a personality test (e.g., the MMPI) prior to medical or surgical treatment and then following patients up at a later time (e.g., immediately after surgery or 6 months later) to determine how personality traits that were identified pretreatment relate to long-term outcome. Several prospective studies have used the MMPI to predict the outcome of low back surgery (Wiltse & Rocchio, 1975; Waring, Weisz, & Bailey, 1976).

Wiltse and Rocchio (1975) used the MMPI, among other psychological tests, to determine whether standardized psychological tests could be used to differentiate those patients who reported pain relief following surgical intervention from those whose symptoms were not relieved. Participants were 130 patients undergoing a surgical intervention that consisted of chemonucleolysis, or chemical ablation of a displaced (herniated) disk. Results indicated that high scores ($T > 75$) on the MMPI Hysteria (Hy) and Hypochondriasis (Hs) scales predicted poorer outcome. The authors recommend that patients with high scores on Hy and Hs and few objective findings should be treated conservatively rather than surgically.

Waring et al. (1976) evaluated 34 patients with low back pain who were admitted to a hospital for surgical treatment. Included in the presurgical evaluation was the MMPI, as well as other measures. Results indicated that the MMPI was not useful in predicting surgical outcome. Instead, surgeons' preoperative ratings of patients' physical findings and emotional readiness for surgery were the best predictors of outcome. In fact, for patients who had a good treatment outcome, T scores of scales Hs, D, and Hy were 62, 62, and 61, respectively, whereas scores for those with a poor treatment outcome were 64 (Hs), 55 (D), and 63 (Hy), resembling a "conversion-V" in pattern but not in magnitude of scale elevations. Problems with this study include the small sample size and selection biases in that the surgeons had most likely determined good surgical candidates prior to hospital admission.

McCreary, Turner, and Dawson (1979) conducted a retrospective study in which they examined personality traits related to the outcome of a conservative pain management program. In this study, personality traits were assessed using the MMPI clinical scales, along with Hanvik's MMPI Low Back Pain scale (1951). Data analysis revealed several relationships between MMPI scales and treatment outcome. Patients scoring low on the Hypochondriasis scale of the MMPI were more likely to show improvement on two of three outcome measures (pain intensity and ability to resume activities). Patients scoring higher on the Depression scale also were more likely to have pain (pain intensity) at follow-up. There were no significant differences on the Hysteria scale with respect to any of the outcome measures. Finally, there was a significant difference on the Low Back Pain scale between those who were more likely to report pain relief and return to normal activities and those who were less likely to report good outcome on the same variables. The authors conclude that, although the MMPI did differentiate between good and poor outcome following conservative treatment, there were "complicated interactions between the types of personality disturbances and various measures of outcome" (McCreary et al., 1979). In addition, they believe that pretreatment personality factors need to be studied to assist in maximizing treatment compliance.

Predicting the Development of Chronic Pain. There has long been debate as to which comes first, the personality traits that lead to chronic pain or chronic pain that leads to certain changes in personality traits. Despite repeated attempts to gain a better understanding of the temporal relationship between personality and chronic pain, this relationship remains enigmatic. A few prospective studies have been conducted.

In a study of acute back pain, Bigos et al. (1991) collected a variety of physical, psychological, and psychosocial measures (including the MMPI) from over 3,000 employees at a Boeing aircraft manufacturing plant. During an approximate 4-year follow-up period, 279 of these employees developed back problems. Data analyses revealed that individuals who scored in the upper quintile on MMPI scale 3 (Hysteria) were 2.0 times more likely to develop back pain than participants scoring low on scale 3. However, the overall elevations on the MMPI scales were lower than those found in other studies of chronic pain. Additionally, scale 4 (*Pd*) and scale 8 (*Sc*), as well as Hanvik's Low Back Pain scale, differentiated those who developed acute low back pain from those who did not develop back pain. Another very important predictor of the onset of back pain was job dissatisfaction.

In another recent prospective study, Hansen, Biering-Sorensen, and Schroll (1995) gave the MMPI to a cohort of approximately 400 Danish men and women over a 20-year period. The MMPI was given to participants at ages 50 and 60 at the time of their health examinations. Participants were questioned about the presence or absence of back pain during the following 10-year interval (between ages 50–60 years and 60–70 years). Results indicated that MMPI scale elevations on *Hs, D,* and *Hy* at ages 50 and 60 were associated with low back pain during the following decade. In addition, elevated MMPI scores at age 60 were associated with back pain during the preceding decade, from ages 50–60. These results are interesting in that they suggest a relationship between certain personality traits and the development of pain complaints. However, a number of limitations make it difficult to interpret the findings. First, no attempt was made to document or control for the participants' physical status. Patients having more physical findings might simply be more prone to focus on their somatic complaints. Second, no attempt was made to explain observed changes in the MMPI over time in the sample. Thus the study does not provide a definitive test of which factor came first, the back pain or the MMPI elevations. Most important, although the MMPIs of patients with low back pain were statistically significantly higher than those of patients without back pain, they were still within the normative range ($T < 70$) and therefore not clinically significant.

Gatchel, Polatin, and Mayer (1995) systematically compared the ability of the MMPI, the Structured Clinical Interview for DSM-III-R (SCID; Spitzer, Williams, Gibbon, & First, 1988), and the Structured Clinical Interview for DSM-III-R Personality Disorders (SCID-II; Spitzer et al. 1988) to predict subsequent pain and disability status. Participants were 421 patients who were recruited within 6 weeks of pain onset and administered a variety of measures, including the MMPI, SCID, and SCID-II. All participants were then contacted at a 1-year follow-up, at which time their job status was classified as either "working/in school," "not working due to pain," or "not working-unrelated to pain." Data analyses were conducted to determine the degree to which scores on the MMPI and SCID measures predicted disability outcome at follow-up. Results demonstrated that participants who initially scored higher on MMPI scale 3 were much more likely to be disabled from work than subjects scoring low on this scale. Other predictors related to employment status included gender, filing of workers' compensation or personal injury claims, and initial scores on a pain and disability measure. Regression analyses revealed that the MMPI scale 3 scores, combined with these other predictors, correctly classified outcome for over 90% of patients treated. Interestingly, Gatchel et al. (1995) found that major psychopathology, such as depression and substance abuse, was not predictive of outcome. Unfortunately, this study did not report the results of the SCID-II. Gatchel et al. believe their study supports the belief that the chronicity of pain disability results in psychopathology, rather than the psychopathology resulting in the chronic pain disability, and they point out the need for early psychosocial intervention to prevent disability from occurring. They also encourage further study to determine the specific emotional and psychosocial events following injury that may result in chronic disability (Gatchel et al., 1995).

Comment. Psychological tests can provide a reliable and standardized way of assessing personality traits in patients with chronic pain. Although a number of psychological tests have been used with chronic pain patients, the MMPI has been the most widely used. Descriptive studies using the MMPI have identified a number of common profile subtypes with a diverse population of patients having chronic pain. Although there is a large body of predictive research on the MMPI and chronic pain, there continues to be great debate as to its predictive utility. Two factors, in particular, have contributed to this debate. First, as we have seen, the results of predictive studies of personality traits in chronic pain patients have been inconsistent. Although some studies have found a relationship between certain personality traits (e.g., hypochondriasis, hysteria, and depression) and treatment outcome, other studies have not found evidence for such relationships. Second, concerns have been expressed that patients having physical findings due to underlying disease or injury may appear to be neurotic on the MMPI because they score high on items that measure somatic focus (e.g., items on the Hysteria and Hypochondriasis scales) (Love & Peck, 1987).

Empirical Studies of Personality Disorders in Chronic Pain Patients

The *Diagnostic and Statistical Manual of Mental Disorders*, fourth edition (DSM-IV; American Psychiatric Association, 1994), lists two criteria that must be satisfied in order to consider personality traits or characteristics severe enough to be a disorder. First, the individual's intrapsychic and interpersonal functioning must be significantly different from that of his or her society or culture. Second, these characteristics must be inflexible and pervasive (Weisberg & Keefe, 1997). Personality disorders, by definition, develop during childhood and become apparent in adolescence or early adulthood (American Psychiatric Association, 1994). They reflect long-standing patterns of maladaptive behaviors, thoughts, and emotions with symptoms severe enough to interfere with the individual's daily functioning. We have recently reviewed the literature on personality disorders and chronic pain (Weisberg & Keefe, 1997). This section, drawing on that review, as well as other material, highlights (1) methods used to diagnose personality disorders, (2) descriptive studies identifying common personality disorders, and (3) predictive studies examining the relationship of personality disorders to the development of chronic pain and treatment outcome.

Methods of Diagnosing Personality Disorders

The most recent versions of the DSM have made considerable advances to improve the methods used to describe, quantify, and diagnose personality disorders since the original *Diagnostic and Statistic Manual of Mental Disorders* (DSM-I; American Psychiatric Association, 1952) was published. Since the third edition (DSM-III; American Psychiatric Association, 1980) each version has outlined specific criteria that an individual must meet in order to be diagnosed with a particular personality disorder. Since the DSM-III (APA, 1980), personality disorders are diagnosed on Axis II of a five-axis system. Table 4.1 highlights the major areas of dysfunction observed in the DSM-IV (American Psychiatric Association, 1994) personality disorders.

Since the advent of the DSM-III, new semistructured interviews have been developed to assist in the diagnosis of both clinical disorders and personality disorders in psychiatric research (for a complete review, see Weisberg & Keefe, 1997). Traditionally, diagnosis of personality disorders was made by a mental health clinician who conducted

TABLE 4.1. DSM-IV Axis II Personality Disorders

	Intrapsychic function/affect	Interpersonal function	Defense mechanisms	Cognition/reality testing
Paranoid PD	Unable to accept responsibility, tense, restricted affect	Suspicious, mistrustful, hypersensitive	Projection, occasional ideas of reference	Concrete, suspicious, distorted
Schizoid PD	Restricted affect	Withdrawn, aloof	Intellectualization, splitting	Good abstraction, intact reality testing
Schizotypal PD	Out of touch with own affect, constricted, anhedonia	Poor, inappropriate interpersonal relations	Paranoid, suspicious	Magical thoughts, perceptual aberrations, may have breaks with reality under stress
Antisocial PD	Seemingly unaware of affect	Unable to conform to social norms, superficially charming, manipulative	Impulsivity	Good reality testing, sometimes heightened
Borderline PD	Unstable affect, poor self-image, free-floating anxiety	Tumultuous relations, overvalues/devalues others	Projection, splitting, devaluation, omnipotence	Impulsivity, poor reality testing at times
Histrionic PD	Poorly modulated affect, insecure with oneself	Attention-seeking, dramatic	Repression, conversion, dissociation	Impaired under stress, vague, global, impressionistic
Narcissistic PD	Grandiose sense of self, fragile self-esteem	Exploitative of others	Entitlement	Fantasies of success, beauty, brilliance. No psychotic thinking
Avoidant PD	Insecurity	Desires relations but shy, withdrawal at fear of rejection	Vigilance	Good reality testing, occasional cognitive interference
Dependent PD	Self-doubt, insecurity	Subverts own needs to those of others, needs excessive advice and reassurance	Submissive	Difficulty with decision making
Obsessive–compulsive PD	Emotional constriction	Unable to compromise, eager to please authority figures	Repetitive acts, intellectualization	Inflexible thought pattern, ruminative, overcontrol, detail-oriented

Note. Adapted from Weisberg and Keefe (1997). Copyright 1997 by W. B. Saunders Company. Adapted by permission.

a clinical interview with the patient or by self-report measures, with their inherent limitations. Unfortunately, interrater reliability is often poor when using clinical interviews, as demonstrated in the few studies that used clinical interviews to diagnose personality disorders (Weisberg & Keefe, 1997). Until the introduction of the DSM-III, the criteria for diagnosing personality disorders had not been adequately standardized. However, with the advent of the DSM-III, a number of semistructured interview techniques have been developed and used in psychiatric research. In contrast to a structured interview, which does not permit follow-up questions to be asked, a semi-structured interview consists of predetermined questions with additional inquiry depending on the patient's response to the structured questions. Each of the structured questions has been demonstrated to have high factor loadings on specific DSM criteria. Scores are given to each response based on the degree of certainty the trained rater has about the criteria being met. From this template, diagnoses are derived.

There are a number of semistructured interview schedules currently being used in psychiatric research. In addition to the commonly used SCID and SCID-II previously discussed in Gatchel et al. (1995), the Semistructured Interview for DSM-IV Personality Disorders (SIDP-IV; Pfohl, Blum, & Zimmerman, 1995) and the Personality Disorder Evaluation (PDE; Loranger, Lehmann-Susman, Oldham, & Russakof, 1985) have been used frequently. All have adequate interrater reliabilities and construct validity. Unfortunately, they are time-inefficient (often taking many hours to complete and score) and psychologically invasive in that they inquire about the entire range of cognitive, behavioral, interpersonal, and intrapsychic function. For these reasons, at present they are not routinely used in the clinical setting. However, a number of studies have recently been conducted that may yield sufficient information to develop briefer, less invasive measures. In some cases, brief screening measures already exist and are in use in psychiatric research, although their utility has yet to be thoroughly documented (Weisberg & Keefe, 1997).

Descriptive Studies

Several studies have attempted to examine the prevalence of personality disorders in chronic pain populations. When evaluating the results of these studies, it is important to bear in mind that overall base rates for all of the personality disorders among the U.S. population range are unknown but believed to be relatively low, from 0.5% for paranoid and avoidant personality disorder to 2–3% for histrionic and antisocial personality disorder (cited in Gatchel, Garofalo, Ellis, & Holt, 1996). Table 4.2 summarizes the results of empirical studies of the prevalence of personality disorders in chronic pain patients.

Reich, Tupin, and Abramowitz (1983) conducted the first study that used a semistructured interview to diagnose personality disorders. Participants included 43 chronic pain patients who underwent a 2-hour interview, which was based on flow sheets derived from the DSM-III listing of personality disorders. According to a table in their article, results demonstrated that 20 of the 43 participants (47%) met criteria for Axis II personality disorders. Histrionic ($n = 6$) and dependent ($n = 5$) personality disorders were the most common diagnoses noted, although there were discrepancies between the above figures cited in the table and in the text (Histronic = 5; Dependent = 4). A wide range of personality disorders was identified, with 7 of the 12 possible disorders represented.

Large (1986) examined personality disorder diagnoses of 50 patients who presented with chronic pain at the Auckland Pain Clinic in New Zealand. Participants underwent a 1½- to 2-hour interview that yielded information for diagnosing DSM-III personality disorders. Consistent with the inherent difficulties of personality diagnosis, reliability was in the low to moderate range (kappa = .27–.46). The authors explain that the criteria for agreement for the personality disorders were quite stringent (i.e., examiners must agree on a specific diagnosis, rather than on a broad class of personality diagnoses) and that this stringent criterion may have resulted in relatively low reliability. Results demonstrated that 40% (20 patients) met criteria for a personality disorder. Mixed personality disorder was the most common diagnosis ($n = 11$), followed by histrionic personality disorder ($n = 3$). Within the group of patients having mixed personality disorder, dependency traits were the most common, noted in 10 of the 11 patients. These findings appear consistent with early psychodynamic literature previously reviewed in this chapter that suggested that dependency and hysterical personalities were overrepresented in the chronic pain population.

Reich and Thompson (1987) studied personality disorder clusters in chronic pain patients. Psychiatric studies of personality disorders have demonstrated that there is moderate overlap of various DSM-III personality disorders (Widiger,

TABLE 4.2. Prevalence of Personality Disorder Diagnosis in Chronic Pain Patients

	Reich, Tupin, & Abramowitz (1983)	Large (1986)	Fishbain, Goldberg, Meagher, Steele, & Rosomoff (1986)	Polatin, Kinney, Gatchel, Lillo, & Mayer (1993)	Gatchel, Garofalo, Ellis, & Holt (1996)[a]	Weisberg, Gallagher, & Gorin (1996)
Participants	n = 43	n = 50	n = 283	n = 200	n = 50	n = 55
Diagnostic measure	Flow sheet interview	Maudsley-style	2-hour semistructured	SCID-II	SCID-II	Longitudinal
Reliability	None reported	Kappa = .46	None reported	Kappa = .63 (n = 20)	None reported	Kappa = .52 (n = 10)
Axis II disorders (total)	47%	40%	59%	51%	None reported	31%
Paranoid PD			3%	33%	18%	2%
Schizoid PD	2%		2%	4%		2%
Schizotypal PD	5%			4%	2%	4%
Histrionic PD	14%	6%	12%	4%	8%	
Antisocial PD				5%		
Narcissistic PD	2%	4%	2%	5%		2%
Borderline PD	7%	2% (traits)	1%	15%	10%	13%
Avoidant PD		2%		14%	4%	
Dependent PD	12%	2% (traits)	17%	3%		
Obsessive–compulsive PD		8% (traits)	7%	6%	10%	11%
Passive–aggressive PD[b]	4%	4%	15%	12%	6%	2%
Self-defeating PD[b]				10%	4%	7%
Mixed PD[b]	5%	22%				
PD not otherwise specified (DSM-IV)			2%	2%	2%	27%

Note. Adapted from Weisberg and Keefe (1997). Copyright 1997 by W. B. Saunders Company. Adapted by permission.

[a]Based on chronic TMD patients only.

[b]DSM-III-R passive–aggressive, self-defeating, and mixed categories.

Trull, Hurt, Clarkin, & Frances, 1987) and have therefore suggested the use of broader clusters to denote personality characteristics. There are three clusters, which have been demonstrated by factor analysis and were outlined in the DSM-III. Cluster A (Odd/Eccentric) consists of the paranoid, schizoid, and schizotypal personality disorders; Cluster B (Dramatic/Emotional) consists of the borderline, histrionic, and narcissistic personality disorders; and Cluster C (Anxious/Avoidant), the avoidant, dependent, obsessive–compulsive, and passive–aggressive personality disorders. Odds ratios were used to compare the prevalence of these personality disorders in three groups of individuals: patients suffering chronic pain, psychiatric patients applying for disability benefits, and psychiatric patients undergoing mental competency hearings (Reich & Thompson, 1987). All patients were given semistructured interviews for both Axis I (clinical disorders) and Axis II (personality disorders) DSM-III diagnoses. Patients were placed in one of the three clusters based on their personality disorders. When a patient met criteria for personality disorders on different clusters, he or she was placed in the cluster that best reflected the most severe symptom. Results indicated that, on average, patients with chronic pain were more likely to have a diagnosable personality disorder than were patients undergoing mental competency hearings. Thirty-seven percent of the chronic pain patients met diagnostic criteria for personality disorder, compared to 11.8% of patients undergoing mental competency hearings. In addition, chronic pain patients were most likely to have personality disorders in Cluster C (Anxious/Avoidant). The chronic pain patients were also more likely than patients undergoing mental competency hearings to have peronality disorders in Cluster B. These results suggest that a relatively high level of personality disorders is found in chronic pain patients and that the most frequently occuring of these are the personality disorders that reflect behaviors related to the anxious/avoidant cluster.

The first large-scale study of personality disorders in chronic pain patients was conducted at the University of Miami Comprehensive Pain and Rehabilitation Center by Fishbain, Goldberg, Meagher, Steele, & Rosomoff (1986). Participants were 283 chronic pain patients who were given a 2-hour semistructured interview that yielded DSM-III (American Psychiatric Association, 1980) personality disorder diagnoses. The interview criteria were based on the DSM-III guidelines, and the interview was conducted in the manner originally recommended by DSM-III (D. Fishbain, personal communication, 1994). Fifty-nine percent of chronic pain patients met criteria for a personality disorder diagnosis. Dependent personality disorder was most frequently diagnosed (17.4%), followed by passive–aggressive (14.9%), histrionic (11.7%), and obsessive–compulsive personality disorder (6.7%). This study examined males and females separately and found that significantly more males met criteria for paranoid and narcissistic personality disorder. In contrast, females met criteria for histrionic personality disorder more often than males. This study is important because it was the first to use rigorous operational criteria to make DSM-III Axis I and Axis II diagnoses in patients having chronic pain (Weisberg & Keefe, 1997). Although it did not use a standardized semistructured interview, it was one of the first studies to include lifetime occupational and social history information when determining Axis II personality diagnosis.

Polatin, Kinney, Gatchel, Lillo, and Mayer (1993) conducted one of the most methodologically sophisticated studies of personality disorders in chronic pain patients. Participants included 200 chronic pain sufferers who underwent structured interviews at the time of entry into a comprehensive pain and rehabilitation program. The Structured Clinical Interview for DSM-III-R (SCID and SCID II; Spitzer et al., 1988) was used to interview patients. This instrument evaluates current and lifetime incidence of both Axis I and Axis II disorders. The study used a version of the SCID designed for nonpsychiatric patients that was administered by experienced raters who obtained excellent reliability (kappa = .905–1.00) on Axis I. The SCID-II interview was used to diagnose personality disorders. Interview questions on this measure are based on the patient's self-report of 120 items derived from DSM-III-R personality disorder criteria. Consistent with the literature, diagnostic reliability for the Axis II personality disorders (kappa = .632), although sufficient, was lower than that for Axis I. Results demonstrated that 98% of the chronic pain patients met criteria for at least one lifetime Axis I diagnosis. With the exception of 97% of patients who met criteria for somatoform pain disorder, major depression was the most common lifetime (64%) and current (45%) Axis I diagnosis. This study also examined the incidence of Axis I disorders that developed after the onset of pain and found that all of the patients with somatoform pain disorders and 29% of the patients with major depression developed these disorders after pain onset. Data analysis of Axis II revealed that 51% of patients met criteria for one personality disorder and 30% met criteria for more than one personality disorder. Paranoid personality disorder was the most common Axis II diagnosis (33%) followed by borderline (15%), avoidant (14%) and passive–aggressive (12%) personality disorders.

In another study, Gatchel et al. (1996) used the SCID and SCID-II to diagnose DSM-III-R (American Psychiatric Association, 1987) Axis I and Axis II disorders in 51 patients with acute and 50 patients with chronic temporomandibular joint disorders (TMD). Results demonstrated that, overall, patients with chronic TMD had higher rates of Axis I disorders than those with acute TMD. Anxiety disorders were most commonly diagnosed in the acute patients (52.9%), whereas affective (depressive) disorders were most common in the chronic patients (78%), followed by somatoform disorder (50%). Chronic TMD patients had greater prevalence of Axis II disorders than did acute patients, although the difference was statistically insignificant. The most common Axis II disorder in the chronic TMD patients was paranoid personality disorder (18%), followed by both obsessive-compulsive personality disorder (10%) and borderline personality disorder (10%).

Weisberg, Gallagher, and Gorin (1996) recently presented data on personality disorders in 55 chronic pain patients evaluated and treated in a comprehensive pain and rehabilitation center. Their study used retrospective longitudinal data that included a clinical interview and treatment outcome, family, and self-report data to diagnose personality disorders. Results indicated that 31% of their participants met criteria for a personality disorder. The most frequent diagnosis was personality disorder not otherwise specified (27%), which is used when an individual meets incomplete criteria for two or more personality disorders. The next most common diagnosis was borderline personality disorder (13%), followed by dependent personality disorder (11%). These authors suggested further research on the same paticipants, to include blind semistructured interviews for the purpose of comparing diagnoses obtained through longitudinal chart review with a valid, reliable interview schedule. The authors argued that a brief, reliable screening measure used at the clinical evaluation may help to guide treatment decisions, thereby improving outcome.

Vittengle, Clark, Owen-Salters and Gatchel (in press) have recently completed a study in which they investigated personality characteristics dimen-sionally and personality disorders (DSM-III-R) categorically in chronic pain patients (n = 125) and normal controls (n = 75). In a subset, they assessed personality both before and 6 months after treatment in a functional restoration program. Measures included the MMPI, SCID-II, and the Schedule for Nonadaptive and Adaptive Personality (SNAP; Clark, 1993), a 375-item multiple-choice instrument that assesses 3 temperament dimensions and 12 personality dimensions (for further information, see Vittengle et al., in press)

Results of the SCID were similar to the other semistructured interview studies (Polatin et al., 1993; Gatchel et al., 1996). The chronic pain patients demonstrated a higher frequency of eight personality disorders (paranoid, schizotypal, narcissistic, borderline, avoidant, dependent, passive-aggressive, and self-defeating) than the comparison group. In those patients assessed pre- and posttreatment (n = 56), paranoid, obsessive-compulsive, passive-aggressive, and self-defeating personality disorders decreased significantly from pretreatment, a result which seems antithetical to the DSM definition of personality disorders as lifelong and stable over time.

On the SNAP, pain patients scored significantly higher than the comparison group on 3 of 6 validity scales (Rare Virtues, Deviance, Invalidity Index) and on 12 of 15 trait scales (Negative Temperament, Mistrust, Manipulativeness, Aggression, Self Harm, Positive Temperament, Exhibitionism, Entitlement, Detachment, Disinhibition, Impulsivity, Workaholism). There were no significant differences on scales measuring Eccentric Perceptions, Dependency, or Propriety. Statistically significant decreases pre- to posttreatment were obtained on scales assessing Desirable Response Inconsistency, Invalidity Index, Aggression, and Workaholism.

The MMPI found significant differences between the patient and comparison groups on all scales except scale 9 (Ma). Pre- to posttreatment decreases were significant on scales 3 (Hy) and scale 10 (Si).

Overall, the results of this study demonstrate greater stability of dimensional personality traits pre- to posttreatment (MMPI and SNAP) than of categorical personality disorders assessed with the SCID II. The authors cite regression to the mean or the "arbitrary nature" of diagnostic cutting points inherent in categorical diagnoses as possible explanations for changes pre- to posttreatment. A third explanation, not cited by the authors, is that of our previously hypothesized diathesis–stress model of personality disorders (Weisberg & Keefe, 1997). Finally, the SCID II may be limited in its test–retest reliability in the pain population.

Predictive Studies

In a recent investigation of the role of clinical (Axis I) and personality (Axis II) disorders, Gatchel and his colleagues (Gatchel, Polatin, Mayer, & Garcy, 1994) compared pretreatment SCID and SCID-II diagnoses of 152 patients who returned to work with those who failed to return to work following a functional restoration program. Consistent with other studies (Fishbain et al., 1986; Polatin et al., 1993), 58% of patients met criteria for an Axis II personality disorder. The most common personality disorders found in both groups (those returning and those not returning to work) were paranoid personality disorder, passive-aggressive personality disorder, and borderline personality disorder. There were no significant differences between both groups on any of the personality disorders. More important, there were no significant differences in the prevalence of either Axis I or Axis II disorders between the patients who successfully returned to work and those who did not return to work. The authors believe this study demonstrates that if treatment addresses both clinical psychiatric symptoms and personality issues, psychopathology need not interfere with successful outcome, including returning to work.

CLINICAL AND RESEARCH ISSUES

Several conclusions can be made based on our review of the literature. First, the assessment of personality can be useful in identifying personality traits and personality disorders that may potentially influence the course and treatment of chronic pain. Pain treatment programs are likely to improve treatment outcome when they account for individual personality differences in treatment decisions. Second, personality disorders occur at a higher rate in the chronic pain population than in the general population. It has long been observed that chronic pain patients have psychiatric comorbidity that includes both clinical symptoms, such as depression and anxiety, and personality traits and disorders; however, a causal relationship between personality traits or disorders and chronic pain has yet to be established. Many scholars and researchers have posited that certain personality styles, such as histrionic, dependent, and depressive traits, predispose an individual to the development of chronic pain disorders. More recently, however, there is increasing evidence that the occurrence of an acute episode of pain and the resulting emotional and psychosocial consequences may account for various forms of psychopathology often seen in the chronic pain population—most notably depressive and anxiety disorders on Axis I and, on Axis II, dependent, histrionic, and passive-aggressive personality disorders. Although it is antithetical to the concept of a "long-standing, lifelong pattern" required by the DSM for the diagnosis of personality disorders, we have proposed elsewhere a diathesis–stress model (Weisberg & Keefe, 1997) in which certain traits that are normally under control of the individual's defensive structure become exacerbated under the stress of an acute injury or insult to the individual and that, when poorly managed, result in a personality disorder. One yet-to-be-published study (Vittengle et al., in press) appears to support the diathesis–stress model of personality disorders (Weisberg & Keefe, 1997). Following treatment that has increased function as a primary goal, stress is likely to decrease. In these cases, individuals who met the criteria for personality disorders prior to treatment may still possess the criterion traits but to a lesser extent than required for a categorical diagnosis. Only further large-scale prospective studies similar to the Bigos et al. (1991) study will be able to shed light on the causal nature of these difficult conditions.

Personality must be assessed in the context in which it is demonstrated. The following case exemplifies the importance of understanding context and not overpathologizing personality disorders. Early in the career of one of us (Weisberg), a patient presented with complaints that he was being watched and videotaped constantly. Rather than finding corroboratory evidence of paranoid personality disorder, investigation revealed that his story was, in fact, true. The insurance company handling his case was following him and videotaping him. Might this be the sort of stress that would result in an underlying diathesis being expressed? Only with an open approach that views the individual as psychologically healthy "until proven otherwise" will we ever be able to assess and treat these individuals appropriately. Until such a time as a brief, reliable personality disorder screening measure is demonstrated to have validity and reliability in the chronic pain population, clinicians are encouraged to do a thorough assessment of psychosocial factors both before and after the onset of pain.

As we discussed in our recent article (Weisberg & Keefe, 1997), the pain clinician should bear in mind that a diagnosis of personality disorders should only be used when it guides treatment decisions, such as providing structure and substance to the treatment team. As an alternative to personality disorder diagnosis, Kahana and Bibring (1964) proposed diagnostic categories, which, they clearly stated, do not represent personality disorders. Their system of delineating personality types has as its goal helping the medical physician understand the needs, the meanings of illness, and the coping styles of his or her patient (Weisberg & Keefe, 1997). It has been used in a number of medical settings to assist physicians in assessment and treatment. The reader is encouraged to review their classic article for further information (Kahana & Bibring, 1964). Inappropriate or overdiagnosis of a patient can be both stigmatizing and detrimental to an individual; we must be reminded to "first do no harm." Furthermore, obtaining historical family, work, and social histories, such as was done by Fishbain and colleagues (1986), is necessary in order to establish the temporal relationship between personality and pain.

SUMMARY

In this chapter we have attempted to outline the important contributions of personality, individual differences, and psychopathology to chronic pain. For over 100 years, personality has been theorized, researched, and understood as playing an important role in the presentation of the chronic pain patient. We have traced the psychodynamic, trait theory, and biopsychosocial roots of the role personality plays in chronic pain and have reviewed major psychometric instruments and studies that have attempted to determine the psychological profile and treatment course of the pain patient. Although some studies found specific traits to exist (i.e., conversion-V), other studies refuted those results. We have also discussed the difference between personality traits and characteristics and personality disorders. There have been relatively few studies that examined personality disorders per se. Those that have been conducted demonstrated a significantly greater incidence of personality disorders in the chronic pain population when compared to epidemiological base rates. The question of which occurs first, the personality or the pain, has begun to be studied. Although some studies have been conducted that examine

the incidence and prevalence of personality disorders in chronic pain and some prospective studies relate MMPI personality characteristics to acute pain, no truly prospective studies have been conducted to evaluate the role of personality disorders in the development and/or maintenance of chronic pain. We have suggested elsewhere that the diathesis–stress model may explain the high rates of personality disorders noted both clinically and in research (Weisberg & Keefe, 1997). Until such time as prospective studies shed additional light on this subject, the clinician is encouraged to thoroughly assess personality and psychopathology as early as possible in the onset of pain and to address these issues therapeutically in an effort to prevent patients from becoming dependent on inappropriate treatmet and angry and rejecting of appropriate assistance and to maximize the individual strengths of the patient in the treatment process.

ACKNOWLEDGMENT

Preparation of this chapter was supported in part by Grant Nos. AR 44064 and AR 42261 from the National Institute of Arthritis and Musculoskeletal and Skin Diseases (NIAMS) and by a grant from the Arthritis Foundation to Francis J. Keefe.

REFERENCES

American Psychiatric Association. (1952). *Diagnostic and statistical manual of mental disorders* (1st ed.). Washington, DC: Author.

American Psychiatric Association. (1980). *Diagnostic and statistical manual of mental disorders* (3rd ed.). Washington, DC: Author.

American Psychiatric Association. (1987). *Diagnostic and statistical manual of mental disorders* (3rd ed., rev.). Washington, DC: Author.

American Psychiatric Association. (1994). *Diagnostic and statistical manual of mental disorders* (4th ed.). Washington, DC: Author.

Armentrout, D., Moore, J., Parker, J., Hewett, J., & Felts, C. (1982). Pain-patient MMPI subgroups: The psychological dimensions of pain. *Journal of Behavioral Medicine, 5*, 201–211.

Banks, S. M., & Kerns, R. D. (1996). Explaining the high rates of depression in chronic pain: A diathesis–stress framework. *Psychological Bulletin, 119*(1), 95–110.

Bigos, S. J., Battie, M. C., Spengler, D. M., Fisher, L. D., Fordyce, W. E., Hansson, T. H., Nachemson, A. L., & Wortley, M. D. (1991). A prospective study of work perceptions and psychosocial factors affecting the report of back injury. *Spine, 16*(1), 1–6.

Blumer, D., & Heilbronn, M. (1982). Chronic pain as a variant of depressive disease: The pain-prone disorder. *Journal of Nervous and Mental Disease, 170*(7), 381–394.

Bond, M. R. (1971). The relation of pain to the Eysenck Personality Inventory, Cornell Medical Index and the Whiteley Index of Hypochondriasis. *British Journal of Psychiatry, 119,* 671–678.

Bond, M. R., & Pearson, I. B. (1969). Psychological aspects of pain in women with advanced cancer of the cervix. *Journal of Psychosomatic Research, 13,* 13–19.

Bradley, L., Prokop, C., Margolis, R., & Gentry, W. (1978). Multivariate analyses of the MMPI profiles of low back pain patients. *Journal of Behavioral Medicine, 1,* 253–257.

Breuer, J., & Freud, S. (1957). *Studies on hysteria.* (J. Strachey, Ed. and Trans.). New York: Basic Books. (Original work published 1893–1895)

Butcher, J. N., Dahlstrom, W. G., Graham, J. R., Tellegen, A. M., & Kaemmer, B. (1989). *MMPI-2: Manual for the administration and scoring.* Minneapolis: University of Minnesota Press.

Clark, L. A. (1993). *Schedule for Nonadaptive and Adaptive Personality (SNAP).* Minneapolis: University of Minneapolis Press.

Costa, P. T., Jr., & McCrae, R. R. (1985). *The NEO personality inventory manual.* Orlando, FL: Psychological Assessment Resources.

Deardorff, W. W., Chino, A. F., & Scott, D. W. (1993). Characteristics of chronic pain patients: Factor analysis of the MMPI-2. *Pain, 54,* 153–158.

Engel, G. L. (1959). "Psychogenic" pain and the pain-prone patient. *American Journal of Medicine, 26,* 899–918.

Engel, G. L. (1977). The need for a new medical model: A challenge for biomedicine. *Science, 196*(4286), 129–136.

Fishbain, D. A., Goldberg, M., Meagher, B. R., Steele, R., & Rosomoff, H. (1986). Male and female chronic pain patients categorized by DSM-III psychiatric diagnostic criteria. *Pain, 26,* 181–197.

Flor, H., & Turk, D.C. (1984). Etiological theories and treatments for chronic back pain: I. Somatic models and interventions. *Pain, 19,* 105–121.

Flor, H., Turk, D. C., & Birbaumer, N. (1985). Assessment of stress-related psychophysiological reactions in chronic back pain patients. *Journal of Consulting and Clinical Psychology, 53*(3), 354–364.

Gatchel, R. J., Garofalo, J. P., Ellis, E., & Holt, C. (1996). Major psychological disorders in acute and chronic TMD: An initial examination. *Journal of the American Dental Association, 127,* 1365–1374.

Gatchel, R. J., Polatin, P. B., & Mayer, T. G. (1995). The dominant role of psychosocial risk factors in the development of chronic low back pain disability. *Spine, 20*(24), 2702–2709.

Gatchel, R. J., Polatin, P. B., Mayer, T. G., & Garcy, P. D. (1994). Psychopathology and the rehabilitation of patients with chronic low back pain. *Archives of Physical Medicine and Rehabilitation, 75,* 666–670.

Gentry, W. D., Shows, W. D., & Thomas, M. (1974). Chronic low back pain: A psychological profile. *Psychosomatics, 15,* 174–177.

Gough, H. E. (1946). Diagnostic patterns on the Minnesota Multiphasic Personality Inventory. *Journal of Clinical Psychology, 2,* 23–37.

Hansen, F. R., Biering-Sorensen, F., & Schroll, M. (1995). Minnesota Multiphasic Personality Inventory profiles in persons with or without low back pain: A 20-year follow-up study. *Spine, 20*(24), 2716–2720.

Hanvik, L. J. (1951). MMPI profiles in patients with low back pain. *Journal of Consulting Psychology, 15,* 350–353.

Hathaway, S. R., & McKinley, J. (1943). *Minnesota Multiphasic Personality Inventory.* Minneapolis: University of Minnesota Press.

Kahana, R. J., & Bibring, G. L. (1964). Personality types in medical management. In N. Zinberg (Ed.), *Psychiatry and medical practice in a general hospital.* New York: International Universities Press.

Large, R. G. (1986). DSM-III diagnoses in chronic pain: Confusion or clarity? *Journal of Nervous and Mental Disease, 174*(5), 295–303.

Loranger, A. W., Lehmann-Susman, V., Oldham, J., & Russakof, L. M. (1985). *Personality Disorder Examination (PDE): A structured interview for DSM-III-R personality disorders.* White Plains, NY: New York Hospital-Cornell Medical Center, Westchester Division.

Love, A. W., & Peck, C. L. (1987). The MMPI and psychological factors in chronic low back pain: A review. *Pain, 28,* 1–12.

McCrae, R. R. (1991). The five-factor model and its assessment in clinical settings. *Journal of Personality Assessment, 57*(3), 399–414.

McCrae, R. R., & Costa, P. T., Jr. (1987). Validation of the five-factor model of personality across instruments and observers. *Journal of Personality and Social Psychology, 52,* 81–90.

McCreary, C., Turner, J., & Dawson, E. (1977). Differences between functional versus organic low back pain patients. *Pain, 4,* 73–78.

McCreary, C., Turner, J., & Dawson, E. (1979). The MMPI as a predictor of response to conservative treatment for low back pain. *Journal of Clinical Psychology, 3*(2), 278–284.

Pfohl, B., Blum, N., & Zimmerman, M. (1995). *Structured Interview for DSM-IV Personality Disorders.* Iowa City: University of Iowa.

Polatin, P. B., Kinney, R. K., Gatchel, R. J., Lillo, E., & Mayer, T. G. (1993). Psychiatric illness and chronic low-back pain. *Spine, 18*(1), 66–71.

Reich, J., & Thompson, D. (1987). DSM-III personality disorder clusters in three populations. *British Journal of Psychiatry, 150,* 471–475.

Reich, J., Tupin, J. P., & Abramowitz, S. I. (1983). Psychiatric diagnosis of chronic pain patients. *American Journal of Psychiatry, 140*(11), 1495–1498.

Spitzer, R. L., Williams, J. B., Gibbon, M., & First, M. B. (1988). *Structured Clinical Interview for DSM-III-R.* New York: New York State Psychiatric Institute.

Sternbach, R. A. (1974). *Pain patients: Traits and treatment.* New York: Academic Press.

Sternbach, R. A., Wolf, S. R., Murphy, R. W., & Akeson, W. H. (1973a). Aspects of chronic low back pain. *Psychosomatics, 14,* 52–56.

Sternbach, R. A., Wolf, S. R., Murphy, R. W., Akeson, W. H. (1973b). Traits of pain patients: The low-back "loser." *Psychosomatics, 14,* 226–229.

Szasz, T. S. (1957). *Pain and pleasure: A study of bodily feelings.* London: Tavistock.

Turk, D. C., & Flor, H. (1984). Etiological theories and treatment for chronic back pain: II. Psychological models and interventions. *Pain, 19,* 209–233.

Vittengle, J. R., Clark, L. A., Owen-Salters, E., & Gatchel, R. J. (in press). Diagnostic change and personality stability following functional restoration treatment in a chronic low back pain patient sample. *Assessment.*

Wade, J. B., Dougherty, L. M., Hart, R. P., & Cook, D. B. (1992). Patterns of normal personality structure among chronic pain patients. *Pain, 48,* 37–43.

Waring, E. M., Weisz, G. M., & Bailey, S. I. (1976). Predictive factors in the treatment of low back pain by surgical intervention. In J. J. Bonica & D. Albe-Fessard (Eds.), *Advances in pain research and therapy* (Vol. 1). New York: Raven Press.

Weisberg, J. N., Gallagher, R. M., & Gorin, A. (1996, November). *Personality disorder in chronic pain: A longitudinal approach to validation of diagnosis.* Poster presented at the Fifteenth Annual Scientific Meeting of the American Pain Society, Washington, DC.

Weisberg, J. N., Gorin, A., Drozd, J., & Gallagher, R. M. (1996, August). *The relationship between depression and psychophysiological reactivity in chronic pain patients.* Poster presented at the Eighth World Congress on Pain, Vancouver, BC, Canada.

Weisberg, J. N., & Keefe, F. J. (1997). Personality disorders in the chronic pain population: Basic concepts, empirical findings and clinical implications. *Pain Forum, 6*(1), 1–9.

Widiger, T. A., Trull, T. J., Hurt, S. W., Clarkin, J., & Frances, A. (1987). A multidimensional scaling of the DSM-III personality disorders. *Archives of General Psychiatry, 44,* 557–563.

Wiltse, L. L., & Rocchio, P. D. (1975). Preoperative psychological tests as predictors of success of chemonucleolysis in the treatment of the low back syndrome. *Journal of Bone and Joint Surgery, 57*(A), 478–483.

Chapter 5

The Role of Emotion in Pain

MICHAEL E. ROBINSON
JOSEPH L. RILEY III

Current conceptualizations of pain recognize that it is a multidimensional construct with both sensory and affective components (International Association for the Study of Pain [IASP], 1979). People who experience chronic pain also experience a wide range of associated emotions (Gaskin, Greene, Robinson, & Geisser, 1992). The most complete picture of individuals who experience clinical pain conditions necessitates an understanding of the rich emotional experience that may accompany and contribute to the pain condition. The purpose of this chapter is to review the role of negative emotion in the experience of pain. We will focus our attention on the broad categories of depression, anxiety, and anger. There are several issues and controversies surrounding the role of negative emotion in pain that we will discuss. These include (1) the prevalence of negative emotion in patients with pain conditions, (2) the measurement of negative affect in pain conditions, (3) the role of negative emotion in disability and outcomes, (4) causal relationships between pain and negative affect, and (5) models incorporating negative emotion and pain.

PREVALENCE OF NEGATIVE EMOTION IN CHRONIC PAIN

Depression has probably been the emotion to receive the most empirical investigation. A number of excellent reviews of the relationship between chronic pain and depression have been published

(Banks & Kerns, 1996; Romano & Turner, 1985). Differences in the definition of depression, populations sampled, and measurement issues have resulted in considerable variability of prevalence, with estimates ranging from 10% to 100% (Banks & Kerns, 1996). Despite the inconsistency in the absolute prevalence of depression, the estimates have almost universally indicated higher rates of depression in patients with chronic pain when compared to the general population (Banks & Kerns, 1996). Banks and Kerns' comparisons of the prevalence of depression in chronic pain with rates in other medical conditions suggest that chronic pain sufferers may have higher rates, though the authors are cautious about drawing definite conclusions from the literature. Depression prevalence estimates of 30–54% in clinic-based chronic pain samples with depression clearly indicate that depression is a significant issue in pain sufferers (Banks & Kerns, 1996).

Because of the larger range of anxiety diagnoses, less consistency regarding prevalence rates is available from the literature. Nonetheless, the role of anxiety in pain has received a considerable amount of study (McCracken, Gross, Aikens, & Carnrike, 1996; Brown, Robinson, Riley, & Gremillion, 1996; Asmundson, Jacobson, Allerdings, & Norton, 1996). Asmundson et al. (1996) found that 17.8% of their sample of chronic musculoskeletal pain patients met DSM-IV criteria for a current anxiety disorder. Atkinson, Slater, Patterson, Grant, and Garfin (1991) compared patients with low back pain to a matched sample of pain-free men and found that the chronic pain groups had significantly higher lifetime prevalence rates of major anxiety disorder (30.9% vs. 14.3%). Fishbain, Goldberg, Maegher, and Steele (1986) also reported high levels of anxiety disorders in their sample of chronic pain patients. Data from the Health Science Center of the University of Florida indicate that patients with a variety of chronic pain conditions report anxiety levels significantly greater than published norms (Gaskin et al., 1992; Brown et al., 1996; Holzberg, Robinson, Geisser, & Gremillion, 1996). These studies have also shown that a significant amount of the variance in pain report can be explained by anxiety (Brown et al., 1996; Holzberg et al., 1996). McCracken et al. (1996) found that anxiety accounted for 16 to 54% of the variance in pain report, disability, and pain-related behavior. Although the diagnostic variability within this area makes definitive statements about prevalence difficult, the data are clear that anxiety plays a strong role in the experience of clinical pain.

A particular interest has been developed in an anxiety-related construct that a number of authors have termed "fear/avoidance" (Asmundson, Norton, & Allerdings, 1997; McCracken, Gross, Sorg, & Edmands, 1993; Waddell, Newton, Henderson, Somerville, & Main, 1993). This construct is based on learning theory models of the acquisition and maintenance of pain behaviors, one of which is the avoidance of painful activities. This avoidance of activity is postulated to result in chronic pain syndromes characterized by a cycle of decreased activity, deconditioning, loss of self-efficacy, fear, and negative affect, leading to further avoidance of pain-related activity (Asmundson et al., 1997). One line of research has employed an instrument (the Pain Anxiety Symptoms Scale, or PASS) based on a conceptualization of this construct that includes fearful appraisals and cognitive, behavioral, and physiological components of pain-related anxiety (McCracken, Zayfert, & Gross, 1992; McCracken et al., 1993). This construct, or components of it, has been related to other diagnostic categorizations of patients with pain (Asmundson et al., 1997), to level of disability due to pain, and to physical performance measures (McCracken et al., 1993).

Another more specific anxiety disorder, posttraumatic stress disorder (PTSD), has been shown to have particular relevance to patients who are injured in traumatic fashion and also to relate to a number of key outcome variables in a sample of chronic pain patients (Geisser, Roth, Bachman, & Eckert, 1997).

Compared to anxiety and depression, anger has received far less attention in the pain literature. Fernandez and Turk (1995) reviewed the limited literature on anger in chronic pain conditions and noted that several authors have investigated the co-occurrence of anger and the related construct of hostility in pain conditions (Kerns, Rosenberg, & Jacob, 1994; Schwartz, Slater, Birchler, & Atkinson, 1991; Kinder & Curtiss, 1988; Gaskin et al., 1992; Taylor, Lorentzen, & Blank, 1990). However, little published evidence is available to ascertain the prevalence of anger as a clinically significant diagnosis in patients with chronic pain. Unlike other negative affective states, anger lacks the specific diagnoses that would make prevalence estimates easier to obtain. Data from our tertiary care site (Gaskin et al., 1992; Brown et al., 1996) indicate that patients with chronic pain report levels of anger significantly higher than the published norms on the State–Trait Anger Expression Inventory (Spielberger, 1985). Although the scope of anger as a diagnostic entity remains unclear, the consequences of anger in patients with pain appear to be significant and to contribute to treatment obstacles and other negative affective experiences (Fernandez & Turk, 1995; Holzberg et al., 1996; Brown et al., 1996).

MEASURING NEGATIVE EMOTION IN PATIENTS WITH PAIN CONDITIONS

Several authors have questioned the prevailing practices of assessing depression in patients with chronic pain because of overlap in somatic symptoms (Rodin & Voshart, 1986; Cavanaugh, 1984; Buckelew, DeGood, Schwartz, & Kerler, 1986; Banks & Kerns, 1996; Geisser, Roth, & Robinson, 1997). Particular concerns have been raised about the use of self-report measures of depression in individuals with chronic pain (Novy, Nelson, Berry, & Averil, 1995; Williams & Richardson, 1993; Geisser, Roth, & Robinson, 1997). Factor analytic studies of the Beck Depression Inventory (BDI; Novy, Nelson, Berry, & Averil, 1995a; Williams & Richardson, 1993) confirm a somatic factor in that particular instrument that might yield artifactually high levels of depression in patients with chronic pain due to somatic symptoms of the pain condition. Geisser, Roth, and Robinson (1997) compared the BDI, the Center for Epidemiological Studies Depression Scale (CES-D), and depression diagnoses from DSM-IV structured interviews. Discriminant analysis indicated that the BDI and

CES-D measures significantly predicted DSM-IV diagnoses for depression, though slightly higher cutoffs than typically reported on the BDI and CES-D were optimal. Of particular interest was another set of analyses in which the authors removed the somatic items from the BDI and repeated the discriminant analysis with no decrement in the classification of depression as made by DSM-IV structured interview. Holzberg et al. (1996) also showed an 80% concordance rate between the BDI and Research Diagnostic Criteria (RDC) for depression that is consistent with the Geisser, Roth, and Robinson (1997) results and suggests that the concerns about somatic symptom overlap between depression and chronic pain are not empirically founded.

There has been less focus in the literature on the symptom overlap between anxiety and pain conditions, though a number of studies have demonstrated a physiological factor in many measures of anxiety used in the assessment of pain conditions (Larsen, Taylor, & Asmundson, 1997; McCracken et al., 1996; McCracken et al., 1992; Krishnan et al., 1985). In the general anxiety literature, anxiety is commonly defined as having three components: cognitive, physiological, and behavioral/motoric (Lang, 1968). The physiological arousal associated with anxiety has several symptoms that overlap with various pain-related symptoms (i.e., muscle tension, autonomic arousal). The same concerns raised earlier about the assessment of depression apply to the assessment of anxiety, though there have been no direct tests of the hypotheses that chronic pain symptoms artifactually increase the diagnosis of anxiety conditions (Fishbain et al, 1986).

Compared to depression and anxiety, there have been virtually no studies directly concerned with the issue of symptom overlap between anger and chronic pain. However, psychophysiological investigations of anger clearly indicate a somatic component—or at least a physiological response to anger (Stemmler, 1989) that suggests that the same issues of symptom overlap that plague anxiety and depression investigations may also be problematic for the assessment of anger in pain conditions. Fernandez and Turk (1995) review the physical health consequences of anger, which indicate that anger has a significant effect on the pathophysiology of a number of physiological systems. This suggests that the same dilemma is present for diagnosing clinically significant anger in patients with pain.

In addition to the symptom-overlap concerns between pain and negative affect, there are concerns that anxiety, anger, and depression correlate strongly enough with each other to represent a higher order factor (Brown et al., 1996) that perhaps represents psychological distress. A number of studies that have employed measures of more than one type of negative affect invariably show a correlation between the affective measures (Gaskin et al., 1992; Brown et al., 1996; Holzberg et al., 1996; Wade, Price, Hamer, & Schwartz, 1990). Regression analyses with other variables have shown that both within and across studies, separate variance is accounted for by each of the negative affect constructs, although the variance accounted for is rarely impressively large for any single affect construct. Brown et al. (1996) have demonstrated that the three affective measures (anger, anxiety, and depression) form a single affective distress factor when employed in structural equation modeling approaches with chronic pain. Although correlation among measures does not necessarily mean that depression, anger, and anxiety lack construct validity, it does make the measurement of these constructs more difficult in a population that has a high likelihood of their co-occurrence. The experience of chronic pain has far-reaching effects, including financial stressors, concerns for health, loss of role identity, legal complications, and loss of avocational and vocational involvement, all of which can differentially affect an individual and manifest itself in varying amounts of each negative emotion. Negative emotion, like pain, is multivariate, with the expectation that its components are likely to intercorrelate (Gracely, 1992). The utility of assessing each component of negative affect, in comparison to an approach that measures a more global psychological distress construct, remains to be fully understood.

The relatively consistent intercorrelations between these constructs may be due to other factors in addition to the overlap of legitimate symptoms of each. Holroyd et al. (1996) have highlighted the significance of method variance in the self-report of pain that may also be represented in the measurement of negative affect, especially when assessed with similar approaches. A related issue is the face validity of most of the measures of negative affect reported and used in the pain literature. This face validity and susceptibility to response set is one possible contributor to the intercorrelation between measures of negative affect and other key variables (Robinson et al., 1997).

NEGATIVE EMOTION AS PREDICTOR OF PAIN, DISABILITY, AND OUTCOME

As previously mentioned, a number of studies have shown a concurrent relationship between negative emotion and levels of pain in correlational designs (Gaskin et al., 1992; Brown et al., 1996; Holzberg et al., 1996; Brown, 1990). Other studies have shown that negative affect is a significant negative predictor with respect to spine surgery outcome (Riley, Robinson, Geisser, Wittmer, & Graham-Smith, 1995; Uomoto, Turner, & Herron, 1988; Junge, Dvorak, & Ahrens, 1995; Hasenbring, Marienfeld, Kuhlendahl, & Soyka, 1994), multidisciplinary treatment for pain (Swimmer, Robinson, & Geisser, 1992; Brennan, Barrett, & Garretson, 1986), and conservative therapies (Gerke, Richards, & Goss, 1989). Burchiel et al. (1995) indicated that level of depression was a significant negative predictor of outcome following spinal cord stimulator surgery for chronic low back pain. Others have suggested that negative affect may mediate the relationship between pain, impairment, and disability (Banks & Kerns, 1996). Holzberg et al. (1996), using a path analytic approach, demonstrated that the self-report of dysfunction/disability was directly influenced by negative affect, whereas pain level did not have a direct effect on self-report of function consistent with the hypotheses posed by Banks and Kerns (1996).

A number of investigators have demonstrated that the chronicity of an injury is predicted by measures of negative affect (Gatchel, Polatin, & Kinney, 1995). Klenerman et al. (1995) demonstrated that fear-avoidance alone accounted for a 66% correct classification of which acutely injured back pain patients would become chronic at a 12-month follow-up. Main and Watson (1992) have developed a short assessment method that employs measures of psychological distress as a screening device specifically aimed at predicting treatment outcome. Patient care cost and health care utilization has also been associated with negative affect in the general population (Byrne, 1996) and in chronic pain patient samples (Engel, Von Korff, & Katon, 1996). These studies, taken in toto, demonstrate that the co-occurrence of negative affect, whether causally linked to injury status or a consequence of injury, are predictive of a number of key variables, including treatment efficacy and health care costs.

NATURE OF THE RELATIONSHIP BETWEEN NEGATIVE EMOTION AND CHRONIC PAIN

The clinical studies reviewed herein have shown that chronic pain and negative emotion are frequently associated, with comorbidity documented to a varying degree depending on the specific pain condition, clinical sample studied, and dimension of negative emotion measured. With few longitudinal studies to address the question of the temporal relationship between pain and emotion, there is considerable debate as to the true nature of this association. However, theories that postulate the nature of these relationships can generally be expressed in four different statements: (1) negative emotion increases somatic sensitivity; (2) negative emotion causes some pain; (3) negative emotion can result from the experience of chronic pain; and (4) pain and negative emotion are concomitant constructs because of similar biological foundations (Brown, 1990; Banks & Kerns, 1996; Fishbain, Cutler, Rosomoff, & Rosomoff, 1997).

Negative Emotion Increases Sensitivity

The first hypothesis states that the experience of negative emotion increases or maintains the report of chronic pain through some sensory process such as enhanced sensitivity to pain. According to the gate control theory (Melzack & Wall, 1965), an individual's physiological perception of pain is modulated by his or her emotions and cognition, with depression and pain modulated by a similar process in the periaqueductal grey area of the dorsal horn. Evidence to support this hypothesis is provided by mood induction studies that have shown increased reporting of aches and pains (Salovey & Birnbaum, 1989) and decreased tolerance for experimentally induced pain (Zelman, Howland, & Cleeland, 1991). Depressed patients also tend to interpret events negatively and are more likely to interpret a given sensation as painful (Pennebaker, 1982). However, Geisser, Gaskin, Robinson, & Greene (1993) failed to find a relationship between the BDI and pain threshold or pain tolerance in a patient sample from an arthritis and fibromyalgia support group, using a cold pressor paradigm.

Pain Is Caused by Negative Emotions

Some authors have argued that chronic pain is due to an underlying depressive disorder, particularly when adequate physical findings or satisfactory diagnosis of somatization disorder (Dworkin & Gatlin, 1991; Kellner, 1985) are not present. Blumer and Heilbronn (1981), citing associations between past or family history of depressive disorder, proposed that chronic pain reflects a manifestation of a muted depressive state. They defined a pain-prone disorder that was associated with specific clinical, psychodynamic, and genetic characteristics.

The psychodynamic view of intractable chronic pain assumes that pain is a symptom of an underlying problem; however, the underlying problem is thought to be unconscious psychic conflict. In this model, pain can be considered a conversion symptom for individuals who have dealt with guilt over anger by "atoning" with pain (Engle, 1959). Emotional pain, often experienced in childhood through the association of pain with important formative emotional experiences, is displaced into the body, where it is more acceptable (Engle, 1959). Thus pain helps to avoid even more unpleasant feelings. However, Gamsa (1994), in her review, concluded that the psychodynamic literature fails to provide support for the hypothesis that childhood emotional problems generate and perpetuate chronic pain.

It has also been speculated that stress-related anxiety and, to a lesser extent, anger may be responsible for the development and maintenance of musculoskeletal disorders. Consistent with psychophysiological models of pain, increased somatic reactivity such as increased skeletal muscle tension (Flor & Turk, 1989) may lead to pain. Variants of this model have been described as the "stress–hyperactivity–pain theory" (Ohrbach & McCall, 1996). For example, Burns, Wiegner, Derleth, Kiselica, and Pawl (1996) found that anger-induced stress produced increased muscle tension, which predicted greater pain severity in chronic back pain patients. This effect was specific to anger in that a measure of depression that was significantly correlated with pain was not associated with increased muscle reactivity. Inhibition of negative emotion has also been suggested in the etiology of chronic pain through increased autonomic and central nervous system activity, which in turn weakens the cognitive process that promotes health, resulting in sleep disturbance, elevation in cortisol levels, and increased health care utilization (Fernandez & Turk, 1995).

Negative Affect Occurs as a Result of Chronic Pain

This hypothesis suggests that negative emotion is a frequent psychological reaction to chronic pain. This suggestion has intuitive appeal, considering the physical and social limitations the experience of chronic pain can place on an individual. This implies the existence of unique cognitive and/or behavioral responses to pain that have a tendency to develop into depressive symptomatology. A number of cognitive processes have been implicated in the risk for negative emotion in chronic pain patients, including attributional style (Love, 1988), catastrophizing cognition (Geisser, Robinson, Keefe, & Weiner, 1994), negative self-image (Holzberg, Robinson, & Geisser, 1993), and beliefs about pain (Williams, Robinson, & Geisser, 1994), although causality cannot be inferred from these correlational studies. Consistent with behavioral models of depression, increased pain and related somatic symptoms would reduce the ability to engage in activities that had been sources of positive reinforcement in the past. In addition, these activities are now accompanied by pain and are, therefore, aversive. The chronic pain patient then reduces his or her range of instrumental activities further because of physical impairment or fear of pain and further injury. A reciprocal cycle of reduced reinforcement, reduced activity, somatic symptoms, and depression (Haythornthwaite, Sieber, & Kerns, 1991) is initiated. Banks and Kerns (1996) provide an excellent review of the major cognitive-behavioral models of depression in the context of chronic pain and propose a diathesis-stress framework for the development of depression in this population.

Pain and Negative Emotion Are Concomitant

This hypothesis posits that pain and negative emotion occur simultaneously because of similar biological mechanisms. Serotonin and norepinephrine are thought to play a role in the development of depression and the modulation of pain. That individuals suffering either pain or depression respond to administrations of tricyclic antidepressants is frequently cited as evidence for common biological mechanisms (Max, 1995). The investigation of depressed individuals or patients experiencing chronic pain has shown that they also frequently share other physiological markers, such as reduction in rapid-eye-movement (REM) sleep, an increase in plasma cortisol, a pathological dexamethasone test, and low 5-hydroxyidoleacetic acid (5-HIAA) levels in the cerebrospinal fluid (Diener, van Schayck, & Kastrup, 1995; Ward, 1982).

EVIDENCE FOR A TEMPORAL RELATIONSHIP BETWEEN NEGATIVE MOOD AND PAIN

Several studies have been published using longitudinal methodology. Unlike correlational studies, they allow temporal and directional inferences about the nature of the relationship between negative emotion and pain.

The earliest study we found was performed by Moldofsky and Chester (1970) using a sample of 16 patients suffering rheumatoid arthritis who were staying in a rheumatic disease unit. Moldofsky and Chester performed what they described as a longitudinal psychosomatic study, collecting measures of joint pain and responses to adjectives describing emotional states twice daily for an average of 36 days. They observed two distinct subgroups, each with different patterns of pain and negative emotion. The first group was characterized by increases in pain that were preceded by elevations in anxiety and hostility (anger). The second group displayed an inverse temporal relationship between pain and a hopelessness/helplessness dimension. These groups were not different in age, duration of illness, radiographic joint changes, functional disability, or medication usage. Although this study is limited in that it followed changes over a relatively short period of time and used an inpatient population, it does suggest the existence of subgroups with differential relationships between pain and dimensions of negative emotions.

Atkinson et al. (1991) assessed lifetime prevalence and premorbid risk of a psychiatric disorder using the NIMH Diagnostic Interview Schedule, a DSM-III-based structured interview. They studied a sample of male chronic low back pain patients attending a primary care clinic at a Veterans Administration Medical Center (VAMC). They determined that, of this sample, 32% had experienced a previous major depressive disorder and 31% had qualified for a diagnosis of major anxiety disorder. They then compared the temporal relationship between these psychiatric disorders and the date of onset of chronic pain. For major depressive disorder, they found that 42% experienced onset of depression before the onset of pain

and 58% experienced onset of depression after onset of chronic pain. With regard to anxiety disorder, 47% were determined to have experienced onset of anxiety before the onset of pain and 53% to have experienced onset of anxiety after onset of chronic pain. They noted that 15% of the patients endorsed the onset of primary depression less than 2 years prior to pain onset. The authors acknowledged several limitations to this study. These included the bias from a sample of VAMC males and the retrospective nature of the design, even though the study included the control of a validated and reliable structured interview. Atkinson and associates (1991) concluded that this study supports the notion of postpain mood disorder, although it also suggests that psychiatric disorders frequently precede onset of chronic pain.

Von Korff, Le Resche, and Dworkin (1993), using a 3-year prospective design, examined whether the onset of five common pain symptoms were associated with baseline depressive symptoms. The participants were 1,016 members of a large northwestern health maintenance organization. Depression was assessed with the Symptom Checklist 90 depression subscale. Patients with scores in the top 10% were categorized as severe and those scoring between 10% and 20% as moderate based on general population norms. The analysis showed that over the period of 3 years the onset risk for headache and chest pain for individuals with moderate or severe depression ranged from 1.7 to 5.0. Baseline depressive symptoms were not predictive of the occurrence of back pain, abdominal pain, or temporomandibular joint pain. However, no consistent effect for severity of depression was observed. In addition, because this effect was not observed across pain conditions, it is difficult to make inferences about a specific effect of depressive symptoms on pain. They also noted that presence of a pain condition at baseline was a more consistent predictor of subsequent pain onset than depressive symptoms.

The link between migraine headaches and major depression was tested by Breslau, Davis, Schultz, and Peterson (1994). They used Cox-proportional hazards models with data collected in a 3.5-year longitudinal design with a sample of 1,007 young adults from a large health maintenance organization. Depression was assessed using the NIMH Diagnostic Interview Schedule. They found that the relative risk for major depression associated with prior migraine was 3.2 and that the relative risk of migraine associated with previous major depression was 3.1. They concluded that their results suggest a bidirectional influence of depression and migraine headaches. Although migraine headaches could be considered a somewhat unique variant of chronic pain, similar factors may operate in the temporal relationship between negative emotion and other pain conditions.

Leino and Magni (1993) studied 607 Finnish industrial workers, assessing the relationship between symptoms of distress and musculoskeletal symptoms on three occasions at 5-year intervals. They found that general emotional distress scores from an earlier assessment were positively related to self-report of musculoskeletal symptoms. However, distress was predictive of later clinical findings only for men. When the direction of the analysis was reversed, none of the musculoskeletal symptoms were predictive of later depressive symptoms. Leino and Magni acknowledged that a drawback of this study was that the measure of emotional distress was not a clinical measure but a composite of 7 items representing depressive symptoms from a 36-item questionnaire on mental well-being. Nevertheless, the strengths of this study are that it is prospective in nature and that it does not suffer from the inherent sampling bias of clinical populations.

Brown (1990) addressed the issue of the temporal relationship between pain and depression using structural equation modeling with latent variables. He used a sophisticated cross-legged prospective design with data collected in two sets over three 6-month intervals. This strategy allowed for the control of previous levels of pain and depression in the analysis. The data was collected using a mailed questionnaire from 243 patients diagnosed with rheumatoid arthritis. With depression from the previous period controlled, the cross-time regression path for pain predicting depression was positive and modest in magnitude for the second 12-month period but not for the first 12-month period. Pain was not predicted by prior episodes of depression when the effect of previous pain was removed. Correlations between latent variables of depression and pain were positive and moderate in magnitude for all time periods. Brown (1990) pointed out that this study does not address issues related to time of onset or recurrence of depression but rather to exacerbation of depressive symptoms following pain episodes. A particular strength of this study was that subjects were not currently seeking treatment and were not experiencing elevated levels of pain; therefore, the combination of design and analysis allows for the inference of causality over time.

Magni, Moreschi, Rigatti-Luchini, and Merskey (1994) used epidemiological methodology to test for a directional effect of depressive symptoms on musculoskeletal pain and vice versa. The data from a general population sample of 2,324 participants collected by the U.S. National Center for Health Statistics were used. They operationalized chronic pain as pain that was experienced for most of a day for at least 1 of the past 12 months. Depression was assessed using the CES-D. Magni et al. found that participants reporting chronic pain were 2.85 times more likely to report depression at follow-up 8 years later, whereas the risk ratio for the prediction of chronic pain from depressive symptoms was 2.14. Their results suggest that hypotheses about whether chronic pain causes depression or depression causes chronic pain may not be mutually exclusive. They speculated that depression may be more predictive of some pain conditions and that certain pain conditions may be more likely to predict depressive symptoms. Limitations of this study include the inability to determine whether depression or pain symptoms were continuous or intermittent across the 8–year duration of the study.

Given the differences in sampling populations (clinical, VAMC primary care, health maintenance organization, general population), pain syndromes (arthritis, back, abdominal, temporomandibular joint, chest, migraine headache, or mixed etiology), dimension of negative emotion measured (usually depression), measurement intervals (1 day, 6 months, 3–8 years), and methodology (mailed questionnaire or clinical examination), these results cannot be compared directly and discussed in terms of replication. Rather, if a pattern emerges, showing that negative emotion precedes pain onset/exacerbation or pain onset/exacerbation precedes negative emotion, the validity of the effect should be considered in terms of its broad occurrence across populations, settings, and methods. If one uses box-score methodology, the following patterns occur: Four studies found results indicating effects in both directions; one study found only that pain predicted negative emotion; one study found only that negative emotion predicted pain; and one study found that negative emotions predicted pain but did not test for a relationship in the other direction. When the studies are interpreted in this manner, it is clear that the causal path is not unidirectional and that all of the above hypotheses may have merit. Pain precedes negative emotion for some individuals, negative emotion precedes pain for other individuals, and, given the high rate of co-occurrence, the common substrate hypothesis seems plausible. However, the complex nature of the human experience suggests that the effects of pain and emotion are probably not entirely direct but are mediated by a number of biological and psychosocial variables. Cohen and Rodriguez (1995) proposed and discussed theoretical models of biological, behavioral, cognitive, and social pathways that link affective disturbances and physical disorders. They emphasized the bidirectional nature of these pathways in the development and maintenance of affective and physical disorders.

POSSIBLE MEDIATORS BETWEEN PAIN AND NEGATIVE MOOD

Given the probability that the relationship between pain and negative emotion are not entirely direct, what are the variables that promote their comorbidity? It is also likely that the influence of these variables may differ in degree across dimensions of negative emotion (depression, anxiety, and anger). There are several constructs in the chronic pain literature that are known to be associated with pain and emotion and that may account, in part, for the comorbidity of pain and negative emotion. We will briefly describe four such constructs: somatization, catastrophizing cognition, perceptions of life control, and social support/interpersonal relationships.

Somatization

Somatization has been defined as the predisposition to amplify physiological sensations or the misclassification of symptoms of emotional arousal. It has been argued that with chronic pain, there may be a sensitizing effect to physiological events that heightens bodily awareness (Barsky, Goodson, & Lane, 1988). Several researchers have found that chronic pain patients blur painful and nonpainful experiences and interpret a wide variety of experience in terms of pain, particularly affective distress (Dworkin, Wilson, & Masson, 1994). Cultural factors and medical/social institutions that selectively focus on physical symptoms at the expense of accompanying psychological distress may also be involved (Dworkin et al., 1994).

Using a path model, Geisser, Gaskin, Robinson, & Greene (1993) found that a measure of somatic focus mediated the relationship between

depression and the sensory component of the McGill Pain Questionnaire. They did not find this relationship for the affective or evaluative components of pain. The authors stated that their results are consistent with Field's neurobiological model of pain, which suggests that the patient's tendency to focus on somatic symptoms activates pain facilitation neurons, which cause the perception of the stimulus to be greater. The general picture emerging is that somatization is related to both pain symptoms and depressive complaints.

Catastrophizing

Catastrophizing is a cognitive process characterized by negative expectations about future outcomes and lack of confidence (Sullivan & D'Eon, 1990). In the chronic pain literature, catastrophizing is thought to be a unique aspect of pain-related negative cognition and is typically measured with the Coping Strategies Questionnaire (Rosensteil & Keefe, 1983; for revised scoring see Riley & Robinson, 1997). There has been some debate as to whether catastrophizing and depression are distinct constructs (Jensen, Turner, Romano, & Karoly, 1991); however, cognitive models of depression view negative cognition as distinct from, but related to, symptoms of depression (Beck, 1976).

Geisser, Robinson, Keefe, and Weiner (1994) found that a measure of catastrophizing mediated the relationship between depression and the affective and evaluative dimension of pain but not the sensory aspect. Although their path analytic methodology did not allow them to determine directionality, this study provided evidence that catastrophizing was a separate construct from depression and an important variable in understanding the relationship between pain and negative emotion.

Social/Interpersonal Factors

The increased risk for the occurrence of negative emotion in chronic pain patients may be due, in part, to the effects of a patient's social interactions and interpersonal relationships. The occurrence and severity of depression that occurs in physical disorders such as chronic pain are associated with lack of social support (Rodin, Cravin, & Littlefield, 1991). In addition, marital dissatisfaction and conflict have been linked to poor patient adaptation to chronic pain. For example, Faucett (1994) found that increased depression was associated with more severe pain, greater conflict about pain, and less social support. She speculated that interpersonal conflict increases the risk of depressive symptoms in chronic pain patients. The data also suggested that these relationships are different across sex. Trief, Carnrike, and Drudge (1995) studied the relationship between the family environment and depression in 70 chronic low back pain patients. Their data showed that depression was associated with perception of social support and quality of the family environment. They interpreted their findings as suggesting that "low social support is linked to and may be a risk factor for depression in chronic pain" (p. 233).

Life Control and Interference

A decline of perceived control has been shown to mediate the relationship between pain and depression in two studies. Rudy, Kerns, and Turk (1988) tested a model of depression secondary to pain based on cognitive-behavioral theories. They used structural equation modeling and latent variables to model the perception of loss of life control and interference of pain in life activities as mediators of the effects of pain on depression. The observed data closely fit the theoretical model and provided support for a mediated model with depression secondary to pain. This suggested that pain did not initiate the depressive symptoms. In a similar study, Turk, Okifuji, and Scharff (1995) tested the role of these same cognitive appraisal variables as mediators in the development of emotional distress in a model similar to that used in the Rudy et al. (1988) study. They tested this model across two samples representing different stages of life by dividing their sample at the 70-year mark ($n = 27$ for participants 70 years old and older and $n = 73$ for participants 69 years old and younger). In the younger sample, life control and interference mediated the association between pain and depressive symptoms, replicating the earlier study. However, in the older sample, pain was directly associated with depressive symptoms, even when the cognitive appraisal variables were controlled, and the relationship remained strong. This finding emphasizes that the effects of mediators may differ across populations.

One must always be cautious of the inference of directionality. These studies were not longitudinal, and therefore, if not theory-driven, it makes as much sense to turn the analysis in the opposite direction with similar results. Nevertheless, these studies, in combination with the longitudinal studies reviewed, emphasize that the causal relationships between pain and negative emotion are complex, are likely to be bidirectional, and may involve multiple feedback loops (Cohen & Rodriguez, 1995).

FUTURE DIRECTIONS, OR WHERE TO GO FROM HERE?

Measurement Repair

To what extent do depression, anxiety, and anger overlap? Is the overlap different across pain syndromes, sex, place in the health care system (primary vs. tertiary care), and duration of pain (e.g., patients became angry and anxious and then with longer pain duration, depressed?), and how does this relate to the way we measure emotion? Do these affects represent a higher order factor of negative emotion, or are the causal and mediated relationships sufficiently different to warrant their consideration as separate, distinct constructs? For example, the dimensions of negative emotion have both shared and distinct components. Depression and anxiety share an emotional-distress component but differ on physiological arousal. How do these emotions relate to the experience of chronic pain? Most studies consider depression; only a few have considered anger.

A related issue arises with respect to the operationalization of negative emotional states. Consider the potential influence on pain report of (1) an anxious state, or transient fluctuations in anxiety; (2) an anxious trait, or an individual difference associated with cognitive and behavioral styles; and (3) a clinical diagnosis of an anxiety disorder (Cohen & Rodriguez, 1995). Different researchers have defined their emotion constructs differently. This tendency clearly has the potential to increase inconsistency between studies and laboratories.

Example of Empirical Analysis

There are many methods by which empirical studies can help us better understand the dimensions of negative emotions, their interrelationships, and their association with pain. Below we present an analysis that addresses the following measurement issues using data from a sample of 169 female facial pain patients evaluated in our clinic.

To what extent do composite measures of depression, anxiety, and anger differ from empirical factors of negative emotion? Do composite measures obscure unique associations between empirical factors of negative emotion and pain and related dysfunction?

We performed an item-level, principal-axis factor analysis on three measures of negative emotion, the BDI, the State–Trait Anxiety Inventory (STAI), and State–Trait Anger Expression Inventory (STAXI), frequently used in research with chronic pain patients. Our analysis found eight distinct factors that accounted for 62% of the total variance (see Table 5.1). With the exception of the Anergia and Failure/Hopelessness factors, factors comprised items within a standardized measure, suggesting relative homogeneity of item content.

We then compared the predictive utility of the "unidimensional" composite measures with the factors across measures of pain and functioning. To accomplish this, we performed eight stepwise multiple regression analyses, entering predictor variables (composite scale scores or factor scores) simultaneously against measures of pain (affective and sensory dimensions of the McGill Pain Questionnaire; MPQ) and functioning (Multidimensional Pain Inventory [MPI] life interference and activity subscales).

Associations with Pain. First, we regressed the MPQ affective score on the eight factor scores. Anergia ($R^2 = .16$), Feelings of Hostility ($R^2 = .06$), and Positive Affect ($R^2 = .06$) contributed significantly to the variance explained (R^2 for the model $= .28$). Then we regressed the MPQ sensory score on the eight factor scores. Only Anergia ($R^2 = .10$) and Feelings of Hostility ($R^2 = .03$) contributed significantly to the variance explained (R^2 for the model $= .13$). When we regressed the affective and sensory dimensions of the MPQ on unidimensional measures of negative emotion (BDI, STAI, and STAXI), we found that the BDI was the only significant unidimensional predictor (affective score, R^2 for the model $= .31$; sensory score, R^2 for the model $= .15$).

Associations with Functioning. Results of regressing the MPI life interference subscale score on the eight factor scores showed that Anergia ($R^2 = .30$), Positive Affect ($R^2 = .13$), and Feelings of Hostility ($R^2 = .07$) contributed significantly to the variance explained (R^2 for the model $= .50$). When we regressed the MPI activity subscale score on the eight factor scores, Troubling Thoughts ($R^2 = .05$)

and Aggression ($R^2 = .04$) contributed significantly to the variance explained (R^2 for the model $= .09$). When we regressed the measures of functioning on the unidimensional measures of negative emotion, we found that the BDI was the only significant predictor of life interference (R^2 for the model $= .40$) and that none of the measures contributed significantly to the variance of physical functioning.

The results demonstrate that the predictive power of anger (STAXI) and anxiety (STAI) is obscured by the association of the BDI with the dependent variables. When using factor scores, components of depression (Anergia), anxiety (Positive Affect), and anger (Feelings of Hostility) are all significant predictors of unique variance in the dependent variables.

The dimensions of negative emotion have been hypothesized to have shared and distinct components. For example, depression and anxiety are thought to share a cognitive component but to differ on physiological arousal. Do they?

We perform principal-axis factor analysis on the eight factor scores used in the preceding analysis to examine whether composite dimensions (shared components) could be identified. We also included the MPQ affective, evaluative, and sensory scores to test for factor discrimination (see Table 5.2).

Shared and Distinct Components. We found four dimensions accounting for 54% of the total variance, which we labeled as somatic, positive emotion, negative emotion, and anger and hostility. Interestingly, the Anergia factor (primarily BDI items) and the pain measures grouped together on the somatic dimension, highlighting the problems in measuring depression in a chronic pain sample (Williams & Richardson, 1993). Also of interest is the hypothesized shared cognitive component of depression and anxiety formed by the Failure/Hopelessness (BDI) and Troubling Thoughts (STAI) factors.

What about Measurement Error and Method Variance?

Multiple regression and between-group tests of variance make the assumption that measurement instruments are void of measurement error. The use of methodology with latent variables allows the identification (or at least an estimate) of measurement error (Hoyle, 1991; Hoyle & Smith, 1994).

TABLE 5.1. Item–Factor Loading Matrix

Item source	Item wording	Factor loading
F1 Positive Affect		
STAI 30	I am happy.	.82
STAI 36	1 am content.	.81
STAI 33	I feel secure.	.80
STAI 27	1 am calm, cool, and collected.	.75
F2 Feelings of Hostility		
STAXI 6	I am mad.	.87
STAX19	1 am burned up.	.82
STAXI 3	I feel angry.	.82
STAXI 10	I feel like swearing.	.78
F3 Anger Expression		
STAXI 13	1 am a hotheaded person.	.81
STAXI 12	I have a fiery temper.	.78
STAXI 16	I fly off the handle.	.76
STAXI 11	I am quick-tempered.	.70
F4 Troubling Thoughts		
STAI 37	Unimportant thoughts run through my mind.	.65
STAI 38	I take disappointments so keenly that I can't put them out of my mind.	.62
STAI 31	I have disturbing thoughts.	.58
STAI 40	I get in a state or turmoil as I think over my recent concerns and interests	.57
F5 Anergia		
BDI 15	It takes extra effort to do something.	.67
BDI 17	I get tired easily.	.65
BDI 16	I don't sleep as well as I used to.	.54
STAI 26	I feel rested.	-.52
F6 Failure/Hopelessness		
BDI 3	I feel like a failure.	.68
BDI 7	1 am disappointed with myself	.65
STAI 25	I feel like a failure.	.57
F7 Slighted by Others		
STAXI 20	I feel infuriated when I do a good job and get a poor evaluation.	.78
STAXI 18	It makes me furious when I am criticized in front of others.	.54
STAXI 15	I feel annoyed when I am not given recognition for doing good work.	.63
F8 Aggression		
STAXI 8	I feel like hitting someone.	.63
STAXI 5	I feel like breaking things.	.62
STAXI 7	I feel like banging on the table.	.62

TABLE 5.2. Composite Factor Matrix

Dimension	Somatic	Negative cognition	Positive emotion	Anger expression
MPQ–Affective	.84			
MPQ–Evaluative	.80			
MPQ–Sensory	.81			
BDI–Anergia	.65			
BDI–Hopelessness		.76		
STAI–Troubling Thoughts		.67		
STAI–Positive Affect			.79	
STAXI–Feelings of Hostility			−.55	
STAXI–Slighted by Others				.78
STAXI–Anger Expression				.49
STAXI–Aggression			−.42	.55

As mentioned previously (Holroyd et al., 1996), there is likely to be unknown method variance across dimensions of negative emotion or across a family of measurement instruments that may be interpreted as associations between actual constructs. Using multitrait, multimethod methodology would help in answering this question, as would latent variable analysis.

Improved Methodology (and Lack of Programmatic Research)

Our review of the literature suggests that there has been little systematic, programmatic research in the area of negative emotion and pain. Those areas that have been systematic appear to be focused on one dimension of negative affect (i.e., depression) to the exclusion of others. A more systematic approach, employing the statistical control of separate dimensions (in the absence of experimental manipulation of affect) while building on the results of previous studies, is likely to yield a more complete understanding of this area.

Lack of Theory-Driven Models

There is a need for models with empirically testable, falsifiable relationships. Several researchers have suggested that structural equation modeling provides an appropriate research methodology within which specific hypothesized relationships can be tested (Bentler & Stein, 1992; Hoyle & Smith, 1994; Novy, Nelson, Frances, & Turk, 1995b). For programmatic research to succeed, it must be theory-driven, with competing theories allowing for the elimination of unsupported theories.

The Presence of Subgroups

The study by Moldofsky and Chester (1970) and a number of cluster analytic studies that have grouped chronic pain patients on their psychosocial responses to pain (Bradley et al., 1978; Riley, Robinson, Geisser, & Wittmer, 1993; Turk & Rudy, 1988; Jamison, Rock, & Parris, 1988) suggest the existence of relatively homogeneous subtypes of chronic pain patients. It is possible that patients can be characterized into subtypes based on their experiences of depression, anxiety, and anger. It seems likely that if emotional distress is considered to be a multidimensional construct (i.e., depression, anger, anxiety), then one could characterize individuals on the relative contribution of each of these components to their pain experiences. The existence of distinct subgroups could be one explanation for inconsistencies in the literature and lack of closure on the relationship between pain and emotion.

In summary, it appears certain that pain is strongly associated with negative emotion. There are literally thousands of published articles on the relationship between chronic pain and emotion. There is evidence that negative emotions co-occur with pain conditions and that individuals in chronic pain have on average greater levels of negative emotions. The data are mixed on the causal relationships between pain and emotion, though some evidence suggests that the relationship can be causal, reactive, and perhaps recursive in different individuals or groups of individuals. Despite the large body of literature, much is left to be understood about the complex relationship between pain and emotion. We have attempted to outline additional work that might increase our understanding of this important area.

REFERENCES

Asmundson, G. J., Jacobson, S. J., Allerdings, M. D., & Norton, G. R. (1996). Social phobia in disabled workers with chronic musculoskeletal pain. *Behaviour Research and Therapy, 34*, 939–943.

Asmundson, G. J., Norton, G. R., & Allerdings, M. D. (1997). Fear and avoidance in dysfunctional chronic back pain patients. *Pain, 69*, 231–236.

Atkinson, J. H., Slater, M. A., Patterson, T. L., Grant, I., & Garfin, S. R. (1991). Prevalence, onset, and risk of psychiatric disorders in chronic pain patients: A controlled study. *Pain, 45*, 111–121.

Banks, S. M., & Kerns, R. D. (1996). Explaining high rates of depression in chronic pain: A diathesis–stress framework. *Psychological Bulletin, 119*, 95–110.

Barsky, A. J., Goodson, D. J., & Lane, R. S. (1988). The amplification of somatic symptoms. *Psychosomatic Medicine, 50*, 510–519.

Beck, A. T. (1976). *Cognitive therapy and the emotional disorders.* New York: International Universities Press.

Bentler, P. M., & Stein, J. A. (1992). Structural equation models in medical research. *Statistical Methods in Medical Research, 1*, 159–181.

Blumer, D., & Heilbronn, M. (1981). The pain prone patient: A clinical and psychological profile. *Psychosomatics, 22*, 395–402.

Bradley, L. A., Prokop, C. K., Margolis, R., & Gentry, W. D. (1978). Multivariate analysis of the MMPI profiles of low back pain patients. *Journal of Behavioral Medicine, 1*, 253–272.

Brennan, A. F., Barrett, C. L., & Garretson, H. D. (1986). The prediction of chronic pain outcome by psychological variables. *International Journal of Psychiatry in Medicine, 16*, 373–387.

Breslau, N., Davis, G. C., Schultz, L. R., & Peterson, E. L. (1994). Migraine and major depression: A longitudinal study. *Headache, 12*, 387–393.

Brown, F. F., Robinson, M. E., Riley, J. L., & Gremillion, H. A. (1996). Pain severity, negative affect, and microstressors as predictors of life interference in TMD patients. *CRANIO, 14*, 63–70.

Brown, G. K. (1990). A causal analysis of chronic pain and depression. *Journal of Abnormal Psychology, 99*, 127–137.

Buckelew, S. P., DeGood, D. E., Schwartz, D. P., & Kerler, R. M. (1986). Cognitive and somatic item response pattern of pain patients, psychiatric patients, and hospital employees. *Journal of Clinical Psychology, 42*, 852–859.

Burchiel, K. J., Anderson, V. C., Wilson, B. J., Denison, D. B., Olson, K. A., & Shatin, D. (1995). Prognostic factors of spinal cord stimulation for chronic back and leg pain. *Neurosurgery, 36*, 1101–1111.

Burns, J. W., Wiegner, S., Derleth, M., Kiselica, K., & Pawl, R. (1996). Linking symptom-specific physiological reactivity to pain severity in chronic low back pain patients: A test of mediation and moderation models. *Health Psychology, 16*, 319–326.

Byrne, B. (1996). Generalized anxiety and mixed anxiety-depression: Association with disability and health care utilization. *Journal of Clinical Psychiatry, 57*, 86–91.

Cavanaugh, S. V. (1984). Diagnosing depression in the hospitalized patient with chronic medical illness. *Journal of Clinical Psychiatry, 45*, 13–17.

Cohen, S., & Rodriguez, M. S. (1995). Pathways linking affective disturbances and physical disorders. *Health Psychology, 14*, 374–380.

Diener, H. C., van Schayck, R., & Kastrup, O. (1995). Pain and depression. In B. B. Bromm & J. E. Desmedt (Eds.), *Pain and the brain: From nociception to cognition.* New York: Raven Press.

Dworkin, S. F., & Gatlin, M. J. (1991). Clinical aspects of depression in chronic pain patients. *Clinical Journal of Pain, 7*, 79–94.

Dworkin, S. F., Wilson, L., & Masson, D. L. (1994). Somatizing as a risk factor for chronic pain. In R. C. Grzesiak & D. S. Ciccone (Eds.), *Psychological vulnerability to chronic pain.* New York: Springer.

Engel, C. C., Von Korff, M., & Katon, W. J. (1996). Back pain in primary care: Predictors of high health-care costs. *Pain, 65*, 197–204

Engle, G. L. (1959). Psychogenic pain and the pain-prone patient. *American Journal of Medicine, 26*, 899.

Faucett, J. A. (1994). Depression in painful chronic disorders: The role of pain and conflict about pain. *Journal of Pain and Symptom Management, 9*, 520–526.

Fernandez, E., & Turk, D. C. (1995). The scope and significance of anger in the experience of chronic pain. *Pain, 61*, 165–175.

Fishbain, D. A., Cutler, R., Rosomoff, H. L., & Rosomoff, R. S. (1997). Chronic pain-associated depression: Antecedent or consequence of chronic pain? A review. *Clinical Journal of Pain, 13*, 116–137.

Fishbain, D. A., Goldberg, M., Meagher, B. R., & Steele, R. (1986). Male and female chronic pain patients categorized by DSM-III psychiatric diagnostic criteria. *Pain, 26*, 181–197

Flor, H., & Turk, D. C. (1989). Psychophysiology of chronic pain: Do chronic pain patients exhibit symptom-specific psychophysiological responses? *Psychological Bulletin, 105*, 215–259.

Gamsa, A. (1994). The role of psychological factors in chronic pain: I. A half century of study. *Pain, 57*, 5–15.

Gaskin, M. E., Greene, A. F., Robinson, M. E., & Geisser, M. E. (1992). Negative affect and the experience of chronic pain. *Journal of Psychosomatic Research, 36*, 707–713.

Gatchel, R. J., Polatin, P. B., & Kinney, R. K. (1995). Predicting outcome of chronic back pain using clinical predictors of psychopathology: A prospective analysis. *Health Psychology, 14*, 415–420.

Geisser, M. E., Gaskin, M. E., Robinson, M. E., & Greene, A. F. (1993). The relationship of depression and somatic focus to experimental and clinical pain in chronic pain patients. *Psychology and Health, 8*, 405–415.

Geisser, M. E., Robinson, M. E., Keefe, F. J., & Weiner, M. L. (1994). Catastrophizing, depression and the sensory, affective, and evaluative aspects of chronic pain. *Pain, 59*, 79–83.

Geisser, M. E., Roth, R. S., Bachman, J. E., & Eckert, T. A. (1997). The relationship between symptoms of post-traumatic stress disorder and pain, affective disturbance and disability among patients with accident and non-accident related pain. *Pain, 66*, 207–214.

Geisser, M. E., Roth, R. S., & Robinson, M. E. (1997). Assessing depression among persons with chronic pain using the Center for Epidemiological Studies-Depression Scale and the Beck Depression Inventory: A comparative analysis. *Clinical Journal of Pain, 13,* 163–170.

Gerke, D. C., Richards, L. C., & Goss, A. N. (1989). Discriminant function analysis of clinical and psychological variables in temporomandibular joint pain dysfunction. *Australian Dental Journal, 34,* 44–48.

Gracely, R. H. (1992). Evaluation of multi-dimensional pain scales. *Pain, 48,* 297–300.

Hasenbring, M., Marienfeld, G., Kuhlendahl, D., & Soyka, D. (1994). Risk factors of chronicity in lumbar disc patients: A prospective investigation of biologic, psychologic, and social predictors of therapy outcome. *Spine, 19,* 2759–2765.

Haythornthwaite, J. A., Sieber W. J., & Kerns, R. D. (1991). Depression and the chronic pain experience. *Pain, 46,* 177–184.

Holroyd, K. A., Talbot, F., Holm, J. E., Pingel, J. D., Lake, A. E., & Saper, J. R. (1996). Assessing the dimensions of pain: A multitrait-multimethod evaluation of seven measures. *Pain, 67,* 259–265.

Holzberg, A. D., Robinson, M. E., & Geisser, M. E. (1993). The relationship of cognitive distortion to depression in chronic pain: The role of ambiguity and desirability in self-ratings. *Clinical Journal of Pain, 9,* 202–206.

Holzberg, A. D., Robinson, M. E., Geisser, M. E. & Gremillion, H. A. (1996). The effects of depression and chronic pain on psychosocial and physical functioning. *Clinical Journal of Pain, 12,* 118–125.

Hoyle, R. H. (1991). Evaluating measurement models in clinical research: Covariance structure analysis of latent variable models of self-conception. *Journal of Consulting and Clinical Psychology, 59,* 67–76.

Hoyle, R. H., & Smith, G. T. (1994). Formulating clinical research hypothesis as structural equation models: A conceptual overview. *Journal of Consulting and Clinical Psychology, 62,* 429–440.

International Association for the Study of Pain (Subcommittee on Taxonomy). (1979). Pain terms: A list with definitions and notes on usage. *Pain, 6,* 249–252.

Jamison, R. N., Rock, D. L., & Parris, W. C. V. (1988). Empirically derived Symptom Checklist-90 subgroups of chronic pain patients. *Journal of Behavioral Medicine, 11,* 147–157.

Jensen, M. P., Turner, J. A., Romano, J. M., & Karoly, P. (1991). Coping with chronic pain: A critical review of the literature. *Pain, 47,* 249–283.

Junge, A., Dvorak, J., & Ahrens, S. (1995). Predictors of bad and good outcomes of lumbar disc surgery. A prospective clinical study with recommendations for screening to avoid bad outcomes. *Spine, 20,* 460–468.

Kellner, R. (1985). Functional somatic symptoms and hypochondriasis. *Archives of General Psychiatry, 42,* 821–833.

Kerns, R. D., Rosenberg, R., & Jacob, M. C. (1994). Anger expression and chronic pain. *Journal of Behavioral Medicine, 17,* 57–67.

Kinder, B. N., & Curtiss, G. (1988). Assessment of anxiety, depression, and anger in chronic pain patients: Conceptual and methodological issues. In C. D. Spielberger & J. N. Butcher (Eds.), *Advances in personality assessment.* Hillsdale, NJ: Erlbaum.

Klenerman, L., Slade, P. D., Stanley, I. M., Pennie, B., Reilly, J. P., Atchison, L. E., Troup, J. D., & Rose, M. J. (1995). The prediction of chronicity in patients with an acute attack of low back pain in a general practice setting. *Spine, 20,* 478–484.

Krishnan, K. R. R., France, R. D., Pelton, S., McCann, U. D., Davidson, J., & Urban, B. J. (1985). Chronic pain and depression: I. Classification of depression in chronic low-back pain patients. *Pain, 22,* 279–287.

Lang, P. J. (1968). Fear reduction and fear behavior: Problems in treating a construct. *Research in Psychotherapy, 3,* 90–102.

Larsen, D. K., Taylor, S., & Asmundson, G. J. (1997). Exploratory factor analysis of the Pain Anxiety Symptoms Scale in patients with chronic pain complaints. *Pain, 69,* 27–34.

Leino, P., & Magni, G. (1993) Depressive and distress symptoms as predictors of low back pain, neck-shoulder pain, and other musculoskeletal morbidity: A 10-year follow-up of metal industry employees. *Pain, 53,* 89–94.

Love, A. W. (1988). Attributional style of depressed chronic low back patients. *Journal of Clinical Psychology, 44,* 317–321.

Magni, G., Moreschi, C., Rigatti-Luchini, S., & Merskey, H. (1994). Prospective study on the relationship between depressive symptoms and chronic musculoskeletal pain. *Pain, 56,* 289–297.

Main, C. J., & Watson, P. J. (1992). Screening for patients at risk of developing chronic incapacity. *Journal of Occupational Rehabilitation, 5,* 207–217.

Max, M. B. (1995). Pain and depression. In B. B. Bromm & J. E. Desmedt (Eds.), *Pain and the brain: From nociception to cognition.* New York: Raven Press.

McCracken, L. M., Gross, R. T., Aikens, J., & Carnrike, C. L. M. (1996). The assessment of anxiety and fear in persons with chronic pain: A comparison of instruments. *Behaviour Research and Therapy, 34,* 927–933.

McCracken, L. M., Gross, R. T., Sorg, P. J., & Edmands, T. A. (1993). Prediction of pain in patients with chronic low back pain: Effects of inaccurate prediction and pain-related anxiety. *Behaviour Research and Therapy, 31,* 647–652.

McCracken, L. M., Zayfert, C., & Gross, R. T. (1992). The Pain Anxiety Symptoms Scale: Development and validation of a scale to measure fear of pain. *Pain, 50,* 67–73.

Melzack, R., & Wall, P. D. (1965). Pain mechanisms: A new theory. *Science, 150,* 971–979.

Moldofsky, H., & Chester, W. J. (1970). Pain and mood patterns in patients with rheumatoid arthritis: A prospective study. *Psychosomatic Medicine, 32,* 309–318.

Novy, D. M., Nelson, D. V., Berry, L. A., & Averil, P. M. (1995a). What does the Beck Depression Inventory measure in chronic pain?: A reappraisal. *Pain, 61,* 261–270.

Novy, D. M., Nelson, D. V., Frances, D. J., & Turk, D. C. (1995b). Perspectives of chronic pain: An evaluative comparison of restrictive and comprehensive models. *Psychological Bulletin, 118,* 238–247.

Ohrbach, R., & McCall, W. D. (1996). The stress-hyperactivity-pain theory of myogenic pain. *Pain Forum, 5,* 51–66.

Pennebaker, J. W. (1982). *The psychology of physical symptoms.* New York: Springer.

Riley, J. L., & Robinson, M. E. (1997). The Coping Strategies Questionnaire: Five factors or fiction? *Clinical Journal of Pain, 13,* 156-162.

Riley, J. L., Robinson, M. E., Geisser, M. E., & Wittmer, V. (1993). Multivariate cluster analysis of the MMPI-2 in chronic low-back pain patients. *Clinical Journal of Pain, 9,* 248-252.

Riley, J. L., Robinson, M. E., Geisser, M. E., Wittmer, V. T., & Graham-Smith, A. (1995). The relationship between MMPI-2 cluster profiles and surgical outcome in low-back pain patients. *Journal of Spinal Disorders, 8,* 213-219.

Robinson, M. E., Myers, C., Sadler, I. J., Riley, J. L., Kvaal, S. A., & Geisser, M. E. (1997). Bias effects in three common self-report assessment measures. *Clinical Journal of Pain, 13,* 74-81.

Rodin, G., Craven, J., & Littlefield, C. (1991). Depression in the medically ill: An integrated approach. New York: Brunner/Mazel.

Rodin, G., & Voshart, K. (1986). Depression in the medically ill: An overview. *American Journal of Psychiatry, 143,* 696-705.

Romano, J. M., & Turner, J. A. (1985). Chronic pain and depression: Does the evidence support a relationship? *Psychological Bulletin, 97,* 18-34.

Rosenstiel, A. K., & Keefe, F. J. (1983). The use of coping strategies in chronic low back pain patients: Relationship to patient characteristics and current adjustment. *Pain, 17,* 33-44.

Rudy, T. E., Kerns, R. D., & Turk, D. C. (1988). Chronic pain and depression: Toward a cognitive-behavioral meditation model. *Pain, 35,* 129-140.

Salovey, P., & Birnbaum, D. (1989). Influence of mood on health-relevant cognitions. *Journal of Personality and Social Psychology, 57,* 539-551.

Schwartz, L., Slater, M. A., Birchler, G. R., & Atkinson, J. H. (1991). Depression in spouses of chronic pain patients: The role of patient pain and anger, and marital satisfaction. *Pain, 44,* 61-67.

Spielberger, C. D. (1985). State–Trait Anger Expression Inventory Professional Manual. Odessa, FL: Psychological Assessment Resources.

Stemmler, G. (1989). The autonomic differentiation of emotions revisited: Convergent and discriminant validation. *Psychophysiology, 26,* 617-632.

Sullivan, M. J. L., & D'Eon, J. L. (1990). Relation between catastrophizing and depression in chronic pain patients. *Journal of Abnormal Psychology, 99,* 260-263.

Swimmer, G. I., Robinson, M. E., & Geisser, M. E. (1992). The relationship of MMPI cluster type to pain coping strategy and treatment outcome. *Clinical Journal of Pain, 8,* 131-137.

Taylor, A. G., Lorentzen, L. J., & Blank, M. B. (1990). Psychologic distress of chronic pain sufferers and their spouses. *Journal of Pain and Symptom Management, 5,* 6-10.

Trief, P. M., Carnrike, C. L. M., & Drudge, O. (1995). Chronic pain and depression: Is social support relevant? *Psychological Reports, 76,* 227-236.

Turk, D. C., Okifuji, A., & Scharff, L. (1995). Chronic pain and depression: Role of perceived impact and perceived control in different age cohorts. *Pain, 61,* 93-101.

Turk, D. C., & Rudy, T. E. (1988). Toward an empirically derived taxonomy of chronic pain patients: Integration of psychological assessment data. *Journal of Consulting and Clinical Psychology 56,* 233-238.

Uomoto, J. M., Turner, J. A., & Herron, L. D. (1988). Use of the MMPI and MCMI in predicting outcome of lumbar laminectomy. *Journal of Clinical Psychology, 44,* 191-197.

Von Korff, M., Le Resche, L., & Dworkin, S. F. (1993). First onset of common pain symptoms: A prospective study of depression as a risk factor. *Pain, 55,* 251-258.

Waddell, G., Newton, M., Henderson, I., Somerville, D., & Main, C. (1993). A Fear-Avoidance Beliefs Questionnaire (FABQ) and the role of fear-avoidance beliefs in chronic low back pain and disability. *Pain, 52,* 157-168.

Wade, J. B., Price, D. D., Hamer, R. M., & Schwartz, S. M. (1990). An emotional component analysis of chronic pain. *Pain, 40,* 303-310.

Ward, N. G. (1982). Pain and depression. In J. J. Bonica (Ed.), *The management of pain* (2nd ed.). London: Lea & Febiger.

Williams, A. C., & Richardson, P. H. (1993). What does the BDI measure in chronic pain? *Pain, 55,* 259-266.

Williams, D. A., Robinson, M. E., & Geisser, M. E. (1994). Pain beliefs: Assessment and utility. *Pain, 59,* 71-78.

Zelman, D. C., Howland, E. W., & Cleeland, C. S. (1991). The effects of induced mood on laboratory pain. *Pain, 47,* 105-111.

Chapter 6

Pain and Stress: A New Perspective

RONALD MELZACK

The neuromatrix theory of pain (Melzack, 1989, 1990, 1991, 1992, 1995) proposes that pain is a multidimensional experience produced by character-istic "neurosignature" patterns of nerve impulses generated by a widely distributed neural network—the "body-self neuromatrix"—in the brain. These neurosignature patterns may be triggered by sensory inputs, but they may also be generated independently of them. Pains that are evoked by noxious sensory inputs have been meticulously investigated by neuro-scientists, and their sensory transmission mecha-nisms are generally well understood (see Melzack & Wall, 1996). In contrast, chronic pain syndromes, which are often characterized by severe pain asso-ciated with little or no discernible injury or pathol-ogy, remain a mystery. The neuromatrix theory of pain, however, provides a new conceptual framework that is consistent with recent clinical evidence. It proposes that the output patterns of the neuromatrix activate perceptual, homeostatic, and behavioral pro-grams after injury or pathology or as a result of multiple other inputs that act on the neuromatrix.

Pain, then, is produced by the output of a widely distributed neural network in the brain rather than directly by sensory input evoked by injury, in-flammation, or other pathology. The neuromatrix, which is genetically determined and modified by sensory experience, is the primary mechanism that generates the neural pattern that produces pain. Its output pattern is determined by multiple influences, of which the somatic sensory input is only a part, that converge on the neuromatrix.

We are so accustomed to considering pain as a purely perceptual phenomenon that we have ig-nored the obvious fact that injury also disrupts the body's homeostatic regulation systems, thereby producing stress and initiating complex programs to restore homeostasis. By recognizing the role of the stress system in pain processes, the scope of the puzzle of pain is greatly expanded, and new pieces of the puzzle provide valuable clues in our quest to understand chronic pain.

THE STRESS SYSTEM

Hans Selye (1950), who founded the field of stress research, studied stress as a biological response to a wide range of stressors. They include physical injury, infection, and other pathology, as well as psychological stressors such as the loss of a job or the death of a friend. Recently, stress has been defined (Chrousos, 1992) as a state of threatened homeostasis—that is, a disruption by stressors of physiological processes such as blood sugar level and body temperature that are normally maintained at a fixed, delicately balanced set point.

The disruption of homeostasis by a stressor, either physical or psychological, activates pro-grams of neural, hormonal, and behavioral activ-ity aimed at restoring homeostasis. The particu-lar programs that are activated are selected from a genetically determined repertoire of programs (which have been modified by events such as earlier exposure to stress) and are influenced by the extent and severity of the perceived stress.

Given the multiplicity of interacting neural and hormonal factors that contribute to homeostasis, it is not surprising that programs to rein-state homeostasis may go awry. The consequence is a variety of stress-related disorders, which include several chronic pain syndromes (Chrousos, 1992; Chrousos & Gold, 1992; Sapolsky, 1992). It is important, therefore, to examine the hypothesis that stress may produce the conditions that give rise to some forms of chronic pain.

When injury occurs, sensory information is projected rapidly to the brain, and, in parallel with the neuromatrix activities that usually lead to pain perception (Melzack, 1991, 1995), the stress system (Figure 6.1) initiates the complex sequence of events to restore biological homeostasis. Activities

in the injured tissues produce cytokines, which are complex molecules produced by the interaction of transformed white blood cells known as macrophages and injured tissues. These cytokines are released within seconds after injury and take part in producing a local inflammatory response. Within minutes, cytokines such as gamma-interferon, interleukins 1 and 6, and tumor necrosis factor enter the bloodstream and travel to the brain, where they breach the blood–brain barrier at specific sites and have an immediate effect on hypothalamic cells (Sapolsky, 1992). The cytokines, together with the perception of pain—a stressor—rapidly begin a sequence of activities aimed at the release and utili-

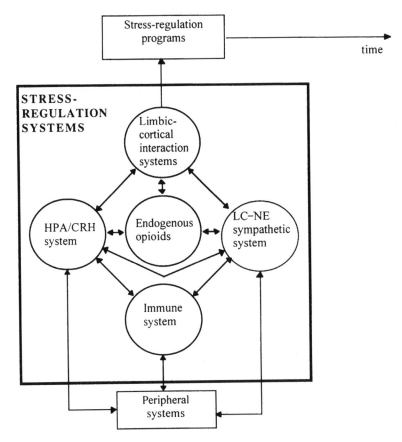

FIGURE 6.1. Components of the stress-regulation systems and their interactions. In the HPA (hypothalamic-pituitary-adrenal) system, the paraventricular nucleus of the hypothalamus, during a stressful event, produces CRH (corticotropin-releasing hormone), which activates the pituitary to produce adrenocorticotropic hormone (ACTH) that, in turn, acts on the adrenal cortex to produce cortisol in humans and corticosterone in animals. The LC–NE (locus coeruleus–norepinephrine)-sympathetic system in the brainstem has descending and ascending projections. Both of these systems interact with the immune, opioid, and limbic-cortical systems. A more detailed schematic figure, which depicts many of the components of the systems and their interactions, is presented by Chrousos and Gold (1992).

zation of glucose for necessary actions such as the repair of tissues and "fight or flight" responses to survive the threat to the body–self.

Cytokines that penetrate the hypothalamus activate the hypothalamic–pituitary–adrenal (HPA) system, in which corticotropin-releasing hormone (CRH) produced in the hypothalamus is released into the local bloodstream that carries it to the pituitary. There, the CRH causes the release of adrenocorticotropic hormone (ACTH) and other substances (Sapolsky, 1992; Chrousos, 1992). The ACTH then activates the adrenal cortex to release cortisol (in humans; corticosterone in animals), which plays a powerful role in the stress response.

At the same time that the HPA system carries out these processes, the autonomic system is activated: The powerful locus coeruleus–norepinephrine (LC–NE)-sympathetic system in the brainstem acts upward on neural mechanisms throughout the brain and, via hypothalamic and other limbic areas, downward through the descending autonomic (sympathetic and parasympathetic) nervous system (Chrousos, 1992). During the stress response, the sympathetic system predominates and produces readiness of the heart, blood vessels, and other viscera for complex action programs to respond appropriately to the stressor and to reinstate homeostasis.

As the stress response continues, it has a powerful impact on multiple additional systems. The immune system is suppressed, and major portions of the limbic system (mesocorticolimbic areas, as well as the amygdala and hippocampus), which play a role in emotional, motivational, homeostatic, and cognitive processes, are activated. Furthermore, the endogenous opioids, such as endorphin, are released within minutes. Their initial function may be primarily to inhibit or modulate the release of cortisol (Chrousos, 1992; Sapolsky, 1992). This highly simplified description does not include multiple other neural and hormonal systems and the complex interactions among them that take part in the stress response (Chrousos, 1992). Figure 6.1 provides a schematic representation of the major components that make up the stress system and their interactions.

The stress and pain-perception systems, therefore, possess overlapping mechanisms. Injury produces information that feeds into the body–self neuromatrix that generates the output patterns that comprise the neurosignature for the perception of the extent and severity of the injury and concurrently activate the appropriate action patterns to be chosen from the available pool (Melzack, 1995).

This output, together with information generated by the neuromatrixes that receive inputs from the other sensory and cognitive systems, acts on the stress-regulation mechanisms that are part of the system—the HPA and LC–NE-sympathetic systems—and determines whether or not pain will be experienced or suppressed. It is well known (Melzack, Wall, & Ty, 1982; Melzack & Wall, 1996) that people who undergo severe injury may not feel any pain for as long as hours, even days, afterward. Because the stress system requires about 1–4 minutes to be activated, the endorphin and other opioid substances released by stressors cannot be the determinant of the complete suppression of pain after injury. Rather, the neuromatrixes that generate sensory-discriminative and evaluative information regarding the state of the body and the circumstances of injury (for example, an injury in an automobile accident or a gash made in the leg of a zebra by a hungry lion) determine the initial activation or suppression of the pain, inflammation processes, and immune systems (Sapolsky, 1992).

Prolonged activation of the stress-regulation systems produces breakdown of muscle, bone, and neural tissue. Excessively long or intense activation of these systems, therefore, can have disastrous consequences. They may set the stage for fibromyalgia, osteoporosis, and other chronic pain syndromes (Chrousos & Gold, 1992).

To recapitulate, the HPA and LC–NE-sympathetic systems are activated by perceived pain or other forms of stress on the basis of sensory and cognitive input to the body–self neuromatrix. At the same time, when injury or other pathology occurs, cytokines are released into the bloodstream and are carried to the hypothalamus, where they act directly on the HPA and LC–NE-sympathetic systems, the two major pillars of the stress system. Activation of the stress system also influences several other powerful systems, including the immune system, the endogenous opiates, and major portions of the limbic system (mesocorticolimbic areas, as well as the amygdala and hippocampus). All of these systems interact with each other and are characterized by multiple checks and balances (Chrousos & Gold, 1992; Fuchs & Melzack, 1996, 1997; Fuchs, Kerr, & Melzack, 1996; Harbuz & Lightman, 1992; Lariviere, Fuchs, & Melzack, 1995; Sapolsky, 1992). It is not surprising, then, to find great variability among studies. Nevertheless, particular effects of the stress system are firmly established.

The inhibitory effect of cortisol on the immune system and the serious effects of prolonged immune suppression are fully documented (Chrousos, 1992; Sapolsky, 1992). The opiates appear to modulate the effects of cortisol, but their full function is not understood. The programs aimed at a return to homeostasis are only partly known; their relation to chronic pain must, because of our lack of knowledge, be surmised.

PROGRAMS INVOLVING THE CORTISOL SYSTEM

Cortisol, together with the activation of the sympathetic system, sets the stage for the stress response. Cortisol plays an essential role because it is responsible for producing and maintaining high levels of glucose for the response. At the same time, cortisol is potentially a highly destructive substance because, to ensure a high level of glucose, it breaks down the protein in muscle and inhibits the ongoing replacement of calcium in bone. It can also have a marked deleterious effect on neurons in the hippocampus (Sapolsky, 1996). As a result, if the output of cortisol is prolonged, excessive, or abnormally patterned, it may produce destruction of muscle, bone, and neural tissue and produce the conditions for many kinds of chronic pain.

The deleterious effect of aging on hippocampal neurons is particularly serious because the hippocampus acts as a natural brake on cortisol release. As aging proceeds, therefore, cortisol is released in larger amounts, producing a cascading destructive effect (Sapolsky, 1992) that could contribute to the increase of chronic pain problems known to occur among older people.

It is possible that any site of increased cytokine activity and inflammation, including sites of strain, sprain, or spasm of muscles and tendons, could become the focus of cortisol action and muscle destruction. This could mark the beginning of trigger zones at sites that tend to become inflamed due to minor injury (Sola, 1994) and may become particularly vulnerable to cortisol's destructive effects. The breakdown of muscle protein could also be the basis for fibromyalgia and other muscle pains. At the same time, calcium replacement in bone is inhibited (Sapolsky, 1992). If the inhibition is prolonged, it may become the basis of osteoporosis, which may produce deformities and fractures, particularly of the vertebrae and hip, that are often extremely painful.

The cortisol output by itself may not be sufficient to cause chronic pain problems but rather provides the background conditions so that other contributing factors may, all together, produce them. Estrogen levels, genetic predispositions, and psychological stresses derived from social competition and the hassles of everyday life may act together to influence the effects of cortisol on the target organs.

A high proportion of cases of chronic back pain may be due to more subtle causes (Jayson & Freemont, 1995). The perpetual stresses and strains on the vertebral column (at discs and facet joints) produce greatly increased vascularization and fibrosis of the area. As a result, there is a release of substances such as bradykinen that are known to produce inflammation and pain into local tissues and bloodstream. As a result, the whole HPA cascade may be triggered repeatedly.

The effect of stress-produced substances—such as cortisol and noradrenalin—at sites of minor lesions and inflammation may, if it occurs often and is prolonged, activate a neuromatrix program that anticipates increasingly severe damage and attempts to counteract it. The program to reduce strain and inflammation could generate the neurosignature for pain, which induces rest, the repair of injured tissues, and the restoration of homeostasis.

This speculation is supported by strong evidence. Chrousos and Gold (1992) and Tsigos and Chrousos (1994) have documented the effects of dysregulation of the cortisol system, to which they attribute fibromyalgia, rheumatoid arthritis, and chronic fatigue syndrome (which is often painful). They propose, on the basis of experimental data, that they are associated with *hypo*cortisolism—that is, reduced release of cortisol during stress. However, hypocortisolism may also reflect a higher level of utilization and metabolism of cortisol, which may appear as a depletion due to prolonged stress. Indeed, an important problem that requires investigation is the effect of a prolonged series of brief stresses—that is, brief spurts of hypo- or hypercortisolism over a long period of time—compared to prolonged, continuous stress. Whatever the mechanism, myopathy, bone decalcification, fatigue, and accelerated neural degeneration during aging are produced by prolonged exposure to stress.

A better understanding of the multiple modulation effects among the components of the stress system, as well as the effects of long durations of abnormal patterns of secretion of cortisol, may reveal the underlying interactional mechanisms (Chrousos & Gold, 1992; Sapolsky, 1992). For example, the endogenous opioids that are released by stress produce a further reduction in cortisol output. Cortisol levels are also decreased by sympathetic activity. The temporal patterns of output of different substances may determine hypo- versus hypercortisolism and, therefore, the resultant painful conditions. Diabetes mellitus, especially with diabetic neuropathy, is associated with *hyper*cortisolism (Tsigos & Chrousos, 1994). Research is therefore especially needed to investigate these deleterious effects on tissues in relation to pain.

PROGRAMS INVOLVING THE IMMUNE SYSTEM

A major effect of stress is the suppression of the immune system, which normally attacks invading bacteria, viruses, and other foreign substances (Steinman, 1993). However, this suppression may induce the immune system to attack the body itself, which would produce autoimmune diseases, many of which are also chronic pain syndromes. A possible mechanism is that prolonged suppression may result in dangerous levels of infection and an accumulation of toxins. Conceivably, the release from suppression may lead to a rebound excessive autoimmune response.

Concurrently with the suppression of the immune response, stress also suppresses the perception of pain and inflammation at the site of injury. The value of suppressing pain is clear: A wounded zebra, for example, needs to run from an attack-ing lion, and pain, as well as inflammation, would hamper running speed and could lead to death (Sapolsky, 1992). However, this suppression of pain, inflammation, and immune-system activity could also produce increased levels of tissue damage and infection. The suppression of pain may persist for hours, sometimes days, yet the pain returns (Fuchs, Kerr, & Melzack, 1996; Fuchs & Melzack, 1997; Melzack, Wall, & Ty, 1982), indicating that the mechanisms that produce pain and inflammation remain intact. It is possible, therefore, that the immune system may rebound with excessive vigor.

Consequently, the initially protective mechanisms may produce autoimmune diseases that are associated with significant levels of pain (Table 6.1). Some are also categorized as chronic pain syndromes—such as Crohn's disease, multiple sclerosis, rheumatoid arthritis, scleroderma, and lupus (Merskey & Bogduk, 1994).

The mechanisms that relate immune suppression to chronic pain are not understood. One possibility is that immune suppression, which prolongs the presence of dead tissue and invading bacteria and viruses, could produce a greater output of cytokines, with a consequent increase in cortisol release and its destructive effects. Another possibility, as I have already suggested, is that prolonged immune suppression may give way to a rebound excessive immune response that may lead

TABLE 6.1. Autoimmune Diseases with a Prominent Pain Component and Painful Diseases with a Suspected Autoimmune Component

Autoimmune diseases with a prominent pain component	Painful diseases with a suspected autoimmune component
Autoimmune arthropathy: rheumatoid synovitis	Endometriosis
Autoimmune polyneuropathies	Fibromyalgia
Dermatomyositis	Osteoarthritis
Inflammatory bowel diseases (Crohn's disease; ulcerative colitis)	
Inflammatory myopathy	
Insulin-dependent diabetes (diabetic neuropathy and pseudo-tabes lightening pains)	
Interstitial cystitis	
Mixed connective tissue disease (polyarthritis; diffuse scleroderma; trigeminal neuropathy)	
Multiple sclerosis	
Polymyositis	
Rheumatoid arthritis	
Scleroderma	
Sjögren's syndrome	
Systemic lupus erythematosus	
Systemic sclerosis	

to autoimmune disease and chronic pain syndromes. Thorough investigation may provide valuable clues for understanding at least some of the chronic pain syndromes that perplex us and are beyond our control. For example, it is well known that estrogen promotes the release of the cytokine gamma-interferon, which in turn produces increases in cortisol output, as well as autoimmune diseases (Steinman, 1993). This may explain why more females than males suffer from most kinds of chronic pain, as well as painful autoimmune diseases such as multiple sclerosis and lupus.

In general, more women than men have autoimmune diseases and chronic pain syndromes (Table 6.2). Among the 5% of adults who suffer from an autoimmune disease, two out of three are women. Pain syndromes also show sex differences, as Berkley (1997) has argued, with the majority prevalent in women and a much smaller number prevalent in men. Of particular importance are the increases and decreases in chronic pain among women concurrently with changes in estrogen output as a function of age. The relationship between autoimmune diseases and some forms of chronic pain leads to a search for possible causes. It is well known that estrogen produces an increase in cor-

tisol levels for a brief period prior to menstruation. If this happens each month, the repetitive pattern could produce a cumulative destructive effect. Because these differences are small, they tend to be discounted, but they should not be. Abnormal patterns of cortisol release may produce myopathy, osteoporosis, neural dysfunction during aging, and autoimmune diseases (Sapolsky, 1992).

However, the role of estrogen in stress-regulation programs is obviously very complex. Estrogen has been implicated by Steinman (1993) as playing a role in several autoimmune syndromes, whereas Chrousos (1992) and Sapolsky (1992) believe that there is not sufficient free estrogen to have a significant effect on stress-dysregulation syndromes. Estrogen, in fact, presents a paradox: It increases the output of cortisol, which diminishes calcium replacement, yet estrogen replacement therapy after menopause is widely used to prevent osteoporosis. It is possible, though unlikely, that estrogen plays only a minor role in stress-related dysfunctional syndromes. It is more likely that its effects are modulated, inhibited, or facilitated by genetic determinants or other concurrently circulating hormones such as vasopressin, as well as by the levels of estrogen receptors and

TABLE 6.2. Sex Prevalence of Various Painful Disorders

Female prevalence	Male prevalence	No sex prevalence
Atypical facial pain (odontalgia) (F>>M)	Ankylosing spondylitis (9:1)	Acute herpes zoster
Burning tongue syndrome (F>M)	Cluster headache (9:1)	Chronic gastric ulcer
Chronic tension headache (1.5:1)	Hemophilic arthropathy (M>>F)	Cluster-tic syndrome
Fibromyalgia syndrome (7:1)	Postherpetic neuralgia (M>F)	Crohn's disease
Interstitial cystitis (10:1)	Posttraumatic headache (M>F)	Thoracic outlet syndrome
Irritable bowel syndrome (5:1)		
Migraine with aura (2:1)		
Migraine without aura (7:1)		
Multiple sclerosis (2:1)		
Raynaud's disease (5:1)		
Rheumatoid arthritis (F>M)		
Scleroderma (3:1)		
Systemic lupus erythematosus (9:1)		
Temporomandibular joint disorder (F>M)		
Tic douloureux (2:1)		

<table>
<tr><td colspan="2" align="center">Age-dependent sex differences</td></tr>
<tr><td>Gout (after age 60)</td><td>Erythromelalgia (over age 50)</td></tr>
<tr><td>Livedo reticularis (under age 40)</td><td>Gout (before age 60)</td></tr>
<tr><td>Osteoarthritis (after age 45)</td><td>Osteoarthritis (before age 45)</td></tr>
<tr><td>Reflex sympathetic dystrophy (under age 18 [6:1] and after age 50)</td><td></td></tr>
</table>

Note. The ratios shown in parentheses are the best estimates available in Merskey and Bogduk (1994) or Wall and Melzack (1994). The "greater than" sign (> or >>) is used when ratios are not available. Adapted from Berkley (1997). Copyright 1997 by *Behavioral and Brain Sciences.* Adapted by permission. Additional information from Merskey and Bogduk (1994).

even the patterns of change of all of these factors. It is also possible that, under some conditions, estrogen may have an inhibitory effect on the cascade of events that leads to stress-related syndromes. Clearly, this is a potentially important field for research, with many tantalizing clues.

Three additional clues reveal the relationship between stress and chronic pain. First, in addition to a higher incidence of autoimmune diseases and chronic pain syndromes, women also have a disproportionately higher incidence (3:1) of depression, which is strongly influenced by stress. Second, as we have seen, antidepressants are often highly effective for the treatment of chronic pain. Third, antidepressants act on the hippocampus, which acts as a brake on cortisol release during stress. Smith (1991) has made a strong argument that macrophages such as interleukin-1 provoke depression. Because the hippocampus plays a powerful role in the affective dimension of pain and acts as a brake on stress, the effect of antidepressants on the neural activity of the hippocampus would be expected to modify the output neurosignature pattern and influence both pain and depression.

PROGRAMS INVOLVING HOMEOSTATIC REGULATION

Pain and other stressors produce changes in every physiological activity that is under homeostatic control, such as blood pressure, blood sugar level, and body temperature. A major stressor produces marked changes in one or more of these activities, and homeostatic programs are activated to bring about a return to normal set-point levels. The relationship between pain sensitivity and several homeostatic physiological activities provides valuable evidence that the body–self neuromatrix contains programs that exert a continuous influence on pain sensitivity in order to maintain homeostatic equilibrium. At least, this is a reasonable assumption. Consider the following examples.

Hypertension and Pain

It is now well established (France & Ditto, 1996) that chronic hypertension is associated with decreased sensitivity to pain. The current explanation is that baroreceptors are stimulated by increased blood pressure to bring about a reduction in pain sensitivity. However, in place of this stimulus–

response interpretation, it is more plausible to propose a genetically determined neuroendocrine program that regulates both hypertension and pain. The decreased sensitivity to pain, I assume, decreases the possibility that severe pain will raise blood pressure to dangerous levels that threaten survival of the body-self. Hypertensive people are less sensitive to pain in a variety of experimental and clinical situations. Remarkably, even the adult children of hypertensive parents who show no signs of hypertension are also less sensitive to pain. This points to a genetically determined program that is influenced by the concurrent genetic predisposition to hypertension and its potential danger to survival. The neuroendocrine program, the evidence suggests, produces a continuously lowered sensitivity to pain.

Further evidence (reviewed by France & Ditto, 1996) supports this concept. Hypertensive people who were placed on antihypertensive medication for 3 months showed significant decreases in blood pressure but no significant change in pain sensitivity. Lowered pain sensitivity, evidently, was maintained by a mechanism independently from the hypertension, although the strong link between the two has been confirmed by a large number of excellent studies. Interestingly, specially bred hypertensive rats also show, as early as 3 weeks of age, a decreased sensitivity to pain that precedes the later development of elevated blood pressure. It is reasonable, then, to propose a genetic mechanism for a neuroendocrine program that anticipates the development of hypertension and maintains a decreased sensitivity to pain in order to prevent bombardment of the brain when injury occurs, thus diminishing pain, stress, and a consequent reflex increase in blood pressure.

Blood Sugar Levels and Pain

Remarkably, lower pain sensitivity is also found in patients with anorexia nervosa and bulimia nervosa and in subjects who restrain their food intake (Lautenbacher, Pauls, Strian, Pirke, & Krieg, 1990; Krieg, Roscher, Strian, Pirke, & Lautenbacher, 1993; Faris et al., 1992). The reduction in sensitivity to heat pain and pressure pain is assumed to be due to an increase in blood sugar and appears to occur after acute rather than persistent episodes of diminished food intake and hypoglycemia (Krieg et al., 1993). Reduced pain sensitivity did not occur after a 3-week diet period, even though the diet resulted in substantial weight loss

(Lautenbacher et al., 1991). In contrast, participants—diabetic or nondiabetic—who receive transfusions of glucose show an increased sensitivity to pain (Morley, Mooradian, Levine, & Morley, 1984). Similar increased pain sensitivity was found in diabetic patients (Morley et al., 1984) and diabetic rats (Lee & McCarthy, 1992). Thye-Rønn et al. (1994) administered transfusions of glucose in a double-blind study and confirmed that there is a significant increase in sensitivity to pressure pain. Interestingly, diabetics who also had high blood pressure showed lower pain sensitivity than diabetics without hypertension, suggesting that the high blood pressure decreases the tendency by diabetics to show increased sensitivity to pain.

Why should there be a relationship between blood sugar levels and sensitivity to pain? It is conceivable that metabolic programs in the homeostatic regulation system have evolved so that, in conditions of low blood sugar availability, the sensory gates to noxious stimuli are relatively closed, decreasing perceived pain, stress, and metabolic demands. However, the programs act rapidly to reinstate normal pain sensitivity when homeostasis is achieved. It is interesting that the neural program permits hyperglycemia to increase pain sensitivity above normal baseline levels, so that after eating, when blood sugar levels are elevated, the organism is more likely to be activated by injury, thereby counteracting the tendency to drowsiness and loss of alertness that often occur after eating.

Brain Temperature and Pain

A major aim of homeostatic programs after moderate to severe injury is to prevent large increases in brain metabolism and the consequent rise in brain temperature produced by injury from reaching dangerous levels. It is a fact that a rise in brain temperature of a few degrees produces convulsions, and a few degrees more results in death. To achieve the goal of maintaining brain temperature within a narrow range, a number of strategies are available to the brain: (1) decrease of brain activity by direct neural inhibition or by the local constriction of blood vessels; (2) dilation of blood vessels in the brain to increase blood flow to remove the heat produced by brain metabolism; (3) decrease of blood flow to sensory nerves (which may destroy them); and (4) the destruction of transmitting nerve cells (apoptosis) by commands from program centers.

Inhibition of activity in widespread areas of the brain, including portions of the visual system,

may be induced by cutaneous stimulation (such as rubbing the skin) under particular conditions (light anesthesia) (Melzack & Casey, 1967; Melzack, Konrad, & Dubrovsky, 1968, 1969). The mechanisms that underlie this inhibition are not known. The large decrease (and occasional increase) in metabolic activity reflect both neural metabolic changes and blood flow. The inhibition, moreover, may persist for long durations after brief periods of stimulation. The brain, therefore, possesses a system capable of exerting strong widespread inhibition that is normally held under control but is available as a program to modulate brain metabolism.

Recent evidence using elegant brain imaging techniques supports the concept of inhibition of brain metabolism during pain. Jones and his colleagues (Di Piero et al., 1991) found that patients with severe, persistent pain due to cancer showed a significantly *lower* level of blood flow in the thalamus compared to pain-free control subjects. Even more impressive is the fact that a cordotomy (which cuts the sensory pathways from the cancerous areas to the thalamus) produced relief of pain and a striking *increase* in blood flow to the thalamus until local temperatures reached normal levels. A further recent study (Canavero et al., 1993) found that two patients with central pain syndromes showed a decrease of blood flow in the parietal lobe, with still further decreases after nonpainful stimulation. These results provide powerful evidence that pain is associated with a homeostatic *decrease* in blood flow in a major sensory transmission relay, which returns to normal, higher levels when pain is relieved. This may seem anomalous, but it is consistent with the idea of long-term homeostatic programs that prevent an excessive increase in brain temperature.

The dilation or constriction of blood vessels to the brain is a well-known accompaniment of the sequence of events that occurs during most migraines. Migraines are subjectively undesirable but represent a powerful program by which the brain, because of a perceived threat, can diminish activity in a large part of the brain and, by inducing pain, can force the organism to rest and decrease all inputs to the brain.

The possible strategy of prolonged, reduced blood flow to nerves and apoptosis ("suicide") of neurons in response to the anticipated danger of a rise in brain temperature may seem drastic, but it is a reasonable strategy for coping with a perceived threat of a prolonged rise in brain temperature that could eventually produce convulsions and incapacitate an animal seeking to escape a deadly predator. Apoptosis of neurons could occur at any level—in the brain itself, in the cord, and in peripheral nerves. It could explain spontaneous neuropathies (as a program gone wrong) or diabetic or other neuropathies related to conditions involving abnormal stimulation of peripheral nerves. For example, because the lower limbs in diabetics may develop circulation problems that would produce massive input and pain, the brain may activate an anticipatory program to destroy the potentially offending nerves by restricting blood flow to them or by apoptosis. Misinformation, misinterpretation of information, or misresponse to information could all lead to inappropriate spontaneous neuropathy. Apoptosis, in this case, is akin to the immune system behaving inappropriately and producing some of the autoimmune diseases.

IMPLICATIONS OF STRESS REGULATION

By unifying the perceptual and stress systems involved in pain, we immediately expand our available knowledge related to pain and open the door to new therapies. Our present understanding of receptor and spinal mechanisms, which is the basis of the gate control theory of pain (see Melzack & Wall, 1996) and its more recent extensions (Melzack, 1971; Melzack & Casey, 1968), is not diminished. Rather, the data and the gate control theory now fit into the broader framework of the neuromatrix theory of pain.

Unity of Perceptual and Stress Mechanisms of Pain

The intimate relationship between the perceptual and stress systems is not surprising. The limbic system, which receives the projections of the medial sensory transmission pathways, is the neural substrate of the affective–motivational dimension of pain (Dennis & Melzack, 1977; Melzack & Casey, 1968), and a portion of the system, including the hypothalamus, is an integral part of the stress system. The two systems are so interdependent that they should be considered as components of a single system (Figure 6.2). This close relationship is further indicated by observations that pain exhibited by rats in the formalin test is abolished by a lesion of the medial projection system at the level of the thalamus but is unaffected by a lesion of the lateral sys-

tem at the same level (McKenna & Melzack, 1994). The lateral system has the important role of conveying precise information to the body–self neuromatrix and generates the information needed for the localization and evaluation of the input. Both kinds of information are projected to the limbic system, which is prepared to generate the affective–motivational response to perceived injury and stress. We now have a new conceptual model of the brain in which limbic structures, the cerebral cortex, and all major components of the stress system play key roles. The new concept has important implications for the study of pain.

Rationale of Pain Therapies

First, let us look at therapies that make sense within the framework of the new concept. For example, tricyclic antidepressant drugs relieve some forms of chronic pain even though the pain is not caused by depression. However, cytokines, particularly interleukin-1, alpha-interferon, and tumor necrosis factor, have been shown to produce the symptoms of major depression (see Smith, 1991), and they also activate the stress system, which may produce the basis for chronic pain syndromes. Conceivably, antidepressants may act on hormones and neurotransmitters, such as noradrenalin and serotonin, that play a role in both depression and pain. Smith (1991) also notes that major depression is as much as two to three times more common among women than men. Moreover, estrogen increases the production of cytokines, which produce an almost fourfold increase in cortisol production. Rheumatoid arthritis, which is associated with dysregulation of cortisol output, also has a female:male ratio in young adults of 5:1. After age 60, this ratio drops to 2:1, and major depression also drops dramatically in women after age 65 (from 5.8% in women aged 18–44 to 1.6% in women over 65). Because migraine, lupus, and a variety of stress- and immune-system diseases also show female:male ratios that range from 2:1 to 9:1, it is reasonable to assume that a large number of chronic pain syndromes, as well as depression, are linked to the stress regulation systems.

A variety of well-known facts that had no place in the Cartesian paradigm now have plausible, meaningful roles. For example, the high rate of pain relief after lesions of the pituitary in cancer patients now becomes comprehensible (Miles, 1994), because the pituitary is a major link in the HPA system. This dramatic relief is reported by patients

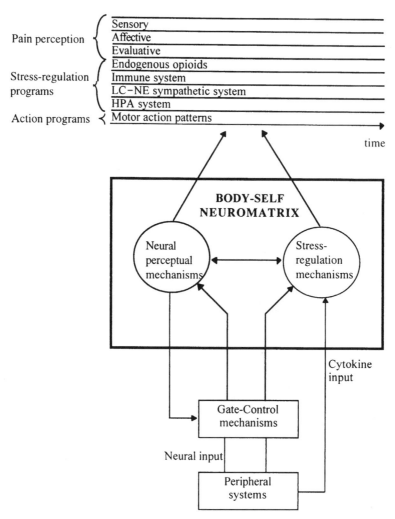

FIGURE 6.2. Components of the neuromatrix theory of pain. The body–self neuromatrix comprises (1) neural perceptual mechanisms and (2) the stress-regulation system. Neural perceptual mechanisms incorporate the mechanisms of the gate control theory (see Melzack & Wall, 1996), as well as the conceptual model of parallel distributed processing systems described by Melzack and Casey (1968). The stress system comprises the component systems and their interactions shown schematically in Figures 6.1 and 6.2. Both parts—perceptual and stress systems—produce actions and perceptions that persist in time and are shown as a vivigram of the components of the action systems. Also shown is the perceptual experience produced concomitantly with the action system activities by the output neurosignature patterns generated by the body–self neuromatrix. The influences of other sensory and cognitive processes on the generation of the neurosignature are not shown.

with hormone-related cancers but also occurs in a variety of non-hormone-related chronic pains. Lesions of the hypothalamus can also produce relief of some kinds of chronic pain (Bouckoms, 1994). Even the excellent pain-relieving effects of lesions of the cingulate cortex and cingulum bundle (Bouckoms, 1994) become comprehensible in view of their strategic location as part of the limbic system and, therefore, of the stress/immune systems.

The neuromatrix theory of pain also fits with observations that a program involving steroid injections can have powerful pain-relieving effects (Kozin, McCarty, Sims, & Genant, 1976; Kozin, Ryan, Carerra, Soin, & Wortmann, 1981). These effects cannot be attributed simply to the local control of inflammation. Steroid injections for reflex sympathetic dystrophy (RSD) can have very dramatic effects, revealing mechanisms that must involve widespread neural, adrenergic, and hormonal mechanisms. The effects of steroids on rheumatoid arthritis may be explained in terms of the dysfunctional HPA system in these patients. But the excellent effects of steroids on RSD cannot be so easily explained. Steroids are potentially dangerous substances, yet they can dramatically relieve pain. Conceivably, as we learn more about augmenting steroids with other substances that are part of the whole stress system, we will learn to do even better. This approach toward controlling the stress system has, I believe, tremendous potential. There is, to be sure, the complexity of the inhibitory, excitatory, and modulatory interactions. But research will undoubtedly reveal them, and our armamentarium for pain therapy will be greatly enriched.

Genetic Determinants of Chronic Pain

Genetic predisposition may contribute to the development of chronic pain syndromes or other illnesses that have a prominent pain component. In the case of multiple sclerosis, for example, a genetic factor appears to be involved (Steinman, 1993): If one member of a set of monozygotic twins has multiple sclerosis, there is one chance in three that the other twin will also develop it. Table 6.3 lists several pain syndromes which may have a genetic contribution.

Genes and sensory inputs may both play synergistic roles in determining the development of a chronic pain syndrome. Consider the following study: Mayeux et al. (1995) and Mayeux (1996) examined the risk of developing Alzheimer's disease in elderly people who had sustained a head injury and possessed the gene known as apolipoprotein-epsilon 4. They found that a tenfold increase in the risk of Alzheimer's disease was associated with both apolipoprotein-epsilon 4 and a history of traumatic head injury, compared with a twofold increase in risk with apolipoprotein-epsilon 4 alone. Head injury in the absence of an apolipoprotein-epsilon 4 allele did not increase risk. These data imply that the biological effects of head injury may increase the risk of Alzheimer's disease but only through a synergistic relationship with apolipoprotein-epsilon 4. In other words, after a physical head injury, the gene may turn a normal repair process into a step toward disease of far greater complexity.

It is reasonable to suspect a similar synergistic relationship between other genes and physical injuries or illnesses as a causal factor in some chronic pain syndromes. For example, multiple sclerosis—which has a prominent pain component—has been shown to have a genetic contribution and often appears a few weeks after a routine illness. These combinations merit further investigation in the attempt to understand chronic pain syndromes. Many syndromes, such as reflex sympathetic dystrophy, causalgia, postherpetic neuralgia, or diabetic peripheral neuropathy, develop in some people and not others, even though the nerve injury is apparently the same in both groups. Why should two people receive virtually identical gunshot wounds, yet one develops horrible, persistent burning pain and the other heals without any subsequent pain? Or why should two people have the same degree of diabetes, yet one person develops peripheral neuropathy and the other does not? Conceivably, a genetic predisposition exerts a synergistic effect together with sensory input following an injury. This hypothesis is highly speculative but merits consideration.

Psychological Contributions to Pain

The place of psychological factors in producing pain and relieving it is clear. Cortisol is released by either psychological stress or physical injury, and Sapolsky (1992) has proposed that the cumulative release of pulses of cortisol is a major determinant of pathology. All psychological stresses may contribute to the neuroendocrine processes that give rise to pain syndromes, and psychological therapies that control stress ultimately affect cortisol release and, therefore, influence the development of chronic pain. A decrease in cortisol output by psychological therapy may not by itself be sufficient to produce a major reduction in pain, but it should be part of multiple therapies that can have additive effects in decreasing the destructive effects of cortisol.

Each kind of stressor can produce physiological effects that are additive with the effects of other stressors. The patterns of stress responses, moreover, may vary for each (Sapolsky, 1992). It is important, therefore, in the context of injury and pain, to recognize that the stress effects of an injury can vary, in severity and pattern, as a function of other stresses, such as loss of self-esteem, employment, or other security symbols.

Individual variation in response to injury or other stresses may be influenced by the enhancement of a given stress by (1) other concurrent stress, (2) the cumulative effect of prior stresses (determined partly by their pattern of appearance),

TABLE 6.3. Pain Syndromes That May Have a Genetic Contribution

Clinical syndrome	Proposed mechanism
Ankylosing spondylitis (Calin & Elswood, 1989; Strosberg, Allen, Calabro, & Harris, 1975)	Familial genetic predisposition. HLA genotype is implicated, and teenagers develop back pain.
Ankylosing spondylitis and coexisting rheumatoid arthritis (Tan, Caughey, & Jugusch, 1983)	Both diseases were found in a patient who had the associated HLA genes.
Back pain (Bengtsson & Thorson, 1991)	In a monozygotic and dizygotic twin study, twin concordance regarding back pain is considerably higher in MZ than DZ twins.
Congenital insensitivity to pain (Landrieu, Said & Allaire, 1990; Larner, Moss, Rossi, & Anderson, 1994)	Inherited abnormalities of peripheral sensory nerves, autonomic nervous system, and/or central nervous system
Degenerative disk disease (Simmons, Guntupalli, Kovalski, Braun, & Seidel, 1996)	Familial predisposition compared to controls; family history: 44.6% versus 25.4%; spinal surgery: 18.5% versus 4.5%
Diskogenic low back pain (Postacchini, Lami, & Pugliese, 1988)	Strong familial predisposition suggests genetic and environmental factors.
Herniation of a lumbar disk in patients younger than 21 years old (Varlotta, Brown, Kelsey, & Golden, 1991)	32% had a positive family history compared with 7% in the control group.
Familial amyloidotic polyneuropathy (Fujitake, Horii, Tatsuoka, Funauchi, & Saida, 1991)	Familial genetic predisposition
Familial coinciding trigeminal and glossopharyngeal neuralgia (Knuckey & Gubbay, 1979)	Familial genetic predisposition
Familial myalgia and cramps (Gospe et al., 1989; Lazaro, Rollinson, & Fenichel, 1981)	Autosomal dominant inheritance
Familial rheumatoid arthritis (Wolfe, Kleinhekel, & Khan, 1988)	Familial genetic predisposition
Familial spinal canal stenosis (Yasuda et al., 1986)	Autosomal dominant disorder
Familial trigeminal neuralgia (Kirkpatrick, 1989)	Family of three nontwin sisters with middle-age onset of classic, severe trigeminal neuralgia
Familial visceral myopathy (Rodrigues, Shepherd, Lennard-Jones, Hawley, & Thompson, 1989)	Autosomal dominant mode of inheritance
Fibromyalgia (Neeck & Riedel, 1994)	Malfunctioning muscle metabolism; defective absorption of tryptophan from the gut, producing decreased serotonin, thereby dysregulating sleep and sensory neural transmission
Hereditary neuralgic amyotrophy (Arts et al., 1983)	Four-generation family is described.
Hereditary sensory neuropathy with neurotrophic keratitis (Donaghy et al., 1987)	Autosomal recessive disorder; loss of small myelinated fibers
Hereditary sensory radicular neuropathy (Shahriaree, Kotcamp, Sheikh, & Sajadi, 1979)	Autosomal dominant
Hereditary spastic paraplegia (Schady & Sheard, 1990; Serena, Rizzuto, Moretto, & Arrigoni, 1990)	Found in 23 patients in 14 families
Migraine (Stewart, Lipton, & Liberman, 1996)	Prevalence differences in Caucasian, African, and Asian women (20.4%; 16.2%; 9.2%) and men (8.6%; 7.2%; 4.2%). Race-related differences in genetic vulnerability.
Multiple sclerosis (Steinman, 1993)	If multiple sclerosis is diagnosed in one monozygotic twin, the other twin has one chance in three of also developing multiple sclerosis.
Osteoarthritis (Hochberg, 1991)	Hereditary defects in type II collagen predispose to early osteoarthritis.

(cont.)

TABLE 6.3. (*cont.*)

Clinical syndrome	Proposed mechanism
Osteoarthritis in women (Spector, Cicuttini, Baker, Loughlin, & Hart, 1996)	Twin study: genetic influence ranging from 39–65%
Primary dysmenorrhea (Silberg, Martin, & Heath, 1987)	Monozygotic and dizygotic twin study; evidence of genes affecting flow and pain
Reflex sympathetic dystrophy (pilot study) (Mailis & Wade, 1994)	Twofold increase in human lymphocyte antigen; is associated with chromosome 6
Sickle cell disease (Gil et al., 1995)	Genetically determined
Rat model of neuropathic pain, revealing genetic determinants (Devor & Raber, 1990; Inbal, Devor, Tuchendler, & Lieblich, 1980)	Different strains of rat show differences in autotomy after denervation of a paw.

Note. This list is tentative due to the small number of studies and the need for replication. Moreover, the extent of the genetic contribution requires further research. Because this field is relatively new, some of the clinical diagnoses and nomenclature overlap, and some have been found in only a single family or even in a single generation. Nevertheless, the studies listed in the table strongly suggest that there is a genetic contribution to several major chronic pain syndromes or diseases with a prominent pain component.

(3) the kinds of concurrent or prior stresses—that is, psychological or physical, and (4) the severity and duration of the stresses.

It is well known that adaptation to repetitive stressors often occurs, so that chronic or repeated stress is frequently associated with normal circulating levels of ACTH and corticosterone (the rat's equivalent of cortisol). There is convincing evidence, however, that the system may become more sensitive to other types of acute stressors during this period. The pituitaries of chronically stressed animals become hypersensitive to the effects of vasopressin, which is an important regulator of pituitary responsiveness to stress (Harbuz & Lightman, 1992).

Studies with animal subjects throw light on these additive effects. Meaney and his colleagues (1993) demonstrated the effects of prenatal stress on HPA function in the adult. Pregnant female rats were subjected to the stress of physical restraint during the third trimester of pregnancy, and the offspring were studied when they were fully mature adults. Interestingly, the effects of prenatal stress were pronounced in female offspring but not in males. The females showed sharply enhanced responses to stress. Similarly, prenatal alcohol intake by the mothers resulted in increased HPA responses to stress in female offspring but not in males. These investigators also found that handling or "gentling" in early postnatal life produced substantial decreases in the response to stress at maturity—a positive effect that occurred in males as well as females. Meaney and his colleagues (1993, p. 83) conclude that "the early environment is able to 'fine-tune' the sensitivity and effi-ciency of certain neuroendocrine systems that mediate the animal's response to stimuli that threaten homeostasis."

The neuromatrix theory, therefore, provides a reasonable mechanism whereby psychological stresses may provide the basis for chronic pain. Stressors have destructive effects on muscle, skeletal, and hippocampal neural tissue, which may become the immediate basis of pain or provide a basis for the devastating effects of later minor injuries in which the severity of pain is disproportionately far greater than would be expected from the injury.

It is possible that psychological stress alone can become a cause of chronic pain because it produces substances that have destructive effects on body tissues. Prolonged stressful events, it is now evident, can leave a memory etched into bone, muscle, and nerve tissue, just as an injury sculpts a neuronal pattern into the neuromatrix. Stress, however, is a subjective experience. Threatening sensory or cognitive events may or may not be perceived as stressors, just as the sensory input from an injury may or may not be perceived as pain. Even when pain is experienced, it may be a stressor if it implies danger and threat to survival of the self, physically or psychologically. In contrast, a major injury may evoke little or no stress if it is perceived as a successful escape from danger, such as a battlefield.

Reflex Sympathetic Dystrophy

The neuromatrix theory of pain also has implications for understanding the origins of reflex sympathetic dystrophy (RSD). It has long been assumed that RSD is primarily a disease of over-stimulation of the sympathetic nervous system. However, it is possible that after a period of time the HPA axis takes over and that the destructive signs observed after several months are the result of dysregulation of the cortisol system rather than the noradrenergic system. This could explain the observation (Hannington-Kiff, 1994) that sympathetic blocks may prevent RSD if administered early in the disease but not if given after the signs are well under way.

Hannington-Kiff (1994) has observed that the "early," mainly autonomic, features are usually clinically obvious by about 3–6 weeks after a minor injury. After this time, major dystrophic changes occur in the skin and nails, with muscle and joint stiffness, skin swelling, excessive heat and sweating, abnormal blood flow and skin color, and abnormal skin sensitivity and pain. At this stage, treatment with sympathetic blocks is rarely effective. The reason may be that the HPA axis has superseded the sympathetic system and now dominates the stress response to the injury that initiated the cascade of events. For this reason, it is possible that psychological stress and stressful events at earlier stages in life contributed to the sequence of events. Current stress also aggravates the course of the disease. This does not mean that RSD is due to "psychogenic" causes. Rather, it may be a stress-related disease, in which all types of stress produce cumulative actions and in which the HPA axis and the destructive effects of cortisol predominate.

These considerations suggest lines of therapy for RSD that differ from those now generally in use. Decreases in stress and manipulation of the HPA component of the stress system are likelier to produce pain relief for these people who suffer so terribly. Kozin (1993) has achieved generally excellent results with RSD patients by using steroid injection therapy, and he notes wistfully that "unlike the interruption of sympathetic pathways, no currently known theoretic mechanisms explain the efficacy of corticosteroids in RSD" (1993, p. 1670). The powerful role of the stress system in chronic pain provides a plausible mechanism.

Predictors of Chronic Pain

A further important feature of chronic pain that implicates the stress system is the fact that the severity of pain during an injury or infection is a major predictor of the occurrence of subsequent persistent pain. Dworkin and Portenoy (1996) have identified six factors that predict those patients with shingles (herpes zoster) who are most likely to develop chronic pain (postherpetic neuralgia) that persists long after the infection has healed. The predictors are: more severe pain during the initial acute stage, greater severity of the infection of the nerve and its effects on the adjacent skin, greater sensory dysfunction of the affected dermatome, greater magnitude and duration of the humoral and immune response during the acute stage, pain in the dermatome before the appearance of the rash (painful prodrome), and fever greater than 38°C during the acute stage. Clearly, these factors include signs of activity of the stress system in addition to the greater pain, which is itself a stressor.

Further evidence of acute pain intensity as a predictor of later persistent pain is the observation by Malenfant et al. (1996) that patients with severe burns who suffer the most intense pain in the initial stages of recovery and healing are the ones most likely to have persistent pain that continues for years after full healing has occurred. Finally, Katz, Jackson, Kavanagh, and Sandler (1996) found that patients with intense pain during the first 2 days after a chest operation (thoracotomy) are much more likely to report persistent chest pain 1½ years after the operation than patients who were pain-free after the operation. Katz concludes that aggressive management of early postoperative pain may reduce the likelihood of long-term post-thoracotomy pain. It is evident, then, that severe pain, which is a powerful stressor, is a major determinant of chronic pain that remains after healing has occurred when there are no obvious physical causes of the severe pain suffered by the patients. The initial pain and stress, it is reasonable to assume, produced changes in both the perceptual and stress systems that contributed to the abnormal output patterns of the body–self neuromatrix.

SUMMARY

In summary, the neuromatrix theory of pain proposes that the neurosignature for pain experience is determined by the synaptic architecture of the neuromatrix, which is produced by genetic and sensory influences. The neurosignature pattern is also modulated by sensory inputs and by cognitive events, such as psychological stress. It may also occur because stressors, physical as well as psychological, act on stress-regulation systems, which may produce lesions of muscle, bone, and nerve tissue, thereby contributing to the neurosignature patterns that give rise to chronic pain. In short, the neuromatrix, as a result of homeostasis-regulation patterns that have failed, produces the destructive conditions that may give rise to many of the chronic pains that so far have been resistant to treatments developed primarily to manage pains that are triggered by sensory inputs. The stress regulation system, with its complex, delicately balanced interactions, is an integral part of the multiple contributions that give rise to chronic pain.

The neuromatrix theory guides us away from the Cartesian concept of pain as a sensation produced by injury, inflammation, or other tissue pathology and toward the concept of pain as a multidimensional experience produced by multiple influences. These influences range from the existing synaptic architecture of the neuromatrix—which is determined by genetic and sensory factors—to influences from within the body and from other areas in the brain. Genetic influences on synaptic architecture may determine—or predispose toward—the development of chronic pain syndromes. Figure 6.3 summarizes the factors that contribute to the output pattern from the neuromatrix that produce the sensory, affective, and cognitive dimensions of pain experience and behavior. We have traveled a long way from the psychophysical concept that seeks a simple one-to-one relationship between injury and pain. We now have a theoreti-

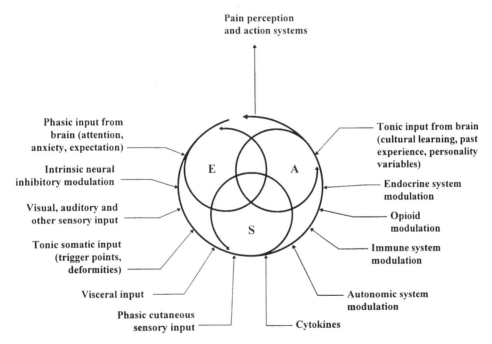

FIGURE 6.3. The body–self neuromatrix. The body–self neuromatrix, which comprises a widely distributed neural network that includes somatosensory, limbic, and thalamocortical components, is schematically depicted as a circle containing smaller parallel networks that contribute to the sensory-discriminative (S), affective-motivational (A), and evaluative-cognitive (E) dimensions of pain experience. The synaptic architecture of the neuromatrix is determined by genetic and sensory influences. The "neurosignature" output of the neuromatrix—patterns of nerve impulses of varying temporal and spatial dimensions—is produced by neural programs genetically built into the neuromatrix and determines the particular qualities and other properties of the pain experience and behavior. Multiple inputs that act on the neuromatrix programs and contribute to the output neurosignature include (1) sensory inputs from somatic receptors (phasic cutaneous, visceral, and tonic somatic inputs); (2) visual and other sensory inputs that influence the cognitive interpretation of the situation; (3) phasic and tonic cognitive and emotional inputs from other areas of the brain; (4) intrinsic neural inhibitory modulation inherent in all brain function; and (5) the activity of the body's stress-regulation systems, including cytokines as well as the endocrine, autonomic, immune, and opioid systems.

cal framework in which a template for the body-self is modulated by the powerful stress system and the cognitive functions of the brain, in addition to the traditional sensory inputs.

The neuromatrix theory of pain—which places genetic contributions and the neural–hormonal mechanisms of stress on a level of equal importance with the neural mechanisms of sensory transmission—has important implications for research and therapy. Some of these have been sketched out here. Others will become evident to endocrinologists and immunologists and, perhaps, to pain specialists with a knowledge of the field of stress. An immediate recommendation is that interdisciplinary pain clinics should expand to include specialists in endocrinology and immunology. Such a collaboration may lead to insights and new research strategies that may reveal the underlying mechanisms of chronic pain and give rise to new therapies to relieve the tragedy of unrelenting suffering.

ACKNOWLEDGMENTS

This study was supported by Grant No. A7891 from the Natural Sciences and Research Council of Canada. I am grateful to Dr. Kirk Osterland for his generous help in developing Table 6.2 and to Dr. Lucy Gagliese, Dr. Ann Gamsa, and Dr. Geoffrey Schultz for their valuable suggestions. Portions of this chapter are derived from a chapter in a forthcoming book.

REFERENCES

Arts, W. F., Busch, H. F., Van den Brand, H. J., Jennekens, F. G., Frants, R. R., & Stefanko, S. Z. (1983). Hereditary neuralgic amyotrophy: Clinical, genetic, electrophysiological and histopathological studies. *Journal of the Neurological Sciences, 62*, 261–279.

Bengtsson, B., & Thorson, J. (1991). Back pain: A study of twins. *Acta Geneticae Medicae et Gemellologiae, 40*, 83–90.

Berkley, K. J. (1997). Sex differences in pain. *Behavioral and Brain Sciences, 20*, 1–10.

Bouckoms, A. J. (1994). Limbic surgery for pain. In P. D. Wall & R. Melzack (Eds.), *Textbook of pain* (3rd ed., pp. 1171–1187). Edinburgh: Churchill Livingstone.

Calin, A., & Elswood, J. (1989). Relative role of genetic and environmental factors in disease expression: Sib pair analysis in ankylosing spondylitis. *Arthritis and Rheumatism, 32*, 77–81.

Canavero, S., Pagni, C. A., Castellano, G., Bonicalzi, V., Bello, M., Duca, S., & Podio, V. (1993). The role of cortex in central pain syndromes: Preliminary results of a long-term technetium-99 hexamethylpropylene-

amineoxine single photon emission computed tomography study. *Neurosurgery, 32*, 185–207.

Chrousos, G. P. (1992). Regulation and dysregulation of the hypothalamic–pituitary–adrenal axis. *Endocrinology and Metabolism Clinics of North America, 21*, 833–858.

Chrousos, G. P., & Gold, P. W. (1992). The concepts of stress and stress system disorders. *Journal of the American Medical Association, 267*, 1244–1252.

Dennis, S. G., & Melzack, R. (1977). Pain-signalling systems in the dorsal and ventral spinal cord. *Pain, 4*, 97–132.

Devor, M., & Raber, P. (1990). Heritability of symptoms in an experimental model of neuropathic pain. *Pain, 42*, 51–67.

Di Piero, V., Jones, A. K. P., Iannotti, F., Powell, M., Perani, D., Lenzi, G. K., & Frackowiak, R. S. J. (1991). Chronic pain: A PET study of the central effects of percutaneous high cervical cordotomy. *Pain, 46*, 9–12.

Donaghy, M., Hakin, R. N., Bamford, J. M., Garner, A., Kirby, G. R., Noble, B. A., Tazir-Melboucy, M., King, R. H. M., & Thomas, P. K. (1987). Hereditary sensory neuropathy with neurotrophic keratitis. *Brain, 110*, 563–583.

Dworkin, R. H., & Portenoy, R. K. (1996). Pain and its persistence in herpes zoster. *Pain, 67*, 241–251.

Faris, P. L., Raymond, N. C., De Zwaan, M., Howard, L. A., Eckert, E. D., & Mitchell, J. E. (1992). Nociceptive, but not tactile, thresholds are evaluated in bulimia nervosa. *Biological Psychiatry, 32*, 462–466.

France, C. R., & Ditto, B. (1996). Risk for high blood pressure and decreased pain perception. *Current Directions in Psychological Science, 5*, 120–125.

Fuchs, P. N., Kerr, B., & Melzack, R. (1996). Delayed nociceptive response following cold-water swim in the formalin test: Possible mechanisms of action. *Experimental Neurology, 139*, 291–298.

Fuchs, P. N., & Melzack, R. (1996). Restraint reduces formalin-test pain but the effect is not influenced by lesions of the hypothalamic paraventricular nucleus. *Experimental Neurology, 139*, 299–305.

Fuchs, P. N., & Melzack, R. (1997). Repeated cold water swim produces delayed nociceptive responses, but not analgesia, for tonic pain in the rat. *Experimental Neurology, 145*, 303–307.

Fujitake, J., Horii, K., Tatsuoka, Y., Funauchi, M., & Saida, K. (1991). Two brother cases of late-onset familial amyloidotic polyneuropathy in Kyoto [in Japanese]. *Rinsho Shinkeygaku [Clinical Neurology], 31*, 184–190.

Gil, K. M., Phillips, G., Webster, D. A., Martin, N. J., Abrams, M., Grant, M., Clark, W. C., & Janal, M. N. (1995). Experimental pain sensitivity and reports of negative thoughts in adults with sickle cell disease. *Behavior Therapy, 26*, 273–293.

Gospe, S. M., Lazaro, R. P., Lava, N. S., Grootscholten, P. M., Scott, M. O., & Fischbeck, K. H. (1989). Familial X-linked myalgia and cramps: A nonprogressive myopathy associated with a deletion in the dystrophin gene. *Neurology, 39*, 1277–1280.

Hannington-Kiff, J. G. (1994). Sympathetic nerve blocks in painful limb disorders. In P. D. Wall & R. Melzack (Eds.), *Textbook of pain* (3rd ed., pp. 1035–1052). Edinburgh: Churchill Livingstone.

Harbuz, M. S., & Lightman, S. L. (1992). Stress and the hypothalamo–pituitary–adrenal axis: Acute, chronic and immunological activation. *Journal of Endocrinology, 134,* 327–339.

Hochberg, M. C. (1991). Epidemiology and genetics of osteoarthritis. *Current Opinion in Rheumatology, 3,* 662–668.

Inbal, R., Devor, M., Tuchendler, O., & Lieblich, I. (1980). Autotomy following nerve injury: Genetic factors in the development of chronic pain. *Pain, 9,* 327–337.

Jayson, M. I. V., & Freemont, A. J. (1995). The role of vascular damage in the development of nerve root problems. In R. M. Aspden & R. W. Porter (Eds.), *Lumbar spine disorders: Current concepts* (pp. 132–144). River Edge, NJ: World Scientific.

Katz, J., Jackson, M., Kavanagh, B. P., & Sandler, A. N. (1996). Acute pain after thoracic surgery predicts long-term post-thoracotomy pain. *Clinical Journal of Pain, 12,* 50–55.

Kirkpatrick, D. B. (1989). Familial trigeminal neuralgia: Case report. *Neurosurgery, 24,* 758–761.

Knuckey, N. W., & Gubbay, S. S. (1979). Familial trigeminal and glossopharyngeal neuralgia. *Clinical and Experimental Neurology, 16,* 315–319.

Kozin, F. (1993). Painful shoulder and reflex sympathetic dystrophy syndrome. In D. J. McCarty & W. J. Koopman (Eds.), *Arthritis and allied conditions* (12th ed., pp. 1643–1676). Philadelphia: Lea and Febiger.

Kozin, F., McCarty, D. J., Sims, J., & Genant, H. (1976). The reflex sympathetic dystrophy syndrome: I. Clinical and histological studies: Evidence for bilaterality, response to corticosteroids and articular involvement. *American Journal of Medicine, 60,* 321–331.

Kozin, F., Ryan, L. M., Carerra, G. F., Soin, J. S., & Wortmann, R. L. (1981). The reflex sympathetic dystrophy syndrome (RSDS): III. Scintigraphic studies, further evidence for the therapeutic efficacy of systemic corticosteroids, and proposed diagnostic criteria. *American Journal of Medicine, 70,* 23–30.

Krieg, J.-C., Roscher, S., Strian, F., Pirke, K.-M., & Lautenbacher, S. (1993). Pain sensitivity in recovered anorexics, restrained and unrestrained eaters. *Journal of Psychosomatic Research, 37,* 595–602.

Landrieu, P., Said, G., & Allaire, C. (1990). Dominantly transmitted congenital indifference to pain. *Annals of Neurology, 27,* 574–578.

Lariviere, W. R., Fuchs, P. N., & Melzack, R. (1995). Hypophysectomy produces analgesia and paraventricular lesions have no effect on formalin-induced pain. *Experimental Neurology, 135,* 74–79.

Larner, A. J., Moss, J., Rossi, M. L., & Anderson, M. (1994). Congenital insensitivity to pain: A 20-year follow up. *Journal of Neurology, Neurosurgery and Psychiatry, 57,* 973–974.

Lautenbacher, S., Barth, K., Freiss, E., Strian, F., Pirke, K.-M., & Krieg, J.-C. (1991). Dieting and pain sensitivity: A validation of clinical findings. *Physiology and Behavior, 50,* 629–631.

Lautenbacher, S., Pauls, A. M., Strian, F., Pirke, K.-M., & Krieg, J.-C. (1990). Pain perception in patients with eating disorders. *Psychosomatic Medicine, 52,* 673–682.

Lazaro, R. P., Rollinson, R. D., & Fenichel, G. M. (1981). Familial cramps and muscle pain. *Archives of Neurology, 38,* 22–24.

Lee, J. H., & McCarthy, R. (1992). Pain thresholds in diabetic rats: Effects of good versus poor metabolic control. *Pain, 50,* 231–236.

Mailis, A., & Wade, J. (1994). Profile of Caucasian women with possible genetic predisposition to reflex sympathetic dystrophy: A pilot study. *Clinical Journal of Pain, 10,* 210–217.

Malenfant, A., Forget, R., Papillon, R., Amsel, R., Frigon, J.-Y., & Choinière, M. (1996). Prevalence and characteristics of chronic sensory problems in burn patients. *Pain, 67,* 493–500.

Mayeux, R. (1996). Reply from the author. *Neurology, 45,* 891–892.

Mayeux, R., Ottman, R., Maestre, G., Ngai, C., Tang, M. X., Ginsberg, H., Chun, M., Tycko, B., & Shelanski, M. (1995). Synergistic effects of traumatic head injury and apolipoprotein-epsilon 4 in patients with Alzheimer's disease. *Neurology, 45,* 555–557.

McKenna, J. E., & Melzack, R. (1994). Dissociable effects of lidocaine injection into medial versus lateral thalamus in tail-flick and formalin pain tests. *Pathophysiology, 1,* 205–214.

Meaney, M. J., Bhatnagar, S., Larocque, S., McCormick, C., Shanks, N., Sharma, S., Smythe, J., Viau, V., & Plotsky, P. M. (1993). Individual differences in the hypothalamic–pituitary–adrenal stress response and the hypothalamic–CRF system. *Annals of the New York Academy of Sciences, 697,* 70–85.

Melzack, R. (1971). Phantom limb pain: Implications for treatment of pathological pain. *Anesthesiology, 35,* 409–419.

Melzack, R. (1989). Phantom limbs, the self and the brain. *Canadian Psychology, 30,* 1–16.

Melzack, R. (1990). Phantom limbs and the concept of a neuromatrix. *Trends in Neuroscience, 13,* 88–92.

Melzack, R. (1991). The gate control theory 25 years later: New perspectives on phantom limb pain. In M. R. Bond, J. E. Charlton, & C. J. Woolf (Eds.), *Proceedings of the Sixth World Congress on Pain* (pp. 9–21). Amsterdam: Elsevier.

Melzack, R. (1992, April). Phantom limbs. *Scentific American, 266,* 120–126.

Melzack, R. (1995). Phantom limb pain and the brain. In B. Bromm & J. E. Desmedt (Eds.), *Pain and the brain: From nociception to cognition* (pp. 73–82). New York: Raven Press.

Melzack, R., & Casey, K. L. (1967). Localized temperature changes evoked in the brain by somatic stimulation. *Experimental Neurology, 17,* 276–292.

Melzack, R., & Casey, K. L. (1968). Sensory, motivational, and central control determinants of pain: A new conceptual model. In D. Kenshalo (Ed.), *The skin senses* (pp. 423–443). Springfield, IL: Thomas.

Melzack, R., Konrad, K. W., & Dubrovsky, B. (1968). Prolonged changes in visual system activity produced by somatic stimulation. *Experimental Neurology, 20,* 443–459.

Melzack, R., Konrad, K. W., & Dubrovsky, B. (1969). Prolonged changes in central nervous system activity produced by somatic and reticular stimulation. *Experimental Neurology, 25,* 416–428.

Melzack, R., & Wall, P. D. (1996). *The challenge of pain* (2nd ed.). London: Penguin Books.

Melzack, R., Wall, P. D., & Ty, T. C. (1982). Acute pain in an emergency clinic: Latency of onset and descriptor patterns. *Pain, 14,* 33–43.

Merskey, H., & Bogduk, N. (1994). *Classification of chronic pain.* Seattle, WA: IASP Press.

Miles, J. (1994). Pituitary destruction. In P. D. Wall &

R. Melzack (Eds.), *Textbook of pain* (3rd ed., pp. 1159–1170). Edinburgh: Churchill Livingstone.

Morley, G. K., Mooradian, A. D., Levine, A. S., & Morley, J. E. (1984). Why is diabetic peripheral neuropathy painful?: The effects of glucose on pain perception in humans. *American Journal of Medicine, 77*, 79–83.

Neeck, G., & Riedel, W. (1994). Neuromediator and hormonal perturbations in fibromyalgia syndrome: Results of chronic stress? *Baillieres Clinical Rheumatology, 8*, 763–775.

Postacchini, F., Lami, R., & Pugliese, O. (1988). Familial predisposition to discogenic low-back pain: An epidemiologic and immunogenetic study. *Spine, 13*, 1403–1406.

Rodgrigues, C. A., Shepherd, N. A., Lennard-Jones, J. E., Hawley, P. R., & Thompson, H. H. (1989). Familial visceral myopathy: A family with at least six involved members. *Gut, 30*, 1285–1292.

Sapolsky, R. M. (1992). Neuroendocrinology of the stress-response. In J. B. Becker, S. M. Breedlove, & D. Crews (Eds.), *Behavioral endocrinology* (pp. 287–324). Cambridge, MA: MIT Press.

Sapolsky, R. M. (1996). Stress, glucocorticoids, and damage to the nervous system: The current state of confusion. *Stress, 1*, 1–19.

Schady, W., & Sheard, A. (1990). A quantitative study of sensory function in hereditary spastic paraplegia. *Brain, 113*, 709–720.

Selye, H. (1950). *Stress.* Montreal: Acta Medical Publisher.

Serena, M., Rizzuto, N., Moretto, G., & Arrigoni, G. (1990). Familial spastic paraplegia with peroneal amyotrophy: A family with hypersensitivity to pyrexia. *Italian Journal of Neurological Sciences, 11*, 583–588.

Shahriaree, H., Kotcamp, W. W., Sheikh, S., & Sajadi, K. (1979). Hereditary perforating ulcers of the foot: Hereditary sensory radicular neuropathy. *Clinical Orthopaedics and Related Research, 140*, 189–193.

Silberg, J., Martin, N. G., & Heath, A. C. (1987). Genetic and environmental factors in primary dysmenorrhea and its relationship to anxiety, depression, and neuroticism. *Behavior Genetics, 17*, 363–383.

Simmons, E. D., Guntupalli, M., Kowalski, J. M., Braun, F., & Seidel, T. (1996). Familial predisposition for degenerative disc disease—A case-control study. *Spine, 21*, 1527–1529.

Smith, R. S. (1991). The macrophage theory of depression. *Medical Hypotheses, 35*, 298–306.

Spector, T. D., Cicuttini, F., Baker, J., Loughlin, J., & Hart, D. (1996). Genetic influences on osteoarthritis in women—A twin study. *British Medical Journal, 312*, 940–943.

Sola, A. E. (1994). Upper extremity pain. In P. D. Wall & R. Melzack (Eds.), *Textbook of pain* (3rd ed., pp. 457–474). Edinburgh: Churchill Livingstone.

Steinman, L. (1993, September). Autoimmune disease. *Scientific American, 269*, 107–114.

Stewart, W. F., Lipton, R. B., & Liberman, J. (1996). Variation in migraine prevalence by race. *Neurology, 47*, 52–59.

Strosberg, J. M., Allen, F. H., Calabro, T. J., & Harris, E. D. (1975). Ankylosing spondylitis in a large kindred: Clinical and genetic studies. *Tissue Antigens, 5*, 205– 212.

Tan, P. L., Caughey, D. E., & Jugusch, M. F. (1983). Genetic predisposition to two rheumatic diseases. *New Zealand Medical Journal, 96*, 422–423.

Thye-Rønn, P., Sindrup, S. H., Arendt-Nielsen, L., Brennum, J., Hother-Nielsen, O., & Beck-Nielsen, H. (1994). Effect of short-term hyperglycemia per se on nociceptive and non-nociceptive threshold. *Pain, 56*, 43–49.

Tsigos, C., & Chrousos, G. P. (1994). Physiology of the hypothalamic–pituitary–adrenal axis in health and dysregulation in psychiatric and autoimmune disorders. *Endocrinology and Metabolism Clinics of North America, 23*, 451–466.

Varlotta, G. P., Brown, M. D., Kelsey, J. L., & Golden, A. L. (1991). Familial predisposition for herniation of a lumbar disc in patients who are less than 21 years old. *Journal of Bone and Joint Surgery, 73*, 124–128.

Wolfe, F., Kleinhekel, S. M., & Khan, M. A. (1988). Familial vs sporadic rheumatoid arthritis: Comparison of demographic and clinical characteristics. *Journal of Rheumatology, 15*, 400–404.

Yasuda, Y., Dokoh, S., Seko, K., Imai, T., Akiguchi, I., & Kameyama, M. (1986). Autosomal dominant osteosclerosis associated with familial spinal canal stenosis. *Neurology, 36*, 687–692.

Chapter 7

Lifespan Developmental Approaches to Pain

GARY A. WALCO
STEPHEN W. HARKINS

Developmental processes are often neglected in the assessment and treatment of pain. Although there is increasing interest in pain among infants and children at one extreme and in pain in the elderly at the other, very little attention has been paid to key aspects of pain that may change over the course of the lifespan. Thus we know very little, for example, about significant aspects of childhood history that may affect pain syndromes in adults, about the long-term prognosis of children and adolescents with chronic pain problems, or about significant events earlier in life that may have an impact on pain in the elderly. The goal of this chapter is to identify themes that may provide some unity in approaches to pain throughout the lifespan.

There has been no organized focus on implementing lifespan developmental approaches to the study of pain. In this chapter, we focus on issues in early development and pain in later life. The issue of the impact of pain in early life on successful adaptation in middle age is not covered in this chapter. The reason is simple—the "adult pain patient" includes all of those from late adolescence to the onset of the later years without discriminating relevant developmental effects over that span. The relationship among developmental factors, adaptation, and pain is an interactive one. We do not know, for example, the impact of pain early in life on individual variables in middle and later life. Lifespan approaches have flourished in other areas of human development and will be beneficial in studying pain.

Developmental sciences highlight two key issues: a focus on change and the study of processes leading to a specific outcome (Baltes, Reese, & Nesselroade, 1977). Although it is clear that pain experiences are subject to change over the course of the lifespan, a number of questions have not been addressed. For example, what are the forces operating to create those changes? What elements are constant over time and which become more variable as a function of aging? How does pain experience affect pain coping in subsequent years? To what degree do models of pain assessment and intervention that have been developed in the "adult" population apply equally over the years from late adolescence to the early elderly years, and to what extent are the principles generalizable to very young or very old patients?

Lifespan developmental approaches involve the study of constancy and change throughout the life course (ontogenesis) from conception to death (Baltes, 1987). In a number of areas, applying lifespan approaches and viewing various clinical phenomena in the context of normal development have been enormously helpful. For example, developmental psychopathology focuses on a longitudinal perspective of various forms of mental illness as they develop and manifest across the life course (Rutter, 1989, 1996; Sroufe, 1997).

The concept of *life course* is central. Its simplest definition is the concrete character of a life in its evolution from beginning to end (Levinson, 1986). *Course* implies a sequence or temporal flow and thus the need to study a life as it unfolds. Foci include stability versus change, continuity versus discontinuity, and orderly progression and stasis versus chaos and fluctuation. *Life* includes many aspects of living that are interwoven to create a larger pattern. Thus intrapsychic phenomena, social relationships, and participation in family and society at large, as well as biological changes, must all be included in this mosaic (Levinson, 1986).

The uniqueness of this approach is demonstrated by the seven elements of lifespan developmental psychology as espoused by Baltes (1987):

1. *Lifespan development.* Ontogenetic development is a lifelong process, and thus no age period holds supremacy in regulating the nature of development.

2. *Multidirectionality.* Diversity or pluralism is found in the directionality of changes, the aggregate of which is ontogeny, even within domains.

3. *Development as gain/loss.* The process of development is not a simple movement toward higher efficacy (what is commonly thought of as "growth"). Rather, development consists of joint occurrences of gain (growth) and loss (decline).

4. *Plasticity.* Depending on life conditions and experiences, individuals' developmental courses may take many forms. The key developmental agenda is the search for the range of plasticities and its constraints.

5. *Historical embeddedness.* Ontogenetic development varies substantially in accordance with historical and sociocultural conditions.

6. *Contextualism as a paradigm.* Individual development can be conceptualized as the outcome of the dialectic of three sources: age-graded, history-graded, and nonnormative factors.

7. *Field of development as multidisciplinary.* Many disciplines (anthropology, biology, sociology, psychology) are concerned with human development. These perspectives are embraced in a comprehensive lifespan developmental model.

Many lifespan developmental issues have already been incorporated into current models of pain assessment and treatment. For example, it has long been recognized that pain is a multidisciplinary problem, requiring input from many medical, psychological, and sociological perspectives (International Association for the Study of Pain, 1994). Historical embeddedness has been addressed, as we have appreciated the impact of cultural background on individuals' pain experiences (Bernstein & Pachter, 1993) and as we may certainly appreciate the changes in the meaning of pain over time within given cultural groups (Rey, 1993).

Other aspects of a lifespan approach would be novel to assess as related to our understanding of pain. For example, are there multidirectional aspects to the development of pain mechanisms and pain experiences across the lifespan? Are there periods of growth and decline in aspects of the pain experience over the life course? Is there plasticity in the nature of pain and its impact over the life course, and if so, what age-graded, history-graded, and nonnormative factors come into play to affect those processes?

Wohlwill (1973) described a methodological approach to the study of developmental issues that may serve as a model to explore the development of pain over the life course. There are five important sequential steps to be invoked. The first is the discovery and synthesis of developmental dimensions. This includes the operational definition of the variable under study and delineation of reliable and valid means of assessing that variable over time. Abstracting uniform and consistent developmental changes from other sources of variation (e.g., situational variables) is central. As related to pain, we must then utilize a definition of the construct that applies throughout the life course and describe common means of gaining data through self-report, behavioral indices, and physiological parameters. Of course, scaling is a major issue because both the subjective experience and the means by which that experience may be expressed will vary over the life course.

The second step is the descriptive study of age changes. This includes both quantitative and qualitative changes. The former focuses on determining the overall direction and form of developmental functions and their parameters. The latter highlights developmental sequences in the appearance of discrete responses over the course of development, along with specification of the forms that these successive responses might take. Often qualitative approaches have incorporated stage models. Wohlwill (1973) is a strong advocate of longitudinal approaches in describing age changes since other means, such as cross-sectional studies, fail to provide adequate continuity. In the case of pain, one would need to study the development of pain mechanisms and pain experience over the life course of individuals. As will be described below, very few studies have utilized longitudinal strategies in assessing pain, and there are far more outcomes in which glimpses of development are gleaned cross-sectionally over some age period.

The third strategy involves the correlational study of age changes. Once variables have been defined and developmental functions plotted, we have only a description of development. By examining temporal correlates to that developmental function, one can begin to understand the mechanisms underlying the observed process. For example, changes in cognition, language, and affect that occur over the course of childhood likely have a strong impact on individuals' subjective pain experiences. We examine these correlates below.

The fourth phase of developmental research is the study of determinants of developmental change. Simply stated, once correlates of developmental change have been delineated, it remains to show causal relationships. This is achieved through the systematic manipulation of variables or by studying temporal relationships among factors to determine the impact on outcomes. In the case of pain research, studies that require active manipulation of factors related to the development of pain systems are done on animals. In addition, however, some clinical situations may be used to document certain outcomes related to the development of pain. Although less amenable to experimenter manipulation (decreased internal validity), such circumstances provide greater ecological (external) validity.

The final step of the process focuses on individual differences. Specifically, the aim is to distinguish individual differences in development from the development of individual differences. In delineating a developmental function, one would observe some average of change over time in a number of individuals. Clearly, however, not every individual will follow precisely the same pattern. Instances in which there are minor variations from the developmental function are deemed to be individual differences in development and typically are not of significant clinical interest. In contrast, there are situations in which individuals deviate from the normal developmental curve in some constant or predictable fashion. That is, there is a stable individual difference in development that persists over time and across circumstances. These differences often are of clinical interest because significant deviations often imply pathological concerns. In con-

sidering issues such as pain threshold, pain tolerance, and pain responsiveness, both as laboratory and clinical phenomena, individual differences play a major role. Accounting for the variance in these observed differences and understanding the causal mechanisms are goals of pain research across the lifespan.

At present, incorporating developmental issues into aspects of pain assessment and management has been done principally in pediatrics and secondarily in geriatrics. Very little work has been done to view pain in a different fashion across the broad range of the "adult" years. If a true lifespan approach is adopted, which makes sense from both theoretical and clinical perspectives, it seems imperative that we begin to focus on themes that are common over the life course. For the purposes of clarity, we will focus on physiological changes associated with the pain experience in the very young and the very old, as well as developmental aspects of cognition and socioemotional issues in those groups.

PAIN IN INFANTS AND CHILDREN

Physiological Development of Pain Networks in the Young

For many years it was believed that infants lacked the neurological mechanisms to experience pain. Recent evidence indicates, however, that nociceptive pathways, although still developing, are in place and functional in even premature neonates (Fitzgerald & Anand, 1993). The peripheral and central nervous system structures involved in nociception develop during the second and third trimesters of gestation (Anand & Carr, 1989). Focus on the development of pain pathways per se is a relatively new endeavor; much has been inferred based on what is known about adult pain systems and the development of critical neuroanatomical substrates in the fetus (Anand & Carr, 1989). In addition, animal models, specifically rat pups, have provided a great deal of the data on the specific biological aspects of pain development (Fitzgerald & Anand, 1993). Although the timetable is compressed, the same developmental progression takes place in both species, and thus reasonable comparisons may be made.

Fitzgerald has conducted a series of studies with rats that map out the essential elements of the developmental neurophysiologic processes related to pain. Peripheral nociceptors, those with both A-delta and C fibers, develop soon after cutaneous axons reach the skin (a process occurring between 7 and 20 weeks gestation in humans), and at birth their function parallels mature nociceptors (Fitzgerald, 1987). Large diameter dorsal root fibers grow into the spinal cord first, followed by small diameter C fibers, a process which occurs just before birth (corresponding to about 24 weeks gestation in humans). There is a discrepancy in developmental patterns between A-delta and C fibers, however (Fitzgerald, 1988). As A-delta fibers grow into the spinal cord, they rapidly produce synaptically evoked activity in dorsal horn cells. C fibers do not produce such activity until the end of the first postnatal week (which roughly translates to several weeks in the human neonate). Thus relatively low-level tactile stimulation may lead to reflexive "pain" responses in young human neonates. In addition, the more typical adult pattern of rapid A-delta firing followed by C-fiber stimulation in response to tissue damage would not be so clear-cut at this stage.

A critical question focuses on the long-term impact of pain experiences early in life. In their discussion of neural development, Anand and Carr (1989) state, "importance of this phase of development in the maturation of the pain system is underscored by the high index of 'brain plasticity' present during this period. Clearly the cellular, synaptic, and molecular mechanisms determining brain plasticity are highest during infancy and early childhood. Painful and other experiences during this period therefore may determine the final architecture of the adult pain system, with subtle and presently undefined characteristics responsible for the clinically evident individual variation" (p. 800).

Fitzgerald and colleagues, through studies with both rats and human neonates, have shed light on this issue. With rats, it was shown that tissue damage in the early postnatal period causes a profound and lasting sprouting response of local sensory nerve terminals (Reynolds & Fitzgerald, 1995). This in turn results in hyperinnervation, which remains evident in adult rats well after the wound has healed. Analyses indicated that both A-delta and C fibers are involved in this process, which may account for the extensiveness of the observed hyperinnervation. The implication is that in the neonatal period, peripheral nerve networks are going through a process of increasing differentiation. When repeatedly insulted with painful stimuli, that process is altered such that lower levels of stimulation potentiate relatively significant nociceptive responses. Indeed, human neonates undergoing repeated heal lancing demon-

strated a similar hyperalgesic response (Fitzgerald, Millard, & McIntosh, 1989).

Other clinical research findings support these concerns. Taddio, Katz, Ilersich, and Koren (1997) focused on reactions to routine vaccination at 4 and 6 months of age among three groups of boys: those who were uncircumcised, those who were circumcised within 5 days of birth using EMLA cream (a topical anesthetic) for pain management, and those who were circumcised with a placebo topical cream. When these children came in for their routine vaccinations, they were videotaped so that a number of pain behaviors could be evaluated, including facial action (brow bulge, nasolabial furrow, eyes squeezed shut) and cry duration, and a visual analogue scale score for pain was assigned. Analyses showed greater pain responses across the board in boys who were circumcised without local anesthesia in contrast to those who were uncircumcised. In addition, visual analogue scores were significantly different between boys circumcised with EMLA versus those with the placebo. Relevant variables, such as temperament, age, weight, time since last feeding, time of last sleep before vaccination, and ingestion of paracetamol, did not correlate with pain indices. Thus early untreated pain experiences appear to sensitize the child to subsequent painful experiences.

Similar possibilities were raised in a study by Walco and colleagues (Walco, Dampier, Hartstein, Djordjevic, & Miller, 1990), who assessed pain threshold values in four groups of children: those with juvenile rheumatoid arthritis (a chronic illness in which chronic pain is a common feature), those with sickle cell disease (a chronic illness in which recurrent episodes of acute pain is a common feature), those with asthma (a chronic illness in which pain is typically not a feature), and healthy controls. Pain threshold was measured in two modalities, direct mechanical pressure stimulation of a digit and circumferential pressure on the upper arm. Results showed that children who experience clinical pain on a regular basis (those with juvenile rheumatoid arthritis and sickle cell disease) had lower pain thresholds than their healthy peers.

Certainly a great deal more research on the development of pain pathways needs to be conducted in order to fully understand these findings. We currently know very little about the development of central components to pain systems, especially in the areas of the thalamus, cortex, and cingulate gyrus of the limbic system. In addition, however, cognitive and affective factors, both of which have their own developmental pathways, play a major role in the pain experience and should be considered.

Cognitive and Emotional Development

Similar to the development of pain networks on a physiological level, both cognition and emotion develop with increasing differentiation and integration. A thorough review of potential cognitive and socioemotional influences on pain is well beyond the scope of this chapter. Thus we will highlight areas in which there has been a specific focus on developmental aspects of pain as related to concept development and to temperament.

It is well known that as children's cognitive abilities increase, their concepts of illness become increasingly differentiated and integrated. Bibace and Walsh (1980) showed that there is a strong relationship between Piagetian cognitive stage and concept of illness. Thompson and Varni (1986) elaborated on this model and discussed the relationship between emerging concepts of illness and related concepts of pain. Although implications for assessment were described, no data were offered demonstrating the precise nature of this relationship.

Ross and Ross (1984) conducted semi-structured interviews with almost 1,000 children between the ages of 5 and 12 years in school, hospital, or clinic settings. Interestingly, they found no age trends in children's pain concepts. Definitions of pain were "unidimensional," as pain was defined in the context of general discomfort or specific pain events. Children failed to comprehend the warning or diagnostic value of pain, and secondary gains or other value of pain were rarely recognized. Specific pain experiences were attributed to immediate causes (e.g., accidents, illness, surgery). Noticeably absent was the notion of pain related to immanent justice; if pain was seen as a punishment, it was in relation to immediate and proximal, not remote, events. Pain descriptors were used meaningfully, and children could recollect various contextual aspects of previous pain experiences.

In contrast, Gaffney and Dunne (1986) showed that children's understanding of pain follows a Piagetian developmental model. They used a sentence completion item of the form "Pain is . . ." in the context of a broader assessment of children between the ages of 5 and 14 years. From the responses, three composite categories were derived that reflected concrete definitions, semi-

abstract definitions, and abstract definitions. Data showed statistically and clinically significant differences as abstraction and generalization increased with age. The authors noted that the three coding categories for definitions of pain correspond to preoperational, concrete operational, and formal operational thought, respectively, and the age distributions observed were consistent with expectations.

In a second study (Gaffney & Dunne, 1987), causality of pain was the focus. Twelve categories were derived, including categories such as illness, malfunction, transgressions involving eating, transgressions involving other activities, transgressions, psychological factors, need states, physiological explanations, and contamination or contagion. Developmental patterns were observed in that the frequency of objective, physical explanations of pain (trauma, malfunction) increased significantly with age, as did abstract, psychological explanations. Physiological explanations were noticeably scarce. The issue of transgression was apparent, as children often attributed pain to carelessness or misdeed. Of note, however, is that the authors viewed these explanations as arising much more from intrinsic processes of cognitive development than from environmental influences, such as attributions made by parents.

We know of no research that specifically examined the relationship between children's understanding of pain and actual clinical pain experiences. However, data from one study appear to support the notion that increasing levels of cognition and awareness, as well as concurrent emotional development, have a significant impact on pain experience. Ilowite, Walco, and Pochaczevsky (1992) used liquid crystal thermography to measure the heat of joints affected by juvenile rheumatoid arthritis in children between the ages of 4 and 16 years. By comparing affected joints with contralateral unaffected joints (or adjacent nonarticular tissue in cases of bilateral disease), they could establish specific values representing changes in temperature due to disease (ΔT). These ΔT values were then correlated with visual analogue scales for pain intensity provided by the patient, parent, and physician. For the latter two, significant correlations were observed, $r = .50$ and $r = .58$, respectively. Although this correlation was also highly significant in younger patients (younger than about 8 years of age), $r = .73$, it was much lower in older patients, $r = .24$. The authors concluded that in older patients, many more variables, including cognitive and emotional processes, come into play and affect subjective pain experiences.

A significant literature exists on the relationship between psychological functioning, personality variables, and aspects of the pain experience in adults (cf. Bradley, Haile, & Jaworski, 1992). In contrast, very little has been published on these elements in children. Increasingly, however, it is becoming recognized that many of the same functional elements that comprise temperamental styles in general may apply to pain as well. Consistent, inherent predispositions underlie and modulate expressions of activity, reactivity, emotionality, and sociability (Goldsmith et al., 1987). Clearly these factors are critical in understanding individual differences in pain response. Recently, attention has been turned to the manner in which temperamental variables affect reactivity and self-regulation, including their relation to self-focus as a coping style for pain (Zeltzer, Bursch, & Walco, 1997). This literature is in its infancy, and laboratory and clinical studies are needed to further delineate specific relationships among temperament, pain responsiveness, and pain coping. Finally, it is clear that affect plays a significant role in the pain experience. Studies comparing the increasing differentiation and integration of affect with elements of the pain experience, including differentiation of those responses, will be extremely helpful.

PAIN IN OLDER ADULTS

Preliminary Considerations

A major challenge in geriatrics is distinguishing between disease and "normal" aging. A number of age-related health problems were, in the past, considered part of "normal aging," not conditions with specific etiologies. This appears to be the case today for chronic pain associated with degenerative musculoskeletal conditions. Discomfort, pain, and suffering associated with degenerative conditions is accepted by many middle-aged and older individuals as a "natural" consequence of growing old, and this belief is too frequently shared by many in the health care delivery system.

Differences between individuals increase with age in the later years of life. This is recognized in adult lifespan research, in which a distinction is made between "young-old," "old," and "old-old" (Neugarten, 1969; Neugarten, Moore, & Lowe, 1965). Young-old are individuals 55 to perhaps 70 years of age. It can even be argued that the "young-old" include those in their mid- and late 40s. The young-old are likely to be healthy, active, and economically advantaged, with satisfying social resources and minimal demand on health care services. The "old" are those between 70 and 85 years of age; as a group, they are characterized by onset of chronic degenerative processes, greater morbidity, and some limitation in activities of daily living compared to the young-old.

The "old-old" consist of persons above 85 years of age. This group is characterized by increasing frailty, frequent use of health care services, and decreased ability to engage in usual and desired activities of daily living. More recently, it has been recognized that it is useful to identify another group consisting of the "oldest-old," those over 95 years of age. The ability to survive to near the upper limit of the human lifespan (approximately 120 to 126 years) with minimal morbidity represents considerable ability to respond at both physiologic and psychosocial levels to life's challenges. Those old-old and oldest-old who are relatively free of chronic illness or dementia represent a group that is likely biologically different from their birth cohort peers who either do not achieve near-centenarian status or who do so with severe infirmity. No systematic research has as yet evaluated the strategies that the old-old and the oldest-old employed for coping with pain over the lifespan or even the epidemiology of pain of the old, the old-old, and the oldest-old.

Psychophysical and Physiological Considerations

Current evidence suggests, in the absence of major insult or injury, that minimal change occurs in nociceptive coding across middle age and into early old age (the young-old). The view that there is a generalized decrease in pain sensitivity with aging or that older adults can endure minor surgical procedures with little or no discomfort is myth. It is likely that unameliorated pain in the middle and later years of life affects physiological processes in a fashion that is similar or parallel to those of biological senescence and thus increases the "rate of aging."

Sensory Changes across the Lifespan

The well-documented and progressive decrements in sensory acuity in the visual (presbyopia: *presby* = old; *opia* = vision) and auditory (presbycusis: *cusis* = hearing) systems represent the onset of old age for the eye and ear. Presbyopia is an age-dependent loss of visual accommodation resulting in a decrease in acuity of near-point vision. Presbycusis is due to loss of specific receptors (hair cells) in the inner ear. It is more pronounced for high frequency sounds, is greater in men than women, is progressive, is associated with decreased ability to identify speech sounds in acoustically noisy environments, and is slightly greater for the left than the right ear. Reduced visual and auditory acuity are almost universal in those above the age of 60 and reach epidemic proportions in those 75 and older. A progressive loss of sensitivity to nociceptive stimuli does not appear to occur with age in the middle and later years of life.

Characterization of changes in the major senses across the adult lifespan has benefited greatly from advances in methods for sensory acuity evaluation. These advances include precise control over physical stimuli, as well as improved methods for quantification of sensation and perception for the major senses. In contrast, the limited and somewhat contradictory findings on age differences in pain perception may well reflect historical limitations in methods for delivery of appropriate stimuli, as well as limitations in use of pain threshold, tolerance, and reaction as psychophysical endpoints (Harkins, 1996; Harkins & Price, 1992; Harkins & Warner, 1980).

Psychophysics and Pain Assessment

The psychophysical evaluation of the effect of age on pain across the lifespan has a history differing considerably from that of almost all other sensory modalities. Although age changes in psychophysiological response to appropriate stimuli presented to the major and to most "minor" sensory modalities have been carefully characterized, this is not true for nociceptive processes, pain perception, and pain-related behaviors. To our knowledge, the complementary and perhaps more important question of the effects of pain on adult development and successful aging has not been well formulated as yet.

There are several reasons for the lag in the understanding of the effects of adult aging on pain and pain on aging. One is due to the precision to which stimuli that activate sensory modalities can be controlled and quantified. For example, in auditory psychophysics, the ease of quantification and control of sound has facilitated the precise definition of presbycusis. In contrast, as noted below, quantification and control of the stimuli that produce pain have been far less precise.

Another reason for the lag is that there has been some confusion as to whether pain operates more as a motivational system or as a sensory modality (Mayer & Price, 1982; Price, 1988; Wall,

1979) and/or whether the pain system is limited to dealing with crude discriminative information only (Mountcastle, 1974; Wall, 1979). There is also the view that pain is a private experience that does not lend itself readily to experimental examination or accurate quantification in clinical settings, and this has dampened the interest of some researchers, including those active in lifespan developmental studies and gerontological research in this area. This view is erroneous.

An additional reason is that it has been assumed by some that age results in loss of pain perception and that older adults with chronic pain complaints are not good candidates for treatment in multidisciplinary pain centers (Harkins, 1996; Sorkin, Rudy, Hanlon, Turk, & Steig, 1990). Such ageist attitudes, combined with the view that pain is not measurable, have limited advances in our understanding of adult developmental factors that influence pain perception and have contributed to unnecessary suffering in one of the most dependent segments of our population—the frail elderly.

A final reason for the lag in understanding of the effects of age on pain perception is that the results of experimental studies of age differences in pain perception in laboratory settings have been contradictory (Harkins & Warner, 1980; Harkins, Kwentus, & Price, 1992; Harkins, Price, Bush, & Small, 1995). This likely reflects choice of methods of stimulation, psychophysical endpoints, and even definition of what represents "aged" subjects (Harkins & Price, 1992).

Fortunately, within the last two decades there has been a resurgence of interest in psychophysical studies of pain. Many of these studies have employed precise contact thermal (Harkins, Price, & Martelli, 1986; Harkins, Davis, Bush, & Kasberger, 1996) or laser (Chakour, Gibson, Bradbeer, & Helme, 1996) stimuli combined with simple but highly informative psychophysical procedures based on magnitude estimation and matching (Marks, 1974; Stevens, 1975; Stevens & Marks, 1971). These methodological advances have led to experimental paradigms that can directly relate neural responses and pain-related behavior to various intensities of suprathreshold painful stimuli and thus allow study of individual differences in pain responses across the lifespan.

Presbyalgos?

If pain sensitivity decreased across the adult lifespan, it would be termed "presbyalgos" (Harkins & Scott, 1996). Changes in most sensory systems in the middle and later years of life appear to follow a pattern reflecting the complexity and metabolic demand of the sensory receptor/transduction system. The more complex the receptor and transduction mechanisms, the more likely that time-dependent, and thus age-related, changes will occur. Changes in the major senses often follow an individual history of long-term exposure to environmental stress (i.e., noise exposure history is related to onset and severity of presbycusis). In more primitive sensory systems, including free nerve endings of the nociceptive system, present evidence points to decreased information processing from cutaneous A-delta Type II mechano-thermal nociceptors but not to C-fiber-mediated cutaneous sensation (Chakour et al., 1996; Harkins et al., 1996), to reduced ability to discriminate pain of low intensity (which may reflect cognitive, not sensory sensitivity, age differences; Harkins, Chapman, & Eisdorfer, 1979; Harkins & Chapman, 1977a, 1977b) to decreased presentation of referred pain as a symptom (see brief review in Harkins et al., 1992), and to reduced negative affect associated with chronic pain (Harkins & Price, 1992; Harkins, 1996) in older adults compared to younger adults. One very preliminary finding also suggests a reduction in slow temporal summation of second pain in older individuals (Harkins et al., 1996).

Response times to onset of first pain have been reported to be slower in older individuals compared to younger individuals following stimulation of the leg but not of the arm. This finding was interpreted as reflecting slowing in conduction properties of A-delta nociceptive afferents and as evidence for selective small fiber peripheral neuropathy in the elderly (Harkins et al., 1996). Other findings indicate that onset of pain sensation as measured by reaction times does not change with age for tooth shock (Harkins & Chapman, 1977a, 1977b) or for sensation of second pain to contact thermal stimulation of either the arm or leg (Harkins et al., 1996). These latter results are most unusual because reaction time slowing is one of the best documented findings in the gerontological literature. The effects of age across the adult lifespan on the nociceptive system are likely quite different from its effects on other sensory systems.

Caveats

Important caveats to the research reviewed here and that summarized recently (Harkins & Scott, 1996) concerning possible characteristics of "presbyalgos" are that all findings are based on cross-sectional

evaluation of individuals under 80 years of age. Cross-sectional studies allow only inferences of group differences and thus interindividual variability. Longitudinal study of pain across the lifespan is lacking, and thus we currently have no information on intraindividual changes in pain responsiveness and behaviors. Cross-sectional research is confounded by birth cohort and thus by social history effects. Psychosocial history can have dramatic effects on pain report and behavior. The importance of the lack of systematic information on individuals over the age of 85 is reflected in the fact that, percentage-wise, this is the fastest growing segment of the population in the more developed countries and also consists of individuals more likely to suffer chronic conditions that are frequently associated with pain. It is in this age group that chronic cognitive disorders that limit the ability to successfully communicate the presence of discomfort, pain, and suffering are greatest. It is also at age 85 and above that age changes may well occur in peripheral and central nociceptive systems. A final definition of presbyalgos remains to be formulated.

Psychosocial Considerations

Lifespan development research explicitly recognizes the importance of psychosocial and cognitive factors on intraindividual formulations of personal plans and reactions to life events, including the perception of and reaction to different types of pain. Although cultural differences in pain behavior illustrate the dramatic impact of social history on expression and response to pain, the impact of personal history, including previous exposure to painful conditions, is poorly defined. Certainly, exposure to pain in specific settings can result in conditioned emotional responses. One only has to interview individuals with needle or dental phobias to understand the impact of setting, situation, and meaning of painful events on emotional distress and suffering.

Some findings indicate that older chronic pain patients report less pain-related negative affect and suffering but not reduced pain intensity compared to younger chronic pain patients (Harkins & Price, 1992). This finding might reflect a generalized reduction in emotionality with age, with intact sensory acuity for pain. Cross-sectional studies do indicate reduced positive and negative affect with age. Longitudinal studies of affect, however, indicate that the cross-sectional age differences are likely due to birth cohort effects and that they therefore reflect social history effects on willingness to endorse affect-loaded items on survey questionnaires (Costa et al., 1987). The fact that older individuals compared to younger ones reported less pain-related suffering under equivalent pain intensity may well result from social history effects. Birth cohort and resulting social history effects can produce "conditioned emotional acceptance" of events. This acceptance occurs within temporal expectancies in relation to "stages" in the lifespan. For example, loss of teeth is historically an accepted part of growing and being old, and the expectancy of tooth loss in old age has a venerable history (see, for example, *As You Like It*, Act II, Scene ii). In fact, recent results indicate that complete loss of teeth is associated with considerable emotional distress and health concern in younger but not in older adults.

Self-report data of edentulousness in the general population of the United States gathered between 1984 and 1986 showed that among more than 9,000 community-dwelling, ambulatory individuals, complete loss of teeth is increasingly common with increasing age. Such loss is, however, not a natural developmental consequence of aging in the later years of life but rather reflects oral hygiene, nutrition, education, and the impact of decay and periodontal disease over the lifespan. The high prevalence of age-related edentulousness in prior generations results in an expectation of tooth loss in later years and thus psychosocial acceptance. Loss of teeth is thus an age-graded event within a social context. Its occurrence in younger individuals is "off-time," unexpected, and thus may be emotionally distressing. The data indicate that younger edentulous individuals report greater health concern and emotional distress than age-matched peers with natural dentition. In contrast, older edentulous individuals do not differ on these variables from age-matched controls with natural dentition (Harkins, Englade, Welleford, & Elliott, 1998).

Across the lifespan, adults react to "their life events in terms of an underlying set of assumptions, expectations, and ideas about what their lives could be" (Whitbourne & Cassidy, 1996, p. 51). As an "off-time" event, complete loss of teeth in younger adults can be a source of health concern and emotional distress (Harkins et al., 1998; Neugarten, 1979). The complete loss of teeth with increasing age, although accepted by previous generations as age-consistent, will change in coming generations due to enhanced oral health care and

education. "Illness itself is a subjective classification; symptoms defined by one group as pathological may be accepted by another as normal and an easily tolerable part of everyday life" (Haber, 1983).

The presence of pain, like the complete loss of teeth, is an accepted part of growing old in the later years of life for many elderly individuals. This will change as pain, both as an acute symptom and as a chronic disease, is better understood and controlled. With improved methods of pain control and education of both the patient and the health care community, acceptance of pain as part of daily living for the elderly, like the acceptance of complete tooth loss, should and hopefully will be challenged more and more.

Quality of Life

The psychological and economic impact of chronic pain on the nation's work force is well documented (Bonica, 1990). The impact of chronic pain on quality of life and on mortality for mostly retired, older adults, however, is not documented. Pain is a major contributor to lowered quality of life, depression, drug misuse and abuse, and failure to thrive in the older, frail adult. Circular reasoning often leads to ascription of older pain patients' distress, negative affect, and depression to "supertentorial," "somatic," and "functional" disorders, when the underlying cause is poorly treated or even untreated and undiagnosed pain. Such patients can reasonably be expected to present with considerable negative affect, low expectation for positive treatment outcome, frustration, and anger.

ARE THE EFFECTS OF PAIN ON DEVELOPMENT MORE IMPORTANT THAN THE EFFECTS OF DEVELOPMENT ON PAIN?

Well-controlled prospective and retrospective studies of the impact of pain on development across the lifespan are lacking. The methods employed in assessment of the impact of pain early in life are not likely to be appropriate for similar study later in life due to the psychosocial and physiological discontinuities between childhood and adulthood. This does not mean that pain early in life has no relevance to the understanding of individual differences in pain across the lifespan, even for centenarians. Rather, it draws attention to the fact that considerable care must be taken in such research. Attention to ecologically valid assessments of individuals' self-reports of pain and its impact across the lifespan are warranted. Lifespan studies should use a combination of qualitative and quantitative methods with the same participants in an effort to better understand and develop assessment tools for measurement of pain, discomfort, and suffering at all life's stages. Causal attribution must rest on well-designed studies that combine not only physiologically relevant questions but also variables related to social history and traits. Such studies will require a willing combination of disciplines and methods.

REFERENCES

Anand, K. J. S., & Carr, D. B. (1989). The neuroanatomy, neurophysiology and neurochemistry of pain, stress, and analgesia in newborns, infants, and children. *Pediatric Clinics of North America, 36,* 795-822.

Baltes, P. B. (1987). Theoretical propositions of life-span developmental psychology: On the dynamics between growth and decline. *Developmental Psychology, 23,* 611-626.

Baltes, P. B., Reese, H. W., & Nesselroade, J. R. (1977). *Life-span developmental psychology: Introduction to research methods.* Monterey, CA: Brooks/Cole.

Bernstein, B. A., & Pachter, L. M. (1993). Cultural considerations in children's pain. In N. L. Schechter, C. B. Berde, & M. Yaster (Eds.), *Pain in infants, children, and adolescents* (pp. 113-122). Baltimore: Williams & Wilkins.

Bibace, R., & Walsh, M. E. (1980). Development of children's concepts of illness. *Pediatrics, 66,* 912-917.

Bonica, J. J. (1990). *The management of pain* (2nd ed.). Philadelphia: Lea & Febiger.

Bradley, L. A., Haile, J. M., & Jaworski, T. M. (1992). Assessment of psychological status using interviews and self-report instruments. In D. C. Turk and R. Melzack (Eds.), *Handbook of pain assessment* (pp. 193-213). New York: Guilford Press.

Chakour, M. C., Gibson, S. J., Bradbeer, M., & Helme, R. D. (1996). The effect of age on A-delta and C-fiber thermal pain perception. *Pain, 64,* 143-152.

Costa, P. T., Jr., Zonderman, A. B., McCrae, R. R., Cornoni-Huntley, J., Locke, B. Z., & Barbano, H. E. (1987). Longitudinal analyses of psychological well-being in a national sample: Stability of mean levels. *Journal of Gerontology, 42,* 50-55.

Fitzgerald, M. (1987). Cutaneous primary afferent properties in the hindlimb of the neonatal rat. *Journal of Physiology, 383,* 79-92.

Fitzgerald, M. (1988). The development of activity evoked by fine diameter cutaneous fibres in the spinal cord of the newborn rat. *Neuroscience Letter, 86,* 161-166.

Fitzgerald, M., & Anand, K. J. S. (1993). Developmental neuroanatomy and neurophysiology of pain. In N. L. Schechter, C. B. Berde, & M. Yaster (Eds.), *Pain in infants, children, and adolescents* (pp. 11-31). Baltimore: Williams & Wilkins.

Fitzgerald, M., Millard, C., & McIntosh, N. (1989). Cutaneous hypersensitivity following peripheral tissue damage in newborn infants and its reversal with topical anaesthesia. *Pain, 39,* 31-36.

Gaffney, A., & Dunne, E. A. (1986). Developmental aspects of children's definitions of pain. *Pain, 26,* 105-117.

Gaffney, A., & Dunne, E. A. (1987). Children's understanding of the causality of pain. *Pain, 29,* 91-104.

Goldsmith, H., Buss, A., Plomin, R., Rothbart, M., Thomas, A., Chess, S., Hinde, R., & McCall, R. (1987). Roundtable: What is temperament?: Four approaches. *Child Development, 58,* 505-529.

Haber, C. (1983). *Beyond sixty-five: The dilemma of old age in America's past.* Cambridge: Cambridge University Press.

Harkins, S. W. (1996). Geriatric pain: Pain perception in old age. *Clinics in Geriatric Medicine, 12,* 435-459.

Harkins, S. W., & Chapman, C. R. (1977a). The perception of induced dental pain in young and elderly women. *Journal of Gerontology, 32,* 428-435.

Harkins, S. W., & Chapman, C. R. (1977b). Age and sex differences in pain perception. In D. J. Anderson & B. Matthews (Eds.), *Pain in the trigeminal region* (pp. 435-441). Amsterdam: Elsevier/North Holland Biomedical Press.

Harkins, S. W., Chapman, L. R., & Eisdorfer, C. (1979). Memory loss and response bias in senescence. *Journal of Gerontology, 34,* 66-72.

Harkins, S. W., Davis, M. D., Bush, F., & Kasberger, J. (1996). Suppression of first pain and slow temporal summation of second pain in relation to age. *Journal of Gerontology: Medical Sciences, 51A,* M260-M265.

Harkins, S. W., Englade, A., Welleford, A., & Elliott, T. (1998). Age graded events and health concern. Manuscript submitted for publication.

Harkins, S. W., Kwentus, J., & Price, D. D. (1992). Pain and suffering in the elderly. In J. J. Bonica (Ed.), *Management of pain* (2nd ed., pp. 552-559). Philadelphia: Lea & Febiger.

Harkins, S. W., & Price, D. D. (1992). Assessment of pain in the elderly. In D. C. Turk & R. Melzack (Eds.), *Handbook of pain assessment* (pp. 315-331). New York: Guilford Press.

Harkins, S. W., Price, D. D., Bush, F., & Small, R. (1995). Geriatric pain. In P. D. Wall & R. Melzack (Eds.), *Textbook of pain* (pp. 769-784). Edinburgh: Churchill Livingstone.

Harkins, S. W., Price, D., & Martelli, M. (1986). Effects of age on pain perception: Thermonociception. *Journal of Gerontology, 41,* 58-63.

Harkins, S. W., & Scott, R. (1996). Pain and presbyalgos. *Encyclopedia of gerontology* (Vol. 2, pp. 247-260). New York: Academic Press.

Harkins, S. W., & Warner, M. (1980). Age and pain. In C. Eisdorfer (Ed.), *Annual Review of Gerontology and Geriatrics* (Vol. 1, pp. 121-131). New York: Springer.

Ilowite, N. T., Walco, G. A., & Pochaczevsky, R. (1992). Pain assessment in juvenile rheumatoid arthritis: Relation between pain intensity and degree of joint inflammation. *Annals of the Rheumatic Diseases, 51,* 343-346.

International Association for the Study of Pain, Task Force on Taxonomy. (1994). *Classification of chronic pain: Descriptions of chronic pain syndromes and definitions of pain terms* (2nd ed.). Seattle, WA: IASP Press.

Levinson, D. J. (1986). A conception of adult development. *American Psychologist, 41,* 3–13.

Marks, L. (1974). *Sensory processes: The new psychophysics.* New York: Academic Press.

Mayer, D. J., & Price, D. D. (1982). A physiological and psychological analysis of pain: A potential model of motivation. In D. W. Staff (Ed.), *The physiological mechanisms of motivation* (pp. 433–471). New York: Springer.

Mountcastle, V. B. (1974). Pain and temperature sensibilities. In V. B. Mountcastle (Ed.). *Medical physiology* (13th ed., Vol. 1, pp. 348–381). St. Louis, MO: Mosby.

Neugarten, B. (1969). Continuities and discontinuities of psychological issues into adult life. *Human Development, 12,* 121–130.

Neugarten, B. (1979). Time, age, and the life cycle. *American Journal of Psychiatry, 136,* 887–894.

Neugarten, B. L., Moore, J. W., & Lowe, J. C. (1965). Age norms, age constraints, and age socialization. *American Journal of Sociology, 70,* 710–717.

Price, D. D. (1988). *Psychological and neural mechanisms of pain.* New York: Raven Press.

Rey, R. (1993). *History of pain* (L. E. Wallace, J. A. Cadden, & S. W. Cadden, Trans.). Paris: Éditions la Découverte.

Reynolds, M. L., & Fitzgerald, M. (1995). Long-term sensory hyperinnervation following neonatal skin wounds. *Journal of Comparative Neurology, 358,* 487–498.

Ross, D. M., & Ross, S. A. (1984). Childhood pain: The school-aged child's viewpoint. *Pain, 20,* 179–191.

Rutter, M. (1989). Pathways from childhood to adult life. *Journal of Child Psychology and Psychiatry, 30,* 23–51.

Rutter, M. (1996). Transitions and turning points in developmental psychopathology: As applied to the age span between childhood and mid-adulthood. *International Journal of Behavioral Development, 19,* 603–626.

Sorkin, B. A., Rudy, T. E., Hanlon, R. B., Turk, D. C., & Steig, R. L. (1990). Chronic pain in old and young patients: Differences appear less important than similarities. *Journal of Gerontology, 45,* P64–P68.

Sroufe, L. A. (1997). Psychopathology as an outcome of development. *Development and Psychopathology, 9,* 251–268.

Stevens, J. C., & Marks, L. E. (1971). Spatial summation and the dynamics of warmth sensation. *Perceptual Psychophysics, 9,* 291–298.

Stevens, S. S. (1975). *Psychophysics: Introduction to its perceptual, neural and social prospects.* New York: Wiley.

Taddio, A., Katz, J., Ilersich, A. L., & Koren, G. (1997). Effect of neonatal circumcision on pain response during subsequent routine vaccination. *Lancet, 349,* 599–603.

Thompson, K. L., & Varni, J. W. (1986). A developmental cognitive-biobehavioral approach to pediatric pain assessment. *Pain, 25,* 282–296.

Walco, G. A., Dampier, C. D., Hartstein, G., Djordjevic, D., & Miller, L. (1990). The relationship between recurrent clinical pain and pain threshold in children. In D. C. Tyler & E. J. Krane (Eds.), *Advances in pain research and therapy: Vol. 15. Pediatric pain* (pp. 333–340). New York: Raven.

Wall, P. D. (1979). On the relation of injury to pain. *Pain, 6,* 253–264.

Whitbourne, S. K., & Cassidy, E. L. (1996). Adaptation. In J. Birren (Ed.), *Encyclopedia of gerontology* (Vol. 1, pp. 65–69). San Diego: Academic Press.

Wohlwill, J. F. (1973). *The study of behavioral development.* New York: Academic Press.

Zeltzer, L., Bursch, B., & Walco, G. (1997). Pain responsiveness and chronic pain: A psychobiological perspective. *Journal of Developmental and Behavioral Pediatrics, 18,* 413–422.

Chapter 8

Sociocultural and Religious Meanings of Pain

DAVID B. MORRIS

> a man cries out he is in pain   we want to say we know
> what that means   what does that mean
>
> how do words refer to sensations   how do we learn the
> meaning of pain
> —DAVID ANTIN, "the black plague" (iii)

PAIN, MEANING, AND BELIEF

Meaning is intrinsic to human pain. Pain, that is, implies continuous processes of nonconscious and conscious interpretation. Why me? Is the pain serious? How long will it last? Whose fault is it? Will I get better? Such questions and their responses may arise well after an initial episode of pain, but meaning is never merely external or added on. Human pain does not exist apart from meaning. Meaning helps to constitute it. We cannot name or begin to discuss the pain we feel except in a natural language fixed at some moment of its historical development that inevitably colors our understanding (Sullivan, 1995). Except for the occasional child raised by wolves, no one experiences pain free from human mediation, including the mediation of our own past experiences. Even the pain of newborns bears the imprint of social structures (such as family or hospital) and of cultural environments (such as an ethnic group or nation) that necessarily surround, shape, and in-

fluence it. Interpretation need not be a conscious, deliberate act. Pain comes to us always already interpreted by the social world we inhabit. We express meanings, moreover, not just in articulate beliefs but through our emotions, behavior, and half-formed attitudes, much as a football player in shrugging off pain silently affirms cultural values associated with courage, sport, loyalty, and maleness. Even the functions of pain—the social or personal uses we make of it—are inseparable from meaning. The Latin root *poena* means punishment, and pain still carries potent links with penalty, discipline, and reproof. Drugs can relieve some kinds of pain while ignoring their implicit or explicit meanings, but meaning does not therefore go away: We merely circumvent it. In difficult cases of chronic pain, ignored beliefs may complicate or entirely undermine effective treatment.

This view is controversial. For three centuries, Western science has maintained the view that pain has no meaning at all. "I have a prejudice against pain," wrote gerontologist Ray Tallis (1991), "believing that, once it has done its job of warning us of danger, it is meaningless." Ironically, the belief that pain is a meaningless alarm bell remains a belief about the meaning of pain—albeit reductive, erroneous, and potentially harmful. Headaches may *seem* meaningless when two aspirin tablets can erase them, but ordinary pain is not identical with meaningless pain. Pain depends not only on neural circuits we share with rats and chimpanzees but also on the complex cognitive processes by which we interpret specific noxious stimuli in specific situations as, for example, ordinary. Recent research challenges the entrenched opinion that pain is merely the result of a neural impulse. Nociception, as Bromm (1995) puts it, is neither a necessary nor a sufficient condition for pain. Chapman (1995) argues that emotion is fundamental to the pain experience rather than a reaction to it. Pain in such revised versions—as it encompasses emotion, perception, and various culturally coded meanings—always implies more than the firing of neurons. The statement that pain has no meaning is more than false. It entangles patients in harm as, unknowingly, they continue to attribute tacit meanings to their pain while believing the erroneous line that pain is meaningless. Gatchel (1996) concludes that, as pain becomes more chronic, psychosocial variables play an increasingly dominant role in maintaining pain behavior and suffering. Effective treatment may require helping patients to confront the harmful meanings they have sealed within their pain.

Research shows that our beliefs have much to do with pain (DeGood & Shutty, 1992). Especially important are beliefs about cause, control, duration, outcome, and blame (Williams & Thorn, 1989; Jensen, Turner, Romano, & Karoly, 1991), as well as beliefs about the need to protect individual identity as it comes under assault by pain (Eccleston, Williams, & Rogers, 1997). Such beliefs affect not only chronic pain but also acute pain and even postoperative pain (Williams, Robinson, & Geisser, 1994; Williams, 1996). Moreover, beliefs about pain are often linked with powerful emotions: anger toward a negligent employer, fear of a catastrophe, hope for financial compensation, love for a hurting or caring spouse. Patients function better who believe they have some control over their pain, who believe in the value of medical services, who believe that family members care for them, and who believe that they are not severely disabled (Jensen & Karoly, 1992). Specific pain beliefs can predict pain intensity (Williams & Keefe, 1991). Shutty, DeGood, and Tuttle (1990),

in a study of 100 patients, show that specific pain beliefs even correlate with treatment outcomes.

In short, pain specialists have been expanding our knowledge of the role played by cognition—which includes meaning—at least since the time Sternbach edited *The Psychology of Pain* (1978). (See also second edition, Sternbach, 1986.) Numerous recent studies explore cognitive influences on pain (Turk, 1996), and such studies strongly suggest that paying attention to meaning and beliefs can have therapeutic benefit in helping to shape individual coping styles. For some researchers, attention to meaning and beliefs ultimately demands revision of the standard biomedical (or disease) model that interprets pain as a meaningless alarm bell, pointing to the need for a new model that we might call, among other names, biocultural (Morris, 1995).

The alarm theory—a version of Descartes's mechanistic analogy that describes pain impulses traveling from the periphery to the brain as if someone pulled on a rope and rang a bell at the other end—ignores biology. Pain, it turns out, is a very poor reporting system (Wall & Jones, 1991). Some fatal diseases reach a crisis long before the alarm goes off, whereas in other cases a feather's touch can trigger nonstop agony. Moreover, pain is a signal we can disarm through discipline or will, as religious mystics and yogis do. Some crucial body parts have no wiring for pain. Brain tissue has all the nociceptors of a grapefruit. The presence or absence of nociceptors is ultimately beside the point. Loeser (1991) in effect summarizes the implications of much recent research on the importance of mind and cognition when he asserts: "The brain is the organ responsible for all pain" (p. 215). "All sensory phenomena, including nociception," he adds, "can be altered by conscious or unconscious mental processes" (p. 216). Or, as my argument (Morris, 1991) put it both literally and metaphorically in describing—throughout human history—the importance of meaning in pain, pain is always in your head.

We do not yet possess a model of pain that fully accounts for the complex role played by meaning and consciousness, but the evidence in favor of such a model is fast accumulating. At the Baylor College of Medicine, 100 paid volunteers were told that the shock they would receive from an electrical stimulator might possibly produce a headache (Bayer, Baer, & Early, 1991). Researchers did not explain that the stimulator, a sham, emitted nothing beyond a low humming sound. The result? Fifty percent of the volunteers reported pain. Chronic low back pain often proves impossible to trace to an organic lesion, such as a prolapsed (or "slipped") disk. Most adults who complain of back pain have lumbar disk disease, but so do many adults without complaints (Jensen et al., 1994). In America, the long-term functioning of patients treated for back pain is similar, whether doctors prescribe medication and bed rest or emphasize self-care and education (Von Korff, Barlow, Cherkin, & Deyo, 1994). The belief that pain is a reliable alarm system justifies countless unnecessary surgeries (the covert belief: "pain means I need an operation"); however, it cannot begin to explain why the two strongest signs predicting that an American worker will develop chronic back pain are job dissatisfaction and unsatisfactory social relations in the workplace (Bigos et al., 1991; Dwyer & Raftery, 1991). It is as if the backs of Americans were wired directly into the sociocultural environment.

Although the role of cultural influences on pain is increasingly acknowledged (Streltzer, 1997), we need an understanding of socioeconomic and religious meanings that looks beyond individual psychology and beyond environmental forces that are restricted mainly to the narrow circle of family or workplace. Pain beliefs reflect shared values and understandings that circulate throughout a specific culture or subculture. One study compared American patients suffering from pain with a group of similar patients in Japan. Japanese patients proved significantly less impaired in psychological, social, vocational, and avocational functioning (Brena, Sanders, & Motoyama, 1990). Low back pain, it appears, means something very different in Japan than in America. In America, it often means that you are thought to be disabled, an official status that may require medical certification and bring a disability payment. It is not clear what low back pain means in Japan, but whatever the eventual explanation—perhaps as basic as the difference between believing oneself disabled and believing oneself impaired—Americans should take it seriously.

It matters greatly how our cultures instruct us, openly or covertly, to think about pain, and the instructions differ greatly. England in the 18th and 19th centuries considered gout—now understood as a congenital form of arthritis—an affliction saturated with moral meaning, in the way that many today regard venereal disease. Gout was a cultural marker, a sign associated with the luxurious lifestyles of the aristocracy and idle rich, as reflected in a lithograph by the English satirist George Cruickshank (1792–1878) (Figure 8.1). The caricatured devil (modestly clad in accordance with

pre-Victorian sensibilities) reflects a weakening of the theological traditions linking pain with divine punishment. In this case, the well-appointed parlor and abundant food, including an exotic pineapple, suggest that pain is now the secular penalty for upper-class self-indulgence. In contrast with the indoor world of gout, the Sakhalin Ainu of Japan suffer from "bear headaches" that resemble the heavy steps of a bear, from "deer headaches" that resemble the lighter steps of a deer, and from the self-explanatory "woodpecker headaches" (Kleinman, Brodwin, Good, & Good, 1992). A strictly biomedical account would hold that pain is pain, no matter what culture it occurs in. Yet headache pain that Americans attribute to stressful lives is not exactly identical with pain that the Sakhalin Ainu experience within an animistic culture in which bear and deer belong to the same spirit realm inhabited by gods, ancestors, and demonic forces. The biology of headache pain may be very similar, but the experience and meaning are worlds apart.

There is no end to the differences uncovered in cross-cultural studies of pain. Anthropologists have long recognized that adolescent rites of passage include pain as a by-product, but Morinis (1985) argues that such pain plays a "central role" in accomplishing the purposes of the initiation. The Bariba people of West Africa, for example, directly link the behavior of young men during painful ritual circumcision to social concepts of shame and honor (Sargent, 1984). Melzack (1973) introduced into discussions of pain the now-familiar and outlawed fertility rites of India, in which young men bless the fields while suspended from flesh-piercing hooks. The traditional Sun Dance of some Native American tribes—where pierced dancers (tied to a ceremonial pole with thongs slipped through cuts in the chest) dance for hours to tear their flesh and break free—also makes pain central to an ordeal in which culture-wide meaning is paramount. Beyond their various ritual meanings, such practices help to emphasize the malleable quality of human pain. Even the mysterious placebo effect—although researchers can replicate it in animals through conditioned reflexes—depends among humans on cultural beliefs that attribute medical power to some specific objects and practices but not to others (Morris, 1997). The power of culturally shaped beliefs, values, and emotions helps explain how pain is subtly reshaped in our own health-managed, whiplash, welfare-state environment. Financial compensation, for example, is well known to complicate treatment for pain (Mendelson, 1992; Guest

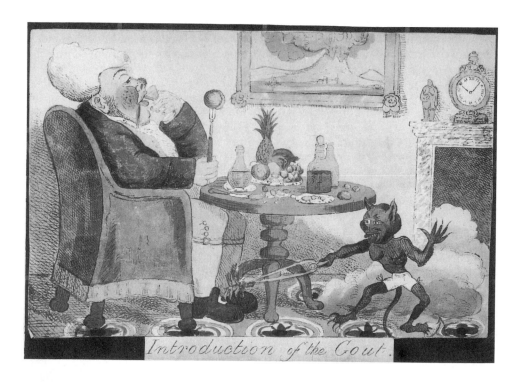

FIGURE 8.1. George Cruickshank. *Introduction of the Gout.* Colored lithograph. 1818. Wellcome Institute Library, London.

& Drummond, 1992). Such are among the adult rites of passage in the West.

The sociocultural and religious meanings of pain invite various forms of study, from anthropological analysis of a specific group (say, Sikhs living in Los Angeles) to vast historical surveys. Medical historian Roy Porter (1994) focuses on a selection of changing historical attitudes toward pain in Western culture, whereas Anderson and Anderson (1994) examine non-Western cultural practices that range from the self-immolation of widows in India to trance-induced surgical anesthesia in Brazil. Other studies throw indirect light on the cultural meanings of pain. Rubin (1976) looks at the conflicts and difficulties endemic among working-class families; Foucault (1977) traces the rejection of corporal punishment as a method of social control; Scarry (1985) offers a rich meditation on pain as underwriting acts of creation or destruction; Rey (1995) describes the historical relation among theories of pain, scientific research, and clinical treatment; and Roy (1992) reviews research into the social context of the chronic pain patient. As such diverse studies suggest, any approach to the meaning of pain will be fragmented

and arbitrary. My preference is to examine sociocultural and religious meanings as they help us consider three issues especially relevant to contemporary pain medicine: suffering, politics, and undertreatment.

RELIGION AND PAIN: THE PROBLEM OF SUFFERING

Almost all major religions address human suffering (Bowker, 1970), but many also address pain, directly or indirectly. The crucial point is that even within a single religion sharp variations exist, both across time and across doctrinal divisions. In pagan thought, at least as far back as the time of Homer, pain was believed to originate with the gods. Although the immediate cause might be a sword or spear, pain was understood as sent by the gods, like the twin serpents dispatched to punish the Trojan priest Laocoön. Pain to the pagan was not a matter of nerves and inner organs, topics on which the ancient Greeks were notoriously vague, but an affliction sent by the gods: It came from outside, like the arrows of Apollo, in punishment or in fulfillment of fate. In Sophocles' tragedy *Philoctetes*, the Greek hero suffers so horribly from a festering snake bite that his friends abandon him on the way to Troy. No one offers a medical explanation of his pain. It is understood rather as a direct result of his crime in violating the sanctuary of a powerful goddess. In his worst episodes of pain, Philoctetes acts as if under assault by an unseen force, much like the science fiction tradition of human bodies invaded by invisible aliens. Although the writings of Hippocrates initiate a far different analysis that points to an eventual scientific account, situating pain within a context of diet, symptoms, and physician–patient relations, a god or an exorcist (not a doctor) is what Philoctetes needs. Obligingly, the demigod Hercules descends at the end of the play to impose a resolution on events that pain has otherwise knotted into intractable tragedy.

Christian thinkers have found numerous, often contradictory, meanings in pain. Pain, for example, can be the result of original sin, a foretaste of damnation, a means of beatific vision, a punishment, a trial, or a sign of divine favor. Medieval Catholicism put major emphasis on the physical suffering of Jesus, a vivid iconography that calls attention to the mystery of a god who took on the pain-prone flesh of man. Later, illustrating the changes in theological temper, the Dutch Protestant engraver Anthonie Wierix (1552–1624) depicts pain as a tool of the devil, no caricature this time, who with his sharp tongs seeks to afflict the believer's heart and turn it away from God (Figure 8.2). Pain here is also depicted as a torment awaiting the soul that heeds the worldly allure of wealth, lust, and power (personified in a richly dressed woman). Several centuries later, in a very different Christian interpretation, Dorothy Wordsworth (1832/1987) describes pain—especially female, domestic pain (Meiners, 1993)—as a wound that God inflicts, lovingly, to humble and to discipline the restless spirit:

> Sickness and sorrow, grief and pain
> Are precious to the humbled soul
> For Mercy wounds with pitying love,
> That can all wayward thoughts control.

Wierix sees pain as an instrument of the devil to turn the soul from God; Wordsworth sees it as an instrument of God to turn the soul from wayward thoughts. These almost opposite views highlight merely two variants in the long history of Christian meditations on the meaning of pain.

Almost all world religions—from Islam and Judaism to Hinduism and Buddhist thought—explore variations in the meaning of pain. The contrasts can grow dizzying: Pain is at some times a means of redemption, at others an absolute evil. A full study would require a treatise in comparative religion, but what matters here is a recognition that theological beliefs can function as (or interfere with) coping mechanisms. The woman who views her pain as "precious" has an incentive to bear it but perhaps also to retain it. The man who views his pain as an instrument of the devil has an incentive to resist it but may also experience the terror of a diabolic attack. Many patients hold religious beliefs bearing directly on the experience of pain, including beliefs that cause them to reject drugs. Treatment that disregards such beliefs overlooks relevant data as surely as if it ignored pulse and respiration. Religious beliefs about pain,

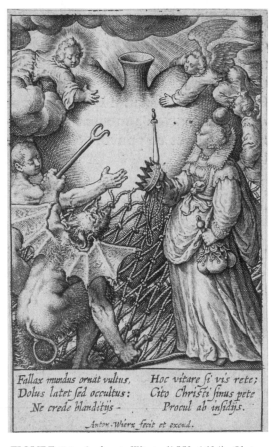

Fallax mundus ornat vultus,
Dolus latet sed occultus:
Ne crede blanditijs —

Hoc vitare si vis rete;
Cito Christi sinus pete
Procul ab insidijs.

Anton. Wierx fecit et excud.

FIGURE 8.2. Anthonie Wierix (1552–1624). *Christ preserves the believer's heart from false worldly decoration, captivity, and pain.* Engraving. Wellcome Institute Library, London.

however, offer more than important information about particular patients. Many religions link pain with a vast and encompassing area that medicine tends to flee: the problem of suffering.

Western medicine for years has delegated (or relegated) suffering to the pastor and chaplain, no doubt because religious language about suffering differs strikingly from the more comfortable scientific, biomedical discourse on pain. The Four Noble Truths of Buddhism, for example, begin with the stark assertion that suffering exists. Unlike medicine, Buddhism takes suffering as the primary fact that must be addressed, and it is in this far wider sense that the Buddha appears to his immediate disciples as a doctor (Danto, 1972). All truth and all remedies, in Buddhism, begin with the fact of suffering. There is much to be learned from this perspective. Suffering and pain are of course conceptually distinct—we can suffer without pain, or be in pain without suffering—but in practice they often overlap and prove inseparable. Once the almost exclusive property of religion, a knowledge of suffering is slowly finding a place within contemporary pain medicine.

What help can religious discussions of suffering offer to pain medicine? First, religious views of suffering reinforce the importance of meaning. Suffering is rarely understood as meaningless affliction. Second, they emphasize the spiritual dimension of human experience. Suffering has something to do with the realm of mind and spirit that Descartes so influentially and disastrously separated from a knowledge of pain. Third, they insist on the need to look beyond anatomy and physiology. The Second Noble Truth of Buddhism asserts that the cause of suffering is human "craving" (which might translate loosely as unfulfilled desire). From a Buddhist perspective, an account of suffering that fails to consider unfulfilled desire cannot address the deepest sources of human affliction. Fourth, religious views of suffering remind us that the tools and techniques of modern pain medicine are often designed to yield quantifiable data. A pain medicine attuned to suffering must invent new tools and techniques. It may at times find music therapy more powerful than analgesics, quality-of-life measures more important than algometers. Finally, religious views remind us that suffering is always more than a private matter between the individual and God. It involves other people (spouse, child, parent, friend, neighbor, boss) and often exists within the context of larger social and historical actions, much as victims of the Nazi Holocaust suffered within the encompassing, intersecting narratives of communities, nations, races, and peoples.

The most important change in recent discussions of suffering is this emphasis on social and cultural contexts. Cassell (1991) argued that suffering constituted a threat to the integrity or wholeness of personhood—as redefined by the networks of one's significant social relationships. Cherney, Coyle, and Foley (1994) apply and extend a similar conception to the specific experience of the advanced cancer patient. Meanwhile, from the perspective of anthropology, Kleinman, Das, and Lock (1997) edit a collection that explores what they call "social suffering," a concept that embraces essays on Holocaust testimony, political widowhood in South Africa, and the role of Maoism in modern China. As such work suggests, suffering is always more than the private and personal existential experience that influential modern thinkers have led us to consider it. Chapman and Gavrin (1993) make a good start at sketching a biology of suffering, but they rightly insist that a biological account alone is insufficient. The recent emphasis on public, shared, social dimensions of suffering offers pain specialists an opportunity to enter into a discussion—with direct benefit to patients—that no longer need be an exclusive topic of religious discourse.

Gustavo Gutiérrez (1973; 1987), the Peruvian founder of Liberation Theology, gives another turn to the idea that individual pain and suffering make sense only within a social context. Liberation Theology asserts as a founding principle that Christianity recovers its true vocation in a concern for the poor. Poverty, however, is for Gutiérrez not a matter of income. In the cramped Lima slums where he carries on his work as a priest, Gutiérrez sees systematic social injustice. The poor, in an age-old resignation, often understand their misery as God's will, but Gutiérrez sees rather the oppression of the weak by a wealthy and powerful elite (including at times leaders of his own Roman Catholic Church). God's will, for Gutiérrez, includes the directive that we oppose injustice and defend the defenseless. Thus the suffering and pain that occupy a major place in his writing are not understood as medical problems. The biomedical account of tissue damage, from his point of view, remains willfully blind to the larger social narrative of oppression that creates the pain and suffering of the poor. It is not opioids he seeks but a society in which the systematic oppression of the poor gives way to justice. Gutiérrez is unwelcome in certain circles within the Church, and his example shows how serious attention to sociocultural and religious meanings could lead away from the clinic and onto the barricades. Clinicians may decide to ignore sources of pain and suffering that fall outside the expertise of the clinic, but such a decision will be uninformed if it ignores what Gutiérrez and other religious leaders (from Gandhi to Martin Luther King, Jr.) tell us. The clinic ultimately does not exist in a neutral space of research and treatment but within the social world which its patients also inhabit.

CULTURE AND MEANING: THE POLITICS OF PAIN

The threshold at which laboratory-induced pain becomes unbearable varies among different cultures (Melzack & Wall, 1988), and culture, as we have seen, also influences the highly variable meanings we attribute to pain. Painful (sometimes fatal) clitoridectomies inflicted upon girls in some parts of Africa suggest how far meanings embraced by one culture may prove alien or incomprehensible to another. In popular songs, Western societies relentlessly associate pain with bourgeois romance: hurts so good, as one rocker puts it. Medicine normally takes no notice of such meanings, even in such bizarre cases as those of the sexual underground of sadomasochism or of the teenage girls who repeatedly cut their skin. Indeed, under normal circumstances meaning seems so invisible that it is simply disregarded.

Pain and Ethnicity

Although the meanings attributed to pain often remain tacit, implicit, and nearly invisible, there is good evidence of distinctive ethnic variations in the experience of pain (Zborowski, 1969; Wolff, 1985; Greenwald, 1991; Bates, Edwards, & Anderson, 1993), including variations in the meanings that pain comes to bear. We do not know enough, however, about how ethnicity and nationality influence pain. When asked about basic activities and mood, cancer patients in China, in the United States, in the Philippines, and in France showed marked similarities in how they responded to pain at moderate levels of intensity, suggesting the value of simple standardized scales for measuring pain across culturally different groups (Cleeland et al., 1996). On the other hand, the MMPI reveals differences among pain patients that follow ethnic lines (Nelson, Novy, Averill, & Berry, 1996), and ethnic differences—or, rather, the beliefs that a physician holds about ethnicity—have been shown to affect the amount of narcotic prescribed for patient-controlled analgesia in a postoperative population (Ng, Dimsdale, Rollnick, & Shapiro, 1996). In increasingly multicultural societies, ethnic stereotypes are more than usually inaccurate, especially when applied to second- or third-generation immigrants. Cultural contexts can override beliefs associated with ethnic identity, as Furnham and Malik (1994), for example, showed in a study that compares middle-aged native Britons with middle-aged Asian immigrants to Britain. In their beliefs about depression, middle-aged Asian immigrants differed significantly not only from native Britons but also from young Asian immigrants. In effect, older Asian immigrants preserved the beliefs of their homeland, whereas younger immigrants assimilated the cultural attitudes and practices of native Britons. We need similar cross-generational studies to show how far a majority culture can override pain beliefs associated with ethnic minorities.

The cultural power to impose or to override beliefs is implicitly and sometimes overtly political. Politics, as I will use the term, has to do with social power. Asad (1983) described how pain served in medieval judicial torture as a means of defining truth, but Scarry (1985) argues that torture today employs pain less to extract truth or information—since interrogation is often absent or irrelevant—than to demonstrate the absolute power of whatever regime or terrorist group employs it. Whipping or maiming is still a legal punishment in some non-Western nations, noticed mainly when inflicted on Westerners. For centuries, however, the infliction of pain was a legitimate expression of royal or national power in Europe, and the whipping post remained an official (if seldom used) punishment in the state of Delaware until 1972. Yet the political implications of pain often operate in subtler or unnoticed ways. Kleinman (1992) described how survivors of China's Cultural Revolution used chronic pain both as a rhetoric of complaint and as a means of resisting the diffused control of the Communist state. Contemporary statistics on spouse abuse and on child abuse suggest that the most insidious politics of pain has simply shifted its location to the veiled interior of the American family.

A politics of pain holds clear implications for medicine when we consider the worldwide distribution of morphine. In Mexico the likelihood that a cancer patient will receive morphine for pain is almost zero, whereas patients in developed English-speaking countries—Britain, Canada, and the United States—get, at least by contrast, generous amounts (Figure 8.3). Although morphine is not expensive in Mexico, its use accounts for only 1% of worldwide consumption. The reason for this sparing medical usage has much to do with problems concerning international traffic in illicit drugs. Dr. Allende Pérez, director of the pain clinic at Mexico's National Cancer Institute, says that "Mexican bureaucrats would rather just restrict the use of morphine altogether and avoid problems" (DePalma, 1996). In effect, the action of bureaucrats carries an implicit meaning: that the pain of Mexican patients is less important than political pressures (largely applied by the United States) to restrict drug trafficking. Mexican patients suffering from cancer may not know that their unrelieved pain bears a political meaning, but it does. It is worth remembering that morphine is least available in the developing countries such as Mexico that will see an enormous increase in population during the next decades.

The history of pain suggests that it is normally the least powerful groups in any culture whose pain is disregarded, often with scientific rationale. In England the insane were locked up naked in dank cells by 18th-century doctors who believed that the mad were insensitive to pain. Laborers were long thought to possess "coarse" nerves that freed them from the pain felt by upper-class men and women with more "refined" nervous systems. In 19th-century America, black women were the subject of medical experiments conducted without anesthesia by doctors who argued that blacks do not feel pain. In the middle of the 20th century, surgery on infants was conducted without anesthesia partly because surgeons mistakenly believed that undeveloped nervous systems prevented infants from experiencing pain. Unfortunately, groups in power can find whatever reasons they need for believing that people without power do not feel the pain of painful events. We are assured that the botched executions of recent years—one sent flames from the head of an electrocuted man—represent painless technical glitches. A skeptic would see condemned prisoners as simply one more powerless minority whose pain is unacknowledged or scientifically denied because, socially, it does not count.

Any serious inquiry into the sociocultural meanings of pain needs to ask what we know about groups currently on the margins of power: women,

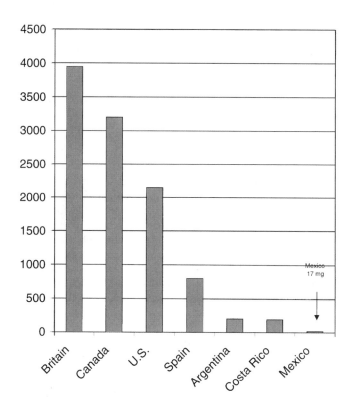

FIGURE 8.3. Morphine usage. Amount of morphine prescribed in 1994, in milligrams per 100,000 people. Source: University of Wisconsin Pain Research Center.

blacks, gays, children, the elderly, the dying. It is not surprising that knowledge is scarce. Evidence from Medicare beneficiaries shows that race and income have "substantial effects" on mortality and on the use of medical services (Gornick et al., 1996). We have little knowledge, however, about pain in black communities. One study in North Carolina found that only 51% of blacks—compared with 73% of whites—saw a physician after chest pain (Strogatz, 1990), which suggests a relationship among race, beliefs, and access to medical care. What pain means to blacks in America, however, especially to blacks from differing socioeconomic groups, is a matter of guesswork. At a metropolitan university hospital, I have heard passionate discussion among staff about blacks with sickle cell disease who come to the emergency room seeking pain relief. Some white staff members reportedly interpret such requests as a covert effort to obtain narcotics for sale or for illicit use. If true, what sickle cell pain means to poor urban blacks is that they come under automatic suspicion. An open discussion of this issue seems taboo. It is clear we need serious studies to know whether and how the racism still prevalent in America affects medical treatment for pain among minority groups.

Pain and Gender

Women make up the majority of chronic pain patients. It is unclear whether this gender imbalance means that women face greater risk of chronic pain or simply use health care services more often (Weir, Browne, Tunks, Gafni, & Roberts, 1996). Recent research has shown that women have a distinctive biological relationship to pain: The class of kappa-opioids, for example, works twice as well for women as for men (Gear et al., 1996). Migraine affects about 6% of men and 15% to 18% of women (Lipton & Stewart, 1997), and the diminished frequency of migraines during pregnancy suggests to some researchers a connection with estrogen. Biological differences between men and women, however, do not completely account for asymmetries in the experience of pain. Unruh (1996) in a major review concludes that women are more likely than men to experience a variety of recurrent pains, to report more severe levels of pain, more frequent pain, and pain of longer duration. The presentation of pain in a health care setting, the study contends, is affected in multiple and complex ways by "gender differences in the construction of meaning" (p. 158).

How might the meaning of pain differ for women? The prominent role of women as over-extended caregivers in chaotic families might help account for their risk of the pain associated with what is sometimes called somatization disorder. (Robins et al., 1984, put the female/male ratio at 10:1.) Coryell and Norten (1981) and Morrison (1989) observed that women diagnosed with somatization disorder are more likely to report childhood sexual abuse than are women with mood disorders. Another study found a significantly higher rate of severe lifetime sexual trauma in women with irritable bowel syndrome than in women with the clearly organic disorder inflammatory bowel disease (Walker, Katon, Roy-Byrne, Jemelka, & Russo, 1993). Women are certainly overrepresented among battered spouses, a circumstance in which pain often coincides with emotional trauma. The significance of gender in the experience of pain, however, is clearest in retrospect. The unequal social position of women is doubtless reflected in the historical Western epidemic of hysteria, in which pain—often without a clear organic source—was a prominent symptom. What did it mean for a 19th-century woman to experience pain of uncertain origin? It meant that male doctors automatically regarded her as hysterical (that is, weak, overemotional, perhaps mendacious, and certainly prone to imaginary ailments). It is not entirely clear what it means to be a woman today suffering from pain of uncertain origin, but beliefs associated with gender differences continue to affect clinical decisions concerning pain (Vallerand, 1995).

Pain in Children and AIDS Patients

There have been large gains recently in the understanding and treatment of pain among two neglected minority groups: children and patients with AIDS. Pediatric pain units have made special efforts to overcome inherent limitations in language skills and in experience common among children. They have also begun to address the special fears that children feel. McGrath (1993) has emphasized that meaning and emotion play a distinctive role in the child's experience of pain, but we need to know more about the possible failures of meaning: moments when pain seems not just inexpressible but incomprehensible. The situation of patients with AIDS is somewhat similar. The social stigma widely and early attached to AIDS—regarded as a disease not only of gays but also of (impoverished black) Haitians and of (illicit) intravenous drug users—indelibly marked the experience of patients (Herek & Capitanio, 1993). Now heterosexual women make up an increasing percentage of AIDS patients, and women face the added burden of living with AIDS in a culture that mistakenly thinks it is a disease mainly affecting gay males. Pain intensity among ambulatory AIDS patients in New York City is associated with gender and race (Breitbart, McDonald, et al., 1996), which clearly suggests sociocultural forces at work. Patients with AIDS also face an increased likelihood of pain-related suffering. Here too we need to know more about how sociocultural meanings linked with AIDS—from deserved misfortune to divine punishment for sin—affect individual patients and about where their experience of pain may at times run up against the limits of what is comprehensible.

Pain in the Elderly

Old age holds pejorative, if not actually stigmatized, meanings in a youth-oriented consumer culture in which individual worth is often equated with good looks, vigor, and economic productivity (Featherstone & Wernick, 1995). Although the meanings of old age have grown somewhat confused as advertisers now court elderly consumers by marketing TV images of golden-age sex and adventure, confused meanings hold a potential to affect the distinctive pain of the elderly no less than pejorative meanings do. The groundbreaking book *Pain in the Elderly* includes a helpful chapter by Roy, Thomas, and Cook (1996) on sociocultural influences, but the subject cries out for additional research. During pauses in a radio interview, the engineer told me that her elderly parents had nearly wrecked their long marriage over pain. Her mother believed that pain signified serious health problems, whereas her father regarded it as a nuisance of aging. Her mother worried about her own pain and about her husband's, too (which irritated him); her father dismissed not only his pain but also his wife's (which outraged her). He thought she was a nag, she thought he was a brute, and the war of contrary meanings dragged on. The erroneous belief that pain has no meaning cannot explain the dynamics of their sabotaged relationship. It also cannot give us any information about the difficulties and losses unique to old age that may complicate the pain of elderly patients.

THE MEANINGS OF UNDERTREATMENT

There is no more powerless, marginalized individual in American culture than the dying patient. It is thus hardly shocking to learn the results of the multimillion-dollar SUPPORT (SUPPORT Principal Investigators, 1995) study of seriously ill hospitalized patients. According to family members, 50% of conscious patients who died in the hospital spent at least half their time in moderate to severe pain. After investigators spent 6 months improving communication among the medical staffs, a follow-up study showed no improvement in the treatment of pain. Specialists may rightly criticize a measurement of pain that relies on family members rather than on patients, but by any measure the lack of improvement is disturbing. The American Pain Society Quality of Care Committee (1995) reports a similar absence of improvement despite "decades of effort" spent providing clinicians with information about analgesics. Among ambulatory patients with AIDS, Breitbart and his colleagues (Breitbart, Rosenfeld, et al., 1996) find an "alarming degree" of undertreatment for pain. The dying of course are not singled out for neglect: Atkinson (1996) discusses the long-standing undertreatment of pain in children and infants. We must ask, however, what it might mean that in the face of regular warnings—and despite plentiful analgesics—health care workers continue to undertreat patients with pain, including even the vulnerable population of dying patients who will end their lives in needless, valueless suffering.

French historian Roselyn Rey (1995), noting a general impression that medicine does not sufficiently take pain into account, observes that health care workers are subject to the same political, religious, and ideological currents as the rest of society. We must thus question, she argues, the social conditions under which medicine is practiced. This approach seems sound. Health professionals work in an environment in which decisions are made under sociocultural pressures that often have little to do with the well-being of an individual patient. Joranson (1994) reviews evidence suggesting that health care reinbursement policies (especially "caps" on prescription drugs) limit access to pain medications. Hill (1993) has argued that federal and state drug enforcement agencies—along with state licensing and disciplinary boards—inhibit adequate pain treatment by means of the fear they inspire among health care professionals over unwarranted discipline and prosecution. Half of the Wisconsin physicians who responded to a survey incorrectly answered questions on the regulation of controlled substances and indicated they would alter their prescribing practice due to concerns about regulatory scrutiny (Weissmann, Joranson, & Hopwood, 1991). It remains to be seen, however, whether new reimbursement policies, new laws, and new attitudes toward licensing, disciplinary action, and drug enforcement can reverse habitual medical undertreatment, which is only in part the result of insurance, laws, and government.

One possible benefit of renewed attention to the sociocultural and religious meanings of pain would be an emphasis on the ethical—rather than merely on the regulatory or clinical—implications of undertreatment. Religious and social traditions have long recognized that pain raises serious moral issues, yet this recognition has not found adequate expression within clinical medicine or within its companion discipline of bioethics. While Hill (1995) rightly focuses on the institutional guidelines and review processes needed to combat the long-standing neglect and medical myths that prevent patients from receiving adequate pain medication, such pragmatic institutional changes are not enough. Rich (1997) argues that the undertreatment of pain also constitutes a major ethical failure: a failure that bioethics has so far been unable to recognize and to address. Fortunately, failure to address the moral dimensions of undertreatment may have started to face challenge. Edmund D. Pellegrino (1998), distinguished physician, educator, and philosopher of medicine, has recently insisted, in a discussion of emerging ethical issues in palliative care, that not to relieve pain optimally is "tantamount to ethical and legal malpractice" (p. 1521).

Meanwhile, the conditions under which medicine is practiced today include, as Rey has indicated, a context of explicit and implicit beliefs that health care workers share with their surrounding culture. Sullivan and Loeser (1992) have argued that if physicians certify or rate a disability, the act of fixing and defining disability at a specific level can "convey a message" to the patient that rehabilitation is over and that an impairment is considered permanent. Our surrounding culture conveys implicit messages or meanings not only about disability but also about certain classes of drugs. Opiophobia is the name that Morgan (1989) gives to the widespread American fear of narcotic pain relievers. The Mayday Fund (1993) surveyed 1,000 American adults and found that people would rather bear pain than take action to relieve it. A full 82% of Mayday respondents agreed with the erroneous statement that "It is easy to get addicted to pain medication." Americans believe, according to the same survey, both that analgesics are overused and that more should be done to alleviate pain. The confusions and errors radiate in many directions but are important finally because—in adding up to a very mixed message about the importance of pain—they underlie and exonerate the continuing systemic medical acceptance of undertreatment.

What to do? Specialists must continue to educate colleagues about harmful and erroneous pain beliefs in order to change the culture of medicine. One neglected medical resource is nationwide public education—an effort to address a wider audience about cultural beliefs that directly and indirectly influence how we think about pain. Patients who know more about pain will be less prey to harmful myths. Medical staff who deal with well-informed patients—patients who know the minuscule odds of hospital addiction, who know the difference between addiction and dependence, who know their right to adequate pain relief—will be less likely to undertreat them. In a campaign that could be (I imagine) generously financed by the pharmaceutical industry, crucial facts about pain could be televised as public service announcements and prominently posted in medical settings. Especially important is recognition— by health care professionals and by the public—that pain is inseparable from the meanings we attribute to it. Today pain, like most symptoms, is automatically inscribed within a medical–scientific tradition that too often ignores the impact of meaning. Health care professionals need at least an acquaintance with the important nonmedical—sociocultural and religious—traditions through which meanings are historically constructed and deconstructed (Bruns, 1992). Such traditions influence both patients and the caregivers who seek to help them, with or without a knowledge of meanings.

ACKNOWLEDGMENTS

David Antin, "the black plague," (iii, lines 1-4), Selected Poems: 1963-1973. Selections from Selected Poems: 1963-1973: © 1991 by David Antin. "the black plague," Selected Poems: 1963-1973 (Los Angeles: Sun & Moon Press, 1991). Reprinted by permission.

Dorothy Wordsworth, "Lines Intended for Edith Southey's Album" (1832). Reprinted courtesy Wordsworth Trust, Dove Cottage, Grasmere, United Kingdom.

REFERENCES

American Pain Society Quality of Care Committee. (1995). Quality improvement guidelines for the treatment of acute pain and cancer pain. *Journal of the American Medical Association, 274*(23), 1874–1880.

Anderson, R. T., & Anderson, S. T. (1994). Culture and pain. In *The puzzle of pain* (pp. 120–138). (F. A. Djité-Bruce, Trans.) New York: Gordon & Breach Arts International.

Antin, D. (1991). *Selected poems: 1963–1973.* Los Angeles: Sun and Moon Press.

Asad, T. (1983). Notes on body pain and truth in medieval Christian ritual. *Economy and Society, 12*(3), 287–327.

Atkinson, L. (1996). Pain management for children and infants. *Contemporary Nurse, 5*(2), 64–70.

Bates, M. S., Edwards, W. T., & Anderson, K. O. (1993). Ethnocultural influences on variation in chronic pain perception. *Pain, 52*(1), 101–112.

Bayer, T., Baer, P. E., & Early, C. (1991). Situational and psychophysiological factors in psychologically induced pain. *Pain, 44*(1), 45–50.

Bigos, S. J., Battié, M. C., Spengler, D. M., Fisher, L. D., Fordyce, W. E., Hansson, T. H., Nachemson, A. L., & Wortley, M. D. (1991). A prospective study of work perceptions and psychosocial factors affecting the report of back injury. *Spine, 16*(1), 1–6.

Bowker, J. (1970). *Problems of suffering in religions of the world.* Cambridge: Cambridge University Press.

Breitbart, W., McDonald, M. V., Rosenfeld, B., Passik, S. D., Hewitt, D., Thaler, H., & Portenoy, R. K. (1996). Pain in ambulatory AIDS patients: I. Pain characteristics and medical correlates. *Pain, 68*(2–3), 315–321.

Breitbart, W., Rosenfeld, B. D., Passik, S. D., McDonald, M. V., Thaler, H., & Portenoy, R. K. (1996). The undertreatment of pain in ambulatory AIDS patients. *Pain, 65*(2–3), 243–249.

Brena, S. F., Sanders, S. H., & Motoyama, H. (1990). American and Japanese low back pain patients: Cross-cultural similarities and differences. *Clinical Journal of Pain, 6*(2), 118–124.

Bromm, B. (1995). Consciousness, pain, and cortical activity. In B. Bromm & J. D. Desmeldt (Eds.), *Pain and the brain: From nociception to cognition* (pp. 35–59). New York: Raven Press.

Bruns, G. L. (1992). *Hermeneutics ancient and modern.* New Haven: Yale University Press.

Cassell, E. J. (1991). *The nature of suffering and the goals of medicine.* New York: Oxford University Press.

Chapman, C. R. (1995). The affective dimension of pain: A model. In B. Bromm & J. D. Desmeldt (Eds.), *Pain and the brain: From nociception to cognition* (pp. 283–301). New York: Raven Press.

Chapman, C. R., & Gavrin, J. (1993). Suffering and its relationship to pain. *Journal of Palliative Care, 9*(2), 5–13.

Cherney, N. I., Coyle, N., & Foley, K. M. (1994). Suffering in the advanced cancer patient: A definition and taxonomy. *Journal of Palliative Care, 10*(2), 57–70.

Cleeland, C. S., Nakamura, Y., Mendoza, T. R., Edwards, K. R., Douglas, J., & Serlin, R. C. (1996). Dimensions of the impact of cancer pain in a four country sample: New information from multidimensional scaling. *Pain, 67*(2–3), 267–273.

Coryell, W., & Norten, S. G. (1981). Briquet's syndrome (somatization disorder) and primary depression: Comparison of background and outcome. *Comprehensive Psychiatry, 22*(3), 249–256.

Danto, A. (1972). *Mysticism and morality: Oriental thought and moral philosophy.* New York: Basic Books.

DeGood, D. E., & Shutty, M. S. (1992). Assessment of pain beliefs, coping, and self-efficacy. In D. C. Turk & R. Melzack (Eds.), *Handbook of pain assessment* (pp. 214–234). New York: Guilford Press.

DePalma, A. (1996, June 19). For Mexicans, pain relief is a medical and political issue. *New York Times,* p. A6.

Dwyer, T., & Raftery, A. E. (1991). Industrial accidents are produced by social relations of work: A sociological theory of industrial accidents. *Applied Ergonomics, 22*(3), 167–178.

Eccleston, C., Williams, A. C. de C., & Rogers, W. S. (1997). Patients' and professionals' understandings of the causes of chronic pain: Blame, responsibility and identity protection. *Social Science and Medicine, 45*(5), 699–709.

Featherstone, M., & Wernick, A. (1995). Introduction. In M. Featherstone & A. Wernick (Eds.), *Images of aging: Cultural representations of later life* (pp. 1–15). New York: Routledge.

Foucault, M. (1977). *Discipline and punish: The birth of the prison.* (A. Sheridan, Trans.) New York: Pantheon Books. (Original work published 1975)

Furnham, A., & Malik, R. (1994). Cross-cultural beliefs about "depression." *International Journal of Social Psychiatry, 40*(2), 106–123.

Gatchel, R. (1996). Psychological disorders and chronic pain: Cause-and-effect relationships. In R. J. Gatchel & D. C. Turk (Eds.), *Psychological approaches to pain management: A practitioner's handbook* (pp. 33–52). New York: Guilford Press.

Gear, R. W., Miaskowski, C., Gordon, N. C., Paul, S. M., Heller, P. H., & Levine, J. D. (1996). Kappa-opioids produce significantly greater analgesia in women than in men. *Nature Medicine, 2*(11), 1248–1250.

Gornick, M. E., Eggers, P. W., Reilly, T. W., Mentnech, R. M., Fitterman, L. K., Kucken, L. E., & Vladeck, B. C. (1996). Effects of race and income on mortality and use of services among medicare beneficiaries. *Journal of the American Medical Association, 335*(11), 791–799.

Greenwald, H. P. (1991). Interethnic differences in pain perception. *Pain, 44*(2), 157–163.

Guest, G. H., & Drummond, P. D. (1992). Effect of compensation on emotional state and disability in chronic back pain. *Pain, 48*(2), 125–130.

Gutierrez, G. (1973). *A theology of liberation.* (C. Inda and J. Eagleson, Trans.) Maryknoll, NY: Orbis Books. (Original work published 1971)

Gutiérrez, G. (1987). *On Job: God-talk and the suffering of the innocent* (M. J. O'Connell, Trans.). Maryknoll, NY: Orbis Books. (Original work published 1985)

Herek, G. M., & Capitanio, J. P. (1993). Public reactions to AIDS in the United States: A second decade of stigma. *American Journal of Public Health, 83*(4), 574–577.

Hill, C. S., Jr. (1993). The negative influence of licensing and disciplinary boards and drug enforcement agencies on pain treatment with opioid analgesics. *Journal of Pharmaceutical Care in Pain and Symptom Control, 1*(1), 43–62.

Hill, C. S., Jr. (1995). When will adequate pain treatment be the norm? *Journal of the American Medical Association, 274*(23), 1881–1882.

Jensen, M. C., Brant-Zawadzki, M. N., Obuchowski, N., Modic, M. T., Malkasian, D., & Ross, J. S. (1994). Magnetic resonance imaging of the lumbar spine in people without back pain. *New England Journal of Medicine, 331*(2), 69–73.

Jensen, M. P., & Karoly, P. (1992). Pain-specific beliefs, perceived symptom severity, and adjustment to chronic pain. *Clinical Journal of Pain, 8*(2), 123–130.

Jensen, M. P., Turner, J. A., Romano, J. M., & Karoly, P. (1991). Coping with chronic pain: A critical review of the literature. *Pain, 47*(3), 249–283.

Joranson, D. E. (1994). Are health-care reimbursement policies a barrier to acute and cancer pain management? *Journal of Pain and Symptom Management, 9*(4), 244–253.

Kleinman, A. (1992). Pain and resistance: The delegitimation and relegitimation of local worlds. In M.-J. D. Good, P. E. Brodwin, B. J. Good, & A. Kleinman (Eds.), *Pain as human experience: An anthropological perspective* (pp. 169–197). Berkeley, CA: University of California Press.

Kleinman, A., Brodwin, P. E., Good, B. J., & Good, M.-J. D. (1992). Pain as human experience: An introduction. In M.-J. D. Good, P. E. Brodwin, B. J. Good, & A. Kleinman (Eds.), *Pain as human experience: An anthropological perspective* (pp. 1–28). Berkeley, CA: University of California Press.

Kleinman, A., Das, V., & Lock, M. (1997). Introduction. *Social suffering* (pp. ix–xxvi). Berkeley, CA: University of California Press.

Lipton, R. B., & Stewart, W. F. (1997). Prevalence and impact of migraine. *Neurologic Clinics, 15*(1), 1–13.

Loeser, J. D. (1991). What is chronic pain? *Theoretical Medicine, 12*(3), 213–225.

Mayday Fund. (1993). *Presentation of findings.* Washington, DC: Mellman-Lazarus-Lake.

McGrath, P. A. (1993). Psychological aspects of pain perception. In N. L. Schechter, C. B. Berde, & M. Yaster (Eds.), *Pain in infants, children, and adolescents* (pp. 39–63). Baltimore: Williams & Wilkins.

Meiners, K. T. (1993). Reading pain and the feminine body in Romantic writing: The examples of Dorothy Wordsworth and Sara Coleridge. *Centennial Review, 37*(3), 487–512.

Melzack, R. (1973). *The puzzle of pain.* New York: Basic Books.

Melzack, R., & Wall, P. (1988). *The challenge of pain* (2nd ed.). New York: Viking Penguin.

Mendelson, G. (1992). Compensation and chronic pain. *Pain, 48*(2), 121–123.

Morgan, J. P. (1989). American opiophobia: Customary underutilization of opioid analgesics. In C. S. Hill, Jr., & W. S. Fields (Eds.), *Advances in pain research and therapy* (Vol. 11, pp. 181–189). New York: Raven Press.

Morinis, A. (1985). The ritual experience: Pain and the transformation of consciousness in ordeals of initiation. *Ethos, 13*(2), 150–174.

Morris, D. B. (1991). *The culture of pain.* Berkeley, CA: University of California Press.

Morris, D. B. (1995). Pain and its meaning: A biocultural model. In A. H. White & J. A. Schofferman (Eds.), *Spine care* (Vol. 1, pp. 496–508). St. Louis, MO: Mosby.

Morris, D. B. (1997). Placebo, pain, and belief: A biocultural model. In A. Harrington (Ed.), *The placebo effect: An interdisciplinary exploration* (pp. 187–207). Cambridge, MA: Harvard University Press.

Morrison, J. (1989). Childhood sexual histories of women with somatization disorder. *American Journal of Psychiatry, 146*(2), 239–241.

Nelson, D. V., Novy, D. M., Averill, P. M., & Berry, L. A. (1996). Ethnic comparability of the MMPI in pain patients. *Journal of Clinical Psychology, 52*(5), 485–497.

Ng, B., Dimsdale, J. E., Rollnick, J. D., & Shapiro, H. (1996). The effect of ethnicity on prescriptions for patient-controlled analgesia for post-operative pain. *Pain, 66*(1), 9–12.

Pellegrino, E. D. (1998). Emerging ethical issues in palliative care. *Journal of the American Medical Association, 279*(19), 1521–1522.

Porter, R. (1994). Pain and history in the western world. In *The puzzle of pain* (F. A. Djité-Bruce, Trans.) (pp. 98–119). New York: Gordon & Breach Arts International.

Rey, R. (1995). *The history of pain* (L. E. Wallace, J. A. Cadden, & S. W. Cadden, Trans.). Cambridge, MA: Harvard University Press. (Original work published 1993)

Rich, B. A. (1997). A legacy of silence: Bioethics and the culture of pain. *Journal of Medical Humanities, 18*(4), 233–259.

Robins, L. N., Helzer, J. E., Weissman, M. M., Orvaschel, H., Gruenberg, E., Burke, J. D., Jr., & Regier, D. A. (1984). Lifetime prevalence of specific psychiatric disorders in three sites. *Archives of General Psychiatry, 41*(10), 949–958.

Roy, R. (1992). *The social context of the chronic pain sufferer.* Toronto: University of Toronto Press.

Roy, R., Thomas, M., & Cook, A. (1996). Social context of elderly chronic pain patients. In B. R. Ferrell & B. A. Ferrell (Eds.), *Pain in the elderly* (pp. 111–117). Seattle: IASP Press.

Rubin, L. B. (1976). *Worlds of pain: Life in the working-class family.* New York: Basic Books.

Sargent, C. (1984). Between death and shame: Dimensions of pain in Bariba culture. *Social Science and Medicine, 19*(12), 1299–1304.

Scarry, E. (1985). *The body in pain: The making and unmaking of the world.* New York: Oxford University Press.

Shutty, M. S., Jr., DeGood, D. E., & Tuttle, D. H. (1990). Chronic pain patients' beliefs about their pain and treatment outcomes. *Archives of Physical Medicine and Rehabilitation, 71*(2), 128–132.

Sternbach, R. A. (Ed.). (1978). *The psychology of pain.* New York: Raven Press.

Sternbach, R. A. (Ed.). (1986). *The psychology of pain* (2nd ed.). New York: Raven Press.

Streltzer, J. (1997). Pain. In W.-S. Tseng & J. Streltzer (Eds.), *Culture and psychopathology: A guide to clinical assessment* (pp. 87–100). New York: Brunner/Mazel.

Strogatz, D. S. (1990). Use of medical care for chest pain: Differences between blacks and whites. *American Journal of Public Health, 80*(3), 290–294.

Sullivan, M. D. (1995). Pain in language: From sentience to sapience. *Pain Forum, 4*(1), 3–14.

Sullivan, M. D., & Loeser, J. D. (1992). The diagnosis of disability: Treating and rating disability in a pain clinic. *Archives of Internal Medicine, 152*(9), 1829–1835.

SUPPORT Principal Investigators. (1995). A controlled trial to improve care for seriously ill hospitalized patients. *Journal of the American Medical Association, 274*(20), 1591–1598.

Tallis, R. (1991, May 1). Terrors of the body. *Times (London) Literary Supplement*, pp. 3–4.

Turk, D. C. (1996). Biopsychosocial perspective on chronic pain. In R. J. Gatchel & D. C. Turk (Eds.), *Psychological approaches to pain management: A practitioner's handbook* (pp. 3–32). New York: Guilford Press.

Unruh, A. M. (1996). Gender variations in clinical pain experience. *Pain, 65*(2–3), 123–167.

Vallerand, A. H. (1995). Gender differences in pain. *Image: Journal of Nursing Scholarship, 27*(3), 235–237.

Von Korff, M., Barlow, W., Cherkin, D., & Deyo, R. A. (1994). Effects of practice style in managing back pain. *Annals of Internal Medicine, 121*(3), 187–195.

Walker, E. A., Katon, W. J., Roy-Byrne, P. R., Jemelka, R. P., & Russo, J. (1993). Histories of sexual victimization in patients with irritable bowel syndrome or inflammatory bowel disease. *American Journal of Psychiatry, 150*(10), 1502–1506.

Wall, P. D., & Jones, M. (1991). *Defeating pain: The war against a silent epidemic*. New York: Plenum Press.

Weir, R., Browne, G., Tunks, E., Gafni, A., & Roberts, J. (1996). Gender differences in psychosocial adjustment to chronic pain and expenditures for health care services used. *Clinical Journal of Pain, 12*(4), 277–290.

Weissmann, D. E., Joranson, D. E., & Hopwood, M. B. (1991). Wisconsin physicians' knowledge and attitudes about opioid analgesic regulations. *Wisconsin Medical Journal, 90*(12), 671–675.

Williams, D. A. (1996). Acute pain management. In R. J. Gatchel & D. C. Turk (Eds.), *Psychological approaches to pain management: A practitioner's handbook* (pp. 55–77). New York: Guilford Press.

Williams, D. A., & Keefe, F. J. (1991). Pain beliefs and the use of cognitive-behavioral coping strategies. *Pain, 46*(1), 185–190.

Williams, D. A., Robinson, M. E., & Geisser, M. E. (1994). Pain beliefs: Assessment and utility. *Pain, 59*(1), 71–78.

Williams, D. A., & Thorn, B. E. (1989). An empirical assessment of pain beliefs. *Pain, 36*(3), 351–358.

Wolff, B. B. (1985). Ethnocultural factors influencing pain and illness behavior. *Clinical Journal of Pain, 1*(1), 23–30.

Wordsworth, D. (1987). Lines intended for Edith Southey's album. In S. M. Levin, *Dorothy Wordsworth and Romanticism* (pp. 215–218). New Brunswick, NJ: Rutgers University Press. (Original work published 1832)

Zborowski, M. (1969). *People in pain*. San Francisco: Jossey-Bass.

Chapter 9

Medicolegal Aspects of Pain: The Nature of Psychological Opinion in Cases of Personal Injury

CHRIS J. MAIN

As the Western world has become increasingly litigious, events previously attributed to misfortune or bad luck are no longer accepted with equanimity. This trend has been particularly apparent in the field of personal injury. If negligence is established, the claimant (or plaintiff) may be entitled to damages, under a number of headings such as pain, suffering, loss of amenity, costs of care, and loss of earnings through inability to work.

Medicolegal issues have had an increasingly important influence on the practice of medicine itself over the last 2 decades. The soaring number of claims for medical negligence and the considerable rise in the number of lawyers specializing in malpractice bear testimony to fundamental changes in the way society views the nature of injury and the role of medicine. Ongoing litigation will affect the doctor's assessment of the patient and possibly the decision to offer treatment. Patients have increasingly high expectations of treatment. If results of treatment are not to their satisfaction, they may consider that someone must be at fault. When patients pursue redress, not only the outcome of treatment but also the practice of medicine itself may come under medicolegal scrutiny.

In the field of personal injury, increasing costs of litigation in cases such as whiplash injury and

occupationally related upper-limb disorders have been particularly striking. In the increasingly adversarial climate, the nature of chronic pain and pain-associated incapacity has come under the most detailed examination.

In cases of chronic pain, there are frequently disagreements among orthopedic and neurological specialists about the reasons for continued incapacity. Since the formulation of the gate control theory of pain (Melzack & Wall, 1965), it has been recognized that severity of pain does not bear a simple relationship to the degree of tissue damage. The experience of pain is influenced not only by the amount of tissue damage but also by the way the information is processed when it reaches the brain. A range of psychological factors have been shown to influence the perception of pain. Furthermore, studies of disability (Waddell, Bircher, Finlayson, & Main, 1984) have demonstrated that disability, or limitation in function, is explained by both physical and psychological factors. The later development of the biopsychosocial model of disability (Waddell, 1987) acknowledged the complicated interplay between medical, psychological, and social factors. Scientific developments in the clinical field have begun to influence appraisal of pain and incapacity in the legal context. Psychologically mediated pain-associated incapacity is now being considered as a possible consequence of injury.

PSYCHOLOGICAL AND PSYCHIATRIC OPINION

To the extent that psychological injury is under consideration, either a psychologist or a psychiatrist may be asked to offer an opinion. Sometimes such an opinion may turn out essentially to be an opinion as to whether the symptoms are credible clinically and whether the expert is satisfied therefore that the client is genuine. A general clinical psychologist or psychiatrist may feel able to give such as an opinion. To the extent that psychiatric illness per se is considered to be a major consideration, a psychiatrist may be preferred, and to the extent that psychological dysfunction is the primary focus, a psychologist may be preferred. In practice, there is significant overlap in expertise. Where the issue of psychologically mediated incapacity is concerned, it is important that the professional has expertise specifically in the assessment and treatment of patients with painful injuries. Unless the client has a major psychiatric illness, specialist knowledge of the psychological impact of pain and the development of pain-associated incapacity may be more important than whether the expert is a clinical psychologist or psychiatrist. Currently, it would appear that in matters of chronic pain, specific psychological opinion is becoming increasingly sought.

The psychological expert may be asked to address a number of issues, but the principal questions usually will center on whether or not the person has sustained a psychological "injury" and whether the persistence of pain or pain-associated incapacity is psychologically mediated. The focus of this chapter is on the role of the psychologist as expert witness, within an adversarial legal system in which "no-fault compensation" does not operate.

Caveats

This chapter will not address the nature of psychological opinion in cases of brain injury or child custody. The identification of psychiatric disorder will be addressed only in the context of psychological injury or in terms of alternative causation. The overall focus will be on mechanisms of injury and the development of pain-associated incapacity rather than on the strengths or limitations

of specific measurement instruments or systems of classification.

THE CONTEXT OF MEDICOLEGAL ASSESSMENT

Background

Although there are some differences in the actual operation of the legal systems in the United States and the United Kingdom, they are based essentially on the same principles of justice. In the United Kingdom, evidence is amassed by one branch of the legal profession (solicitors) and presented for adjudication by the other branch (barristers in England, advocates in Scotland). Solicitors act either for the plaintiff (the injured party) or for the defendant. Each side instructs its own barrister. In civil cases, the barristers present their cases to a judge. Usually only in criminal cases is the evidence presented to a jury. In cases of personal injury (PI), the principal role of the psychological expert witness is to give an opinion on the nature of injuries sustained, consider the extent of damages (quantum), and offer a view concerning the future course of the claimed incapacities. The expert may or may not have treated the patient. There are advantages and disadvantages to having treated the client. On the one hand, the expert can be assumed to have detailed knowledge of the client, but on the other hand, he or she may not be considered sufficiently independent to give an unbiased opinion. Psychologists are also asked to reply to reports produced by psychologists on the other side or to defend their own reports against difficulties or weaknesses highlighted by the other. Finally, they may assist the barrister cross-examining the opposing psychologist in court.

In the United States, an expert who has examined a client and prepared a report is termed a "clinical expert" or sometimes a "rebuttal expert." Experts are also employed simply to examine the strengths or weaknesses of the deposition taken from other experts. They are termed "consultant experts." Their focus of inquiry is the quality of the evidence and the credentials of the clinical expert. They do not examine the litigant and do not normally offer opinions specifically on the litigant, except insofar as to offer alternative opinions to those offered.

The purpose of this chapter is to consider the roles of the psychologist as expert witness for the plaintiff or defense (in the United Kingdom). These roles are approximately equal to clinical and rebuttal experts, respectively, in the United States. (The specific role of the consultant expert is discussed in considerable detail by Ziskin [1995] and is not the main focus of this chapter). The term "expert witness" will be used generally to refer to psychologists who have examined a litigant and prepared a report or produced a deposition (whether for the prosecution or the defense).

As experts, these witnesses are entitled to take into account additional evidence (whether scientific or legal) in the formulation of their opinion, rather than simply matters of fact. It must be remembered, however, that "expert witnesses, however skilled and eminent, can give no more than evidence. They cannot usurp the function of the jury, or judge sitting as jury, any more than a technical assessor can substitute his advice for the judgement of the court" (*Davie v. Magistrates of Edinburgh* [1953], cited in Graham Hall & Smith, 1992).

The Nature of Expertise

The primary role of the expert is to provide a professional opinion on the origin, nature, and prognosis of a client's complaints in response to a letter of instruction from a solicitor (whether that of the plaintiff or that of the defendant). It should be noted immediately that the request comes from the solicitor acting on behalf of the client by whom he/she has been instructed and not directly from the client. The client can, and often does, express a view concerning the content of the assessment, but the solicitor is acting essentially on behalf of the court to prepare evidence for consideration by legal counsel in the light of possible submission to court. The role of the expert witness is, therefore, to respond chiefly to the needs of the legal process and only indirectly to the needs of the client, which are not properly a matter of direct concern to the expert witness. The relationship between the client and the medicolegal assessor is therefore radically different from that between patient and doctor. This fact is seldom appreciated by either the client or the expert witness. (In considering final prognosis, it may be relevant to suggest further treatment, but clinical care is not the responsibility of the independent expert.)

The Nature of the Legal Process

The expert's report is presented as part of a body of evidence adduced by the teams of solicitors to prosecute or defend a complaint. It has to be remembered that the system is essentially adversarial. Although a high proportion of cases are settled as a result of negotiation between the two teams of lawyers, the expert witness needs to be mindful that this is not always so. In the case of PI, both the plaintiff and the defendant have a right to an adjudication by a disinterested third party. In the United Kingdom, most cases come under civil litigation and are tried by a judge. In some cases of personal injury (such as injuries following assault), a jury may be involved, as is common in the United States.

In any event, the primary role of the expert witness is to present an opinion not on the "rights or wrongs" of the case, which is properly a matter for adjudication, but on the origin, nature, and likely prognosis of the complaint. The opinion is based on the nature of the specific professional expertise for which the expert has been instructed. Clearly the witness will be expected to have a sound and respected knowledge of the condition in question. The report is subject to scrutiny prior to the disclosure of evidence by the instructing solicitor or at time of deposition; in the event of a trial, it is subject to cross-examination in court. In that context, both the substance of the report and the authority of the expert as evident in his or her defense of the report will have a bearing on the adjudication. The nature of the adjudication (whether by judge or jury) should have no significant bearing on the content of the opinion, although the "courtroom tactics" employed by the lawyers in examination and cross-examination may of course differ. Presentation of evidence is discussed in detail by Ziskin (1995) and is not specifically addressed in this chapter.

The Basis of Expertise

According to Ziskin, "generally an expert is described as one who is so qualified by study or experience that he can form a definite opinion of his own respecting a division of science, branch of art, or department of trade concerning which persons having no particular training or special study are incapable of forming accurate opinions or of deducing correct conclusions" (1995, p. 1).

The matter is not necessarily settled by general academic qualifications or special responsibilities. The consultant expert may have raised doubts not only about the particular expert in terms of knowledge and competency but may also have attacked the scientific and professional basis of his or her opinion. Ultimately it is for the lawyers to identify relevant expertise, and ultimately, according to Graham Hall and Smith (1992), "It is for the Judge to determine whether the witness has undergone such a course of special study, or possesses such experience, as will render him expert in that particular subject" (p. 3).

Clinical Judgment

Any sort of judgment results from a complex decision-making process. Giving an expert opinion in cases of PI is particularly difficult because the "data" may be incomplete or contradictory and may come from a wide variety of sources. Even the best information available, however, may be subject to bias and distortion in how it is represented. Ziskin (1995) has offered a penetrating analysis of psychiatric and psychological judgment in the chapter titled "Challenging Clinical Judgment." Although he is concerned mainly about forensic opinion, parts of his critique have a more general relevance. He compares "clinical judgment," in which a judge collates information "in his head," with "actuarial judgment," in which decision rules derived from empirical data are used to make the judgment. He cites several studies (Dawes, 1989; Sawyer, 1966) that demonstrate clear superiority of actuarial judgment. Sawyer also demonstrated that the combination of clinical judgment with actuarial judgment was in fact *less* accurate then clinical judgment alone. Judges were more accurate when they disregarded interview results. Ziskin observes that "the research suggests that clinicians cannot rely on their own judgment about when to rely on their own judgment" (1995, p. 211). Other skill deficits identified are: disregard of baseline data, failure to analyze covariation, reliance on illusory correlation, selective use of information, and inability to integrate complex information.

In addition to skill deficits, Ziskin (1995) identifies bad judgment habits and biases. These include hindsight bias, in which an accurate appraisal of past events is distorted by the current "mental set" and confirmatory bias. He cites a large number of studies indicative of such bias but integrates them under several headings: favoring initial hypotheses; using double standards of evidence (i.e., using different criteria to appraise different reports); premature closure; and selectivity in data collection. He also addresses specific biases in the forensic area, such as finding psychopathology

where none exists and the effect of preconceived ideas on the witnesses' observation and perception of data (Temerlin & Trousdale, 1969). These biases appear to be of a more general relevance.

Judgment appears to be affected by both intellectual and emotional biases. "Research suggests that problematic judgement practices do not stem from emotional biases alone, but also from faulty approaches to judgement tasks that would not be eliminated even were emotional factors corrected. Thus, even if one believes that an expert has controlled his emotional biases, it is doubtful that it solves the problem of assessment error stemming from faulty judgement practices" (Ziskin, 1995, p. 247). Finally, the "illusion of insight" (or the inability to critically evaluate one's own judgments) and the lack of relationship between confidence and accuracy are addressed.

In conclusion, Ziskin offers a powerful critique of expert clinical judgment. Although many of his specific concerns relate to forensic issues such as the prediction of dangerousness and judgments of malingering, his analysis contains much of relevance to psychological opinion in the context of PI and merits careful study.

The Standing of the Expert

As an expert, the witness will be expected to bear credentials that support the legitimacy of his or her claims to expertise. The standing of the expert certainly will be appraised in terms of clinical familiarity with the injury or incapacity concerned, but the expert must also appear credible, as well as knowledgeable. Credibility will be a function of the expert's professional reputation, current professional standing, and demeanor in the witness box. An important issue is that of the expert's impartiality, which is sometimes difficult to sustain in the adversarial medicolegal process. Indeed, doubt has been expressed about whether any witness can be truly impartial (Slovenko, 1988 cited in Ziskin, 1995). According to Lord Wilberforce: "expert evidence presented to the court should be, and should be seen to be, the independent production of the expert, uninfluenced as to form or content by the exigencies of litigation. To the extent that it is not, the evidence is likely to be not only incorrect, but self-defeating" (*Whitehouse v. Jordan* [1981], cited in Graham Hall & Smith, 1992).

The task confronting the expert witness, therefore, is a complex and highly technical one, yet the basis of the opinion, of course, is clinical. The basis of a witness's expertise lies not only in the elucidation of "facts" to support his or her opinion but also in the authority given to that opinion by his or her familiarity with similar injuries and the usual variation in responses to treatment.

Specific Difficulties in Offering Psychological Opinion in Cases of Personal Injury

From the legal point of view, a clear, specific, and noncontroversial diagnosis is desirable. Advances in clinical research in matters of chronic pain and disability, particularly in the last two decades, have illustrated, however, that the nature of chronic incapacity is more complex than previously believed. In the case of complex personal injuries, it is likely that several different specialists will have been instructed. The psychological report will not simply be viewed in comparison with a psychological report from the other side but will be considered alongside medical reports addressing the physical basis of the injury.

PERSONAL INJURY

The History of Personal Injury Litigation

The nature of current medicolegal practice in the field of PI can be illuminated by considering its historical origins. Although it is possible to find awards of damages for emotional distress as early as the 14th century, a significant increase in PI legislation followed the construction of the railways in the second half of the 19th century. The debate concerning the physical basis of continued incapacity after injury has been described elsewhere (Allen & Waddell, 1989). Of particular relevance to this article is the role of psychological factors. Mendelson (1988) offers a fascinating account of the polarization that developed between those who considered "railway spine" to be due to an "organic" cause and those who viewed the condition as a type of "nervous shock." He also cites Judd, who "clearly expressed the view that 'concussion of the spine' was largely the complaint of 'cheats and frauds,' and that as a consequence 'cities and corporations are robbed of vast sums of money yearly by malingerers, aided by unscrupulous legal talent, and by ignorant or dishonest surgeons" (Mendelson, 1988, p. 6). Mendelson also cites a number of cases in which claims for "nervous shock" in the absence of a concurrent physical injury have been successful but cautions that "In a legal context the phrase 'nervous shock' has been used to refer to identifiable psychiatric illness and not simply to emotional states such as anxiety, sadness or grief and therefore damages can not be obtained for emotional reactions which are not recognised as distinct psychiatric disorders" (1988, p. 11). Although this may have been the case until the mid-1980s, the as yet ill-defined "chronic pain syndrome" now is increasingly referred to in medicolegal reports. According to Mendelson (1992), "the judicial system is paying increasing attention to recent advances in the understanding of mechanisms which determine the experience of pain." In a recent case in the United Kindom (*Bird v. Hussain*, 1993), a patient who developed a chronic pain syndrome after a road traffic accident was awarded general damages of £23,500 specifically for pain, suffering, and loss of amenity, although there was "no recognised organic basis for her continuing symptoms."

This case illustrates that chronic pain in certain circumstances may be considered compensable in its own right and not simply as a mental illness deemed to have resulted from the accident. Because it is now accepted that psychological factors are an important component of chronic pain, it can be argued that psychological features that do not fulfill classical psychiatric criteria are de facto being judged compensable as a feature of chronic incapacity.

"Physical" and "Psychological" Opinion

In many accidents, there is clear and unequivocal evidence of damage, and in such cases an orthopedic, neurosurgical, or neurological opinion may be considered sufficient in the determination of the mechanisms of injury. When the evidence of damage is more equivocal, the symptoms are less specific, and the pattern is more generalized, only a nonspecific diagnosis may be sustainable. In such cases, the appropriate expert may be a specialist in pain management. Such a specialist may come from a variety of professions, such as anesthetists specializing in pain, rheumatologists specializing in rehabilitation, or clinical psychologists with particular expertise in the pain field. The specialist must have both credible experience in working in the field of musculoskeletal incapacity and also have the professional qualifications to offer a particular perspective on injury and resulting incapacity. It has been customary for the opinions of pain specialists to be sought only when the orthopedic evidence is irreconcilable or when the orthopedic specialist is unable to explain the persistence of pain or dysfunction. For complex problems such as "whiplash" injury, the opinion of pain specialists increasingly is becoming sought. Experts differ in the extent to which they are willing to be pressed by lawyers to be specific on such matters. Differences between the opinion of the plaintiff's and defendant's medical experts on these matters frequently lie at the heart of difficulty in resolution of the case. Increasingly, a psychological opinion is sought either to resolve conflicting medical opinion or to consider alternative explanations for the persistence of chronic incapacity.

The Purpose of Psychological Reports in Personal Injury Litigation

In PI, any expert needs to consider the injury in terms of causation (liability) and quantum (damages). More specifically, the expert will be asked to address the nature of the injury or incapacity in terms of the nature of alleged dysfunction or incapacity, the extent to which it is related to the injury in question, and the prognosis.

There are three principal aspects to a psychological report (detailed in the following sections: "Identification of Psychological Injury," "Determination of Psychologically Mediated Chronic Incapacity," and "The Identifying Exaggeration, Faking, and Malingering"). To the extent that opinion is based on the report and behavior of the client, however, issues of credibility or veracity also become important. This topic is also discussed.

Identification of Psychological Injury

Formal diagnosis of mental illness is properly a matter for a psychiatrist. In the context of musculoskeletal injury, the diagnosis of specific recognizable mental illness, such as clinical depression or posttraumatic stress disorder, may be possible on the basis of such identifiable clinical criteria as those recommended in one of the systems of diagnostic classification such as the *International Classification of Diseases* (ICD; World Health Organization, 1992) or the *Diagnostic and Statistical Manual of Mental Disorders* (DSM; American Psychiatric Association, 1994).

Incorporation of psychometric tests is properly a matter for a clinical psychologist. A range of psychometric measures, discussed later, is available.

Both psychiatrists and clinical psychologists may feel entitled on the basis of their professional training and clinical experience to offer a view on aspects of clinical history, symptom presentation, and prognosis. Frequently, psychologists and psychiatrists will come up with similar formulations.

In the case of PI, however, patients frequently do not fulfill criteria for major mental illness yet are distressed and dysfunctional. The experts' credentials as a pain specialist are perhaps more relevant than experience specifically in mainstream psychology or mainstream psychiatry. Familiarity with the psychological effects of persistent pain and pain-associated incapacity are essential in arriving at an expert view of the nature of the personal injury.

Limitations of Psychiatric and Psychological Testimony. Ziskin (1995) challenges the validity of "expertise" principally on two accounts: the scientific basis of the evidence on which the expert relies and the nature of clinical judgment. He then addresses specifically psychiatric and psychological testimony. It should be noted that Ziskin takes the standpoint of the consultant expert (to the noncommitted, he might appear less than "evenhanded"). His attention is directed at both psychiatric and psychological opinion, although several of his more penetrating analyses are directed at forensic issues (such as the evaluation of "dangerousness" and "malingering"). He does not address specifically pain-associated injuries or chronic pain syndromes, but since the opinion may require consideration of possible psychiatric diagnoses or formulations founded on psychometric testing, his analysis is of considerable interest.

Psychiatric Diagnosis and Classification

Psychiatric opinion generally relies primarily on psychiatric diagnosis. Classifying a patient's presenting signs and symptoms in terms of a diagnosis enables comparison of similar individuals, investigation of determinants of illness, and assignment to treatment. Most commonly, classification is offered according to the DSM. Problems with accuracy, reliability, and clinical utility have led to successive modifications of the manual. There have been, so far, five versions of DSM, beginning in 1952 with DSM-I and culminating in the latest, DSM-IV, published in 1994. The system is widely used in clinical psychiatry. DSM can be seen simply as a system of classification that may or may not offer a helpful way of classifying a particular individual's constellation of difficulties. It offers criteria for mental illness against which an individual may be compared. From the legal point of view, there appear to be four main limitations that are relevant. First, it is difficult to identify the scientific basis from which the system has been constructed. It relies on psychopathological theory rather than on a clinically validated classification. Second, there appear to be major problems with the unreliability of psychiatric diagnosis. In one experimental study, it was demonstrated than even with major diagnostic classifications such as schizophrenia (combining the subtypes), there was less than 50% agreement among experienced psychiatrists. Ziskin (1995) reports on a large number of other studies that have been unable to establish sufficient agreement concerning psychiatric diagnosis. Third, there are such major differences between the latest and the earlier versions of DSM that the "evidence base" regarding its clinical utility is hard to interpret. Simply put, an individual may fulfill the diagnostic criteria for a particular disorder in one version of the DSM and fail to fill it in another. Furthermore, some diagnoses have "disappeared," while new ones have emerged. Fourth, and perhaps most important, there appears to be little relationship between diagnosis and objective assessment of psychiatric impairment (Nussbaum, Puig, & Arizaga, 1981–1982) or between awareness of the nature of one's actions and prediction of future behavior. According to Goldstein (1973), "a learned and distinguished body of jurists, legal historians, forensic psychiatrists and other social critics have seriously questioned the wisdom of a growing tendency to attribute to psychiatrists inflated powers of diagnosis and prediction in what is still an uncharted and poorly understood area—the interface of psychiatry, law and society—either past or future behavior" (p. 1134).

Psychometric Tests. There are a vast range of psychological tests available. They vary widely in acceptability from the point of test construction, clinical validity, and predictive utility. Six criteria for acceptability of tests are offered by Ziskin (1995), paraphrased here:

1. Is the test reliable?
2. Is there a true relationship between the test score or sign and criterion of interest?
3. Do positive correlations withstand base rate analysis?
4. Does it produce incremental validity (i.e., does it enhance results)?

5. Has it been standardized for the particular population on which it is being used?
6. Does the test diagnose or predict with reasonable accuracy?

Few tests appear to have a satisfactory scientific basis. Projective tests, such as the Rorschach, the Thematic Apperception Test, the Bender Gestalt Test, and the Draw-a-Person Test, are still used clinically in some countries. Their clinical value is not universally agreed on, and their utility in cases of PI is hard to imagine. It does not seem necessary to discuss them in this chapter.

Personality tests such as the MMPI and the MMPI-2 are commonly used both clinically and legally, particularly in the United States. The test has been the subject of a recent critical evaluation in terms of its structural properties and general clinical validity (Helmes & Reddon, 1993). It has been suggested further that its use in the assessment of pain and pain-associated incapacity requires fundamental reappraisal (Helmes, 1994; Main & Spanswick, 1995a).

Determination of Psychologically Mediated Chronic Incapacity (or Chronic Pain Syndrome)

Some of the current difficulties facing the plaintiff in PI cases involving pain and incapacity are a consequence of a general failure to understand the nature of chronic incapacity. This failure is illustrated by overreliance on an outmoded differentiation of diagnoses into "organic" and "functional" on the one hand and an oversimplistic evaluation of the nature of psychological factors on the other.

The terms "functional overlay" and "illness behavior" are frequently adduced to explain the persistence of pain (and associated incapacity) following injury, particularly when the physical findings are inconclusive. They are often diagnosed "by exclusion," based on the *absence* of conclusive physical findings rather than the *presence* of alternative explanations such as psychological reactions to injury and incapacity. As such, they are frequently employed as "pseudopsychological diagnoses." Ambiguities inherent in the use of such terms as "functional overlay" and "illness behavior" are addressed elsewhere (Main & Spanswick, 1995b).

Studies of chronic pain patients have illustrated the limitations of a simple differential diagnosis into physical or psychological pain (often referred to as "functional" or "organic" in the literature). Theoretically and clinically, questions such as, Is the pain real or imaginary? or Is the pain physical or psychological? are usually meaningless but may have to be addressed to reassure the patient that he or she is being taken seriously. Determinations of the extent to which resultant disability is organic or functional are equally problematic. There are large variations is the responses of individuals to any injury, but deliberate simulation of incapacity or frank exaggeration of symptomatology is rarely found. In arriving at a psychological opinion in cases of PI, it is necessary to assess not only the reported symptoms in terms of pain or distress but also the effects of pain in terms of associated incapacities.

Psychological opinion has to be located within a biopsychosocial perspective (Waddell, 1987) rather than within a narrow medical or psychiatric perspective. During the last 15 years, a considerable quantity of research into the psychology of pain and pain-associated incapacity has been published. The textbooks by Turk and Melzack (1992) and Gatchel and Turk (1996) are excellent sources of detail regarding the nature of psychological factors in pain and in response to treatment. It is possible only to identify a few examples of the sorts of psychological factors that have been identified. They are chosen to illustrate the diversity of psychological aspects of pain.

Early studies into the nature of functional disability demonstrated that distress and pain behavior are more important than long-standing personality traits (Main & Waddell, 1987). The recognition of the importance of cognitive factors (Turk, Meichenbaum, & Genest, 1983) inspired investigations of cognitive factors in adjustment to pain and development of disability. These have been reviewed in detail by DeGood and Shutty (1992). In addition to specific beliefs about pain (such as pain control and self-efficacy), coping strategies (Rosenstiel & Keefe, 1983) have also been investigated. Negative or inappropriate coping strategies have been shown to be of importance not only in adjustment to pain (Turner & Clancy, 1986) but also in the prediction of disability (Burton, Tillotson, Main, & Hollis, 1995). Fear of hurting and harming (Waddell, Newton, Henderson, Somerville, & Main, 1993; Vlaeyen, Kole-Snijders, Boeren, & van Eek, 1995) has recently received attention and has been implicated in the development of guarded movements (Watson, Booker, & Main, 1997). Results from the latter study are consistent with complex psychobiological models linking central psychological characteristics with physiological changes in the nervous system. Even more

complex theoretical models have integrated physical, psychological, and psychophysiological perspectives (Flor, Birbaumer, Schugens, & Lutzenburger, 1992).

Arriving at a psychological opinion, therefore, is a complex task involving the integration of a number of different clinical dimensions. The major focus may rest less on the origin of the pain (which in the case of specific accidents may be relatively unambiguous) and more on the nature of the injury and the components of the resultant incapacity. In arriving at an overall opinion, it is necessary, therefore, to integrate a range of perspectives. Each component of the psychological opinion should if possible be clearly appraised before any attempt is made to integrate the opinion. The principal ingredients of a psychological opinion are presented below.

Major Features of a Psychological Report

A simple structure for a psychological report has been presented by Main and Spanswick (1995b, Table 1). Some general considerations are offered here.

Clinical History and Examination

It is always advisable to take a clear clinical and socioeconomic history not only of the injury and its sequelae but also of the client prior to the injury. There may be an opportunity for corroboration or elaboration on the basis of a separate interview with a spouse or significant other, but the expert has to rely on information given by the client, either in the context of a structured interview or on the basis of some sort of self-report questionnaire or assessment schedule. In the latter cases, however, it is important that such information is elicited from the client at the time of the assessment, lest it could be argued that the responses were not provided by the client. A clinical history will have already been recorded by previous assessors, but the important features may have to be reexamined to determine the client's psychological reaction to the events in question. The psychologist has to construct a profile of the client prior to the injury in question, establish the specific psychological effects of the injury, give the nature of and response to treatment, compare the client's current status with that immediately before the injury, interpret the client's current status, and offer a prognosis in terms of continued pain, suffering, incapacity, and ability to work. In arriving at his or her opinion, the psychologist may be assisted by previous reports and interviews with significant others but should place most emphasis on the clinical interview with the client and the results of formal psychometric testing.

Formal Psychometric and Behavioral Evaluation

A range of psychometric tests and assessment tools is available. A detailed discussion of the use and interpretation of such tests is far beyond the scope of this Chapter, but I will mention a number of tests with which I am familiar for illustrative purposes.

Pain. The psychologist will usually include an assessment of the patient's pain using a questionnaire such as the short-form McGill Pain Questionnaire (Melzack, 1987). It has been claimed that this measure distinguishes sensory from emotional components of pain. Emotional content can also be identified using the Pain Drawing Test (Ransford, Cairns, & Mooney, 1976), but a recent study (Parker, Wood, & Main, 1995) has demonstrated that although patients with clearly abnormal pain drawings are almost always distressed, 50% of distressed patients produce normal pain drawings.

Pain Behavior. Pain behavior may be assessed in a number of ways: by rating scales using self-report data (Turk & Melzack, 1992), by assessing behavioral responses to physical examination (Waddell, McCulloch, Kummel, & Venner, 1980), or by using a videotaped Behavioral Observation Test (Keefe & Hill, 1985). The latter test in particular, however, requires careful training for use in the clinical context, since routine videotaped assessment is not a practical possibility.

Personality Characteristics. The Minnesota Multiphasic Personality Inventory, or MMPI (Hathaway & McKinley, 1983) and MMPI-2 (Butcher, Dahlstrom, Graham, Tellegren, & Kaemmer, 1989), has been widely used, particularly in North America, for the assessment of personality traits. Although its historical pedigree is undeniable, its specific value for clinical assessment has recently been questioned (Main & Spanswick, 1995a). The test is discussed in more detail in a later section.

Distress. Simple measures of distress (comprising assessment of somatic awareness and depressive symptomatology), such as the Distress Risk

Assessment Method (DRAM; Main, Wood, Hollis, Spanswick, & Waddell, 1992) are also available.

Pain and Disability Beliefs. A wide range of tests is available for the assessment of attitudes or beliefs about pain and disability. A wide number of constructs, including locus of control, self-efficacy, and fears of hurting/harming, offer slightly more detailed psychological perspectives. Particularly useful sources are Chapters 7 and 13 in Turk and Melzack (1992).

Cognitive and Behavioral Coping Strategies. Specific cognitive coping strategies should also be assessed. The most widely used questionnaire is the Coping Strategies Questionnaire (CSQ; Rosenstiel & Keefe, 1983). A recent study (Burton et al., 1995) has shown that negative or ineffective coping strategies such as catastrophizing ("fearing the worst") are strongly predictive of poor outcome following treatment.

Identifying Exaggeration, Faking, and Malingering

The extent to which a mental health expert should explicitly offer a view concerning issues of faking, exaggeration, or malingering is a matter of debate. Malingering has been defined medically as "the wilful, deliberate, and fraudulent feigning or exaggeration of the symptoms of illness or injury, done for the purpose of a consciously desired end" (*Dorland's Illustrated Medical Dictionary*, cited in Mendelson & Mendelson, 1993, p. 28)—a narrower definition than the legal one, which is derived from regulations governing military discipline. In general, clinical diagnosis is based on the assumption that the patient is truthful. Furthermore, the clinician has no special expertise in the assessment of veracity. Mendelson and Mendelson (1993) are emphatic that "while the psychiatric expert witness may draw attention to inconsistencies in the history obtained . . . the ultimate veracity of the claimant is for the court to decide" (1993, p. 31). Strictly speaking, assessment of malingering per se is a matter for the court, not an expert witness, because the issue of fraud or deliberate attempt to deceive is a legal rather than a medical matter. According to Mendelson and Mendelson (1993):

> The task of the forensic psychiatric expert witness should be confined to issues of diagnosis of mental disorders, their aetiology, and the degree of psychiatric impairment. The psychiatrist may draw at-

tention to inconsistencies in the history obtained and on mental status examination, poor treatment compliance, and the lack of co-operation or motivation during the course of treatment or rehabilitation programme. However, the specific question of the veracity of the claimant is for the court to decide. (p. 34)

In the field of PI, similar considerations arise in determining the extent to which the claimant is being honest in regard to his or her stated incapacity. Lawyers may put considerable pressure on expert witnesses to identify faking or malingering. Certainly, in formulating an expert opinion, the expert has to decide whether to accept the information given to him or her by the patient. In taking a detailed history and in appraising presenting symptoms, the expert has to rely principally on what the client tells him or her. In PI cases that might involve future loss of earnings, there may be a considerable incentive for a patient to lie. Irrespective of whether the expert has been asked explicitly to address the veracity of the client, truthfulness has to be considered. Simply put, if the client has been giving false information, the opinion may not be sustainable.

Even if lawyers do not attempt to persuade their experts to give a view on malingering, usually the experts are asked to comment on faking (simulation) or exaggeration. Attribution of faking does not necessarily imply perpetration of fraud, but if established in court it will almost certainly damage beyond repair the credibility of the client. The psychologist may reasonably be expected to offer a view of the "credibility" of the client. The opinion may be based on the clinical interview or on more formal assessment measures.

A patient's refusal to cooperate with a clinical interview should be reported, but the interpretation of the behavior should be a matter for the court. Apparent inconsistencies between the interview and information given to previous assessors should be noted but interpreted with caution. Clients are sometimes made nervous and even frightened by medicolegal assessments, particularly if they have been hurt by previous physical examinations or have been upset by dismissive and unsympathetic comments made to them. If the patient is distressed or flustered, the accuracy of his or her self-report may be affected. Inaccuracy in recall of aspects of medical history and salient events is not necessarily suspicious. If exaggeration is identified, it may be either deliberate or unintended. Unconscious exaggeration of symptoms may represent an honest but inaccurate appraisal.

Deliberate exaggeration may be undertaken with a view to either convince or deceive. In summary, the issue of veracity is a complex and difficult area of investigation. The difficulty faces all expert witnesses. It is sometimes assumed that by virtue of their professional background and training, psychologists should be better placed than other experts to address the issue, but in terms of offering a general view, they are in no better position than any other expert. According to Slovenko (1966), "a good poker player probably knows better than a mental health professional whether a person is lying. A psychiatrist is a doctor, not a lie detector" (p. 129). The doctor–patient relationship usually is predicated on the assumption that the patient's complaint is genuine, and the doctor's clinical experience may even be a hindrance in the detection of faking. There is virtually no research in the field of PI on the ability of mental health professionals to detect faking. Most research on clinical judgment concerns psychiatric assessment of patients in forensic settings. Ziskin (1995) references a review article by Schretlen: "The findings suggest that until research validates use of the diagnostic interview for this purpose, it is probably indefensible to render expert testimony regarding the likelihood of malingering without psychological test data bearing on the question" (cited in Ziskin, 1995, pp. 1144–1145).

According to Faust (1995), "some malingerers practice deception for a living, and can easily outmatch the physician who lacks the same type of experience, mental set and willingness for exploitation that sometimes characterise the professional con artist" (p. 259). He concludes that "there seems to be little justification for extreme confidence in our capacity to detect deception" (p. 259).

The issue of faking on formal assessment measures has been addressed from five principal perspectives: diagnostic assessment, psychometric measures, symptom validity testing, behavioral assessment, and psychophysiology ("lie-detection tests").

Diagnostic Assessment. According to the DSM-IV (American Psychiatric Association, 1994), "Factitious disorders are characterized by physical or psychological symptoms that are intentionally produced or feigned in order to assume the sick note" (p. 471). As Mendelson (1988) points out, however, the conceptualization of Factitious Disorders is still far from satisfactory. For the diagnosis to be made, "there is no apparent goal other than to assume the patient role, and there is an 'absence of external incentives for the behavior'" (1988, p. 173). Clearly such a diagnosis is unlikely to be possible in the context of a PI claim.

Detection of Faking by Self-Report Measures and Questionnaires. The use of questionnaires to identify faking in forensic settings has principally involved the detection of neuropsychological abnormalities in cases of head injury. For the purpose of this chapter, attention will be restricted to evaluation of pain and musculoskeletal incapacity.

It has been asserted that people who simulate pain in the back use different pain descriptors (Leavitt, 1985). Such differences are claimed to distinguish patients with clinical pain both from people who simulate pain when it does not exist and from people who consciously augment existing pain. These differences formed the basis of the 103-item Low Back Pain Symptom Checklist used to predict disability through simulation scores based on 13 of the items (Leavitt, 1991). The checklist is purported to simplify the evaluation of psychological disturbance by relying solely on an assessment of pain vocabulary as a clinical marker of psychological disturbance. Somewhat surprisingly, it is claimed that the checklist has the advantage that "it detects pre-existing psychological disturbance in patients with low back pain rather than the milder form of psychological symptoms that may develop in reaction to refractory pain" (Leavitt, 1990, p. 448). The authors do not seem to have considered adequately the complexity of pain and pain assessment. In a study of outcomes of osteopathic treatment for back pain, it was demonstrated that the report of pain is influenced by a range of different psychological factors (Main & Burton, 1995). As far as the detection of faking is concerned, the claims for the discriminative validity of the checklist would seem to rely principally on a comparison between patients with clinical pain and people being asked to simulate or exaggerate pain. It has not been demonstrated convincingly as yet that it can identify conscious simulation with the intention to deceive in a legal situation. Further clarification would seem to be needed before this scale could be recommended as a test of faking.

It has been claimed that neurosis and conscious symptom exaggeration can be differentiated using the Illness Behavior Questionnaire (IBQ; Pilowsky & Spence, 1975). Clayer, Bookless, & Ross (1984) have produced a 21-item Conscious Exaggeration Scale (CE). They compared employees who were asked to imagine an accident and to attempt to convince authorities of serious injury with a comparable group given no such instruction and with a third group of pain patients whose complaint of pain was considered to be neurotically determined. Although the results were interesting, the authors acknowledge the limitations of equating conscious deception with clients attempting to defraud, and recommend further research on this issue.

By far the most widely researched psychometric instrument is the MMPI (Hathaway & McKinley, 1983). The 556 items yield scores on 10 major clinical scales and 3 so-called validity scales. The validity scales include the L scale, which gives a measure of the extent to which the individual is presenting him/herself in the best possible light; the K scale, which is a measure of lack of openness (or defensiveness), and the F scale, which has various interpretations, one of which is that it assesses the tendency to exaggerate or fake disorder. In addition to the original 13 scales, many others have been constructed.

Many studies have attempted to evaluate the use of various cutoffs on the F minus K dissimulation index (Gough, 1950). The scale has been used to detect simulation of psychiatric illness. In one paradigm, scores of individuals instructed to try to fake psychiatric illness are compared with actual scores obtained from several clinical groups. Unfortunately, the discrimination is not perfect, and a significant proportion of genuine profiles can be misinterpreted as faked. The 74-item Dissimulation scale, or Ds (Gough, 1950) offers an additional index of malingering. The later 40-item revision, the Ds-r (Gough, 1954), is apparently more effective. According to Ziskin (1995), a score of 2 standard deviations above the mean misclassifies only 3% of genuine patients, and "in the context of litigation, with its related motives to falsify or exaggerate, such a score should represent strong evidence of malingering" (p. 1159).

The "obvious–subtle" or "subtle–obvious" (O-S or S-O) scale has also been used as an index of dissembling. A set of items clearly indicative of psychopathology constitutes the obvious items, and a set of items not obviously associated with psychopathology but statistically loaded on one of five clinical scales constitutes the subtle items. It is assumed that absence of subtle items may indicate a less-than-genuine profile. Sometimes all three dissimulation indices have been used in combination. The use of these scales is discussed extensively elsewhere (Greene, 1988a, 1988b; Ziskin, 1995).

The original MMPI was developed from items derived originally in the 1940s and 1950s. Significant structural weaknesses in the instrument have since been identified and have resulted in the development of the later MMPI-2 (Butcher et al., 1989). A recent study (Dush, Simons, Platt, Nation, & Ayres, 1994) used the MMPI-2 to compare chronic pain patients in the midst of litigation with a similar group who were not. They selected 10 key MMPI-2 variables a priori and found that litigants were most distinct in endorsing more obvious and fewer subtle symptoms. Assuming there was no unconscious bias in selection of the a priori items and that the items were not directly related to the medicolegal process (and therefore trivially discriminating), then further research would seem to be merited. It would be important to show, using an adequate sample size, that a robust scale could be constructed and that its statistical properties could be confirmed on a further sample. If this could be demonstrated, then the validity of the "scale" for medicolegal purposes could then be properly examined.

There is an inherent attractiveness in being able to detect faking or malingering using a psychometric assessment such as the MMPI, but despite the enthusiasm of Ziskin (1995) and others, it is clear that the research supporting the use of the "faking" scales is based on shaky foundations.

Symptom Validity Testing

Pankratz (1988) has developed procedures for symptom validity testing that have been used to investigate neuropsychological symptoms using a sensory-testing format. The client is asked to make a series of perceptual discriminations using a forced-choice format. The individual's responses are compared with known error rates to determine whether he or she is systematically producing wrong responses. According to Faust (1995):

> The main shortcoming of system validity testing appears to be its limited sensitivity. Although research outcomes vary, in a number of studies a fairly high percentage of simulators (sometimes even the majority) have beaten the method, probably by discerning the underlying design and adjusting their performance accordingly. Also, malingerers may not try to feign gross deficits, and will often not be detected if one requires significantly below chance performance. (p. 261)

Despite Faust's optimism that such procedures are capable of further refinement, it is not easy to see

they could be applied to the investigation of pain-associated incapacity.

Faust (1995) offers some very useful advice, summarized as follows:

1. Do not let subjective confidence be your guide.
2. Consider whether, or to what degree, the examinee has a motive to deceive.
3. Do not depend on interview and medical examination alone, especially with "softer" conditions or evidence, or when the diagnosis rests mainly on self-report.
4. Obtain collateral information.

Behavioral (Nonorganic) Signs and Symptoms

Pain behavior has long been recognized as a concomitant of incapacity (Fordyce, 1976). It can be assessed on the basis of behavioral observation, using rating scales (Richards, Nepomuceno, Riles, & Suer, 1982) or videotaped assessment (Keefe & Hill, 1985), but the behavioral (nonorganic) signs test is perhaps the most widely used in clinical assessment (Waddell et al., 1980). The test is incorporated within the physical examination of the back patient. Eight different variables, grouped into five classes, give an assessment of the patient's psychological response to examination. These behavioral signs are interrelated and correlated with the patient's overall level of distress (Waddell et al., 1984). They form only one part of an overall assessment of the patient and are only clinically interpretable if the score is clearly elevated. The uses and abuses of the behavioral signs in clinical and legal practice has recently been reviewed by Main and Waddell (1998). They conclude:

> behavioural signs may be learned responses to pain which have developed since the original injury, and of which the patient is largely unaware. Even if the behavioural signs are assumed to be under voluntary control, however, and the patient is consciously responding in a guarded manner, it cannot be assumed *de facto* that they are evidence of simulation for the purpose of financial gain. In the first instance the signs should be viewed as an indicator of pain behaviour. Their interpretation should be considered with reference to other psychological and behavioural information. In the absence of distress, fear, mistaken beliefs, maladaptive coping strategies and active attempts to seek treatment, it is perhaps more likely that the signs are evidence of simulation, but the behavioural signs cannot be interpreted in isolation. . . . They are not on their own a test of credibility or veracity. Interpretation of the signs is only

possible within the context of a broader clinical or psychosocial assessment. (p. 2371)

Polygraphy

Because polygraphy purports to offer a method for validating self-report, it will be reviewed briefly here, even though it is not necessarily carried out by psychologists. Despite enthusiastic support among police forces (Nardini, 1987), the use of polygraphy has been trenchantly criticized on both scientific and ethical grounds. The Office of Technology Assessment, in a report to the U.S. Congress, found serious limitations and widely differing results in its review of polygraphy validity and reliability research (Brooks, 1985). Two further major recent reviews in the United Kingdom (Gale, 1988; Levey, 1988) have been even more critical of the reliability, validity, and use of such techniques. It has been argued that polygraphy cannot adequately distinguish fear from guilt (Saxe, 1991) and that it does not adequately distinguish orienting from emotional responses (Horneman & Gorman, 1987). Controlled Question Test (CQT) methodology in particular has been criticized for a general sampling bias (Patrick & Iocono, 1991), with particular susceptibility to false positive errors (McCauley & Forman, 1988). On a more general level, Ben-Shaker & Bar-Hillel (1991) point out that the complexity of the information available to the examiner, coupled with the lack of well-defined quantification and integration rules, allows the examiner to overweigh confirming evidence and to disregard disconfirming cues. Such issues in part have led to specific ethical concerns about the use of polygraphy (Thornton, 1988) and specific trade-union concerns (Jones, 1988). Polygraphy is inadmissible in the U.K. legal system.

Limitations of Expertise

If an expert strays beyond his or her expertise, doubt may be cast on the validity of the rest of his or her testimony. In cases specifically of psychological injury, the only professional boundary likely to be problematic is whether in a particular case a psychological or a psychiatric report is more appropriate. That is matter to be discussed with the trial lawyer. If the expert is reporting on a patient whom he or she has treated, the issue may be simpler to resolve. In cases of pain-associated incapacity, the legitimacy of a psychological opinion itself may be challenged. This should be countered with reference to scientific studies demonstrating the relevance of psychological factors in pain and pain-associated incapacity.

The expert may be asked to address issues of causality, mechanisms of injury, and prognosis. Even though judgment is recognized to be probabilistic, the lawyer may try to persuade the expert to be more precise than he or she is able. Such pressure should be resisted. If there is no sound basis on which to form an opinion, this should be stated. If an expert feels that prognosis in a particular case is uncertain, reference can be made to general statistics regarding the likelihood of various levels of recovery of function. Without specific knowledge of the work situation, unless special expertise in assessment can be demonstrated, a psychologist should be advised not to offer too specific a prognosis.

If challenged about the nature of expert judgment itself, which may be relatively unlikely, it is prudent to acknowledge that all experts are subject to bias; however, the witness should be prepared to defend his or her opinion against the charge of major or systematic bias. Similarly, the "gap" between clinical assessment and future behavior should be acknowledged. Alluding to research studies that demonstrate the relationship between particular psychological features and response to treatment (or prediction of chronic incapacity) may go some way to defend against the charge that diagnosis is irrelevant. It may be that the "gap" represents more of a problem with psychiatric than with psychological testimony, since research is becoming increasingly focused on psychological mechanisms (in relation to the development of chronic incapacity).

CONCLUSIONS AND RECOMMENDATIONS

The clinical importance of psychological factors in chronic pain and pain-associated incapacity is now recognized, and psychological opinion in cases of PI is becoming increasingly sought. It seems at this time that psychological opinion is perhaps less vulnerable than psychiatric opinion in terms of the "gap" between theoretical classification and demonstration of a relationship with pain mechanisms and the development of chronic incapacity, but the ultimate test of such opinion is a legal one. It seems that the evidential base of psychological opinion still needs considerable articulation and development. Particular challenges lie in improving skill in clinical judgment and in reducing bias, but the biggest challenge of all perhaps lies in further clarifying the nature of psychologically mediated chronic incapacity. It might be appropriate, finally, to offer some suggestions for improving the quality of psychological opinion and refining its use in the courtroom.

1. Recognize the difference between a clinical opinion and an expert legal opinion.
2. Expect and prepare for the basis of the opinion to be challenged.
3. Attempt to elicit all available facts before arriving at an opinion.
4. Be prepared to justify one's credentials as a psychological expert in PI.
5. Admit limitations in one's own expertise.
6. Don't be persuaded to alter or adjust opinion unless further facts come to light.
7. Attempt to be truly independent, fair, and impartial.
8. Learn from your mistakes.

Establishment of the psychologist as an expert witness in PI offers a huge challenge. This challenge will only be met if there is a willingness to understand the legal process itself and to attempt to develop the highly technical skills needed to translate a simple clinical opinion that an expert opinion that will assist the court.

ACKNOWLEDGMENTS

I acknowledge a particular debt to J. Ziskin and the fifth edition of his classic three-volume textbook, which has inspired parts of this chapter.

A further acknowledgment to the stimulating research and writing of George and Danuta Mendelson, who inspired a much earlier version of this chapter (Main & Spanswick, 1995b). Thanks is also due to Bill Braithwaite, who assisted with certain points of law. Misrepresentation of the positions of any of the above is unintentional. The opinions expressed in this chapter are mine alone.

REFERENCES

Allen, D. B., & Waddell, G. (1989). An historical perspective on low back pain and disability [Special issue]. *Acta Orthopaedica Scandinavica* (Suppl. 234), 60.

American Psychiatric Association. (1994). *Diagnostic and statistical manual of mental disorders* (4th ed.). Washington, DC: Author.

Ben-Shaker, G., & Bar-Hillel, M. (1991). Misconceptions in Martin and Terris. Predicting infrequent behaviour: Clarifying the impact on false-positive rates. *Journal of Applied Psychology, 78,* 148–150.

Bird v. Hussain. Current Law Yearbook Case 1486 (Leeds High Court 1993).

Brooks, J. (1985). Polygraph testing: Thoughts of a skeptical legislator. *American Psychologist, 40,* 348–354.

Burton, A. K., Tillotson, M., Main. C. J., & Hollis, S. (1995). Psychosocial predictors of outcome in acute and subchronic low back trouble. *Spine, 20,* 722–728.

Butcher, J. N., Dahlstrom, W. G., Graham, J. R., Tellegen, A., & Kaemmer, B. (1989). *Manual for the restandardized Minnesota Multiphasic Personality Inventory: MMPI-2. An administrative and interpretive guide.* Minneapolis: University of Minnesota Press.

Clayer, J. R., Bookless, C., & Ross, M. W. (1984). Neurosis and conscious symptom exaggeration: Its differentiation by the Illness Behavior Questionnaire. *Journal of Psychosomatic Research, 28,* 237–241.

Dawes, R. M. (1989). Experience and validity of clinical judgment: The illusory correlation. *Behavioural Sciences and the Law, 7,* 457–467.

DeGood, D. E., & Shutty, M. S. (1992). Assessment of pain beliefs, coping, and self-efficacy. In D. C. Turk & R. Melzack (Eds.). *Handbook of pain assessment* (pp. 214–234). New York: Guilford Press.

Dush, D. M., Simons, L. E., Platt, M., Nation, P. C., & Ayres, S. Y. (1994). Psychological profiles distinguishing litigating and non-litigating pain patients: Subtle, and not so subtle. *Journal of Personality Assessment, 62,* 299–313.

Faust, D. (1995). The detection of deception. In M. I. Weintraub (Ed.), *Neurologic clinics, malingering and conversion reactions* (pp. 255–265). Philadelphia: Saunders.

Flor, H., Birbaumer, N., Schugens, M., & Lutzenburger, W. (1992). Symptom specific psychophysiological responses in chronic pain patients. *Psychophysiology, 29,* 452–460.

Fordyce, W. E. (1976). *Behavioral methods for chronic pain and illness.* St. Louis, MO: Mosby.

Gale, A. G. (1988). *The polygraph test: Lies, truth and science.* London: Sage.

Gatchel, R. J., & Turk, D. C. (Eds.). (1996). *Psychological approaches to pain management: A practitioner's handbook.* New York: Guilford Press.

Goldstein, R. O. (1973). The fitness factory: 1. The psychiatrist's role in determining competency. *American Journal of Psychiatry, 130,* 1134–1147.

Gough, H. G. (1950). The F minus K dissimulation index for the Minnesota Multiphasic Personality Inventory. *Journal of Consulting Psychology, 14,* 408–441.

Gough, H. G. (1954). Some common misperceptions about neuroticism. *Journal of Consulting Psychology, 18,* 287–292.

Graham Hall, J., & Smith, G. D. (Eds.). (1992). *The expert witness.* Chichester: Barry Rose Law.

Greene, R. L. (1988a). Assessment of malingering and defensiveness by objective personality inventories. In R. Rogers (Ed.), *Clinical assessment of malingering and deception* (pp. 124–158). New York: Guilford Press.

Greene, R. L. (1988b). The relative efficacy of F-K and the obvious and subtle scales to detect overreporting of psychopathology on the MMPI. *Journal of Clinical Psychology, 44*, 152–159.

Hathaway, S. R., & McKinley, J. C. (1983). *Minnesota Multiphasic Inventory Manual.* New York: Psychological Corporation.

Helmes, E. (1994). What type of useful information do the MMPI and MMPI-2 provide on patients with chronic pain? *American Pain Society Bulletin, 4*, 1–5.

Helmes, E., & Reddon, J. R. (1993). A perspective on developments in assessing psychopathology: A critical review of the MMPI and MMPI-2. *Psychological Bulletin, 133*, 453–471.

Horneman, C. J., & Gorman, J. G. (1987). Individual differences in psychophysiological responsiveness in laboratory tests of deception. *Personality and Individual Differences, 8*, 321–333.

Jones, E. A. (1988). American individual rights and an abusive technology: The torts of polygraphing. In A. Gale (Ed.), *The polygraph test: Lies, truth and science.* London: Sage.

Keefe, F. J., & Hill, R. W. (1985). An objective approach to quantifying pain behavior and gait patterns in low back pain patients. *Pain, 21*, 153–161.

Leavitt, F. (1985). Pain and deception: Use of verbal pain measurement as a diagnostic aid in differentiating between clinical and simulated low back pain. *Journal of Psychosomatic Research, 29*, 494–505.

Leavitt, F. (1990). The role of psychological disturbance in extending disability time among compensable back injured industrial workers. *Journal of Psychosomatic Research, 34*, 447–453.

Leavitt, F. (1991). Predicting disability in time using formal low back pain measurement: The low back pain simulation scale. *Journal of Psychosomatic Research, 35*, 599–607.

Levey, A. B. (1988). *Polygraphy: An evaluative review.* London: Her Majesty's Stationery Office.

McCauley, C., & Forman, R. F. (1988). A review of the Office of Technology Assessment report on polygraph validity. *Basic and Applied Social Psychology, 9*, 73–84.

Main, C. J., & Burton, A. K. (1995). The patient with low back pain: Who or what are we assessing? An experimental investigation of a clinical puzzle. *Pain Reviews, 2*, 203–209.

Main, C. J., & Spanswick, C. C. (1995a). Focus article: Personality assessment and the Minnesota Multiphasic Personality Inventory. 50 years on: Do we still need our security blanket? *Pain Forum, 4*(2), 90–96.

Main, C. J., & Spanswick, C. C. (1995b). "Functional overlay," and illness behavior in chronic pain: Distress or malingering? Conceptual difficulties in medicolegal assessment of personal injury claims. *Journal of Psychosomatic Research, 39*(6), 737–753.

Main, C. J., & Waddell, G. (1987). Symposium on measurement. The assessment of pain. *Clinical Rehabilitation, 3*, 267–274.

Main, C. J., & Waddell, G. (1998). Behavioural responses to examination (a re-appraisal of the interpretation of "non-organic signs"). *Spine, 23*, 2367–2371.

Main, C. J., Wood, P. L. R., Hollis, S., Spanswick, C. C., & Waddell, G. (1992). The distress risk assessment method: A simple patient classification to identify distress and evaluate the risk of poor outcome. *Spine, 17*, 42–50.

Melzack, R. (1987). The short form McGill pain questionnaire. *Pain, 30*, 191–197.

Melzack, R., & Wall, P. D. (1965). Pain mechanism: A new theory. *Science, 150*, 971–979.

Mendelson, G. (1988). *Psychiatric aspects of personal injury claims.* Springfield, IL: Thomas.

Mendelson, G. (1992). Guest editorial: Compensation and chronic pain. *Pain, 48*, 121–123.

Mendelson, G., & Mendelson, M. (1993). Legal and psychiatric aspects of malingering. *Journal of Law and Medicine, 1*, 28–35.

Nardini, W. (1987). The polygraph technique: An overview. *Journal of Police Science and Administration, 15*(3), 239–249.

Nussbaum, K., Puig, J. G., & Arizaga, J. R. (1981–1982). Relevance of objective assessment to medical-legal psychiatry. *American Journal of Forensic Psychiatry, 2*, 17–20.

Pankratz, L. (1988). Malingering on intellectual and neuropsychological measures. In R. Rogers (Ed.), *Clinical assessment of malingering and deception* (p. 169). New York: Guilford Press.

Parker, H., Wood, P. L. R., & Main, C. J. (1995). The use of pain drawing as a screening measure to predict psychological distress in chronic low back pain. *Spine, 20*, 236–243.

Patrick C. J., & Iocono, W. G. (1991). A comparison of field and laboratory polygraphs in the detection of deception. *Psychophysiology, 28*, 632–638.

Pilowsky, I., & Spence, N. D. (1975). Patterns of illness behavior in patients with intractible pain. *Journal of Psychosomatic Research, 19*, 279–287.

Richards, J. S., Nepomuceno, C., Riles, M., & Suer, Z. (1982). Assessing pain behavior: The UAB pain behavior scale. *Pain, 14*, 393–398.

Rosenstiel, A. K., & Keefe, F. J. (1983). The use of coping strategies in chronic low back pain patients: Relationship to patient characteristics and current adjustments. *Pain, 17*, 33–34.

Ransford, A. O., Cairns, O., & Mooney, V. (1976). The pain drawing as an aid to the psychological evaluation of patients with low back pain. *Spine, 1*, 127–134.

Sawyer, J. (1966). Measurement and prediction, clinical and statistical. *Psychological Bulletin, 66*, 178–200.

Saxe, L. (1991). Science and the CQT polygraph: A theoretical critique. *International Journal of Physiology and Behavioural Sciences, 26*, 223–231.

Slovenko, R. (1966). Witness, psychiatry and the credibility of testimony. *University of Pennsylvania Law Review, 19*, 2–111.

Temerlin, M. K., & Trousdale, W. W. (1969). The social psychology of clinical diagnosis. *Psychotherapy: Theory, Research and Practice, 6*, 24–29.

Thornton, P. (1988). Lie detection and civil liberties in the UK. In A. Gale (Ed.), *The polygraph test: Lies, truth and science.* London: Sage.

Turner, J. A., & Clancy, S. (1986). Strategies for coping with chronic low back pain: Relationship to pain and disability. *Pain, 24*, 355–364.

Turk, D. C., Meichenbaum, D., & Genest, M. (1983). *Pain and behavioral medicine: A cognitive-behavioral perspective.* New York: Guilford Press.

Turk, D. C., & Melzack, R. (Eds.). (1992). *Handbook of pain assessment.* New York: Guilford Press.

Vlaeyen, J. W. S., Kole-Snijders, A. M. J., Boeren, R. G. B., & van Eek, H. (1995). Psychological factors in low back pain disability. *Clinical Orthopaedics and Related Research, 195,* 178-184.

Waddell, G. (1987). A new clinical method for the treatment of low back pain. *Spine, 12,* 632-644.

Waddell, G., Bircher, M., Finlayson, D., & Main, C. J. (1984). Symptoms and signs: Physical disease or illness behaviour? *British Medical Journal, 289,* 739-741.

Waddell, G., McCulloch, J. A., Kummel, E., & Venner, R. M. (1980). Nonorganic physical signs in low-back pain. *Spine, 5,* 117-125.

Waddell, G., Newton, M., Henderson, I., Somerville, D., & Main, C. J. (1993). A fear avoidance beliefs questionnaire (FABQ) and the role of fear-avoidance beliefs in chronic low back pain and disability. *Pain, 52,* 157-168.

Watson, P. J., Booker, C. K. & Main, C. J. (1997). Evidence for the role of psychological factors in abnormal paraspinal activity in patients with chronic low back pain. *Journal of Musculoskeletal Pain, 5*(4), 41-56.

World Health Organization. (1992). *International classification of diseases* (9th ed.). Geneva: Author.

Ziskin, J. (Eds.). (1995). *Coping with psychiatric and psychological testimony* (5th ed.). Los Angeles: Law & Psychology Press.

Part II

SPECIAL TOPICS
AND POPULATIONS

Chapter 10

Acute Pain (with Special Emphasis on Painful Medical Procedures)

DAVID A. WILLIAMS

It has been known for some time that pain is one of the more common complaints for which people seek medical attention. In any given year, greater than 70% of the adult U.S. population experiences some form of pain (Sternbach, 1986). Pain accompanies many events, including injury, trauma, painful disease, recovery from surgery, and childbirth. Despite extraordinary advances in determining sensory mechanisms underlying pain, the complete phenomena of pain is still poorly understood. This is due largely to a lack of understanding regarding the cognitive and affective components of the pain experience. This chapter explores the fascinating interrelationship between sensation and these more nebulous higher brain functions in the production of acute pain. Examples from the fields of medicine, surgery, and dentistry will underscore the importance of further research in this area.

PAIN: FROM A PHILOSOPHICAL PERSPECTIVE

From as early as 2600 BC, historical accounts document that acute pain was a common and natural part of the human condition (Bonica, 1990). Although there has been consistent acknowledgment of its existence, the meaning of pain has varied considerably throughout recorded history and by culture. Christian societies during the Middle Ages gave pain religious value as a sign of future reward

in heaven. During the Renaissance and Classical periods, pain was valued as a means of compelling the senses to obey reason, of promoting moral progression, and of paying penitence for one's sins. Medical models of the 18th through early 20th centuries viewed pain as a tool for stirring weak or dormant vital forces in the body and was considered necessary for the promotion of healing (Rey, 1993). Current Western societies have adopted a very different view of acute pain. There is currently a trend to view pain as an integral part of the body's multisystem response to stress, as opposed to an independent mechanism dedicated solely to the production of pain sensations (Kehlet, 1986; Ohrbach & McCall, 1996; Page, 1996). This more integrated view suggests that pain can be adaptive in terms of learning to avoid dangerous environmental stressors (Wiertelak et al., 1994), but if left unmanaged, it can promote the advancement of some illnesses (Liebeskind, 1991; Page, 1996).

THEORETICAL MODELS OF PAIN: THE ROLE OF PSYCHOLOGICAL FACTORS

Some early models of pain attempted to identify receptors in the body that were specifically dedicated to pain: Others held that summation of neuronal firing from a variety of sources triggered the sensation of pain. Each theory appeared to be

151

partially supported, but each theory was also incomplete. The confounding observation for most early physiological theories of pain was that the intensity of a painful stimulus did not share a consistent relationship with an individual's experience of pain. In fact, a standardized pain stimulus could produce different levels of pain in two separate individuals or even different levels of pain within the same individual under differing conditions or across different times. Such variability led prominent early physiologists (e.g., Sherrington, 1900) and prominent psychologists (e.g., Strong, 1895) to agree that pain was composed of at least two components: sensory and affective (Bonica, 1990). Rapid advances have been made in support of sensory theories (e.g., labeled line theory; Willis, 1994). Exploration into higher brain mechanisms (e.g., psychological factors) has also continued but at a considerably slower pace. Operationalization of psychological constructs and mapping the effects of higher brain functions onto the descending inhibitory systems represents an exciting but time-consuming area of growth in pain research. This line of research will help to fill in the gaps now present in prominent theories of pain such as the gate control theory (Melzack & Wall, 1982) and theoretical approaches to pain treatment such as the biopsychosocial perspective (Turk, Meichenbaum, & Genest, 1983) and will add additional empirical support to the psychological training guidelines for new practitioners of pain medicine (Fields, 1991).

Although there is apparent consensus that psychological factors are important to the understanding of pain, there exists great confusion among physicians, patients, third-party payers, and even pain researchers as to what constitutes a psychological factor and how psychological factors actually influence pain. Psychological factors can be divided into two types: (1) psychological disorders and (2) psychosocial factors that influence pain. Psychological disorders, such as major depression, anxiety disorders, posttraumatic stress disorder (PTSD), and personality disorders, are diagnosable concerns that can coexist with and negatively affect pain. Treatment of coexisting psychological disorders is highly appropriate because pain and these disorders can exacerbate one another. A person need not be psychologically disturbed, however, for pain to be influenced by psychological factors. Psychosocial factors include but are not limited to ethnic and cultural influences, patient beliefs/attributions about pain, patient expectancies for a given treatment to work, and emotional/stress responses to pain. Such factors are considered normal but nevertheless can profoundly influence how pain is experienced.

THE INTEGRATION OF NOCICEPTION AND HIGHER BRAIN FUNCTIONS IN ACUTE PAIN PERCEPTION

Nociception is considered the first event that occurs in a long cascade of peripheral and central processes that lead to the perception of pain. When a noxious event such as the tearing of tissue occurs, nociceptive nerve endings transduce the noxious event into neural signals that transmit information about the noxious event along a variety of C and A-delta fibers (Torebjork, 1994). These afferent nerve fibers enter the posterior dorsal horn of the spinal cord, where they synapse with the cells of several afferent pain pathways that transmit nociceptive signals to higher brain centers. These afferent pathways include the spinothalamic, spinomesencephalic, spinoreticular, spinolimbic, spinocervical, and postsynaptic dorsal column tracts (Willis & Westlund, 1997). At higher brain centers (e.g., thalamus and cerebral cortex), nociceptive (sensory) signals are integrated with signals from a variety of psychological processes such as emotions, beliefs, expectations, perceived environmental demands, and memories of past painful events (Chapman, 1985; Peck, 1986). The resulting integration is known as the experience of acute pain, and any report of pain offered by the individual will reflect the product of this integration. The psychological factors resident at higher brain centers are thought to be capable of modulating both nociceptor sensitivity and subsequent afferent transmission of sensory signals. The means by which this is accomplished is via the descending analgesic systems. Currently, there are three basic types of analgesia that the body can offer to quiet afferent sensory activity. The most thoroughly studied is the descending endorphin-mediated analgesia system. Starting in the hypothalamus above the periaqueductal gray midbrain region and extending to the dorsal horn of the spinal cord, this system, rich in endogenous opiate-like substances, functions to gate (turn on or off) afferent activity from peripheral nociceptive sites (Bonica, Yaksh, Liebeskind, Pechnick, & De Paulis, 1990; Fields & Basbaum, 1989). This system, facilitated by serotonin and norepinepherine (Besson, 1994), may provide insight into why antidepressants and psychotherapy have been successful in the treatment of pain (Drossman, 1996). The other two types of analgesia come from nonopiately mediated descending systems. One such system follows similar anatomical projections as the opiately mediated system but releases excitatory amino acids that bind with NMDA receptors to dampen afferent sensory signals (Wilcox, 1991). This and the third system are thought to respond to greater pain and more severe stress than the opiately mediated system. The third and least studied system is thought to exist only in females. This system is mediated by estrogen and is hypothesized to have developed in response to the special pain inhibition needs of females during reproductive processes (Mogil, Sternberg, Kest, Marek, & Liebeskind, 1993). Given that all three descending inhibitory systems originate in higher brain structures involved in integrative pain processing, future investigations are likely to find psychological factors to be playing an even more important role in pain than previously suspected.

SPECIFIC PSYCHOSOCIAL FACTORS AND ACUTE PAIN

Clinicians who elicit pain in the course of delivering their services (e.g., dentists, surgeons, obstetricians, gynecologists, nurses, oncologists, general practitioners, etc.) are recognizing the importance of psychosocial factors in delivering satisfactory medical services. For the purposes of this chapter, psychosocial factors will be grouped into those that have a predominantly affective orientation and those that have a predominately cognitive orientation. These two psychosocial components are considered separately here only for convenience; in reality, they are inseparably intertwined in their influence on pain perception. It is also recognized that social, cultural, and behavioral factors are frequently included in discussions of psychosocial factors affecting pain. They will be considered here as well but as secondary overt external factors that influence the more primary covert cognitive/affective processes.

Affect, Stress, and Acute Pain

Tom is undergoing surgery. His peripheral sensory mechanisms are incapable of distinguishing a surgeon's scalpel from the slash of a bear's claw. Physiologically, Tom responds to the violation of his body's integrity as a stressful event. The surgeon's scalpel triggers a cascade of events. Starting with increased sympathetic tone, this cascade can include increased muscle tension; vasoconstriction of the skin, splanchnic region, and nonpriority organs; increased cardiac output; increased blood pressure and viscosity; increased metabolic rate and oxygen consumption; decreased gastric tone and emptying; and decreased urinary tract tone and evacuation. Endocrine and metabolic responses to acute pain tend to mimic the responses seen under conditions of acute stress, including increases in catabolic substances such as adrenocorticotropic hormone (ACTH), cortisol, antidiuretic hormone (ADH), growth hormone (GH), catecholamines, cyclic AMP (cAMP), renin, angiotensin II, glucagon, aldosterone, and IL-1 and decreases in immunological competence and anabolic substances such as insulin and testosterone (Bonica, 1990; Carron, 1989; Dionne, 1992).

Given a defined set of physiological responses to a stressor like surgery, it might be assumed that similar medical procedures would elicit comparable levels of pain in patients undergoing a given procedure. Clinical experience, however, does not support this assumption. Anxiety, depression, anger, and fear are perhaps the four most prominent emotions that affect acute pain. Of these emotions, anxiety has been the best studied for acute pain (Chapman & Turner, 1990; Gil, 1992). Anxiety is associated with increased pain perception, increased risk to physical health, and prolongation of the pain experience. Bonica (Bonica, 1990) cites several examples of how anxiety associated with acute pain can further complicate a clinical picture: (1) Anxiety causes cortically mediated increases in blood viscosity and clotting time, fibrinolysis, and platelet aggregation, leading to increased risk of thromboembolism. (2) Anxiety can cause a 50–200% increase in the neuroendocrine secretion of catecholamines and cortisol, resulting in significant increases in cardiac output, abnormally high sympathetic tone, shock, excessive vasoconstriction, intestinal ischemia, and hypoxic tissue damage. (3) Anxiety also can cause 5- to 20-fold increases in ventilation with the potential of respiratory alkalosis. Additionally, anxiety can lower pain threshold, causing the patient to interpret a variety of sensations as painful, which can limit the physician's ability to complete an invasive procedure (Dworkin, 1967). Although the use of deeper sedation or general anesthesia can be used with highly anxious patients, oversedation is not without risk. The Agency for Health Care Policy and Research (AHCPR; 1992) highlights numerous concerns associated with pharmacological analgesia and sedation, including hypoxemia, nausea, urinary retention, confusion, pruritis, chest wall rigidity, bradycardia, hypotension, oxygen desaturation, hypoxia, apnea, and even death. As several dentists have lamented, "No technique, no devise, no magic solution wil anesthetize patients who are so distraught and upset that they interpret any stimulus as pain" (Walton & Torabinejad, 1992).

In a survey of 500 U.S. households, 77% of adults reported having pain after surgery, with 80% experiencing moderate to extreme pain. Fifty-seven percent cited pain after surgery as their primary fear before surgery (Warfield & Kahn, 1995). What is unknown is whether much of the moderate to extreme pain could have been reduced if presurgical fears had been adequately addressed. Examples highlighting the role anxiety can play on postsurgical pain are numerous. For example, in a recent study of children undergoing surgery, presurgical ratings of anticipatory anxiety were significant predictors of postoperative pain, with greater anxiety being associated with greater pain (Palermo & Drotar, 1996). In a sample of over 700 women who gave birth in England, preoperative anxiety about labor pain was one of the strongest predictors of negative experiences (e.g., pain) during labor, of lack of satisfaction with the birth, and of poor emotional well-being postnatally (Green, 1993). In a review of pain, anxiety, and distress in dental procedures, Litt (1996) found that many medical procedures that are inherently harmless were still associated with great pain and anxiety. The covert characteristics of the individual (e.g., expectations for pain and associated anxiety about the procedure) were more important in determining how aversive the event became than any objective characteristics of the actual procedure. Thus simply controlling the sensory component of pain without attention to anticipatory affect can lead to highly variable management of pain.

It becomes difficult to discuss affective influences on pain without evaluating the origin of those affective responses. Just as two individuals can laugh at or be offended by the same joke, love or hate the same person, or feel honored or burdened at being assigned a task, one's affective response to nociceptive signals is determined in part by one's cognitive interpretation of those signals.

Cognitive Factors Influencing Acute Pain

Nociceptive signals are evaluated against a background of (1) previous experiences with similar signals (memory and learning), (2) current events in the individual's consciousness (attention and discrimination), (3) perceived meaning of the nociceptive signals (appraisal and cultural background), and (4) perceived ability to deal effectively with those signals (expectancy, coping ability, and control). Each cognitive factor has been shown to play an important role in acute pain perception.

Memory

Mary is about to give birth. The nurse asks her to rate her pain on a scale of 0 to 100 points. Mary indicates a "98." Two weeks following the birth of a beautiful baby girl, Mary is asked to recall how much pain she was in just before giving birth. Odds are good that her memory will be inaccurate, but will she be more likely to overestimate or underestimate her pain?

Recall of pain intensity may be underestimated in situations in which positive emotion accompanies the painful event. One such study found deflated pain recall in a group of postpartum mothers who recalled the pain of childbirth as being lower than they had reported it being during the actual birth (Norvell, Gaston-Johansson, & Fridh, 1987). Remembering childbirth as being less painful than it actually was may be adaptive in helping to ensure that reproduction continues, whereas remembering harmful events as being more painful may lead to avoidance of such events in the future. In support of this hypothesis, a subsequent study by the same group of researchers found that expectant mothers (both primiparas and multiparas) tended to have unrealistic expectations about how much pain they would experience during labor. Both groups of mothers, regardless of their prior labor experience, tended to underestimate their actual pain during labor (Fridh & Gaston-Johansson, 1990). Not all studies support the underestimation of pain as being facilitory. Experimental pain studies of the effects of inaccurate pain expectations have suggested that underpredictions of pain can leave patients vulnerable to unpleasant surprise when a procedure is more noxious than anticipated. Such discrepancy between prediction and actual experience can produce fear that disrupts the pain habituation process (Arntz, van den Hout, van den Berg, & Meijboom, 1991). Underprediction of pain based on inaccurate memories may also lead to inadequate preparation on the part of the patient or clinical staff or underutilization of available pharmacological resources.

Overestimation is the more common effect of inaccurate memories for pain. A number of factors have been hypothesized to influence inflated pain recall bias. If pain is high at the time a patient is asked to recall a previous medical procedure such as a dental procedure, the memory of pain associated with the previous dental procedure is likely to be overestimated (Eich, Reeves, Jaegar, & Graff-Radford, 1985). These findings were partially replicated in a similar study using a more general pain sample (Salovey, Smith, Turk, Jobe, & Willis, 1993). Kent (1985) found that recalled pain more closely reflected a rating of predicted pain than the actual pain rating being recalled. This finding underscores again the importance of expectations in determining how a patient will react to pain in the medical setting (Litt, 1996). Redelmeier and Kahneman (1996) found that only the most affectively salient and recently occurring portions of a medical procedure are recalled. In this study, only the moment of worst pain and the final 3 minutes of the procedure were reflected in pain recall. This resulted in an inflated memory of pain intensity for the whole experience. Not all studies concur with the findings that memories for pain are inherently inaccurate. A number of studies have found memories for pain to be relatively accurate (Hunter, Philips, & Rachman, 1979; Salovey et al., 1993; Beese & Morley, 1993) and suggest that recall of pain intensity and the use of relatively simple measures of pain intensity can be obtained and are of clinical value.

When one accesses a memory of pain, the assessment is not only of the sensory component of pain but also of the integrated experience of pain, which includes emotional processing. Two theories dominate the pain memory and recall literature with regard to the role of affect in pain memories: state dependency theory and mood congruency theory. State dependence refers to the tendency for material to be recalled more accurately when there is equivalence between the mood at the time of exposure and mood at the time of recall. Thus if Sally is anxious at the time she reports dental pain but calm at the time she attempts to recall the pain, she is likely to be inaccurate. Some evidence supports state dependency as an influential factor in recall with acute pain (Pearce et al., 1990). Mood congruency refers to the tendency for material to be better recalled if the quality of the material is similar to the mood of the individual at the time of recall (Erskine, Morley, & Pearce, 1990). For example, if a patient is depressed at the time of recall, she is likely to selectively recall negative af-

fect associated with the dental procedure. If, on the other hand, she is chipper at the time of recall, negative aspects of the dental procedure will be less accessible for her to recall, whereas any positive affective experiences that might have occurred will be more readily remembered. Some studies, however, find no influence on recall due to mood (Salovey et al., 1993).

If, indeed, memory for pain is an inaccurate estimation of what was originally experienced, clinicians using recalled pain to guide treatment may be making clinical treatment decisions based on distorted information. Similarly, if pain is recalled as being greater than it was originally, patients' expectations regarding their ability to function with pain may be diminished, the perceived need for medication may be heightened, and fear associated with the procedure may develop. Fear not only can increase immediate pain perception but also can decrease willingness to engage in future potentially painful medical procedures (e.g., dental), with reduced compliance and increased avoidance of needed medical care resulting.

Learning

Little Suzy does not remember ever getting a shot at the doctor's office. Just before seeing the doctor, she witnesses another little girl crying and screaming about having been given a shot. Against a background of no prior information, chances are good that witnessing this other little girl will provide Suzy with information about shots that can influence her own experience when she meets her doctor.

Research findings from the field of social modeling have provided valuable insights into the role of social learning on the experience of acute pain. Early experimental studies demonstrated reduced pain thresholds in response to novel electric shock when the subject was in the presence of another individual who was intolerant of the shock. Conversely, when subjects were in the presence of a model who was tolerant of the shock, pain thresholds were higher (Craig & Weiss, 1971).

In the absence of previous experience with a painful procedure, patients appear to utilize whatever information is available at the time to construct a cognitive/affective framework (schema) for evaluating the novel experience. Input into this framework appears to influence the experience of pain. For example, in a study of hospitalized patients receiving arteriotomies, patients were given one of two suggestions about the sensations associated with the procedure. One condition specifically mentioned pain, whereas the other mentioned coolness and numbness. Significantly reduced pain levels were associated with the suggestions about coolness and numbness (Austan, Polise, & Schultz, 1997). In other studies, children who were candidates for surgical and dental procedures viewed films of peers undergoing the procedure that they would be receiving. Children who saw films showing peers responding to treatment in a competent fashion experienced decreased complications and anxiety with their own procedures (Craig, 1978; Melamed & Siegel, 1975; Melamed, Yurcheson, Fleece, Hutcherson, & Hawes, 1978). In a more recent study, patients who came from families that modeled good pain tolerance showed better tolerance for pain and less severe pain associated with their own medical procedures (Bachiocco, Scesi, Morselli, & Carli, 1993). In a study of two groups of adult patients undergoing minor gynecological surgery, preassessment showed that expectations for procedurally related pain did not differ. However, when one group was given additional accurate preparatory information about their surgery, this group reported lower postsurgical pain intensity ratings. The other group, receiving no accurate information, had posttreatment ratings that were more similar to their original pretreatment expectations (Wallace, 1985).

Previous experience with a specific pain stimulus can influence the current experience of pain. In a study of nonchronic pain patients undergoing thoracic surgery, those patients who had previously been subject to medical pain in the past experienced greater pain intensity postoperatively (Bachiocco, Morselli, & Carli, 1993). The design of this study did not permit analysis of whether this result was due to a sensitizing effect associated with previous pain experiences or to higher pain expectancies tied to upwardly biased memories of previous pain. The study does, however, support the notion that adequate resolution of pain at each medical encounter is important, since future treatment may be influenced by previous experiences with pain. In studies of chronic pain patients exposed to acute experimental cold pressor pain, chronic pain patients demonstrated poorer acute pain tolerance and reported higher acute pain levels than did pain-free patient controls (Brands & Schmidt, 1987). Whereas these findings could have a multitude of explanations, one possibility is that chronic pain patients have learned that pain tends to be intense and enduring. New acute pain stimuli are evaluated against this background, and the resulting

integration of acute pain nociception with past experiences creates a heightened current pain experience. Such a learning process could have profound detrimental implications for the development of additional pain, the exacerbation of pain, and the prospect of managing pain in such patients over a long term. In a particularly intriguing study, dental patients who were anxious and who expected higher pain than they eventually reported were given repeated exposures to a painful dental procedure. With exposure and learning, these patients' expectations for pain lowered and became more consistent with their actual pain reports. Anxious patients, however, required more exposures than less anxious patients, and, over time, anxious patients returned to their original inaccurate level of prediction whe exposures (and thus opportunities for disconfirmation) were less frequent (Arntz, van Eck, & Heijmans, 1990).

Learning may also influence pain perception via classical conditioning. If pain is assumed to be a more general body function that facilitates avoidance of future damaging events, animal models of illness have been used to support the utilitarian role of pain in the avoidance of harmful environmental agents. One such study found that hyperalgesia was specifically elicited by two agents designed simply to produce illness in rats. Hyperalgesia was then conditioned to a taste aversion when the agents were paired with food. The conditioned hyperalgesia was similar in magnitude and duration to that elicited by the pharmacologically induced illness (Wiertelak et al., 1994). Thus both previous experiences with pain and associated environmental events occurring at the time pain is experienced appear to become integrated into the experience of acute pain.

Attention and Discrimination

Tommy is a football player. During the big game of the season, he is tackled roughly and rises slowly after the whistle is blown. He hears his coach say, "Shake it off kid . . . shake it off." Tommy continues to play the rest of the game. Following the game, Tommy learns that he has strained a muscle in his back, and he stays home from school because of pain the whole next week. How is it that pain is experienced as more intense hours after the injury than it was at the time the injury occurred?

"Under certain circumstances, it is important for an organism not to feel pain, for example . . . if you are engaged in a battle, fighting to the death, you don't want to stop to tend to your wounds"

(Liebeskind, quoted in Touchette, 1993). If it is assumed that nociceptive signals must be recognized in order for pain to be experienced in humans, then any process that permits those signals to be ignored, missed, or interpreted as something other than pain is likely to diminish pain. Passive lack of attention or active distraction is likely to function in this way. Support for the utility of distraction as a suppressor of pain perception comes from the experimental pain literature, in which distraction through cognitive tasks or through distracting imagery has been associated with increased pain tolerance (Jaremko, 1978; Kanfer & Goldfoot, 1966; Worthington, 1978; Kanfer & Seidner, 1973; Hodes, Howland, Lightfoot, & Cleeland, 1990; Neumann et al., 1997). Based largely on the findings of these early studies, current nonpharmacological approaches to clinical pain management continue to highlight the importance of distraction techniques (Turk et al., 1983; McGrath & Hillier, 1996; Keefe, 1996; Keefe et al., 1990; ter Kuile, Spinhoven, Linssen, & van Houwelingen, 1996; Lang & Hamilton, 1994). In a study of chronic pain patients, White and Sanders (1986) found that when patients were encouraged to focus on and talk about pain-related content (attention), they had higher pain intensity ratings than similar patients who were encouraged to talk about non-pain-related topics (distraction).

Appraisal and the Meaning of Pain

Sarah and Tracy need to get their blood drawn. Both are being seen by the same phlebotomist. Sarah experiences her blood being drawn as an invasion into the integrity of her body by a stranger. She leaves feeling mildly upset and focused on her aching wrist. Tracy experiences her blood being drawn as a routine medical procedure. She leaves thinking about her bus ride home and barely notices the cotton taped to her wrist. That two individuals can experience the same procedure so differently is not unique to the experience of pain. This relationship has been found for other types of stressors as well and is the reason that work on the appraisal process (Lazarus & Folkman, 1984) is so often considered relevant to understanding cognitive events that determine one's perception of pain. According to theory, once a nociceptive event occurs, the individual makes an appraisal of the event. Primary appraisal typically determines if the nociceptive event is harmful, threatening, or of some benefit. If judged harmful or threatening, a secondary appraisal process helps to determine

if the individual possesses the necessary resources for controlling and dealing with the nociceptive event. If resources are adequate, then appropriate coping can commence and the pain experience can diminish. If resources are inadequate, then affective and stress-related sympathetic arousal act to heighten the perception of pain until appropriate resources for quieting the pain are discovered. If adaptive resources for comfort are not identified, then potentially maladaptive responses such as helplessness and illness behaviors can begin to operate in the person's life. This may result in the pain becoming more chronic (Gatchel, 1996).

Numerous studies on the appraisal of pain (specifically of its threatening or harmful nature) and on specific beliefs about the meaning of pain have been shown to influence perceptions of pain and eventual compliance with pain treatments (Williams & Thorn, 1989; Williams & Keefe, 1991; Williams, Robinson, & Geisser, 1994; Jensen, Turner, Romano, & Lawler, 1994; Jensen & Karoly, 1991). Such beliefs might include a strong conviction that pain and illness encompass all aspects of life (Waddell, Pilowsky, & Bonds, 1989), that pain is mysterious and will be enduring regardless of treatment (Williams & Keefe, 1991), and that a cause and cure must be found for the pain before attempts at functioning are worthwhile (Jensen et al., 1994).

Chapman (1985) explored the potential meanings of pain in the context of surgery. Because surgery by nature is an invasive procedure, one might suspect that it would always be appraised as harmful and be accompanied by anxiety or fear. Of course, this is not the case, as experiences of childbirth provoke vastly different emotional responses than disease-altering forms of surgery. Hypotheses about the impact of "meaning" on subsequent pain and the subsequent need for adequate pain management are presented in Table 10.1. These heuristic insights, although supported anecdotally by clinical examples, are worthy of additional study, as they could provide valuable insight into better ways of evaluating the meaning of pain for a given individual while learning how to better tailor pain management services for diverse surgical interventions.

Cultural Factors

Cultural affiliation has been shown to influence perception and response to both experimental and acute pain in multiple studies (Zborowski, 1952; Lipton & Marbach, 1984; Bates, Edwards, &

TABLE 10.1. The Meaning of Pain and Pain Management Considerations for Surgical Procedures

Purpose of surgery	Likely meaning and management considerations
Restoration of function	Improved well-being leads to positive affect and likelihood of lower pain levels.
Organ donation	Altruism leads to positive affect and heightened self-esteem, with the likelihood of lower pain levels.
Cesarean section (planned child)	Positive affect and plans for a positive future overcome discomfort, with likelihood of adequate pain management following the birth.
Cesarean section (unwanted child)	Negative affect and thoughts of a disrupted future increase the likelihood of inadequate pain management following the birth.
Exploratory surgery	Fear of finding a catastrophic problem, especially when the patient is asymptomatic at preop, increases the likelihood of increased pain. If postoperative findings are bad, pain is likely to be enhanced.
Amputation or mutilating procedure	Even when lifesaving, such a loss is likely to lead to increased pain.

Note. Modified but based on the heuristic work of Chapman (1985) on the meaning of surgery.

Anderson, 1993; Greenwald, 1991). Important ethnic factors include the culture's tendency to be emotionally expressive or stoic, beliefs about the meaning of pain and its controllability, and learned models for illness behaviors that influence how a patient responds to pain. For example, early studies comparing Italian Americans, Jewish Americans, and Anglo-Saxon Americans found that cultural norms for the expression of pain were learned at an early age and resulted in differences between these groups in later life. The Italian American group was characterized as being interested in immediate pain relief, the Jewish American group as being interested in the meaning of the pain and its future implications, and the Anglo-Saxon American group as being generally less expressive about pain and more emotionally withdrawn (Zborowski, 1952). A study with similar findings (Sternbach & Tursky, 1965) compared responses to a standardized experimental stimulus in a sample of housewives representing four different cultural backgrounds: They included Anglo-Saxon, Irish, Italian, and Jewish women. Pain thresholds did not differ between groups, but tolerances did differ, with Italian women having the lowest tolerance for pain. Like the earlier study by Zborowski, differences between the four groups centered on attitudes toward pain, with stoic or neutral responses being characteristic of the Irish and Anglo groups. Diminished reactivity was found in the Jewish sample, as they tended to minimize the significance of the

experimental pain stimulus with reference to the future. The Italian women were more reactionary to the pain, with their orientation being more attentive and focused on the immediacy of the pain (Sternbach & Tursky, 1965). A more recent, mixed-gender study of 543 acute postoperative dental pain patients evaluated pain in Asian, African American, European, and Latino patients. Patients of European descent reported significantly less severe pain than the African American or Latino groups. The Asian group was not significantly different from the European group (Faucett, Gordon, & Levine, 1994).

Some investigators believe that ethnic differences are diminishing as assimilation and acculturation produces a blending of cultural influences on pain. Although cultural assimilation may be obscuring sensory differences between cultures, affective differences are still being found in the pain reports of various ethnic groups (Greenwald, 1991). A study by Bates and Edwards (1992) evaluated a sample of 372 chronic pain patients from six ethnic groups to determine what variables best accounted for differences in pain perception across groups. Surpassing genetic influences, behavioral factors, attitudes, psychopathology, socioeconomic status, treatment history, clinical diagnosis, and medication intake, the most salient predictors of differing ethnic pain reports were heritage consistency and a factor related to secondary appraisal—the perceived ability to control the pain.

Expectancy, Coping Ability,
and Perceived Control

Harvey arrived at the dentist's office for a routine cleaning of his teeth. Harvey did not have any abnormalities with his teeth or gums but, unlike most patients, he entered the dentist's office expecting this procedure to be highly painful. Consistent with his expectation, he experienced great pain while having his teeth cleaned.

Once primary appraisal has determined that nociception is harmful or threatening, secondary appraisal must evaluate the available coping resources. Beliefs regarding personal efficacy to cope with and control pain have been associated with numerous studies on reported pain (Jensen, Turner, Romano, & Karoly, 1991).

An example of a pain-specific expectation that can increase one's perception of pain is the belief in the endurance of the pain stimulus. In experimental pain paradigms, faulty assumptions about the assumed duration of pain has influenced pain report in the direction of the faulty assumption even when the actual pain stimulus and duration of pain was held constant. For example, in a normal healthy sample exposed to experimental cold pressor pain, the belief in greater pain duration was associated with increased reported pain intensity. In this study, the actual pain stimulus and the actual duration of pain was identical for all participants at the point of comparison (i.e., 2 minutes), but the participants who believed that the pain trial was fixed to a 3-minute duration reported significantly lower pain ratings than those who believed the duration of the pain trial was open-ended (Williams & Thorn, 1986). To insure that these results were stable, this study was replicated in a second experimental pain study using an ischemic pain stimulus (Thorn & Williams, 1989).

Numerous studies have already been described that underscore how expectations become integrated with other cognitive and affective factors that eventually determine the actual pain a patient reports. One additional study of note evaluated expectancies in a heterogeneous sample of 126 postsurgical patients in an attempt to identify, from among a field of variables, which ones were most strongly associated with pain. Variables included self-control expectancies, previous pain behavior, familial pain tolerance, personality, locus of control, and expected ability to cope with pain. Of these variables, the secondary appraisal, "expected ability to cope with pain," was the most strongly associated with the total pain experience (e.g., intensity and duration) (Bachiocco, Scesi, et al., 1993). Enhancing the perception of control and the perception of ability to cope with pain continues to be the target of clinical investigations into improved pain management. Although more and more is being learned about what cognitive and emotional factors may exacerbate acute pain (e.g., catastrophizing, anxiety, fear, etc.), far less is known about which coping strategies consistently improve acute pain control. The major exception to this observation is the use of the relaxation response in acute pain management.

COGNITIVE/AFFECTIVE APPROACHES TO ACUTE PAIN MANAGEMENT

A subset of medical procedure candidates will enter treatment already possessing cognitive and affective strengths in managing their pain (Buckelew et al., 1992). Others may require brief intervention to diminish the complications that can accompany undermanaged pain. The AHCPR (1992) guidelines for acute pain management suggest that such interventions be used with the following types of patients: (1) those who find such interventions appealing, (2) those who could benefit from reducing or avoiding a pharmacological approach, (3) those who express fear or anxiety not due to a psychiatric condition, (4) those who will need to endure a prolonged painful procedure or prolonged postoperative recovery, and (5) those who have incomplete pain relief following appropriate pharmacological intervention. The goals of interventions targeting the cognitive/affective components of pain have changed little over the past 10 years (Chapman & Turner, 1986). They include (1) increasing the patient's knowledge about the procedure, (2) increasing a sense of control over the pain experience and the medical procedure, and (3) enhancing the patient's ability to quiet affective responses to pain that augment the body's general response to stress.

Increasing patients' knowledge about pain and medical procedures can help to reduce appraisals of threat and harm. By diminishing such appraisals, the associated affective responses (e.g., fear, anxiety, worry) are less likely to occur and are less likely to exacerbate the pain experience. The use of patient education in this prophylactic fashion has been recommended for acute pain services (Waldman, 1992).

Many patients are abandoning the passive role of leaving care up to their doctors and are becoming educated consumers of health services. Medical textbooks, education classes, and the Internet are increasingly popular sources of consumer information about the procedures they will be experiencing. The quality and accuracy of this information (particularly from the Internet), however, is highly variable and, unfortunately, can introduce the very fears that patient education was supposed to diminish. Therefore, clinicians need to remain current not only about the latest scientific knowledge but also about the potential misinformation that patients may be bringing into the treatment setting. Like the experimental studies already described, this misinformation can heighten fear and, therefore, pain.

The ability to diminish affective sympathetic arousal is a powerful self-management tool and can greatly contribute to a sense of control over pain and painful medical procedures. One low-tech procedure that accomplishes all of the above quickly and effectively is the relaxation response. The relaxation response can directly reduce peripheral muscular responses that contribute to some forms of pain, as well as reduce more general components of sympathetic nervous system arousal. The focus of relaxation strategies on pleasant or neutral experiences additionally serves as a distraction that diminishes the ability of cognitive and affective factors to influence nociceptive signals. The relaxation response is the most widely studied psychological intervention for postoperative pain and comes in a wide variety of forms. Some of these forms include progressive muscle relaxation (Jacobson, 1938), brief relaxation (McCaffery & Beebe, 1989), the minitrip (Williams, 1996), visual imagery (Turk et al., 1983), biofeedback (Schwartz & Associates, 1995), hypnosis (Hilgard & Hilgard, 1975), anodyne imagery (Lang & Hamilton, 1994), and music-assisted relaxation (Locsin, 1981). A recent National Institutes of Health (NIH) consensus panel evaluated the evidence for relaxation training as a treatment for pain and concluded that sufficient evidence existed to recommend its use (N.I.H. Technology Assessment Panel, 1996). To date, however, although the general concept of relaxation is recommended, no one specific form of relaxation training has been determined consistently superior to any other approach.

CONCLUSIONS

This chapter has reviewed some of the theories and some of the evidence highlighting the influential role of cognitive and affective factors in acute pain. Given the evidence that cognitive and affective factors influence pain, it is surprising that more emphasis has not been placed on assessment and treatment of these factors in medical settings in which acute pain is common. Consideration of acute pain control should target both sensory and psychological components of the experience, since pain is an integration of both elements. Frequently, however, psychological treatment of pain is limited to the comorbid psychological disturbances, a focus which, as stated, is appropriate for that subset of pain cases but misses the point that psychosocial factors are operating in all instances of pain. This does not mean that everyone with pain will require intervention. Again, the term "psychological" should not connote weakness or pathology; in fact, some individuals will enter treatment with psychosocial strengths that predispose them to deal effectively with pain. At a minimum, acute pain services should screen for both sensory and psychosocial components of pain and should possess the *ability* to briefly intervene in pain-specific psychosocial issues (in appropriate cases) should they be identified. Assessment and intervention for the psychosocial components of pain should no longer be lumped together with the mental health treatment of comorbid psychological disorders; rather, consideration of psychosocial factors should be an integral aspect of competent medical management of the acute pain experience.

REFERENCES

Agency for Health Care Policy and Research (AHCPR). (1992). *Acute pain management: Operative or medical procedures and trauma* (Clinical Practice Guideline No. 1). Rockville, MD: U.S. Department of Health and Human Services.

Arntz, A., van den Hout, M. A., van den Berg, G., & Meijboom, A. (1991). The effects of incorrect pain expectations on acquired fear and pain responses. *Behaviour Research and Therapy, 29*(6), 547–560.

Arntz, A., van Eck, M., & Heijmans, M. (1990). Predictions of dental pain: The fear of any expected evil, is worse than the evil itself. *Behaviour Research and Therapy, 28*(1), 29–41.

Austan, F., Polise, M., & Schultz, T. R. (1997). The use of verbal expectancy in reducing pain associated with arteriotomies. *American Journal of Clinical Hypnosis, 39*(3), 182–186.

Bachiocco, V., Morselli, A. M., & Carli, G. (1993). Self-control expectancy and postsurgical pain: Relationships to previous pain, behavior in past pain, familial pain tolerance models, and personality. *Journal of Pain and Symptom Management, 8*(4), 205–214.

Bachiocco, V., Scesi, M., Morselli, A. M., & Carli, G. (1993). Individual pain history and familial pain tolerance models: Relationships to post-surgical pain. *Clinical Journal of Pain, 9*(4), 266–271.

Bates, M. S., & Edwards, T. (1992). Ethnic variation in the chronic pain experience. *Ethnicity and Disease, 2,* 63–83.

Bates, M. S., Edwards, W. T., & Anderson, K. O. (1993). Ethnocultural influences on variation in chronic pain perception. *Pain, 52,* 101–112.

Beese, A., & Morley, S. (1993). Memory for acute pain experiences is specifically inacccurate but generally reliable. *Pain, 53,* 183–189.

Besson, J. M. (1994). The pharmacology of pain: Twenty-five years of hope, despair, and hope. In G. F. Gebhart, D. L. Hammond, & T. S. Jensen (Eds.), *Proceedings of the Seventh World Congress on Pain* (pp. 23–39). Seattle: IASP Press.

Bonica, J. J. (1990). History of pain concepts and theories. In J. J. Bonica (Ed.), *The management of pain* (pp. 2–17). Philadelphia: Lea & Febiger.

Bonica, J. J., Yaksh, T., Liebeskind, J. C., Pechnick, R. N., & DePaulis, A. (1990). Biochemistry and modulation of nociception and pain. In J. J. Bonica (Ed.), *The management of pain* (pp. 95–121). Philadelphia: Lea & Febiger.

Brands, A. M., & Schmidt, A. J. (1987). Learning processes in the persistence behavior of chronic low back pain patients with repeated acute pain stimulation. *Pain, 30*(3), 329–337.

Buckelew, S. P., Conway, R. C., Shutty, M. S., Lawrence, J. A., Grafing, M. R., Anderson, S. K., Hewett, J. E., & Keefe, F. J. (1992). Spontaneous coping strategies to manage acute pain and anxiety during electro-diagnostic studies. *Archives of Physical Medicine and Rehabilitation, 73*(6), 594–598.

Carron, H. (1989). Extension of pain relief beyond the operating room. *Clinical Journal of Pain, 5*(Suppl.), S1–S4.

Chapman, C. R. (1985). Psychological factors in postoperative pain. In G. Smith & B. G. Covino (Eds.), *Acute pain* (pp. 22–41). Boston: Butterworths.

Chapman, C. R., & Turner, J. A. (1986). Psychological control of acute pain in medical settings. *Journal of Pain and Symptom Management, 1*(1), 9–20.

Chapman, C. R., & Turner, J. A. (1990). Psychologic and psychosocial aspects of acute pain. In J. J. Bonica (Ed.), *The management of pain* (pp. 122–132). Philadelphia: Lea & Febiger.

Craig, K. D. (1978). Social modelling influences on pain. In R. A. Sternbach (Ed.), *The psychology of pain* (pp. 73–109). New York: Raven Press.

Craig, K. D., & Weiss, S. M. (1971). Vicarious influences on pain threshold determinations. *Journal of Personality and Social Psychology, 19,* 53–59.

Dionne, R. A. (1992). New approaches to preventing and treating postoperative pain. *Journal of the American Dental Association, 123*(6), 27–34.

Drossman, D. A. (1996). Chronic functional abdominal pain. *American Journal of Gastroenterology, 91,* 2270–2281.

Dworkin, S. F. (1967). Anxiety and performance in the dental environment: An experimental investigation. *Journal of the American Society of Psychosomatic Dentistry and Medicine, 14,* 88–102.

Eich, E., Reeves, J. L., Jaegar, B., & Graff-Radford, S. B.

(1985). Memory for pain: Relation between past and present pain intensity. *Pain, 23,* 375–379.

Erskine, A., Morley, S., & Pearce, S. (1990). Memory for pain: A review. *Pain, 41,* 255–265.

Faucett, J., Gordon, N., & Levine, J. (1994). Differences in postoperative pain severity among four ethnic groups. *Journal of Pain and Symptom Management, 9*(6), 383–389.

Fields, H. L. (1991). *Core curriculum for professional education in pain.* Seattle: IASP Press.

Fields, H. L., & Basbaum, A. I. (1989). Endogenous pain control mechanisms. In R. D. France & K. R. R. Krishnan (Eds.), *Textbook of pain* (pp. 206–217). Edinburgh: Churchill Livingstone.

Fridh, G., & Gaston-Johansson, F. (1990). Do primiparas and multiparas have realistic expectations of labor? *Acta Obstetrica et Gynecologica Scandinavica, 69*(2), 103–109.

Gatchel, R. J. (1996). Psychological disorders and chronic pain: Cause-and-effect relationships. In R. J. Gatchel & D. C. Turk (Eds.), *Psychological approaches to pain management: A practitioner's handbook* (pp. 33–52). New York: Guilford Press.

Gil, K. M. (1992). Psychological aspects of acute pain. In R. S. Sinatra, A. H. Hord, B. Ginsberg, & L. M. Preble (Eds.), *Acute pain: Mechanisms and management.* St. Louis, MO: Mosby.

Green, J. M. (1993). Expectations and experiences of pain in labor: Findings from a large prospective study. *Birth, 20*(2), 65–72.

Greenwald, H. P. (1991). Interethnic differences in pain perception. *Pain, 44,* 157–163.

Hilgard, E. R., & Hilgard, J. R. (1975). *Hypnosis in the relief of pain.* Los Altos, CA: Kaufmann.

Hodes, R. L., Howland, E. W., Lightfoot, N., & Cleeland, C. S. (1990). The effects of distraction on responses to cold pressor pain. *Pain, 41*(1), 109–114.

Hunter, M., Philips, C., & Rachman, S. (1979). Memory for pain. *Pain, 6,* 35–46.

Jacobson, E. (1938). *Progressive relaxation.* Chicago: University of Chicago Press.

Jaremko, M. E. (1978). Cognitive strategies in the control of pain tolerance. *Journal of Behavior Therapy and Experimental Psychiatry, 9,* 239–244.

Jensen, M. P., & Karoly, P. (1991). Control beliefs, coping efforts, and adjustment to chronic pain. *Journal of Consulting and Clinical Psychology, 59*(3), 431–438.

Jensen, M. P., Turner, J. A., Romano, J. M., & Karoly, P. (1991). Coping with chronic pain: A critical review of the literature. *Pain, 47*(3), 249–283.

Jensen, M. P., Turner, J. A., Romano, J. M., & Lawler, B. K. (1994). Relationship of pain-specific beliefs to chronic pain adjustment. *Pain, 57*(3), 301–309.

Kanfer, F. H., & Goldfoot, D. A. (1966). Self-control and tolerance of noxious stimulation. *Psychological Reports, 18,* 79–85.

Kanfer, F. H., & Seidner, M. L. (1973). Self control: Factors enhancing tolerance of noxious stimulation. *Journal of Personality and Social Psychology, 25,* 381–389.

Keefe, F. J. (1996). Cognitive behavioral therapy for managing pain. *Clinical Psychologist, 49,* 4–5.

Keefe, F. J., Caldwell, D. S., Williams, D. A., Gil, K. M., Mitchell, D., Robertson, C., Salutario, M., Nunley, J., Beckham, J., Crisson, J. E., & Helms, M. (1990). Pain coping skills training in the management of osteoarthritic knee pain: A comparative study. *Behavior Therapy, 21,* 49-62.

Kehlet, H. (1986). Pain relief and modification of the stress response. In M. J. Cousins & G. D. Phillips (Eds.), *Acute pain management* (pp. 49-75). New York: Churchill Livingstone.

Kent, G. (1985). Memory for dental pain. *Pain, 21,* 187-194.

Lang, E. V., & Hamilton, D. (1994). Anodyne imagery: An alternative to IV sedation in interventional radiology. *American Journal of Radiology, 162,* 1221-1226.

Lazarus, R. R., & Folkman, S. (1984). *Stress, appraisal, and coping.* New York: Springer.

Liebeskind, J. C. (1991). Pain can kill [Editorial]. *Pain, 44*(1), 3-4.

Lipton, J. A., & Marbach, J. J. (1984). Ethnicity and the pain experience. *Social Science Medicine, 19*(12), 1279-1298.

Litt, M. D. (1996). A model of pain and anxiety associated with acute stressors: Distress in dental procedures. *Behaviour Research and Therapy, 34,* 459-476.

Locsin, R. G. (1981). The effect of music on the pain of selected post-operative patients. *Journal of Advanced Nursing, 6,* 19-25.

McCaffery, M., & Beebe, A. (1989). *Pain, clinical manual for nursing practice.* St. Louis, MO: Mosby.

McGrath, P. A., & Hillier, L. M. (1996). Controlling children's pain. In R. J. Gatchel & D. C. Turk (Eds.), *Psychological approaches to pain management: A practitioner's handbook* (pp. 331-370). New York: Guilford Press.

Melamed, B. G., & Siegel, L. J. (1975). Reduction of anxiety in children facing hospitalization and surgery by the use of film modelling. *Journal of Consulting and Clinical Psychology, 43,* 511-521.

Melamed, B. G., Yurcheson, R., Fleece, E. L., Hutcherson, S., & Hawes, R. (1978). Effects of film modelling on the reduction of anxiety-related behaviors in individuals varying in level of previous experience in the stress situation. *Journal of Consulting and Clinical Psychology, 46,* 1357-1367.

Melzack, R., & Wall, P. D. (1982). *The challenge of pain.* New York: Basic Books.

Mogil, J. S., Sternberg, W. F., Kest, P., Marek, P., & Liebeskind, J. C. (1993). Sex differences in the antagonism of swim-induced analgesia: Effects of gonadectomy and estrogen replacement. *Pain, 53,* 17-25.

N.I.H. Technology Assessment Panel. (1996). Integration of behavioral and relaxation approaches into the treatment of chronic pain and insomnia. *Journal of the American Medical Association, 276,* 313-318.

Neumann, W., Kugler, J., Pfand-Neumann, P., Schmitz, N., Seelbach, H., & Kruskemper, G. M. (1997). Effects of pain-incompatible imagery on tolerance of pain, heart rate, and skin resistance. *Perceptual and Motor Skills, 84*(3, Part 1), 939-943.

Norvell, K. T., Gaston-Johansson, F., & Fridh, G. (1987). Remembrance of labor pain: How valid are retrospective pain measures? *Pain, 31,* 77-86.

Ohrbach, R., & McCall, W. D. (1996). The Stress-Hyperactivity-Pain theory of myogenic pain: Proposal for a revised theory. *Pain Forum, 5*(1), 51-66.

Page, G. G. (1996). The medical necessity of adequate pain management. *Pain Forum, 5*(4), 227-233.

Palermo, T. M., & Drotar, D. (1996). Prediction of children's postoperative pain: The role of presurgical expectations and anticipatory emotions. *Journal of Pediatric Psychology, 21*(5), 683-698.

Pearce, S. A., Isherwood, S., Hrouda, D., Richardson, P. H., Erskine, A., & Skinner, J. (1990). Memory and pain: Tests of mood congruity and state dependent learning in experimentally induced and clinical pain. *Pain, 43,* 187-193.

Peck, C. L. (1986). Psychological factors in acute pain management. In M. J. Cousins & G. D. Phillips (Eds.), *Acute pain management* (pp. 251-274). New York: Churchill Livingstone.

Redelmeier, D. A., & Kahneman, D. (1996). Patients' memories of painful medical treatments: Real-time and retrospective evaluations of two minimally invasive procedures. *Pain, 66,* 3-8.

Rey, R. (1993). *History of pain.* Paris: Editions La Decouverte.

Salovey, P., Smith, A. F., Turk, D. C., Jobe, J. B., & Willis, G. B. (1993). The accuracy of memory for pain: Not so bad most of the time. *American Pain Society Journal, 2*(3), 184-191.

Schwartz, M. S., & Associates. (1995). *Biofeedback: A practitioner's guide* (2nd ed.). New York: Guilford Press.

Sherrington, C. S. (1900). Cutaneous sensations. In E. A. Schafer (Ed.), *Textbook of physiology* (pp. 920-1001). Edinburgh: Pentland.

Sternbach, R. A. (1986). Pain and "hassles" in the United States: Findings of the Nuprin pain report. *Pain, 27,* 69-80.

Sternbach, R. A., & Tursky, B. (1965). Ethnic differences among housewives in psychosocial and skin potential responses to electric shock. *Psychophysiology, 1,* 241-246.

Strong, C. A. (1895). The psychology of pain. *Psychological Reviews, 2,* 329.

ter Kuile, M. M., Spinhoven, P., Linssen, A. C., & van Houwelingen, H. C. (1996). Cognitive coping and appraisal processes in the treatment of chronic headaches. *Pain, 64*(2), 257-264.

Thorn, B. E., & Williams, G. A. (1989). Goal specification alters perceived pain intensity and tolerance latency. *Cognitive Therapy and Research, 13,* 171-183.

Torebjork, E. (1994). Nociceptor dynamics in humans. In G. F. Gebhart, D. L. Hammond, & T. S. Jensen (Eds.), *Proceedings of the Seventh World Congress on Pain* (pp. 277-284). Seattle: IASP Press.

Touchette, N. (1993). Estrogen signals a novel route to pain relief. *Journal of NIH Research, 5,* 53-58.

Turk, D. C., Meichenbaum, D., & Genest, M. (1983). *Pain and behavioral medicine: A cognitive-behavioral perspective.* New York: Guilford Press.

Waddell, G., Pilowsky, I., & Bonds, M. R. (1989). Clinical assessment and interpretation of abnormal illness behavior in low back pain. *Pain, 39,* 41-53.

Waldman, S. D. (1992). Acute and postoperative pain: Management from a primary care perspective [Special issue]. *Postgraduate Medicine,* 5-18.

Wallace, L. M. (1985). Surgical patients' expectations of pain and discomfort: Does accuracy of expectations minimize post-surgical pain and distress? *Pain, 22*(4), 363-373.

Walton, R. E., & Torabinejad, M. (1992). Managing local anesthesia problems in the endodonic patient. *Journal of the American Dental Association, 123,* 97-102.

Warfield, C. A., & Kahn, C. H. (1995). Acute pain management: Programs in U.S. hospitals and experiences and attitudes among U.S. adults. *Anesthesiology, 83*(5), 1090-1094.

White, B., & Sanders, S. H. (1986). The influence on patients' pain intensity ratings of antecedent reinforcement of pain talk or well talk. *Journal of Behavior Therapy and Experimental Psychiatry, 17*, 155–159.

Wiertelak, E. P., Smith, K. P., Furness, L., Mooney-Heiberger, K., Mayr, T., Maier, S. F., & Watkins, L. R. (1994). Acute and conditioned hyperalgesic responses to illness. *Pain, 56*(2), 227–234.

Wilcox, G. L. (1991). Excitatory neurotransmitters and pain. In M. R. Bond, J. E. Charlton, & C. L. Woolf (Eds.), *Proceedings of the Sixth World Congress on Pain* (pp. 97–117). Amsterdam: Elsevier.

Williams, D. A. (1996). Acute pain management. In R. J. Gatchel & D. C. Turk (Eds.), *Psychological approaches to pain management: A practitioner's handbook* (pp. 55–77). New York: Guilford Press.

Williams, D. A., & Keefe, F. J. (1991). Pain beliefs and the use of cognitive-behavioral coping strategies. *Pain, 46*, 185–190.

Williams, D. A., Robinson, M. E., & Geisser, M. E. (1994). Pain beliefs: Assessment and utility. *Pain, 59*, 71–78.

Williams, D. A., & Thorn, B. E. (1986). Can research methodology affect treatment outcome?: A comparison of two cold pressor test paradigms. *Cognitive Therapy and Research, 10*, 539–546.

Williams, D. A., & Thorn, B. E. (1989). An empirical assessment of pain beliefs. *Pain, 36*, 351–358.

Willis, W. D. (1994). Central plastic responses to pain. In G. F. Gebhart, D. L. Hammond, & T. S. Jensen (Eds.), *Proceedings of the Seventh World Congress on Pain* (pp. 301–324). Seattle: IAPS Press.

Willis, W. D., & Westlund, K. N. (1997). Neuroanatomy of the pain system and of the pathways that modulate pain. *Journal of Clinical Neurophysiology, 14*(1), 2–31.

Worthington, E. I. (1978). The effect of imagery content, choice of imagery content, and self-verbalization on the self-control of pain. *Cognitive Therapy and Research, 2*, 225–240.

Zborowski, M. (1952). Cultural components in responses to pain. *Journal of Social Issues, 8*, 16–30.

Chapter 11

Low Back Pain: An Epidemic in Industrialized Countries

JOHN PAUL GAROFALO
PETER POLATIN

Lower back pain (LBP) is a health condition that is currently taking a significant toll on the U.S. health care system, as well as on the personal lives of individuals who suffer from such problems. It is has been estimated that 1 in 25 people will change his or her work because of LBP or will retire early due to disability stemming from low back problems (Taylor, 1976); a high percentage of American adults suffering from LBP attribute this condition to an occupational injury. LBP is proving to be a major medical condition that is pervasive in other industrialized countries as well, with a growth rate that could be described as "epidemic" in nature (Frymoyer, 1991). Back pain has been found to be the most expensive benign condition in industrialized countries, while representing the primary cause of disability in persons under the age of 45 (Mayer, 1991; Mayer & Gatchel, 1988). In fact, $16 billion of the estimated $27 billion annual medical care for musculoskeletal pain in the United States is directed towards the treatment of LBP, of which approximately one-half is consumed by surgical treatment (Holbrook, Grazier, Kelsey, & Stauffer, 1984; Mayer, 1991; Mayer & Gatchel, 1988). Clearly, these projective costs are indicative of a medical condition of a refractory nature that seems to be absorbing a significant amount of the nation's health care resources.

Despite the overarching influence of LBP, both on a societal and individual level, there is still no identifiable cause for its onset or its recurrence. Nonetheless, new technology has furthered the understanding of LBP and the identification of pain sources, as well as neurophysiological mechanisms of nociception (Mayer, 1991). The objective of this chapter is to provide a cogent discussion of the factors that are believed to contribute to its high incidence in Western industrialized countries and in particular occupational settings. Although there is general agreement among researchers and clinicians that exposure to a combination of occupational risk factors may render certain individuals more susceptible to musculoskeletal pain, it is clear that there is no single causal relationship. In addition to the physical factors, psychological and social variables also have an impact on the expression of back pain.

THE IMPACT OF LOW BACK PAIN ON THE UNITED STATES

An estimated 2–5% of the adult U.S. population has a disabling LBP condition at any given time (Andersson, 1979; Klein, Jensen, & Sanderson, 1984; Frymoyer & Cats-Baril, 1987), and 80% of people will experience low back problems at one

164

point in their lives. Once an episode of LBP has occurred, recurrences are reported to occur in between 30% and 70% of patients (Garg & Moore, 1992a). The incidence of LBP among men and women appears to be equal. Garg and Moore (1992a) report that women are at higher risk for work-related back problems, as well as for filing workers' compensation claims, when their jobs require heavy physical labor. MacDonald et al. (1997), however, found that most injured workers with one or more additional claims were young males.

Epidemiological studies have independently documented that LBP is an international problem of immense proportion (Berkowitz, Johnson, & Murphy, 1976; Howard, Brehm, & Nagi, 1980; Mayer, 1991; U.S. Department of Health and Human Services, 1987). Spine injuries, in general, lead to spiraling treatment costs in workers' compensation systems (Webster & Snook, 1994). Current prevention programs do not appear to have decreased the incidence of LBP injuries in industrial populations. The prevalence of LBP and LBP disability in nonindustrial settings has not been well studied (Honeyman & Jacobs, 1996), but it is in the industrial arena that costs to society have been defined.

LOW BACK PAIN
IN OTHER COUNTRIES

Cross-cultural comparisons were made among LBP patients being treated at specialized pain treatment centers in several countries, including the United States, Mexico, Japan, Italy, and New Zealand (Sanders et al., 1992). Although the degree of disruption resulting from LBP was high among all the respondents, American patients reported the greatest level of impairment in all areas of life functioning. It is not known whether this is due in part to cultural factors or if it is suggestive of an undefined genetic difference. Other cross-cultural comparisons have revealed that experiences of back problems were reported less frequently in Hong Kong than in Britain (Lau et al., 1996). Although Hong Kong respondents tended to be shorter and engaged in heavy lifting less often than British respondents, these differences did not fully account for the varying incidence rates. Lau et al. (1996) speculated further that cultural factors may contribute to the differences reported in that individuals from Hong Kong may have a higher threshold for reporting pain symptoms.

A survey in a Nordic sample of more than 2,000 individuals found that 60–65% of 30- to 50-

year-old men and women reported a lifetime prevalence of low back problems, and 44–54% reported LBP in the last year (Leboeuf-Yde, Klougart, & Lauritzen, 1996). However, Mayer (1991) reported that only 25–40% of lost time in Scandinavia is due to LBP, compared to 90% of lost time in the United States. What makes this finding even more peculiar is that the costs of medical resources and disability payments are reportedly greater in Northern European countries in which the socialized economies do not emphasize the distinction between compensable and noncompensable pain to the extent done in the United States (Mayer & Gatchel, 1988).

PREVALENCE RATES FOR VARIOUS
OCCUPATIONAL SETTINGS
IN INDUSTRIALIZED SOCIETIES

One of the earliest studies that examined the rates of LBP in the work environment took place during the 1950s. Hult (1954) compared prevalence rates of LBP among different subsets of workers. Sixty percent of forest workers reported having LBP at the time of the study or having a history of LBP. Pain symptoms generally began after the age of 30. Although the frequency of LBP was comparable for both heavy labor and lighter jobs, heavy labor workers were more at risk to have disability as a result of LBP. Hult (1954) found that the rates of industry-related LBP were greater than in the general population.

Since then, a number of investigators have targeted the work environment to better assess the rate of LBP according to vocation and to advance the understanding of the contributing mechanisms of LBP among different occupational subsets. Burton, Tillotson, Symonds, Burke, and Mathewson (1996) surveyed LBP in a large sample of police officers; the investigators were attempting to identify potential risk factors that may contribute to the high rate of first-onset and recurrent back problems. The wearing of body armor, weighing approximately 20 pounds (8.5 kg), increased the likelihood of first-onset LBP far in excess of other risk factors, including vehicular exposure and sports activities. However, the chronicity of the condition appeared to be more attributable to psychological factors such as the stressful nature of being a police officer rather than to physical demands of the job alone. Absenteeism stemming from LBP was not fully accounted for by the wearing of body armor, but police officers wearing body armor who also acknowledged having difficulties at work had higher rates of absenteeism than armored officers who did not report work-related grievances.

There has been general agreement that nursing is a high-risk profession for LBP. It has been reported that a significantly high proportion of nurses take 4 weeks off work per year because of low back problems (Smedley, Egger, Cooper, & Coggon, 1995). Among the 1,616 female nurses surveyed, 60% of the respondents reported a lifetime prevalence of LBP, and 45% reported LBP in the preceding 12-month period. Hignett (1996) found that 40–50% of nurses experienced low back problems in the previous year, and 35–80% reported a history of LBP. Occupational risk factors associated with LBP in nurses included frequency of lifting and manually moving patients between bed and chair (Garg & Owen, 1992; Smedley, Egger, Cooper, & Coggon, 1995), particularly in home care settings (Knibbe & Friele, 1996).

A number of studies have examined prevalence rates of LBP in various industrial settings in which heavy labor is merely one component of the individual's daily routine. A survey administered to over 400 steelworkers revealed that low back, neck, and shoulder pains were the most commonly reported symptoms (Hildebrandt, Bongers, Dul, Van Dijk, & Kemper, 1996). Suadicani, Hansen, Fenger, and Gyntelberg (1994) found that 51% of 469 employees at another steel plant experienced LBP during the preceding 12 months. The majority of workers attributed their back problems to heavy and frequent lifting. In a sample of male coal miners, it was found that 56% of those surveyed experienced LBP during the preceding year (Agius et al., 1994). Thirty-four percent of the respondents had experienced their first episode of back pain during the previous year, and 69% of the respondents reported a lifetime prevalence of LBP.

In a 12-year follow-up study, 366 middle-aged farmers were surveyed by telephone (Manninen, Rhiihimaki, & Heliovaara, 1995). Approximately 13% of the respondents complained of LBP in the past year. Farmers who were free of low back problems were found to have a better prognosis than those who reported one episode of back pain. Simply stated, initial pain proved to be the best predictor of future pain. The authors also noted that smokers in this sample were more likely to report LBP than nonsmokers. This commonly reported association between a history of habitual cigarette smoking and LBP will be discussed later in this chapter.

Not all epidemiological studies attribute the high rates of low back problems to heavy labor; in fact, a commonly reported origin of such pain is linked to sitting. Self-reported LBP has been found to be as prevalent among sedentary workers as among manual workers (Burton, 1997). Approximately 66% of the employees of a pharmaceutical company reported a significant level of LBP in the preceding year (Rotgoltz, Derazne, Froom, Grushecky, & Ribak, 1992); the majority of these worked in the packing department. A higher rate of back problems was noted in employees who had chairs that were found to be ergonomically unfit. Sitting, lifting, and longer tenure in the packing department were associated with increased LBP. Among 6,000 employees of a chemical manufacturing company, 35.4% reported back pain during the preceding year (Burchfiel, Boice, Stafford, & Bond, 1992), with an additional association with sitting.

Bigos, Battie, Spengler, et al. (1992) prospectively followed 3,020 employees of a Boeing-Everett aircraft manufacturing plant to assess risk factors that predispose workers to file industrial back injury claims. Acute back problems were reported by 279 participants. A history of medical treatment proved to be the only physical variable predictive of LBP. Other nonphysical variables shown to be predictive of future back pain included job task dissatisfaction and psychological distress.

In a cross-sectional study of approximately 700 workers from a machine-building factory in Russia, 48.2% of the respondents reported a lifetime prevalence of LBP, and 31.5% reported having experienced LBP during the preceding year, point prevalence was 11.5% (Toroptsova, Benevolenskaya, Karyakin, Sergeev, & Erdesz, 1995). Low back complaints from workers increased with age but were typically limited in duration. According to Toroptsova et al. (1995), the duration of the pain episode was less than 2 weeks in 88.2% of the respondents, and only 1.8% reported pain persisting more than 12 weeks. An association between LBP and the frequency of bending was found.

Van Doorn (1995) examined the extent of low back disability retrospectively among Dutch dentists, veterinarians, physicians, and physical therapists. Out of 1,119 claims filed between 1977 and 1989, 839 claimants had LBP. The presence of psychosocial distress at the onset of disability was associated with prolonged duration of low back problems. Furber et al. (1992) surveyed the prevalence of LBP in French physicians. Approximately 32% of the respondents reported experiencing LBP in the preceding 12 months, and 62% of the respondents reported a lifetime prevalence of low back problems. When queried about the origin of their pain, the majority of respondents linked their symptoms to occupationally related behaviors, including bending, sitting for extended periods of time, and posture.

Jefferson and McGrath (1996) administered a self-report questionnaire in an aircraft engine factory to measure the incidence rate among 306 employees. Approximately 69% of the respondents reported LBP in the preceding year. However, when occupational health records were reviewed, it was revealed that only 27% of the respondents actually complained of LBP and that only 2.3% experienced absenteeism due to back problems. In addition, Jefferson and McGrath (1996) reported that the level of LBP was associated with the level of neck and peripheral joint pain; this may indicate over-reporting of LBP symptoms. These findings suggest that a self-report questionnaire may not be sufficient in identifying a clinical level of back pain; instead, an accurate and thorough assessment of back pain incidence in the workplace will require reviewing other records (see Table 11.1).

NORMAL COURSE OF TREATMENT

The course of LBP is usually benign. One-half of patients suffering from LBP will return to full functioning within 2 weeks; 70% will recover in 1 month; and approximately 90% will recover within 3 to 6 months (Mayer & Gatchel, 1988). Nevertheless, 30–70% of people suffering from LBP will experience a recurrence of three or more episodes (Benn & Wood, 1975). The age of onset is often in the mid- to late 20s, and the risk of experiencing LBP increases with age. Patients remaining symptomatic after 6 months have a much poorer prognosis, with diminished levels of occupational and social functioning (Mayer, 1991). The majority of this group will remain disabled after 1 and 2 years. Chronicity of pain is less dependent on medical than on psychosocial factors.

The course of treatment for back pain typically begins with the patient seeking immediate relief for his or her pain from a primary care provider. Spontaneous recovery or early intervention helps the majority of patients by leading to a successful outcome. Immediately following an injury, passive treatment modalities are typically directed toward controlling the pain symptoms (Polatin & Mayer, 1995). It is at this point that the majority of patients experience both full relief of their pain and a complete recovery from the injury. However, for the patients whose pain symptoms do not subside, the processes of deconditioning and disability reinforced by secondary gain are beginning. The desire to avoid pain leads to reduced physical activity and results in joints becoming progressively stiffer and muscles becoming weaker.

When pain persists beyond the initial 4 weeks, secondary care programs are recommended to correct early deconditioning. Mobilization, strengthening, and work simulation, with the objective of having the patient practice typical work demands and develop a greater endurance to fatigue and pain, facilitate the return to work. Although psychosocial intervention is offered during this phase of treatment, it is typically not integrated into secondary care rehabilitation programs.

Tertiary care is recommended for the 5–8% of patients who did not benefit from secondary care and remain symptomatic and disabled beyond 4 to 6 months after injury. Factors associated with poor treatment outcome in secondary care include noncompliance, financial reward, litigation, high

TABLE 11.1. Incidence of LBP in the Workplace

Occupation	Lifetime	1-year	Study
Forest rangers	60%	—	Hult (1954)
Nurses	60%	45%	Smedley et al. (1995)
	80%	50%	Hignett (1996)
Steel workers	—	51%	Suadicani, Hansen, Fenger, & Gyntelberg (1994)
Aircraft workers	—	69%	Jefferson & McGrath (1996)
Machinery workers	48%	32%	Toroptsova, Benevolenskaya, Karyakin, Sergeev, & Erdesz (1995)
Coal miners	69%	56%	Agius et al. (1994)
Farmers	—	13%	Manninen, Rhiihimaki, & Heliovaara (1995)
Pharmaceutical workers	—	66%	Rotgoltz, Derazne, Froom, Grushecky, & Ribak (1992)
Chemical manufacturing workers	—	35%	Burchfiel, Boice, Stafford, & Bond (1992)
Physicians	62%	32%	Furber et al. (1992)

levels of psychological distress, and inhibited function (Mayer et al., 1995). Tertiary care tends to offer a higher level of intensity than either primary or secondary care and effects improvement in a subgroup of chronic pain patients that seems treatment-resistant. Functional restoration represents a tertiary care approach in which chronic LBP patients are treated with physical and occupational therapy within an interdisciplinary cognitive-behavioral model, utilizing quantification of function to document physical improvement (Polatin & Mayer, 1995).

Definitive treatment beyond primary care should be initiated quickly if patients fail to improve within the first few weeks after injury, for there is a decreased likelihood of returning to work as the duration of sick leave increases (Valat, Goupille, & Vedere, 1997).

PHYSICAL FACTORS

Individuals in jobs requiring manual labor, including heavy lifting, bending, and twisting, are at an increased risk for low back problems (Bombardier, Kerr, Shannon, & Frank, 1994; Marras et al., 1995; Schierhout, Meyers, & Bridger, 1995). Trunk extensor weakness in a worker with a physically demanding job contributes further to this injury risk (Cady, Bischoff, O'Connell, Thomas, & Allan, 1979; Garg & Moore, 1992a; Mayer, Gatchel, et al., 1985; Mayer, Smith, Keeley, & Mooney, 1985).

Past methods of measuring physical workload have included self-reports, observation, recording muscle activations, and estimated spinal loads (Wells et al., 1997). Despite its frequent use, the least accurate and most unreliable form of assessment is self-report questionnaires. There is a need for an assessment instrument capable of measuring physical concomitants of LBP. Knibbe and Friele (1996) found that the majority of disabling LBP cases were attributable to a high physical workload. Burdorf, van Riel, van Wingerden, and Snijders (1995) examined the relationship between trunk muscle strength and the occurrence of LBP in steelworkers with a high physical workload. Workers with low back problems demonstrated a lower trunk muscle performance than workers without a history of LBP, so that trunk extensor weakness may be predictive of LBP.

However, there has been a recent shift from static models of spinal loading to dynamic models to account for the high rates of LBP (Burton, 1997;

Marras et al., 1995). Marras et al. (1995) studied 400 industrial jobs in 50 varied industries and found that a combination of five trunk motion and workplace factors predicted both medium and high risk for the development of lower back problems. As these workplace factors (lifting frequency, load moment, trunk lateral velocity, trunk twisting, velocity, and trunk sagittal angle) increased in magnitude, the risk for LBP increased proportionally. Conversely, as the magnitude of these factors decreased, the risk for LBP decreased by a factor of 10. This supports the belief that changes in the work setting can influence the incidence of developing LBP.

There is a clear association between heavy manual labor and musculoskeletal problems. However, individuals whose job duties do not require heavy manual tasks also report a high rate of LBP compared to the general population. Posture, age, smoking, and other physical markers have all been implicated in LBP (Garg, 1992; Leboeuf-Yde, 1995; Mayer, 1991). Risk assessment studies of physical labor focus on single manual activities such as pulling, lifting, carrying, lowering, and pushing. Lifting is an example of a task that is seen as the triggering event leading to LBP (Bigos et al., 1986; Andersson, 1981). Posture and plane of activity in multiple sequential tasks may influence safety with even relatively light loads, thereby increasing injury risk (Garg, 1992). Even when light loads require lifting, certain postures can lead to a high level of tension in the muscles. Therefore, the safe weight of a load depends both on the capacity of all the muscles involved in lifting to develop sufficient muscle strength and on the body maintaining appropriate postural balance (Garg, 1992). Few studies have investigated the risk of combining these tasks, and those that have typically have subdivided combination tasks into single tasks. The use of single tasks to estimate the risk of combination tasks results in unacceptable risk errors of manual handling tasks (Straker, Stevenson, & Twomey, 1996).

Perhaps one of the most agreed on but least understood individual risk factors outside the occupational environment for developing LBP is habitual cigarette smoking. A number of epidemiological studies, both prospective and retrospective, agree on the existence of a strong association between smoking and LBP (Deyo, 1991; Deyo & Bass, 1989; Kelsey et al., 1984; Harreby, Kjer, Hesselsoe, & Neergaard, 1996; Leboeuf-Yde, 1995). Jamison, Stetson, and Parris (1991) reported that out of a sample of 250 patients with low back problems, 54% smoked cigarettes on a regular basis.

The pathogenesis is still poorly understood, but Deyo (1991) suggested that (1) increased coughing leads to elevated disc pressure and risk of herniation and (2) nicotine can cause vasoconstriction that will interfere with discal metabolism.

Other investigators have found a particularly significant association between back problems and seated work (Andersson & Ortengren, 1974; Pope, 1991). According to Pope (1991), this link is due to fixed posture in jobs that require a great deal of sitting. The unused muscles may experience atrophy, which will subsequently lead to deconditioning accompanied by pain.

Physical factors are not predictive of LBP but rather of disability from low back pain and of high compensation cost (Garg & Moore, 1992a). According to Burton (1997), achieving successful rehabilitation through ergonomic intervention as dictated by biomechanical factors has failed to receive universal support. This suggests that definitive treatment needs to incorporate strategies to deal with all the factors associated with LBP (Bigos & Andary, 1991; Burton, 1997). Table 11.2 lists the physical factors associated with LBP.

PSYCHOSOCIAL FACTORS

Psychosocial factors are believed to be important determinants of LBP onset, response to treatment, and chronic disability (Gatchel, 1996). The gate control theory marks one of the earliest attempts to integrate physical and psychological factors into a conceptual model of chronic pain (Melzack & Wall, 1965). The mediation of pain perception is explained by central nervous system mechanisms and psychological factors, such as mood and cognitive style, through excitatory and inhibitory influences of modulating ascending and descending nerve fiber pathways (Turk, 1996).

Depressive symptoms are frequently observed in LBP patients, including feelings of despair, anhedonia, insomnia, appetitive disturbance, and anergia. Other emotional distress symptoms associated with LBP include hysteria, hypochondriasis, somatization, and substance and alcohol abuse. The Minnesota Multiphasic Personality Inventory (MMPI) is a standardized psychological test that is very sensitive to these symptoms and has been useful for documenting them in chronic pain patients (Garg & Moore, 1992b; Gatchel, Polatin, Mayer, & Garcy, 1994).

In chronic pain patients, attempts to maintain a previous level of physical activity sometimes produce pain. The patient may, in turn, experience feelings of anxiety coupled with a pattern of pain-avoidance behavior, resulting in decreased participation in physical activity (Troup & Slade, 1985). This "pain behavior" becomes pathological if it persists and may lead to increased anxiety and hypervigilance (Rainville, Ahern, Phalen, Childs, & Sutherland, 1991).

TABLE 11.2. Physical Factors Associated with LBP

Physical factor	Study
High physical workload	Knibbe & Friele (1996)
Heavy lifting, bending, twisting	Bombardier, Kerr, Shannon, & Frank (1994)
	Schierhout, Meyers, & Bridger (1995)
Prolonged sitting	Andersson & Ortengren (1974)
	Pope (1991)
Dynamic tasks	Marras et al. (1995)
Trunk extensor weakness	Cady et al. (1979)
	Garg & Moore (1992a)
	Mayer, Gatchel, et al. (1985)
	Mayer, Smith, et al. (1985)
	Burdorf, van Riel, van Wingerden, & Snijders (1995)
Age	Garg (1992)
Posture	Garg (1992)
	Mayer (1991)
Smoking	Leboeuf-Yde (1995)
	Deyo (1991)
	Deyo & Bass (1989)
	Kelsey et al. (1984)
	Harreby, Kjer, Hesselsoe, & Neergaard (1996)

Individuals with job dissatisfaction are more apt to report LBP (Bigos et al., 1991; Bigos, Battie, Spengler, et al., 1992; Frymoyer et al., 1980). The negative quality of attitudes and beliefs is believed to influence the occupational functioning of the individual. Higher rates of absenteeism in one group of workers was associated with negative beliefs regarding the working environment as compared to another group with lower rates of absenteeism (Symonds, Burton, Tillotson, & Maia, 1996). Specific attitudes identified involve resentment regarding the work demands of the position and negative relationship with the supervisor (Hales & Bernard, 1996).

Social factors associated with an increased incidence of LBP include a low level of education, language difficulties, low income, and family problems (Valat, Goupille, & Vedere, 1997; Toroptsova et al., 1995). LBP often has little to do with the demands of the job but instead appears to be more related to compensation and disability (Magora & Taustein, 1969; Bergquist-Ulman & Larson, 1977; Rowe, 1983). Compensation, particularly when dispensed in lump sum claims, was associated with increased incidence and duration of back pain (Greenough, 1993). Disability compensation, if comparable to the employee's salary prior to his or her health problems, will likely serve as a disincentive to return to work (Garg & Moore, 1992a). The fear of injury and of losing financial compensation, coupled with job dissatisfaction, are likely factors in influencing the patient's motivation to return to work (Turk, 1996). Van Doorn (1995) conducted a retrospective study of 1,000 disability claimants and found that the risk was greater for claiming low back disability if a higher rate of insured daily compensation was accessible. A deferred period of 14 days or more decreased the incidence of claiming low back disability.

For some LBP patients, being sick enables them to renounce a previous caretaker role imposed by personal and/or family dysfunction (Parsons, 1958). The patient's family may experience high levels of stress because of the patient's low back problems (Barnes, 1991; Payne & Norfleet, 1986), and may inadvertently play a role in maintaining the pain experience (Barnes, 1991). In these situations, part of the overall treatment strategy will be to teach the family members how not to reinforce the patient's dysfunctional "pain behaviors."

A conceptual model developed at the Center for Occupational Rehabilitation at the University of Rochester Medical Center predicates that the return to work is influenced by multiple factors (Feuerstein & Zastowny, 1996). Using an integrated approach to work disability, the "Rochester Model" directs clinical evaluations, identifies obstacles interfering with work return, develops interventions, and provides rehabilitative services. The strength of the model resides in its ability to address the physical and psychosocial components and their interactions, including physical faculties that are affected at work, and overt or underlying psychological distress (i.e., fear of returning to work, fear of losing financial compensation). The LBP patient is treated by a multidisciplinary team, with the objective of identifying and removing barriers to return to work. The evaluation process comprises several components, including symptom identification, assessment of level of function, ergonomic job analysis, and assessment of other workplace factors. A successful treatment outcome is defined as the return to work, improved pain management, and increased social functioning. Table 11.3 lists some psychosocial factors associated with LBP.

BIOPSYCHOSOCIAL MODEL

The biopsychosocial model focuses on the dynamic interplay between the biological, psychological, and social dimensions that seem to perpetuate chronic pain (Turk, 1996). Whereas biological factors are believed to initiate a physical disturbance, psychological factors appear to influence pain perception and experience, and social factors mediate the behavior exhibited by the patient in response to the pain. Stress can indeed influence hormonal levels and immune function by way of biological pathways (Andersen, Kiecolt-Glaser, & Glaser, 1994; Flor, Turk, & Birbaumer, 1985; Turk, 1996), contributing to chronic illness, as well as to emotional distress. As a result, the patient may have decreased motivation to participate in exercise or work behavior that would prevent atrophy of an injured area (Gatchel, 1996; Rainville et al., 1992). The subsequent decrease in physical capacity may then pose a threat to the emotional well-being of an individual and may lead to further psychological distress (Gatchel, Baum, & Krantz, 1989). The symptoms may acquire the significance of demonstrating a sense of helplessness with the intent of securing assistance or release from responsibilities from an external source (i.e., amplification of physical and/or emotional symptoms as a result of secondary gain issues).

TABLE 11.3. Psychosocial Factors Associated with LBP

Psychopathology	Study
Pain avoidance	Gatchel, Polatin, Mayer, & Garcy (1994)
Job dissatisfaction	Troup & Slade (1985)
	Rainville, Ahern, & Phalen (1992)
Negative work attitudes	Symonds, Burton, Tillotson, & Maia (1996)
	Hales & Bernard (1996)
Lower socioeconomic status	Bigos, Hansson, et al. (1991)
	Bigos, Hansson, et al. (1992)
	Frymoyer et al. (1980)
Compensation	Magora & Taustein (1969)
	Bergquist-Ulmann & Larson (1977)
	Rowe (1983)
	Greenough (1993)
	Garg & Moore (1992a)
Fear of reinjury	Turk (1996)
Wish to be cared for	Parsons (1958)
Family dynamics	Payne & Norfleet (1986)
	Barnes (1991)

THE NEED FOR PREVENTION

The essential component of any effective treatment modality is a comprehensive understanding of a disorder's etiology. Consequently, a shift from curative efforts toward preventative strategies is beginning to dominate the current direction of research with regard to LBP (Bigos & Battie, 1987). There are three levels of prevention recognized by treatment teams: primary, secondary, and tertiary. Whereas primary prevention techniques try to reduce the incidence of the disorder prior to its onset, secondary prevention strives to implement a comprehensive intervention early in the development of the disorder (Garg & Moore, 1992b). Tertiary prevention generally involves eliminating or reducing disability and suffering stemming from the disorder (Garg & Moore, 1992b). Past preventive strategies designed to reduce low back problems in the workforce have focused on achieving three primary goals: (1) reducing LBP episodes believed to be initiated by work, (2) reducing LPB-related medical leave, and (3) prolonging the tenure of employees with LBP in their respective industry (Rowe, 1983; Snook, 1978).

There is a range of strategies to decrease the high cost of LBP disability. One can try to develop and improve the capability to identify individuals who are at risk for chronic disability after the onset of LBP (Gatchel, Polatin, & Kinney, 1995; Hazard, 1995). Alternatively, attempts to identify people at risk for LBP prior to employment have received attention in the past 20 years. However, focusing solely on physical factors has its limitations (Bigos, Battie, Fisher, et al., 1992). For example, the lumbosacral roentgenographs as a preemployment screening device to predict acute back injury claims has had little predictive value in identifying individuals who are more likely to file a back injury claim. Strength testing (Garg & Moore, 1992b) could help determine when job requirements exceed the strength capability of the employee, but it has generally failed to curb the cost created by LBP claims.

There has been a shift in focus toward accommodating LBP patients in the workforce, encouraged by the recent Americans with Disabilities Act (ADA; Cross, 1992). It has been hypothesized that redesigning the working environment will not only decrease the risk for developing LBP injuries in workers (Herrin, 1991; Marras et al., 1995) but will also facilitate work return for LBP patients. If the workplace allows for the altering of work task factors that are predictive of low back injury, the risk for developing LBP may decrease (Marras et al., 1995).

According to Burton (1997), however, work restrictions in LBP patients returning to work does not always correlate with reduced symptoms or work absence. For example, interventions such as the use of "back belts" in noninjured workers to prevent LBP actually increases the incidence of low back problems (Minor, 1996). A possible explanation of the reported lack of success may be feelings of vulnerability in LBP patients whose rehabilitation has included work restriction (Burton, 1997). Consequently, the LBP patient may exhibit a greater degree of hesitancy in approaching typical tasks that do not exceed his or her capabilities.

CONCLUSION

LBP is a major health problem in occupational settings, particularly in industrialized societies. Despite the basic assumption that physically taxing work leads to LBP, not all vocations with high physical demands lead to high rates of low back injuries. Understanding the problem requires a biopsychosocial perspective, because a multiplicity of factors influences the onset of LBP and the duration of associated disability. Although physical factors such as trunk extensor strength or previous LBP episodes may provide some indication of individual vulnerability, psychosocial factors such as work satisfaction, emotional distress, and secondary gain are felt to be far more important when attempting to limit disability. Prevention will consist of (1) identifying someone at high risk for a low back injury, (2) predicting who will remain disabled for a long period of time after such an injury, (3) ensuring effective treatment algorithms to get patients back to work as soon as possible, and (4) identifying workplace modifications to prevent injury and enable early work return. The disability experience, with its potential for secondary gain factors that reinforce dysfunction, is a critical area for further study. It is the responsibility of the insurer and the employer as well as the health care provider and all others involved in an occupational health system to strive to provide cost-efficient and compassionate services to the injured worker.

REFERENCES

Agius, R. M., Lloyd, M. H., Campbell, S., Hutchison, P., Seaton, A., & Soutar, C. A. (1994). Questionnaire for the identification of back pain for epidemiological purposes. *Occupational and Environmental Medicine, 51*(11), 756–760.

Andersen, B. L., Kiecolt-Glaser, J. K., & Glaser, R. (1994). A biobehavioral model of cancer stress and disease course. *American Psychologist, 49*(5), 389–404.

Andersson, G. B. J. (1979). Low back pain in industry: Epidemiologic aspects. *Scandinavian Journal of Rehabilitation Medicine, 11*, 163–168.

Andersson, G. B. J. (1981). Epidemiologic aspects of low-back pain in industry. *Spine, 6*, 53–59.

Andersson, G. B. J., & Ortengren, R. (1974). Myoelectric back muscle activity during sitting. *Scandinavian Journal of Rehabilitation Medicine Supplementum, 3*, 73.

Barnes, D. (1991). Social factors affecting back pain. In T. G. Mayer, R. G. Gatchel, & V. Mooney (Eds.), *Contemporary conservative care for painful spinal disorders* (pp. 143–148). Philadelphia: Lea & Febiger.

Benn, R. T., & Wood, P. H. (1975). Pain in the back: An attempt to estimate the size of the problem. *Rheumatology and Rehabilitation, 14*(3), 121–128.

Bergquist-Ullmann, M., & Larson, U. (1977). Acute low back pain in industry. *Acta Orthopaedica Scandinavica, 170*(Suppl.), 1–117.

Berkowitz, M., Johnson, W., & Murphy, E. (1976). *Public policy toward disability*. New York: Praeger Press.

Bigos, S. J., & Andary, M. T. (1991). Practitioner's guide to industrial back problems. *Neurosurgery Clinics of North America, 2*(4), 863–875.

Bigos, S. J., & Battie, M. C. (1987). Acute care to prevent back disability. Ten years of progress. *Clinical Orthopaedics and Related Research, 221*, 121–130.

Bigos, S. J., Battie, M. C., Spengler, D. M., Fisher, L. D., Fordyce, W. E., Hansson, T. H., Nachemson, A. L., & Wortley, M. D. (1991). A prospective study of work perceptions and psychosocial factors: A report of back injury. *Spine, 16*, 1–6.

Bigos, S. J., Battie, M. C., Spengler, D. M., Fisher, L. D., Fordyce, W. E., Hansson, T. H., Nachemson, A., & Zeh, J. (1992). A longitudinal prospective study of industrial back injury reporting. *Clinical Orthopaedics and Related Research, 279*, 21–34.

Bigos, S. J., Battie, M. C., Fisher, L. D., Hansson, T. H., Spengler, D. M., & Nachemson, A. L. (1992). A prospective evaluation of preemployment screening methods for acute industrial back pain. *Spine, 17*(8), 922–926.

Bigos, S. J., Hansson, T., Castillo, R. N., Beecher, P. J., & Wortley, M. D. (1992). The value of preemployment roentgenographs for predicting acute back injury claims and chronic back pain disability. *Clinical Orthopaedics and Related Research, 283*, 124–129.

Bigos, S. J., Spengler, D. M., Martin, N. A., Zeh, J., Fisher, L., Nachemson, A., & Wang, M. H. (1986). Back injuries in industry: A retrospective study: II. Injury factors. *Spine, 11*, 246–251.

Bombardier, C., Kerr, M. S., Shannon, H. S., & Frank, J. W. (1994). A guide to interpreting epidemiologic studies on the etiology of back pain. *Spine, 19*(18S), 2047S–2056S.

Burchfiel, C. M., Boice, J. A., Stafford, B. A., & Bond, G. G. (1992). Prevalence of back pain and joint problems in a manufacturing company. *Journal of Occupational Medicine, 34*(2), 129–134.

Burdorf, A., van Riel, M., van Wingerden, J. P., & Snijders, C. (1995). Isodynamic evaluation of trunk muscles and low-back pain among workers in a steel factory. *Ergonomics, 38*(10), 2107–2117.

Burton, A. K. (1997). Back injury and work loss: Biomechanical and psychosocial influences. *Spine, 22*(21), 2575–2580.

Burton, A. K., Tillotson, K. M., Symonds, T. L., Burke, C., & Mathewson, T. (1996). Occupational risk factors for the first-onset and subsequent course of low back trouble. A study of serving police officers. *Spine, 21*(22), 2616–2620.

Cady, L. D., Bischoff, D. P., O'Connell, E. R., Thomas, P. C., & Allan, J. H. (1979). Strength and fitness and subsequent back injuries in firefighters. *Journal of Occupational Medicine, 21*, 269–272.

Cross, L. L. (1992). Americans with Disabilities Act: Meeting the requirements. *AAOHN Journal, 40*(6), 284–286.

Deyo, R. A. (1991). Historic perspective on conservative treatments for acute back problems. In T. G. Mayer, R. J. Gatchel, & V. Mooney (Eds.), *Contemporary conservative care for painful spinal disorders* (pp. 278–289). Philadelphia: Lea & Febiger.

Deyo, R. A., & Bass, J. E. (1989). Lifestyle and low-back pain: The influence of smoking and obesity. *Spine, 14*, 501–506.

Feuerstein, M., & Zastowny, T. R. (1996). Occupational rehabilitation: Multidisciplinary management of work-related musculoskeletal pain and disability. In R. J. Gatchel & D. C. Turk (Eds.), *Psychological approaches to pain management: A practitioner's handbook* (pp. 458–485). New York: Guilford Press.

Flor, H., Turk, D. C., & Birbaumer, N. (1985). Assessment of stress-related psychophysiological responses in chronic pain patients. *Journal of Consulting and Clinical Psychology, 35*, 354–364.

Frymoyer, J. W. (1991). Epidemiology of spinal disorders. In T. G. Mayer, V. Mooney, & R. J. Gatchel (Eds.), *Contemporary conservative care for painful spinal disorders* (pp. 10–23). Philadelphia: Lea & Febiger.

Frymoyer, J., & Cats-Baril, W. (1987). Predictors of low back pain disability. *Clinical Orthopedics and Related Research, 221*, 88–98.

Frymoyer, J., Pope, M. H., Constanza, M. C., Rosen, J. C., Goggin, J. E., & Wilder, D. G. (1980). Epidemiological studies of low-back pain. *Spine, 5*, 419–423.

Furber, A., Fanello, S., Roquelaura, Y., Lelevier, F., Le Cardinal, S., Penneau-Fontbonne, D., & Renier, J. C. (1992). Lower back pain in physicians: Epidemiological aspects and risk factors. *Revue du Rhumatisme et des Maladies Osteo-Articulaires, 59*(12), 777–783.

Garg, A. (1992). Occupational biomechanics and low-back pain. *Occupational Medicine, 7*(4), 609–628.

Garg, A., & Moore, J. S. (1992a). Epidemiology of low-back pain in industry. *Occupational Medicine, 7*(4), 593–608.

Garg, A., & Moore, J. S. (1992b). Prevention strategies and the low back in industry. *Occupational Medicine, 7*(4), 629–640.

Garg, A., & Owen, B. (1992). Reducing back stress in nursing personnel: An ergonomic intervention in a nursing home. *Ergonomics, 35*(11), 1353–1375.

Gatchel, R. J. (1996). Psychological disorders and chronic pain: Cause-and-effect relationships. In R. J. Gatchel & D. C. Turk (Eds.), *Psychological approaches to pain management: A practitioner's handbook* (pp. 33–52). New York: Guilford Press.

Gatchel, R. J., Baum, A., & Krantz, D. (1989). *An introduction to health psychology* (2nd ed.). New York: McGraw-Hill.

Gatchel, R. J., Polatin, P. B., & Kinney, R. K. (1995). Predicting outcome of chronic back pain using clinical predictors of psychopathology: A prospective analysis. *Health Psychology, 14*(5), 415–420.

Gatchel, R. J., Polatin, P. B., Mayer, T. G., & Garcy, P. D. (1994). Psychopathology and the rehabilitation of patients with low back pain disability. *Archives of Physical Medicine and Rehabilitation, 75*, 666–670.

Greenough, C. G. (1993). A recovery from low back pain: 1–5 year follow-up of 287 injury-related cases. *Acta Orthopaedica Scandinavica, 254*(Suppl.), 1–34.

Hales, T. R., & Bernard, B. P. (1996). Epidemiology of work-related musculoskeletal disorders. *Orthopedic Clinics of North America, 27*(47), 679–709.

Harreby, M., Kjer, J., Hesselsoe, G., & Neergaard, K. (1996). Epidemiological aspects and risk factors for low back pain in 38-year-old men and women: A 25-year prospective cohort study of 640 school children. *European Spine Journal, 5*(5), 312–318.

Hazard, R. (1995). Spine update: Functional restoration. *Spine, 20*, 2345–2348.

Herrin, G. D. (1991). Ergonomic considerations in workplace design and worker selection. In T. G. Mayer, R. J. Gatchel, & V. Mooney (Eds.), *Contemporary conservative care for painful spinal disorders* (pp. 500–521). Philadelphia: Lea & Febiger.

Hignett, S. (1996). Work-related back pain in nurses. *Journal of Advanced Nursing, 23*(6), 1238–1246.

Hildebrandt, V. H., Bongers, P. M., Dul, J., Van Dijk, F. J., & Kemper, H. C. (1996). Identification of high-risk groups among maintenance workers in a steel company with respect to musculoskeletal symptoms and workload. *Ergonomics, 39*(2), 232–242.

Holbrook, T., Grazier, K., Kelsey, J. L., & Stauffer, R. (1984). *The frequency of occurrence, impact, and cost of selected musculoskeletal conditions in the United States.* Chicago: American Academy of Orthopedic Surgeons.

Honeyman, P. T., & Jacobs, E. A. (1996). Effects of culture on back pain in Australian aboriginals. *Spine, 21*(7), 841–843.

Howard, I., Brehm, H., & Nagi, S. (1980). *From social problem to federal programs.* New York: Praeger Press.

Hult, L. (1954). Cervical, dorsal, and lumbar spinal syndromes. *Acta Orthopaedica Scandinavica, 24*, 174.

Jamison, R. N., Stetson, B. A., & Parris, W. C. (1991). The relationship between cigarette smoking and chronic low back pain. *Addictive Behaviors, 16*(3–4), 103–110.

Jefferson, J. R., & McGrath, P. J. (1996). Back pain and peripheral joint pain in an industrial setting. *Archives of Physical Medicine and Rehabilitation, 77*(4), 385–390.

Kelsey, J. L., Githens, P. B., O'Conner, T., Weil, U., Calogero, J. A., Holford, T. R., White, A. A., Walter, S. D., Ostfeld, A. M., & Southwick, W. O. (1984). Acute prolapsed lumbar intervertebral disc: An epidemiological study with special reference to driving automobiles and cigarette smoking. *Spine, 9*, 608–613.

Klein, M., Jensen, R., & Sanderson, L. (1984). Assessment of workers compensation claims for back strain/sprain. *Journal of Occupational Medicine, 26*, 443–448.

Knibbe, J. J., & Friele, R. D. (1996). Prevalence of back pain and characteristics of the physical workload of community nurses. *Ergonomics, 39*(2), 186–198.

Lau, E. M., Egger, P., Coggon, D., Cooper, C., Valenti, L., & O'Connell, D. (1996). Low-back pain in Hong Kong: Prevalence and characteristics compared to Britain. *Journal of Epidemiology and Community Health, 49*(5), 492–494.

Leboeuf-Yde, C. (1995). Does smoking cause low back pain? A review of epidemiologic literature for causality. *Journal of Manipulative and Physiological Therapeutics, 18*(4), 237–243.

Leboeuf-Yde, C., Klougart, N., & Lauritzen, T. (1996). How common is low back pain in the Nordic population?: Data from a recent study on middle-aged general Danish population and four surveys previously conducted in the Nordic countries. *Spine, 21*(13), 1518–1525.

MacDonald, M. J., Sorock, G. S., Volinn, E., Hashemi, L., Clancy, E. A., & Webster, B. (1997). A descriptive study of recurrent low back pain claims. *Journal of Occupational and Environmental Medicine, 39*(1), 35–43.

Magora, A., & Taustein, I. (1969). An investigation of the problem of sick-leave in the patient suffering from low back pain. *Medical Surgery, 38,* 398–408.

Manninen, P., Rhiihimaki, H., & Heliovaara, M. (1995). Incidence and risk factors of low-back pain in middle-aged farmers. *Occupational Medicine, 45*(3), 141–146.

Marras, W. S., Lavender, S. A., Leurgans, S. E., Fathallah, F. A., Ferguson, S. A., Allread, W. G., & Rajulu, S. L. (1995). Biomechanical risk factors for occupationally related low back disorders. *Ergonomics, 38*(2), 377–410.

Mayer, T. G. (1991). Rationale for modern spinal care. In T. G. Mayer, V. Mooney, & R. J. Gatchel (Eds.), *Contemporary conservative care for painful spinal disorders* (pp. 3–9). Philadelphia: Lea & Febiger.

Mayer, T. G., & Gatchel, R. J. (1988). *Functional restoration for spinal disorders: The sports medicine approach.* Philadelphia: Lea & Febiger.

Mayer, T. G., Gatchel, R. J., Kishino, N., Keeley, J., Capra, P., Mayer, H., & Barnett, J., & Mooney, V. (1985). Objective assessment of spinal function following industrial injury: A prospective study with comparison group and one-year follow-up. *Spine, 10,* 482–493.

Mayer, T. G., Polatin, P. B., Smith, B., Smith, C., Gatchel, R. J., Herring, S. A., Hall, H., Donelson, R. G., Dickey, J., & English, W. (1995). Contemporary concepts in spine care rehabilitation: Secondary and tertiary nonoperative care. *Spine, 20*(18), 2060–2066.

Mayer, T. G., Smith, S. S., Keeley, J., & Mooney, V. (1985). Quantification of lumbar function: Part 2. Sagittal plane trunk strength in chronic low-back pain patients. *Spine, 10,* 765–772.

Melzack, R., & Wall, P. D. (1965). Pain mechanisms: A new theory. *Science, 50,* 971–979.

Minor, S. D. (1996). Use of back belts in occupational settings. *Physical Therapy, 76*(4), 403–408.

Parsons, T. (1958). Definitions of health and illness in the light of American values and social structure. In E. G. Jaco (Ed.), *Patients, physicians, and illness* (pp. 3–29). New York: Free Press.

Payne, B., & Norfleet, M. A. (1986). Chronic pain and the family: A review. *Pain, 26*(1), 1–22.

Polatin, P. B., & Mayer, T. G. (1995). Occupational disorders and the management of chronic pain. *Occupational Disorder Management, 27*(4), 881–890.

Pope, M. H. (1991). Physiology and spine mechanics. In T. G. Mayer, R. J. Gatchel, & V. Mooney (Eds.), *Contemporary conservative care for painful spinal disorders* (pp. 278–289). Philadelphia: Lea & Febiger.

Rainville, J., Ahern, D. K., Phalen, L., Childs, L. A., & Sutherland, R. (1992). The association of pain with physical activities in chronic low back pain. *Spine, 17,* 1060–1064.

Rotgoltz, J., Derazne, E., Froom, P., Grushecky, E., & Ribak, J. (1992). Prevalence of low back pain in em-

ployees of a pharmaceutical company. *Israel Journal of Medical Sciences, 34*(2), 129–134.

Rowe, M. L. (1983). *Backache at work.* Fairport, NY: Perington Press.

Sanders, S. H., Brena, S. F., Spier, C. J., Beltrutti, D., McConnell, H., & Quintero, O. (1992). Chronic low back pain patients around the world: Cross-cultural similarities and differences. *Clinical Journal of Pain, 8*(4), 317–323.

Schierhout, G. H., Meyers, J. E., & Bridger, R. S. (1995). Work related musculoskeletal disorders and ergonomic stressors in the South African workforce. *Occupational and Environmental Medicine, 52,* 46–50.

Smedley, J., Egger, P., Cooper, C., & Coggon, D. (1995). Manual handling activities and risk of low back pain in nurses. *Occupational and Environmental Medicine, 52,* 160–163.

Snook, S. H. (1978). The design of manual handling tasks. *Ergonomics, 21,* 963–985.

Straker, L. M., Stevenson, M. G., & Twomey, L. T. (1996). A comparison of risk assessment of single and combination manual handling tasks: 1. Maximum acceptable weight measures. *Ergonomics, 39*(1), 128–140.

Suadicani, P., Hansen, K., Fenger, A. M., & Gyntelberg, F. (1994). Low back pain in steel plant workers. *Occupational Medicine, 44*(4), 217–221.

Symonds, T. L., Burton, A. K., Tillotson, K. M., & Maia, C. J. (1996). Do attitudes and beliefs influence work loss due to low back trouble? *Occupational Medicine, 46*(1), 25–32.

Taylor, D. G. (1976). The costs of arthritis and the benefits of joint replacement surgery. *Proceedings of the Royal Society of London, 192,* 145–155.

Toroptsova, N. V., Benevolenskaya, L. I., Karyakin, A. N., Sergeev, I. L., & Erdesz, S. (1995). "Cross-sectional" study of low back pain among workers at an industrial enterprise in Russia. *Spine, 20*(3), 328–332.

Troup, J., & Slade, P. (1985). Fear avoidance and chronic musculoskeletal pain. *Stress Medicine, 1,* 217–220.

Turk, D. C. (1996). Biopsychosocial perspective on chronic pain. In R. J. Gatchel & D. C. Turk (Eds.), *Psychological approaches to pain management: A practitioner's handbook* (pp. 3–32). New York: Guilford Press.

U. S. Department of Health and Human Services. (1987). *Report of the commission on the evaluation of pain* (SSA Publication No. 64-031). Washington, DC: Social Security Administration, Office of Disability.

Valat, J. P., Goupille, P., & Vedere, V. (1997). Low back pain: Risk factors for chronicity. *Revue du Rhumatisme* (English Edition), *64*(3), 189–194.

Van Doorn, J. W. (1995). Low back disability among self-employed dentists, veterinarians, physicians and physical therapists in the Netherlands: A retrospective study over a 13-year period and an early intervention program with 1-year follow-up. *Acta Orthopaedica Scandinavica, 226*(Suppl.), 1–64.

Webster, B., & Snook, S. (1994). The cost of compensable upper-extremity cumulative trauma disorders. *Journal of Occupational Medicine, 36,* 713–717.

Wells, R., Norman, R., Neumann, P., Andrews, D., Frank, J., Shannon, H., & Kerr, M. (1997). Assessment of physical workload in epidemiological studies: Common measurement metrics for exposure assessment. *Ergonomics, 40*(1), 51–61.

Chapter 12

Workstyle and Work-Related Upper Extremity Disorders

MICHAEL FEUERSTEIN
GRANT D. HUANG
GLENN PRANSKY

Work-related upper extremity disorders (WRUEDs) have become an increasing public health concern in industrialized nations. Symptoms of work-related upper extremity disorders typically include pain, numbness, stiffness, and aching in the finger, wrist, forearm, elbow, upper arm, shoulder, and neck regions (Putz-Anderson, 1988; Rempel, Harrison, & Barnhardt, 1992). These symptoms and disorders have also been linked to exposure to biomechanical stressors such as repetition, awkward postures, excessive force, inadequate work–rest cycles, vibration, and temperature extremes (Armstrong et al., 1993; Ulin & Armstrong, 1992). Should prolonged pain and work disability associated with these disorders occur, several problems can result for the worker, work organization, and society as a whole. Recently, the Bureau of Labor Statistics (1998) reported that in 1996, there were over 425,000 upper-extremity-related occupational illnesses in the United States that involved days away from work. Although there is much controversy as to the etiology of work-related upper extremity disorders/symptoms (Hadler, 1992), research suggests

that a complex interaction among medical, ergonomic, organizational, and psychosocial factors may contribute to the development, exacerbation, and maintenance of these disorders (Armstrong et al., 1993; Chaffin & Fine, 1992; Bernard, 1997).

This chapter will focus on one factor that is not typically addressed in the literature—workstyle, or how an individual worker approaches work. After presenting a background on WRUEDs, we provide the following: an operational definition of the workstyle construct; a review of available research that serves as preliminary support for the emerging construct; and a model proposed to explain the impact of workstyle on the etiology, exacerbation, and maintenance of work-related upper extremity disorders/symptoms. Suggestions for management and prevention, as well as intervention-based research that focuses on workstyle modification, are also presented. Although the workstyle construct as discussed must be considered in light of the complex interaction among medical, ergonomic, and psychosocial factors (Feuerstein, 1991), this chapter does not address the role that ergonomic stressors play in WRUEDs (Armstrong et al., 1993; Stock, 1991). Yet one should bear in mind that certain high-risk workstyles may interact with ergonomic risk factors to increase the likelihood of initiation, exacerbation, and/or maintenance of WRUEDs and concomitant work disability.

The opinions or assertions contained herein are the private ones of the authors and are not to be construed as official or reflecting the views of the Department of Defense or the Uniformed Services University of the Health Sciences.

WORK-RELATED UPPER EXTREMITY DISORDERS

Work-related upper extremity disorders are associated with muscle-, tendon-, and/or nerve-related symptoms and functional limitation in the hands, wrists, elbows, arms, shoulders, and neck (Rempel et al., 1992; Putz-Anderson, 1988). Several terms have been used to describe these symptom clusters and disorders including: cumulative trauma disorders, occupational cervicobrachial disorders, overuse syndromes, regional musculoskeletal disorders, work-related disorders, repetitive strain injuries, and repetitive trauma disorders (Gerr, Letz, & Landrigan, 1991). Caution is advised with the use of such terms, particularly the latter two, because they imply a causal mechanism (i.e., repeated or cumulative trauma) that has not been definitively determined. Common types of WRUEDs include: carpal tunnel syndrome (CTS), tendinitis, tenosynovitis (e.g., de Quervain's disease), lateral epicondylitis, nerve entrapment syndromes, and hand–arm vibration syndrome (Rempel et al., 1992, Gerr et al., 1991). Table 12.1 provides a comprehensive list of upper extremity disorders as proposed by the National Safety Council (1996).

As early as the 1960s, the International Labor Organization Advisory Committee on Salaried and Professional Workers identified "repetition strain injuries" as an occupational disease that was associated with mechanized work (Chatterjee, 1987). In the early 1980s a large number of compensation claims for "repetition strain injuries" associated with the arm and wrist areas were filed in Australia (Hocking, 1987). Some have suggested that these injuries were the consequence of overuse, whereas others have argued that the epidemic was the result of "mass hysteria with an element of band wagoning" (Hagberg, 1996). An increase in the incidence of "repetitive strain injuries" has also been noted in Canada since 1986 (Ashbury, 1995).

Prevalence rates of WRUEDs depend on the occupation, anatomic area, and case definition examined. The Bureau of Labor Statistics (1998) indicated that in the United States, 29,900 (3.6%) work-related cases of carpal tunnel syndrome resulted in days away from work in 1996. Brogmus, Sorock, and Webster (1996) used data from the Bureau of Labor Statistics (BLS) and Liberty Mutual Insurance Company's workers' compensation claims to estimate the frequency of "cumulative trauma disorders of the upper extremities" (CTDUEs). Their findings indicated that the percent of CTDUE workers' compensation claims at Liberty Mutual increased from less than 0.5% in 1986 to approximately 3.5% in 1993. The BLS data on total occupational injuries and illnesses followed a similar trend. In 1986, cases associated with repeated trauma accounted for just under 1% and rose to approximately 4.5% in 1993. It is unclear whether these trends resulted from improved reporting and classification procedures or from a greater awareness of these disorders by health professionals.

Patterns of how work-related upper extremity disorders are presented vary. Some workers may indicate that the particular region affected often feels fatigued. Muscle tension and tenderness have also been reported as symptoms of WRUEDs (Downs, 1997). Other symptoms reported include pain, tingling, and numbness (Szabo & Madison, 1995; Amadio, 1995). Such symptoms may be an indication of a nerve disorder and/or compressive neuropathy (Williams & Westmorland, 1994). Upon physical examination, tenderness, swelling, and crepitations may be found (Williams & Westmorland, 1994; Gerr et al., 1991). Although there are no established criteria for qualifying the presence of symptoms as an upper extremity disorder, it has been suggested that persistence for a week or longer, a frequency of greater than 20 times in 1 year, or both be used (Silverstein, Fine, & Armstrong, 1986). Furthermore, it is important to emphasize that although the majority of individuals with upper extremity disorders continue to work with pain (Feuerstein, Miller, Burrell, & Berger, 1998), for those who lost days because of carpal tunnel syndrome, the average number of lost days was very similar to that for neck/trunk strain claimants, symptoms well known for high levels of work disability (CTS = 84 days; neck/trunk = 100 days).

Upper extremity symptoms may eventually lead to functional limitations and/or work disability of a recurrent or chronic nature. Such disability results when pain reaches the point at which the worker can no longer maintain a productive work schedule. Historically, it has been the role of the psychologist or mental health provider to enter the natural history of the disorder in these latter stages, when chronic pain and disability prevail. Improved understanding of the psychosocial factors that affect fatigue and symptoms (such as pain and functional limitations) early in the course of these disorders should serve as a foundation for the earlier role of psychosocial intervention. Furthermore, such interventions could target the afected worker, the work organization, health care providers, case managers, and others involved in facilitating a safe and successful recovery.

TABLE 12.1. ICD-9 Diagnoses Generally Considered Work-Related Upper Extremity Disorders (WRUEDs)

Diagnosis	ICD-9 Number
Tendon, synovium, and bursa disorders	727
Trigger finger (acquired)	727.03
Radial styloid tenosynovitis (de Quervain's)	727.04
Other tenosynovitis of hand and wrist	727.05
Specific bursitis often of occupational origin	727.2
Unspecified disorder of synovium, tendon, and bursa	727.9
Peripheral enthesopathies	726
Rotator cuff syndrome, supraspinatus syndrome	726.10
Bicipital tenosynovitis	726.12
Medial epicondylitis	726.31
Lateral epicondylitis (tennis elbow)	726.32
Unspecified enthesopathy	726.9
Disorders of muscle, ligament, and fascia	728
Game-Keeper's thumb	728.8
Muscle spasm	728.85
Unspecified disorder of muscle, ligament, and fascia	728.9
Other disorders of soft tissues	729
Myalgia, myositis, fibromyositis	729.1
Swelling of limb	729.81
Cramp	729.82
Unspecified disorders of soft tissue	729.9
Disorders of the cervical region	723
Cervicalgia (pain in neck)	723.1
Cervicobrachial syndrome (diffuse)	723.3
Unspecified neck symptoms or disorders	723.9
Osteoarthritis	715
Mononeuritis of upper limb	354
Carpal tunnel syndrome (median nerve entrapment)	354.0
Cubital tunnel syndrome	354.2
Tardy ulnar nerve palsy	354.2
Lesions of the radial nerve	354.3
Unspecified mononeuritis of upper limb	354.9
Peripheral vascular disease	443
Raynaud's syndrome	443.0
Hand–arm vibration syndrome	443.0
Vibration white finger	443.0

WORKSTYLE: OPERATIONAL DEFINITION

In order to objectively measure and validate a construct such as workstyle, it is essential to provide an operational or working definition. A proposed definition is as follows:

1. Workstyle is an individual pattern of cognitions, behaviors, and physiological reactivity that co-occur while performing job tasks.
2. Workstyle may be associated with alterations in physiological state such that, following repeated elicitation, they can contribute to the development, exacerbation, and/or maintenance of recurrent or chronic musculoskeletal symptoms related to work.
3. An adverse workstyle (i.e., one associated with increased occurrence of work-related upper extremity symptoms) may be evoked by a high work demand (perceived or directly communicated by supervisor) or self-generated by a high need for achievement and/or acceptance. It may also be triggered by fear of job loss, by avoidance of a

job-related negative consequence, or by inadequate and/or improper training. Additional features appear to include a lack of awareness that a particular workstyle might be a potential high-risk behavior and may be self-generated by time pressure.

This definition identifies a style or pattern of behaviors, thoughts, and physiological reactivity evoked in response to a set of work demands. It is possible that as a consequence of some combination of temperament and/or social learning, an employee develops a relatively stable workstyle response characterized by heightened cognitive and/or behavioral and/or physiological reactivity to work demands.

It is hypothesized that an adverse workstyle of sufficient frequency, intensity, and duration may predispose an individual to develop work-related upper extremity symptoms, particularly when coupled with exposure to suspected ergonomic risk factors. It is important to emphasize that there is evidence to suggest that exposure to ergonomic stressors are associated with an increased risk for upper extremity symptoms/disorders irrespective of the workstyle concept (Armstrong et al., 1993). Therefore, it is suggested that a high-risk workstyle may increase exposure to existing biomechanical stressors if it contributes to excessive elevations in force, repetition, awkward posture, and/or prolonged static loading of select muscles in the upper extremities. Workstyle may also lead to inadequate work–rest cycles independent of work station- or work process-related biomechanical stressors. A similar process may exist in the exacerbation of symptoms/disorders as well as the maintenance of episodic or chronic pain and work disability. This current definition of workstyle should serve only as a working definition. It will undoubtedly be refined as additional research on measurement and validation of the concept evolves.

HISTORICAL PERSPECTIVE

The implications of workstyle variations on worker health and safety have been recognized for centuries. Ramazzini (1713/1964) commented on the variation in worker performance of similar tasks and suggested that such workstyles were associated with elevated risk for hand/wrist disorders among those involved in construction, crafting, and scribing. In this chapter, we attempt to delineate the components of workstyle that consist of subtle individual variations in behaviors, cognitions, and

physiological responses that may increase the risk for symptoms and disorders in the upper extremities. An early example of empirical research related to workstyle and upper extremity disorders was reported by Armstrong and Chaffin (1979). In a case–control study of production sewing workers, Armstrong and Chaffin (1979) observed that carpal tunnel syndrome cases demonstrated significantly greater hand forces in all wrist positions than healthy controls. In addition, cases also tended to use a deviated (from neutral) wrist position more frequently than controls when performing similar highly repetitive work tasks. Although these findings do not support the causal role of work methods in carpal tunnel syndrome, they do provide preliminary support for the existence of different work methods or workstyles and their apparent association with a specific WRUED.

Models explaining the role of psychosocial factors in health (e.g., Levi, 1972) are useful for identifying factors that could contribute to the workstyle–WRUEDs link. Specifically, in certain individuals and situations, workstyle may be characterized as a work-related response to stress. The early stress model proposed by Levi (1972) includes the presence of social systems that may be perceived as either threatening or nonthreatening, specific physical and psychosocial stimuli, the individual's psychobiological "program" influenced by early environmental experiences, and genetics that can effect pathogenic mechanisms that serve as precursors to disease and further distress. These factors are modulated by a set of interacting variables such as level of social support or coping skills. The concept of workstyle has certain features in common with the Levi model, as well as with other models of job stress and health. The majority of the occupational stress–health models include a source of stress (e.g., intrinsic to job, role in organization, career development, relationships at work, organizational structure and climate), individual characteristics, symptoms of ill health (individual and organizational), and disease or illness outcomes (Cooper, 1986). The concept of workstyle emerges, in part, from these transactional models of occupational stress and health. The Kahn and Byosiere (1991) framework for the study of stress in organizations provides a useful heuristic for considering the workstyle construct. This model comprises organizational antecedents to stress, such as features of the organization (e.g., size, work schedule, organizational structure); physical and psychosocial stressors in organizational life; perceptions; and cognitions (i.e., appraisal processes). Mediators of stress include responses to stress at the physiological, psychological, and behavioral levels; consequences of organizational stress (e.g., health and organizational effectiveness); and properties of the person and the situation (e.g., supervisor support, psychological coping style). It is important to mention that although numerous models of stress and health exist (Feuerstein, Labbe, & Kuczmierczyk, 1986) and although the construct of workstyle has evolved in part from such models, workstyle should not be conceptualized simply as a response to stress. While workstyle may be triggered or exacerbated by stress and manifest itself as a characteristic response to work with or without the presence of psychosocial stressors, it can also be conceptualized as a relatively stable response to work.

ANECDOTAL EVIDENCE

Interviews with supervisors and employees, as well as observations of workers during workplace "walkthroughs," have suggested to us that one differentiating factor between those who experience symptoms and those who do not may be in *how* they perform their work (i.e., their workstyle). As our group began to formulate this construct, we began to ask the following questions:

1. Could the manner or intensity in which a given individual meets the demands of a work task give rise to increased levels of muscular exertion, excessive force, awkward postures, inadequate work–rest cycles, increased sympathetic nervous system arousal, and muscle tension?
2. If so, could this response contribute to the development, exacerbation, and/or maintenance of upper extremity symptoms/disorders that ultimately lead to prolonged functional decrements and work disability?
3. Could a particular workstyle predispose a worker to WRUEDs?

As workers with WRUEDs were seen in our clinics, we began to observe different patterns of behavior during simulated work tasks and questioned injured workers about their approach to work. A subgroup of individuals presented with an intensity of effort not observed in all patients and rarely observed in chronic occupational low back pain patients. Many of these patients reported that they continued to work with pain for months because of their keen interest in keeping their jobs, need to achieve at work, perception of the

important contribution of their work to the organization, or a strong work ethic. These individuals also tended to report difficulty in pacing their work, as well as a need to consistently perform perfectly. Furthermore, they displayed what appeared to be a heightened behavioral reactivity when performing rehabilitation-related tasks (e.g., exercising), as well as a highly intensive effort and urgency to improve their health in order to return to work as soon as possible. Although these observations only represent anecdotal impressions, they are reported here because we believe that they suggest a pattern of cognitions and behaviors with possible physiological correlates that might help explain the occurrence of some WRUEDs.

EMPIRICAL RESEARCH

The concept of workstyle as a biobehavioral risk factor in the development, exacerbation, and maintenance of work-related upper extremity disorders and disability was first proposed in an earlier chapter (Feuerstein, 1996). However, findings from various epidemiological, laboratory, and outcome studies conducted over the past 20 years provide indirect support for its existence and role in the exacerbation of upper extremity symptoms. The literature on psychosocial factors in WRUEDs is also relevant to workstyle since these factors can increase the likelihood of high-risk workstyle responses.

Epidemiological Studies

Research conducted by the National Institute of Occupational Safety and Health (NIOSH) in the context of two health hazard evaluations identified specific psychosocial factors associated with work-related musculoskeletal symptoms and disorders of the upper limbs, neck, and shoulder regions (NIOSH, 1992). A health hazard evaluation conducted in a large West Coast newspaper (NIOSH, 1993) indicated that 41% of participants had at least one work-related upper extremity disorder. The following factors were associated with the presence of the following work-related musculoskeletal symptoms: *hand/wrist*—more time spent typing on computer keyboards, greater number of hours on deadline, and less support from immediate supervisor; *shoulder*—less participation in job decision making, greater number of years employed by a specific employer, and greater job pressure; *neck*—greater number of hours on deadline, increased work variance (uneven workload during the day), more time on the telephone, and the perception that management does not value the importance of ergonomics. The only variables related to WRUEDs that were identified using a more restrictive case definition of hand/wrist musculoskeletal disorder (positive symptoms and positive physical findings) were female gender and percent of time spent typing on a computer keyboard.

In a study of the prevalence of work-related musculoskeletal disorders in telecommunications workers, 22% met the case definition (Hales et al., 1994). The following psychosocial variables were associated with upper extremity disorders: *hand/wrist*—high information processing demands; *elbow*—fear of being replaced by computers, routine work lacking decision making opportunities, and surges in workload; *shoulder*—fear of being replaced by computers; *neck*—lack of productivity standard, routine work lacking decision making opportunities, fear of being replaced by computers, job requiring a variety of tasks, high information processing demands, and increased work pressure; *upper extremity overall*—fear of being replaced by computers, job requiring a variety of tasks, and increasing work pressure. Increased symptom severity (standardized composite score of frequency, severity, and duration) was associated with the following factors: *hand/wrist*—high information processing demands, uncertainty about job future, routine work lacking decision making opportunities, increasing work pressure, and lack of supervisor support; *elbow*—routine work lacking decision making opportunities, uncertainty about job future, surges in workload, increasing work pressure, and lack of coworker support; *shoulder*—increasing work pressure, overtime in the past year (negative association); *neck*—increasing work pressure and uncertainty about job future. It is important to emphasize that in this study the percent variance accounted for by each of these measures was very modest, ranging from 1% to 3%.

Studies of workers who use a video display terminal have also indicated the involvement of occupational psychosocial factors in work-related upper extremity symptoms/disorders. Using employees from an editorial department of a newspaper (56% response rate), Faucett and Rempel (1994) examined the relationship between self-report of work stress and musculoskeletal symptoms. Forty-two percent of the participants also volunteered to take part in work station evaluations. Findings indicated that lower levels of decision latitude and coworker support significantly contrib-

uted to upper extremity (i.e., hand and arm regions) numbness. Furthermore, employees who reported low decision latitude on the job tended to have more severe upper extremity numbness associated with a less than ideal ergonomic location of the keyboard (i.e., above the elbows). These results, in conjunction with those of other studies (Linton & Kamwendo, 1989; Bammer, 1987; Hales et al., 1994), suggest that there may be an interaction between psychosocial factors (e.g., lack of control and reduction in task diversity) and ergonomic factors experienced by those who work on computers. Subsequently, such an interaction may contribute to increased reports of work-related upper extremity symptoms/disorders.

Although the surveys used in the investigations reviewed herein measure certain workplace psychosocial variables and indicate their association with the presence and/or exacerbation of upper extremity symptoms and disorders, they have not directly addressed the role of workstyle. Feuerstein, Carosella, Burrell, Marshall, and De Caro (1997) conducted a large-scale survey of 1,398 sign language interpreters (58% response rate), a group with a relatively high exposure to biomechanical stressors associated with upper extremity symptoms (Feuerstein & Fitzgerald, 1992; Shealy, Feuerstein, & Latko, 1991). The survey revealed that 20–32% of the respondents reported work-related symptoms depending on anatomic location. Based on a multivariate logistic regression analysis that considered years on the job, work demands, perceived work environment, and workstyle variables, this study found that certification, years worked, physical conditions on the job, constant job pressure, fear of developing a pain problem at work, and a tendency to continue to work with pain to insure quality were associated with the presence of work-related hand/wrist symptoms. The variable "continue to work with pain to insure high quality" is considered be an aspect of workstyle found in those workers who experience increased levels of pain and functional limitation. Those sign language interpreters who continued to expose themselves to repetitive, forceful movements and awkward postures despite pain to insure the quality of their work were more likely to be defined as cases. Although the odds ratio for this variable was modest, this finding provides preliminary support for the need to consider how an individual performs his or her work. It is important to note that other measures of self-reported workstyle included in the survey (e.g., work–rest breaks, "jerky" forceful movements) were not associated with case status for hand/wrist symptoms. In contrast, when factors associated with increased levels of pain and muscular tension at work, as well as the impact of pain on function, were considered, a number of behavioral workstyle variables were associated with exacerbation of pain, muscular tension, and disability.

Data on work demand identification, job stress, and workstyle variables from the Sign Language Interpreter Survey were also analyzed to differentiate cases with partial and full days of lost work related to upper extremity symptoms from cases with no lost time from work (Feuerstein, Carosella, et al., 1997). A discriminant function analysis was conducted on 277 lost-time cases and on a randomly selected group of 277 cases with no lost time. The variables that discriminated lost-time from no-lost-time cases were: high levels of fear of pain related to interpreting, continuing to work in a painful way to insure quality, tendency to view work with a high degree of urgency, higher perceived levels of exertion, lack of control over work, and unpleasant physical conditions at work. The majority of variance in work disability was explained by the combination of the fear of pain related to interpreting and the tendency to continue working in a painful way to insure quality work. Again, these cognitive dimensions of workstyle, where an individual continues to work with pain or tends to drive oneself to insure quality, together with a fear of developing a pain problem at work and perception of minimal control or initiative, appear to contribute to a condition in which work absence is more likely. Measures of self-reported behavioral components of workstyle (e.g., work–rest breaks, moving hands as fast as possible, "jerky" forceful movements) were not associated with time lost from work. As with the prediction of case status described earlier, the absence of significant behavioral findings regarding components of workstyle may have been a consequence of the use of a self-report measure of workstyle behavior in contrast to a direct behavioral observation method, as was used in Feuerstein and Fitzgerald (1992). It may also be possible that the cognitive components of workstyle contribute to time lost from work to a greater degree than the behavioral components. Future research should determine whether differences exist between the behavioral and cognitive components of workstyle across types of work. Additionally, research should also examine the relationship of the behavioral and cognitive components of workstyle to outcomes such as pain and function at work. Such empirical efforts

could further our understanding of the role of workstyle in WRUEDs associated with more common hand-intensive jobs (e.g., computer use, manufacturing).

Observational Research: The Workplace, Laboratory, and Clinic

There have been several attempts to observe the behavioral, cognitive, and physiological dimensions of workstyle either in the natural work environment or during simulated work tasks. A prospective study of work technique and severity of upper extremity disorders was conducted on 96 female electronics manufacturing workers (Kilbom & Persson, 1987) to determine the relationship among disorders, symptoms, and work technique. Disorders in the neck, shoulder, and arm regions, as well as the frequency and severity of symptoms (i.e., pain, ache, and fatigue), were assessed. No participant had been on sick leave for any of the above disorders during the previous year. Participants were followed up at 1 and 2 years with a medical evaluation and an assessment of work technique using the VIRA method, a standardized video protocol for the analysis of postures and movements of the upper arm, head, and shoulder (Persson & Kilbom, 1993). The method was developed to measure short-cycle repetitive work under visual control with the assumption that the hands are held close to the sagittal plane and that no heavy objects are handled. The authors observed a wide variation in work technique in an identical circuit board assembly and soldering task (performed longer than 1 year prior to the study). For example, work cycle time varied considerably across workers and ranged between 4.6 and 9.1 minutes. The total number of changes in posture for each cycle varied between 170 and 452, as did the percentage of work cycle time in different postures (rest > 2 seconds: 4–42%; 0 to 30°: 31–64%; 30 to 60°: 2–43%; > 60°: 0–5%) in response to a standardized work task with a fixed work duration. Work technique predicted progression toward a more severe disorder at any anatomic location at both 1- and 2-year follow-up intervals.

In addition to posture and movement differences between symptomatic and asymptomatic workers, research on musculoskeletal response to standard work tasks (i.e., chocolate packing process) indicated that workers who experience pain, fatigue, and soreness in the neck and/or shoulders demonstrated high static electromyograph (EMG) levels and fewer EMG gaps (periods with contraction levels consistently below 0.5% Maximum Voluntary Contraction (MVC) than asymptomatic workers (Veiersted, Westgaard, & Andersen, 1990). These investigators also observed that workers with a lower frequency of EMG gaps, also in response to a standard work task measured prior to symptom development, were more likely to experience symptoms in the neck and shoulder region (Veiersted, Westgaard, & Andersen, 1993). Given the relatively modest effect of EMG gap frequency, its significance remains unclear. However, the tendency toward emitting fewer of these "unconscious" (i.e., the worker is unaware of the occurrence) EMG gaps to a standardized work task may represent a physiological concomitant of workstyle with potential etiological significance. At present, although these studies suggest the potential of workstyle, it is not possible to determine the relative magnitude of the workstyle effect compared to other determinants, such as ergonomic factors.

In a case–control laboratory analysis of workstyle, Feuerstein and Fitzgerald (1992) compared two groups of professional sign language interpreters (working with pain and working without pain) on measures of repetitiveness of hand/wrist motion, work–rest cycle, postural stress, and smoothness of movement. The two groups were equivalent on age, gender distribution, years of interpreting, and wrist and forearm endurance and flexibility. Participants were exposed to a standardized work task and videotaped. Assessments of rest breaks, hand/wrist deviations per minute from neutral, mean work envelope excursions per minute, frequency of high-impact hand contacts and visual analogue measures of pace of finger/hand movements and smoothness of finger/hand movements were conducted. Findings indicated significant differences between the two groups on rest breaks, hand/wrist deviations, work envelope excursions, and pace of finger/hand movements. Increased pain was associated with an increase in hand/wrist deviation frequency; increased fatigue was associated with fewer rest breaks and an increase in hand/wrist deviations. Decrease in flexibility was associated with an increased work envelope deviation and a higher pace of finger/hand movements. These findings provide further support for the workstyle construct and its relationship to subjective symptoms of pain, fatigue, and decrease in perceived function.

Another source of evidence for the existence of workstyle can be found in the research conducted by Radwin (1992) on psychomotor function in patients with carpal tunnel syndrome. Although this research is directed at the development of innovative functional tests that may be useful in workplace surveillance (Rodriquez, Radwin, & Jeng, 1993), the observations of Radwin (1992) are intriguing as they relate to the workstyle concept. Radwin developed a rapid pinch and release psychomotor task that uses the muscles of the hand innervated by the median nerve. The method uses a strain gauge dynamometer with limited feedback. Participants were instructed to perform a rapid repeated pinch and release task. The strain gauge is repeatedly pinched to a predetermined minimum upper force level (F upper), using the index finger and thumb, and released as rapidly as possible, then to a second predetermined maximum lower force level (F lower). Variables measured were pinch rate, "isometric force control" in terms of overshoot force (F over), and time above the upper force level (T upper). A comparison of CTS cases and controls indicated that the CTS cases generated fewer pinches per second than controls and demonstrated a pattern of overshoot to a greater degree than controls (28.3% MVC in CTS vs. 12% in controls). While higher correlations were observed between nerve conduction findings and pinch speed, a significant correlation between median transcarpal latency and overshoot was also observed. In addition, T upper was positively correlated with both median nerve motor and transcarpal latencies (Rodriquez et al., 1993). This study suggests that a preexisting disease state is associated with a tendency toward generation of excessive force, which in turn might aggravate the disease process.

Studies on disabled keyboard operators, as well as individual differences in key force levels in asymptomatic pianists and computer keyboard operators, provide further support for the emerging construct of workstyle as a factor contributing to WRUEDs. A series of clinical studies of disabled keyboard operators presenting with pain in the forearms, elbows, wrists, shoulders, and hands was reported by Pascarelli and Kella (1993). Through the use of videotaped observations, the authors identified several workstyles that may have contributed to the presenting problems. Specifically, cases with hypermobility of finger joints tended to stiffen the fingers in extension, stabilizing finger joints but making finger flexion more difficult and requiring the wrist to compensate by flexing with each keystroke and extending with each release. These investigators also constructed a taxonomy of "keyboard techniques" based on videotape analysis. It is interesting to note that 14 of the 53 cases (26%) demonstrated a tendency to use the keyboard with considerable "vigor and rapidity." The force generated was associated with a loud clacking noise. They referred to these cases as "clackers" and reported that 71% had evidence of extension and flexion forearm pain, 36% had de Quervain's disease, and 21% were diagnosed with carpal tunnel syndrome. The gender distribution was 33% male and 23% female. Although they did not elaborate, the authors did suggest that these cases had a higher incidence of epicondylitis. It is unfortunate that the authors did not present data on the validity and reliability of the methodology used to assess workstyle or on the "intrinsic ergonomic factors" in order for others to replicate these findings. Additionally, it would have been useful to have comparison data on a population of keyboard operators in order to determine whether "clackers" have higher than expected rates of upper extremity symptoms.

Clinical studies have indicated that instrumental musicians (including pianists) experience a range of upper limb symptoms/disorders (Lambert, 1992; Larsson, Baum, Mudholkar, & Kollia, 1993) assumed to be in part related to technique (Fry, 1986) or workstyle. Investigations of piano keyboard technique provide further support for the existence of workstyle and its possible role in upper limb symptoms. In a study of asymptomatic experienced pianists, Wolf, Keane, Brandt, and Hillberry (1993) identified the presence of individual differences in keyboard technique that resulted in significant variations in force on finger joints and tendons. Using a biomechanical model of force based on free-body equilibrium analysis (Harding, Brandt, & Hillberry, 1989), Wolf and colleagues (1993) calculated force as a function of finger-segment size, finger geometry, angular position of finger, and keystroke force. They also observed considerable variations in magnitude of keystrike force in response to a standard musical passage. Differences between the participants with the lowest and highest mean keystrike force varied by 178% (2.00 N vs. 5.56 N). While a strong inverse relationship between force and years of piano-playing experience was observed, a wide range of keystrike forces was associated with "variations in interpretation" of identical segments of the music. The differences in interpretation of the "work task" may represent a feature of the cognitive dimension of workstyle with direct implications for joint and tendon force. In this study, such workstyle differences were associated with variations in metacarpophalangeal (MP) joint force from 6.94 to 46.59 N between two participants in response to an identical note (note 2). The tendon force coefficient (sum of forces in the three intrinsic tendons of the hand) for note 2 between the same two participants also varied significantly, from 0.32 to 4.88 (13-fold difference).

Although these data are only presented as an example, it is feasible that individual "interpretations of work task" can result in significant variations in the force exerted to perform the task, thus placing the hands at greater risk for overexertion, fatigue, and pain. If this force is repeated over time, such a workstyle may contribute to recurrent or chronic upper extremity symptoms and disorders.

A group of studies indirectly related to the workstyle construct within an office environment was conducted on asymptomatic subjects. These studies were designed to determine whether participants exert more force than necessary to activate computer keys during a keyboarding or typing task (Armstrong, Foulke, Martin, Gerson, & Rempel, 1994; Rempel & Gerson, 1991). Armstrong and colleagues (1994) developed a device to measure keyboard force related to three different desktop personal computer keyboards. The device measures key displacement using a linear voltage differential transformer driven by a rack and pinion system. The findings indicated that peak forces applied by participants were 3.1 times greater than the force required for key activation. In addition, Rempel and Gerson (1991) indicated that an analysis of variance on keyboard × participant × row × finger revealed that the main effects for participant and keyboard explained most of the variation in force. These findings indicate the presence of significant individual differences in the degree of force a person exerts on a keyboard in a standardized typing task. Based on these earlier studies, Feuerstein, Armstrong, Hickey, and Lincoln (1997) conducted an investigation to determine whether individuals with varying levels of work-related upper extremity symptoms generated differential levels of keyboard force in a standard keyboard task. Participants who were equivalent on perceived levels of job stress, years working on keyboards, and other variables assumed to influence task performance completed a typing task while their pain, discomfort, and mood were monitored. Participants were also divided according to a composite symptom severity score. Those who were highly symptomatic generated higher levels of force than the less symptomatic cases during the word processing task. Levels of pain and discomfort increased during the typing task for the highly symptomatic group. The results also indicated that although both groups generated force far beyond that required to operate the keyboard, the highly symptomatic group responded to the task with higher force (i.e., high-risk workstyle) despite greater levels of grip strength in the less symptomatic group.

DOES WORKSTYLE MEDIATE UPPER EXTREMITY SYMPTOMS, DISORDERS, AND DISABILITY?

The research reviewed in the previous sections provides preliminary evidence for the following: (1) workplace stressors, such as job uncertainty, increased work pressure, lack of supervisor/coworker support, surges in workload, and minimal decision making opportunities, are associated with either the presence or exacerbation of work-related upper extremity symptoms/disorders; (2) individual differences in how a worker performs a standard task exist, and these variations are associated with the presence of and/or exacerbation of symptoms, disorders, and neurologic markers of disease; and (3) individual differences have been observed in keyboard force in both asymptomatic and symptomatic subjects, suggesting the potential role of workstyle in the etiology, exacerbation, and/or maintenance of upper extremity symptoms related to computer work.

If workstyle plays a role in the development, exacerbation, and/or maintenance of work-related upper extremity symptoms, disorders, and subsequent disability, how might this process occur? Figure 12.1 illustrates a possible pathway linking exposure to workplace psychosocial stressors, work demands, the evocation of the "high risk" workstyle, and the experience of symptoms, disorders, and disability. The figure also highlights the potential role of ergonomic stressors (work-task- and work-station-related) that may co-occur with psychosocial stressors and high-risk workstyle, as well as the potential interaction of workstyle with ergonomic stressors.

The conceptual framework presented in Figure 12.1 proposes that workstyle may preexist as a characteristic approach to work demands and/or be triggered or exacerbated by the presence of workplace psychosocial stressors and/or increased work demands.

Many factors, such as psychosocial stressors, increased work demands, predisposing temperament, social learning history, and social support, have been demonstrated to affect the response to potential threats (Feuerstein et al., 1986). The proposed model suggests that these factors can exert a modulating effect on cognitive filtering processes that in turn affect the level of perceived distress or threat (Lazarus, 1974; Levi, 1972). An adverse workstyle may represent a learned or overlearned response to work in general and may, therefore, be present at some static or baseline level. How-

ever, it is also possible that the intensity, duration, and/or frequency of the adverse workstyle is influenced by the perceived level of threat. As the psychosocial stressors increase, the frequency, intensity, and duration of the adverse workstyle should also increase.

Workstyle can be divided into three components: behavioral, cognitive, and physiological. Although the existence of each of these components needs to be validated, and although the degree of concordance among these components or dimensions is unclear at present, certain features or dimensions may be more pronounced in a given individual or in response to a specific job task and/or set of workplace psychosocial stressors. Nevertheless, the model assumes that workstyle is composed of each of these dimensions. The behavioral component represents the actual overt manifestations of movement, posture, and activity. These behaviors can set the stage for excessive biomechanical strain of muscles and tendons. The cognitive component of workstyle refers to thoughts, feelings, and appraisals of the situation and the worker's evaluation of the success of any response in terms of reducing threat or enhancing personal sense of achievement regarding work. The final component, physiological, represents the biological changes that accompany the behavioral and cognitive reactions. These changes may include increases in muscle tension, force on tendons, changes in intracarpal tunnel pressure, increased catecholamine release, and stress-induced changes in immune function. Subsequently, recurrent pain, numbness, tingling, inflammation, and decrement in function may arise because these changes are either recurrently evoked, not permitted to recover, or unable to reestablish a homeostatic level. As these changes continue, development of the tendon-related or nerve-entrapment-related disorders can occur and lead to alterations in physical and psychological function and subsequent work disability if left unresolved.

As discussed earlier, a number of psychosocial stressors, such as job uncertainty, increasing work pressure, lack of supervisor and/or coworker support, surges in workload, and minimal decision making opportunities, may serve as precipitators of workstyle. These factors may combine to create a problematic work environment for an individual who is self-driven toward high performance/high achievement. In particular, this person may not receive the latitude or flexibility needed in order to initiate ideas or work processes that are deemed important toward achieving optimal performance. This situation, coupled with minimal support and

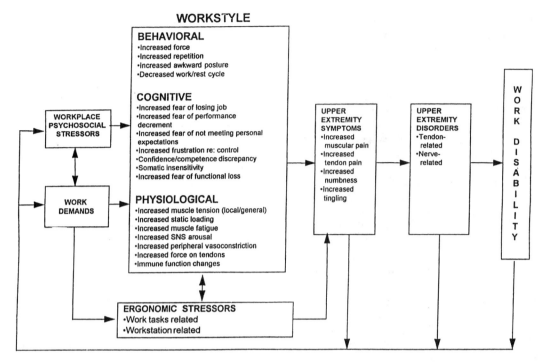

FIGURE 12.1. Potential pathway linking workplace psychosocial stressors, work demands, and ergonomic stressors to work related upper extremity symptoms, disorders and disability. From Feuerstein (1996). Copyright 1996 by Taylor & Francis. Reprinted by permission.

increasing surges in workload, can trigger a high-risk workstyle. This type of individual may continually exert excessive levels of effort, generating significant biomechanical and physiological strain on muscles and tendons and thus increasing the likelihood of symptoms. As symptoms persist and the characteristic workstyle is continuously elicited, along with its concomitant physiological correlates, very little opportunity is available for repair or recovery of tendons and muscles, and the cycle of the behavior pattern and pain continues. Coupled with minimal support, such an individual may resort to his or her primary coping style, which may be to do more work or to continue to persist despite symptoms. This situation could set the stage for continuous exposure to increased or persistent biomechanical strain in the upper extremities, subsequently leading to potential injury and decrement in function.

A tendency to drive oneself despite symptoms is suggested by the research of Reid, Ewan, and Lowy (1991). In an investigation of critical events and perceptions regarding the development of and subsequent evaluation and treatment for "repetition strain injury" (RSI), they studied a group of

52 women who were either currently employed or work-disabled due to RSI. It should be noted that these women worked either in a poultry processing plant or in telecommunications as keyboard operators. The investigators reported that 65% of those interviewed depicted themselves as displaying hardworking habits as part of their premorbid lifestyle.

In a study on psychological factors in carpal tunnel syndrome, Vogelsang, Williams, and Lawler (1994) studied participants with and without CTS who were matched on gender and job duties. These investigators observed that "general musculoskeletal problems" and goal directedness differentiated the two groups. Although it is difficult to ascertain whether or not "goal directedness" is an indication that a person will actually push himself or herself harder at work, the finding provides additional support for the potential role of the tendency to meet deadlines and drive oneself despite pain.

While the research by Reid and colleagues (1991) and Vogelsang and colleagues (1994) used retrospective designs, the findings provide additional support for the hypothesis that a feature of this workstyle may be a heightened tendency to drive or push oneself. Such a tendency, particularly in response to increased work demands, may not allow time to attend to the range of premonitory signs of an impending upper extremity problem. This tendency to drive oneself and to remain preoccupied with the demands of work may also serve to divert attention away from symptoms. Another possibility is that this behavioral style may be associated with an attenuated perceptual sensitivity to symptoms. These potential psychophysiological processes need to be validated scientifically.

It is important to reemphasize that workstyle is not intended to reflect a certain variant of psychopathology but rather a complex multidimensional response to work. With regard to this point, one study investigated the presence of psychopathology among patients with acute and chronic work-related upper limb pain, patients with acute and chronic accident injuries of the upper limbs, and non-injured keyboard operators (Spence, 1990). Comparisons of the accident-injured patients or non-injured controls to the patients with acute and chronic occupational upper limb pain found no differences in measures of depression, anxiety (state and trait), neuroticism, and psychoticism. However, lower levels of extroversion were observed for the chronic accident-injured patients in contrast to the chronic occupational upper limb group.

IMPLICATIONS FOR PRIMARY, SECONDARY, AND TERTIARY PREVENTION

The workstyle construct may provide opportunities to develop comprehensive and potentially more effective approaches to primary, secondary, and tertiary prevention. This section provides some examples of ways in which workstyle evaluation and intervention may be useful in efforts at improving outcomes for WRUEDs. The utility of these suggestions will require evaluation through well-controlled outcome research. They are described to stimulate such research.

The discussion of intervention options related to workstyle is organized around a hazard chain for WRUEDs and disability (Figure 12.2). Each stage in the chain is presented, along with proposed interventions to prevent, reverse progression of early symptoms, treat, or rehabilitate workers with WRUEDs and/or disability. This hazard chain for the development of work-related upper extremity disorders also considers stage of employment. Potential points of intervention are indicated below

the chain and highlighted with arrows. Other interventions, such as engineering and work practice controls, may be far more effective in treating and preventing work-related musculoskeletal disorders than interventions directed at workstyle, and these suggestions require controlled outcome research to justify their utility. The chain assumes that asymptomatic workers are hired into a new job as trainees progressing to become experienced workers. New or experienced workers may report strain in response to work activities. A subset of workers who cannot compensate through alterations in physical capacity or other compensatory avenues progress to experiencing pain. Some workers may identify themselves as injured because of work activities, and some cannot continue to perform all of their work activities at an acceptable level of performance. At this point, the injured worker enters the medical system and undergoes a diagnostic evaluation; he or she may receive medications as well as a prescription for rest and/or physical therapy to relieve symptoms. Those workers with more serious and prolonged problems may also enter a rehabilitation program. Ultimately, the goals of the medical management process include symptom relief, functional restoration of the affected extremities, and return to employment.

There are many points in the hazard chain at which workstyle-related intervention may be of value. Theoretically, employers may be motivated to select workers with low-risk workstyles, perhaps based on observations during work simulation (such as keyboard force measurements during typing tests). The authors are not suggesting the use of such screening, and to our knowledge this approach has not been implemented. Furthermore, the absence of any scientifically demonstrated predictive ability or benefit from workstyle-based preemployment or preplacement selection, as well as the proscription against discriminatory practices as stipulated by the Americans with Disabilities Act (1991), argues strongly against this approach.

Contemporary job design methods that incorporate ergonomics to minimize risk for WRUEDs suggest that workstyle factors could be considered as well. A thorough job analysis could identify factors that might encourage high-risk workstyles, such as open-ended incentive pay systems, excessive time pressure, and lack of supervisory support.

Studies suggest that job-specific workstyles are established within the first two weeks of taking a new job (Veiersted, Westgaard, & Andersen, 1990), identifying a potential window of opportunity to train and reinforce low-risk workstyles. Training

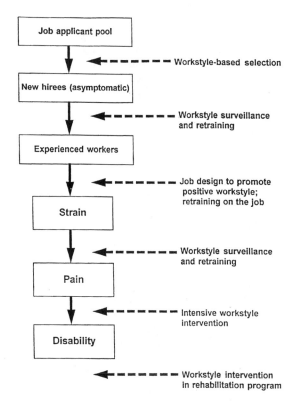

FIGURE 12.2. Workstyle interventions along the hazard chain for WRUEDs.

programs for new employees are typically designed to maximize quality and productivity, implicitly suggesting that trainees should ignore symptoms that appear during the first weeks on the job (Parenmark, Engvall, & Malmkvist, 1988). It is possible that worker education on WRUEDs that focuses on causes and prevention (e.g., the possible role of workstyle in symptom exacerbation) may lead to increased worker attention to high-risk workstyles, as well as to an associated decrease in symptoms. An effect on workstyle and symptoms may also result from systems-level interventions that restructure job tasks, implement total quality management strategies to reduce fear in the workplace (Ryan & Oestreich, 1991), increase sense of control over certain features at work, and train employees in strategies to promote their own musculoskeletal safety and health through ergonomic and personal health initiatives.

In certain workplaces, early identification of workers whose pain or injury is partially workstyle-related may provide opportunities for interventions that can prevent progression to disability. For example, our intervention with sign language interpreters focused on greater awareness and control of high-risk workstyles. Subsequently, the result was a reduction of reported workers' compensation

indemnity and medical costs in the 2 years following its implementation (Feuerstein et al., 1998). Efforts can be directed at reducing the prevalence and magnitude of workplace psychosocial stressors through stress management training (Murphy, 1996), thereby potentially reducing the chance of evoking the high-risk workstyle. Instruction of supervisors and employees in the identification and modification of high-risk components of workstyle, coupled with line supervisor training to facilitate attitude and behavior change regarding musculoskeletal problems, may also prove useful (Linton, 1991).

If high-risk workstyle and symptoms persist, more individualized interventions may be required, including some combination of self-monitoring, cognitive intervention, videotaped feedback, and reinforcement. In addition, behavioral rehearsal and psychophysiological interventions, such as biofeedback and/or relaxation techniques that target specific high-risk muscle groups or that are directed at facilitating a generalized reduction in musculoskeletal and autonomic levels of reactivity, may be utilized (Everly, 1989; Lehrer & Woolfolk, 1993; Schwartz, 1987). The specific interventions used should be based on a comprehensive assessment of the presenting problem, including a determination of the existence of behavioral, cognitive, and psychophysiological components of the high-risk workstyle on an individual and group basis. Such an approach is characteristic of cognitive-behavioral assessment and treatment (Hersen & Bellack, 1985).

To this point, potential worksite-based interventions have been described. However, once workers seek treatment for work-related injuries in the medical system, there may be additional opportunities for more in-depth analyses of workstyles that require modification. Such analyses may help determine what is necessary before a successful return to work is possible. In this regard, job simulation in a controlled environment may provide useful information. On the other hand, failure to elicit symptoms of a high-risk workstyle may only indicate that the critical workplace factors, such as time pressure, incentive pay, reactivity to a certain supervisor, or particular physical demands of the job, have not been adequately simulated.

In summary, the workstyle concept may assist in understanding the complex interaction between ergonomic and psychosocial factors that contribute to upper extremity symptoms and disorders. Although workstyle may be an attractive heuristic for developing interventions, the scientific basis for such approaches has not been well established. Controlled studies on the effects of various interventions that target workstyle and measure effects on symptoms, productivity, lost work time, and workers' compensation costs will be needed to determine the utility and cost-effectiveness of such approaches. Interventions will also need to address cost–benefit. These efforts should be directed at developing approaches that exert minimal interference with ongoing work flow.

FUTURE RESEARCH

The workstyle construct is in its early stages of development. Although the concept has potential for furthering the understanding of the role of biobehavioral factors in the development, exacerbation, and maintenance of work-related upper extremity disorders, much remains to be determined. It is unclear as to whether workstyle acts as a risk factor for WRUEDs. The levels of evidence used to determine the validity of a suspected risk factor can serve as a useful framework for identifying areas requiring future research. Typically, there are eight levels of proof that are used to assess the validity of a suspected risk factor (Gordis,

1996). These criteria are: temporal relationship, strength of association, dose–response relationship, biological plausibility, coherence, consistency with other knowledge, specificity of association, and experimental confirmation.

In order to determine the strength of the effect of workstyle on WRUEDs, a general consensus regarding a working definition of the construct needs to be established. Specific assessment methodologies must be developed and their reliability and validity determined. Further research can determine the specific contribution of workstyle relative to other risk factors. Preliminary findings suggest that certain features of the construct are associated with work-related upper extremity symptoms, disorders, and symptom severity.

Standardized measurement protocols are also critical for determining the consistency of the relationship. The consistency of the association between workstyle and WRUEDs across different types of work (e.g., manufacturing, office) observed by a diverse group of investigators is necessary to determine the robustness of the effect. Specific endpoints (symptoms and disorders) will assist in identifying reliable findings linking workstyle to work-related upper extremity symptoms and disorders.

It is unclear whether workstyle exerts a specific effect on certain symptoms, sets of symptoms, or disorders. Therefore, research that addresses the specificity of workstyle needs to be conducted. Examples of questions that can be investigated include: (1) Does workstyle contribute to symptoms of muscular fatigue in the hands, wrists, forearms, shoulders, and neck in contrast to symptoms of pain, numbness, or tingling in the hands? and (2) Is workstyle a factor in carpal tunnel syndrome but not in lateral epicondylitis? Clearly, answers to such questions concerning specificity should assist in further defining the influence of workstyle.

Determination of the temporal relationship between workstyle and WRUEDs and symptoms is a major criterion for identifying the etiological role of this construct. Prospective longitudinal studies are required to determine the temporal sequence and are particularly critical because one could argue that the observed behavior was a secondary consequence of the symptom or disorder. For example, if excessive keyforce was observed in individuals with WRUEDs or symptoms in contrast to controls, the question remains as to whether or not the increased force was the consequence of the symptoms or the disorder. The symptoms or disorders may have restricted the sensory and/or motor feedback to the fingers, thereby preventing self-regulatory processes that calibrate the force necessary to efficiently operate the keys. Although difficult to conduct, prospective studies are essential to help determine cause–effect relationships. In contrast, to address the role of workstyle in the exacerbation of established symptoms, such designs are not necessary.

The dose–response criteria determines the relationship between levels of workstyle (intensity, frequency, duration) and increased likelihood of occurrence of WRUEDs or symptoms, as well as the relationship between workstyle levels and symptom severity. With regard to symptom severity, there is preliminary evidence indicating that a greater intensity of high-risk workstyle (e.g., higher levels of self-generated force, fewer rest breaks) is associated with a higher level of symptom severity. Determination of dose–response relationships between workstyle and other measures reflecting disease or biologically meaningful endpoints is necessary to further validate the role of workstyle in WRUEDs.

The concept of workstyle has biological plausibility. Increases in biomechanical and psychological strain potentially associated with the high-risk workstyle could contribute to muscular fatigue, pain, tendon strain, and increased sympathetic arousal. In turn, an increased intracarpal tunnel pressure and entrapment of sensory and motor nerves of the hand, as well as psychoneuroimmunologic changes, may result. These items could then contribute to episodic or persistent inflammatory processes (Blair, 1993). Given the role of the central and autonomic nervous systems in immune function and the effect of behavioral and psychosocial factors on the stress response and immune function, this link is plausible (Ader, Felton, & Cohen, 1991). Research on the biochemical correlates of workstyle variations and their relationship to symptoms represents a fruitful area for further research. Psychophysiological reactivity studies (e.g., Moulton & Spence, 1992) on those with and without symptoms, as well as on those with various levels of high-risk workstyle, also are warranted.

The question of whether the link between workstyle and upper extremity symptoms and disorders is consistent with other known data on the natural history and etiology of these problems will need to await further research. Anecdotal evidence suggests that individuals who develop persistent or recurrent pain problems in the upper extremities tend to continue working and persist despite pain. Subsequently, these workers consistently expose themselves to biomechanical stressors that can contribute to the development of a longer term tendon- or nerve-related problem.

In terms of experimental confirmation, there are no randomized outcome studies investigating the effects of modifying workstyle on symptom development or symptom severity. Anecdotal evidence exists to suggest that efforts at modifying workstyle may be related to improved outcomes. A pilot program evaluation (uncontrolled group outcome study), in which workstyle modification represented one component in a multicomponent treatment package, suggested that the approach was associated with decreases in the frequency of accident reports, as well as lost time and medical costs (Feuerstein et al., 1998). Given the nature of this evaluation, it was impossible to determine the specific effects of such an intervention. Future controlled investigations should provide useful information regarding the ability to modify workstyle and the impact of such changes on symptoms and function.

CONCLUSIONS

The problematic nature of work-related upper extremity disorders has served as the impetus for increased research efforts. The National Institute for Occupational Safety and Health (1996) has designated "musculoskeletal disorders of the upper extremities" as a priority research area. Such research continues to support the role of both ergonomic and psychosocial factors in the etiology, exacerbation, and maintenance of this diverse set of symptoms and disorders. However, despite the increased awareness of the involvement of ergonomic and psychosocial factors, there remains a tendency by researchers, clinicians, and policy makers to focus on only one set of factors. We propose the existence of a dimension of work (i.e., the style in which an employee performs a work task) that may help explain how psychosocial factors interact with ergonomic factors in the workplace, thereby contributing to WRUEDs. This concept may help serve as a bridging mechanism linking psychosocial stressors to behavioral and cognitive responses, physiological consequences, and the development, exacerbation, and maintenance of symptoms. Although the workstyle construct requires further validation, it expands the conceptualization of the problem and thus holds potential for the development of innovative prevention, evaluation, and treatment approaches.

Spence, S. H. (1990). Psychopathology amongst acute and chronic patients with occupationally related upper limb pain versus accident injuries of the upper limbs. *Australian Psychologist, 25,* 293–305.

Stock, S. R. (1991). Workplace ergonomic factors and the development of musculoskeletal disorders of the neck and upper limbs: A meta-analysis. *American Journal of Industrial Medicine, 19,* 87–107.

Szabo, R. M., & Madison, M. (1995). Carpal tunnel syndrome as a work-related disorder. In S. L. Gordon, S. J. Blair, & L. J. Fine (Eds.), *Repetitive motion disorders of the upper extremity* (pp. 421–434). Rosemont, IL: American Academy of Orthopaedic Surgeons.

Ulin, S. S., & Armstrong, T. J. (1992). A strategy for evaluating occupational risk factors of musculoskeletal disorders. *Journal of Occupational Rehabilitation, 2,* 35–50.

Veiersted, K. B., Westgaard, R. H., & Andersen, P. (1990). Pattern of muscle activity during stereotypical work and its relation to muscle pain. *International Archives of Occupational and Environmental Health, 62,* 31–41.

Veiersted, K. B., Westgaard, R. H., & Andersen, P. (1993). Electromyographic evaluation of muscular work pattern as a predictor of trapezius myalgia. *Scandinavian Journal of Work, Environment, and Health, 19,* 284–290.

Vogelsang, L. M., Williams, R. L., & Lawler, K. (1994). Lifestyle correlates of carpal tunnel syndrome. *Journal of Occupational Rehabilitation, 4,* 141–152.

Williams, R., & Westmorland, M. (1994). Occupational cumulative trauma disorders of the upper extremity. *American Journal of Occupational Therapy, 48,* 411–420.

Wolf, F. G., Keane, M. S., Brandt, K. D., & Hillberry, B. M. (1993). An investigation of finger joint and tendon forces in experienced pianists. *Medical Problems of Performing Artists, 8,* 84–95.

Chapter 13

Psychological Management of Recurrent Headache Disorders: Progress and Prospects

KENNETH A. HOLROYD
GAY L. LIPCHIK

We highlight the clinical and research developments that have had the greatest impact on the psychological management of recurrent headache disorders in the last 25 years. We also identify current trends we believe will influence clinical practice in this area in the next decade. In looking backward we focus on major developments in diagnosis, epidemiology, and psychological treatment most relevant to the psychosocial focus of this volume. Consequently, we do not discuss important developments in other areas, for example, drug therapy, the medical evaluation of headaches, or our understanding of the pathophysiology of headache disorders. Information on these and other topics can be found in several excellent texts (see Davidoff, 1995; Goadsby & Silberstein, 1997; Lance, 1993; Olesen, Tfelt-Hansen, & Welch, 1993; Rapoport & Sheftell, 1993b). In looking forward we emphasize changes in health care delivery and drug therapy that are currently transforming the environment in which psychological treatments are used. We shift our focus in looking to the future because we suspect the prospects for the psychological management of headache disorders will be influenced more by developments in health care delivery and economics than by traditional psychological research.

CLASSIFICATION AND DIAGNOSIS

By 1980 the limitations of the classification system that had guided clinical diagnosis for 30 years was evident. In an attempt to remedy this problem, the Headache Classification Committee of the International Headache Society (IHS) published an extensive revision of existing classification systems (Olesen, 1988). The IHS revision adopted a format similar to that of the *Diagnostic and Statistical Manual of Mental Disorders* (DSM-IV; American Psychiatric Association, 1994), introducing operational criteria for the diagnosis of each headache disorder. This was an important step in improving the reliability of headache diagnosis, particularly for the most common primary headache disorders, which are diagnosed on the basis of the individual's description of headache characteristics and history, in the absence of positive medical or neurologic findings (see sample criteria in Table 13.1). Poorly defined diagnostic categories such as "mixed" (migraine and tension) headache were eliminated by the committee. Instead, separate diagnoses are made if, at different times, the individual experiences distinguishable headaches, each of which meets a different set of diagnostic criteria.

TABLE 13.1. Diagnostic Criteria for Migraine and Tension-Type Headache

1. Migraine

    1.1. Migraine without aura

        A. At least 5 attacks fulfilling B–D

        B. Headache attacks lasting 4–72 hours (untreated or unsuccessfully treated)

        C. Headache has at least two of the following characteristics:

            1. Unilateral location

            2. Pulsating quality

            3. Moderate or severe intensity (inhibits or prohibits daily activity)

            4. Is aggravated by walking stairs or similar routine physical activity

        D. During headache at least one of the following:

            1. Nausea and/or vomiting

            2. Photophobia and phonophobia

    1.2. Migraine with aura

        A. At least 2 attacks fulfilling B

        B. At least 3 of the following characteristics:

            1. One or more fully reversible aura symptoms indicating focal cerebral cortical and/or brainstem dysfunction

            2. At least one aura symptom develops gradually over more than 4 minutes, or 2 or more symptoms occur in succession

            3. No aura symptom lasts more than 60 minutes. If more than one aura symptom is present, accepted duration is proportionately increased

            4. Headache follows aura with a free interval of less than 60 minutes (it may also begin before or simultaneously with the aura)

2. Tension-type headache

    2.1 Episodic tension-type headache

        A. At least 10 previous headache episodes fulfilling B–D

           Number of days with such headache < 180 per year (< 15 per month)

        B. Headache lasting from 30 minutes to 7 days

        C. At least 2 of the following:

            1. Pressing/tightening (nonpulsating) quality

            2. Mild or moderate intensity (may inhibit but does not prohibit daily activity)

            3. Bilateral location

            4. Is not aggravated by walking stairs or similar routine physical activity

        D. Both of the following:

            1. No nausea or vomiting (anorexia may occur)

            2. Photophobia and phonophobia are absent or one but not the other is present

    2.2 Chronic tension-type headache

        A. Average headache frequency > 15 days per month, 180 per year for 6 months fulfilling B & C

        B. At least 2 of the following:

            1. Pressing/tightening

            2. Mild or moderate severity (may inhibit but does not prohibit daily activity)

            3. Bilateral location

            4. Is not aggravated by walking stairs or similar routine physical activity

        C. Both of the following:

            1. No vomiting

            2. No more than one of the following: nausea, photophobia, or phonophobia

Note. From Headache Classification Committee of the International Headache Society (Olesen, 1988).

The IHS criteria, which were adopted immediately in epidemiological surveys and in clinical trials around the world, appear to have improved the reliability of diagnosis (Granella et al., 1994; Leone, Filippini, D'Amico, Farinotti, & Bussone, 1994) and have facilitated developments in the area of diagnosis, for example, the development of computerized diagnosis (Gobel, 1994; Penzien et al., 1991). Adoption of these criteria by clinicians is proceeding more slowly, particularly in the United States. Nonetheless, the IHS diagnostic criteria are likely to guide headache research and, increasingly, clinical decision making into the next century.

The IHS classification system is not without critics, and a revision is planned by the year 2000. However, this revision will likely involve the refinement of the existing system rather than fundamental changes.

Rebound Headaches

The change in diagnosis that has had the greatest impact on the management of primary headache disorders in the last two decades is the general recognition of "rebound headache," "drug-induced headache" (Diener & Wilkinson, 1988), or, in the IHS classification system, "headache associated with substances or their withdrawal." This relatively new diagnostic category reflects an important insight: that frequent use of prescription or nonprescription analgesic or abortive medications (combination analgesics, opiates, nonopioid analgesics, barbiturates, ergots, and other abortive agents) can both worsen headaches and render headaches refractory to what would otherwise be efficacious drug and nondrug therapies (cf. Diener & Tfelt-Hansen, 1993; Diener & Wilkinson, 1988; Rapoport & Sheftell, 1993a). Because headaches that are aggravated by medication use often can only be effectively managed if intake of the offending medications is reduced or eliminated, recognition of this problem has, in many cases, rendered previously refractory headache problems responsive to treatment.

The International Headache Society (Olesen, 1988) and the Second International Workshop on Drug-Induced Headache (Diener & Wilkinson, 1988) have proposed different operational criteria for drug-induced headache (see Table 13.2). The IHS criteria use the quantity of medication consumed as the primary indicator of problematic use, whereas the Second International Workshop criteria use the number of days medication is consumed as the primary indicator. The Second International Workshop criteria have the advantage that they do not require detailed information about medication consumption that may be difficult to obtain. We suggest that medication overuse be considered as an aggravating factor if an individual meets, or comes close to meeting, the Second International Workshop criteria. Unfortunately, a definitive diagnosis is only possible retrospectively, when headaches initially worsen with the withdrawal of the offending medication and then improve.

Susceptibility to rebound headache varies widely across individuals, so a certain level of medication use that may aggravate headache problems in one person may not have this effect for another individual. "Rebound headaches" appear to occur primarily in individuals who are vulnerable to headache disorders: Daily analgesic use, common in the management of disorders such as arthritis, does not appear to induce headaches de novo in individuals who do not at least have a history of problem headaches. Typically, the patient who is susceptible to drug-induced headaches has a history of intermittent headaches. Headache medications provide only partial or short-lived relief, leading to an increase in medication intake. Over time, increasing medication use transforms intermittent headaches to daily, unremitting headaches that are increasingly refractory to treatment (Matthew, 1990).

Chronic Daily Headaches

The diagnosis of patients with continuous or nearly continuous headaches, sometimes referred to as chronic daily headaches (CDH), continues to stimulate debate (Mathew, 1993; Sanin, Mathew, Belmeyer, & Ali, 1994; Silberstein, Lipton, Solomon, & Mathew, 1994). Data from specialty headache centers in which difficult-to-treat headache problems are frequently seen suggests that 30 to 40% of patients presenting for treatment experience continuous or nearly continuous headaches (Mathew, Reuveni, & Perez, 1987). The majority of these patients report symptoms of both migraine and tension-type headache; a significant proportion also meet diagnostic criteria for drug-induced headache (Matthew, 1990).

Investigators and clinicians are divided into two opposing camps with regard to the diagnosis of these continuous or nearly continuous headaches. Those in one camp assert that a significant portion of continuous headaches evolve from migraine and argue that the IHS classification system, which does not take this "evolutive" history into account, cannot appropriately classify these headaches (Granella et al., 1994; Mathew et al., 1987; Silberstein, Lipton, & Sliwinski, 1996). A new diagnostic category, transformed migraine, has thus been proposed, and several efforts have been made to develop operational criteria for this diagnostic category (Manzoni et al., 1995; Silberstein et al., 1996). The transformation of migraines into near-daily headaches that has been postulated by proponents of the "transformed migraine" diagnosis has been inferred from patients' descriptions of

TABLE 13.2. Diagnostic Criteria for Headaches Aggravated by Chronic Medication Use

IHS criteria[a]	Second International Workshop criteria[b]
Headache characteristics	
1. More than 14 headache days per month	1. More than 20 headache days per month
2. Headache is diffuse, pulsating, and distinguished from migraine by absent attack pattern and/or absent associated symptoms for ergotamine-induced headache	2. Daily headache duration exceeds 10 hours
Relationship to medication use	
1. Ergotamine a. Onset is preceded by daily ergotamine intake (oral 2mg, rectal 1 mg)	1. Intake of analgesics or abortive medication on more than 20 days per month

2. Analgesics
  a. At least 50 grams of aspirin or equivalent per month
  b. At least 100 tablets per month of analgesics combined with barbiturates or other nonnarcotic compounds
  c. Narcotic analgesic use
	2. Regular intake of analgesics and/or ergotamine in combination with barbiturates, codeine, caffeine, antihistamines, or tranquilizers

3. Headache disappears within 1 month after withdrawal of substance	3. Increase in the severity and frequency of headaches after discontinuation of drug intake

[a]Headache Classification Committee of the International Headache Society (Olesen, 1988).
[b]Diener and Wilkinson (1988).

their headache history. However, because migraines are frequently disabling and may be accompanied by dramatic symptoms, migraines are more likely to be remembered than are less disabling tension-type headaches that may have preceded these migraines. We believe creation of a new diagnostic category, based largely on this inferred natural history, should thus await confirmatory findings from systematic longitudinal research.

Investigators and clinicians in another camp contend that there is no convincing evidence that classification of these headaches requires a distinct diagnostic category. Rather, it is asserted that these headaches can be appropriately classified using multiple diagnoses, a procedure which, it is further argued, has the advantage of facilitating effective management because each headache type identified may require a different therapeutic intervention (Olesen & Rasmussen, 1996). Both camps agree that these daily headaches are typically refractory to standard monotherapy with either drug or nondrug therapies and, thus, that understanding these headaches is an important clinical priority.

Developments in Genetics

To date, our understanding of the pathophysiology of primary headache disorders has not led to a biological marker that allows differential diagnosis. Progress has been made in understanding the genetic basis of a relatively rare hereditary form of migraine, family hemiplegic migraine (Ophoff, Terwindt, Vergouwe, Frants, & Ferrari, 1997). Multiple genes appear to be implicated, suggesting that genetic contribution to more common headache disorders will be complex and difficult to unravel. Given the heterogeneity in migraine presentations, this should come as no surprise. Nonetheless, recent developments in genetics hold out the hope that, within the next decade, the classification of headaches could be tied to the underlying pathophysiology of the headache disorder as genotypes underlying different phenotypic headache presentations are identified. This is likely to be the next major development in diagnosis.

EPIDEMIOLOGY AND IMPACT OF HEADACHE

During the past decade, the International Headache Society Criteria for the Classification of Headaches (Oleson, 1988) has become the standard for epidemiological research, eliminating the most significant problem of earlier epidemiological investigations: the use of differing, and often unreliable, case definitions for headache disorders across studies. Thus, the past 10 years have witnessed considerable growth in the availability of accurate information about the prevalence of primary headache disorders. However, information about the impact of headache disorders on individual's lives and the societal costs of headache disorders is just beginning to appear.

We now know that migraine is highly prevalent and is associated with substantial societal and individual burdens (see Table 13.3 for an overview of the epidemiology and impact of migraine). In the United States alone, migraine afflicts 25 to 30 million individuals; of these, 11 million are moderately to severely disabled by their migraine attacks, with disability typically at its maximum during the peak working years (Lipton, Stewart, & Von Korff, 1997). Migraine results in lost labor costs between $6.5 and $17.2 billion annually (Osterhaus, Gutterman, & Plachetka, 1992) with less than half of individuals with migraine accounting for more than 80% of these costs (Lipton et al., 1997). Migraine sufferers report greater impairment in functioning and well-being than patients with other chronic conditions that are generally considered to be more debilitating than migraine, such as type II diabetes and osteoarthritis (Osterhaus, Townsend, Gandek, & Ware, 1994). Despite the significant impact of migraine on the individual and society, most migraine sufferers do not seek treatment, and many of those who do receive suboptimal care (Stang, Osterhaus, & Celentano, 1994).

In comparison to migraine, the epidemiology of tension-type headache has been largely ignored. We currently know that approximately 78% of people experience tension-type headache (TTH) at some time; approximately 14% of the population experiences TTH several times per month, and 3% of the population have a TTH more than half of the time (Rasmussen, Jensen, Schroll, & Olesen,

TABLE 13.3. Overview of Epidemiology of Headache Disorders

Migraine headache

Prevalence: 8 to 14% in developed countries (for review Stewart, Schecter, & Lipton, 1994)
Affects between 12 to 25% of women; 4 to 8% of men (O'Brien, Goeree, & Streiner, 1994; Stewart et al., 1994)
Prevalence peaks between ages 25 and 55 years (Stewart et al., 1994)
In women, prevalence peaks between ages 40 and 45 years (Lipton & Stewart, 1993; O'Brien et al., 1994)
In the United States, more prevalent in low- than in high-income households (Stewart et al., 1992)
In the United States, at least 1 severe attack per month occurs in 60% of women and 50% of men (Lipton & Stewart, 1993)
Causes severe disability in at least one-third of migraine sufferers (Lipton & Stewart, 1993)
One-third of migraineurs cancel family and social activities or require bed rest (Pryse-Philips et al., 1992)
Only about 60% of migraineurs ever seek medical treatment for their headaches (Lipton & Stewart, 1993)
Most common precipitants: Stress and poststress down periods (Rasmussen, 1993)
Comorbid medical disorders: Major depression, anxiety disorders, including panic disorder, and epilepsy (Breslau & Davis, 1992; Breslau et al., 1994; Lipton, Ottman, Ehrenberg, & Hauser, 1994)

Episodic tension-type headache

Prevalence of ETTH: 35 to 86% of women; 29 to 69% of men (Rasmussen et al., 1991; Schwartz, Stewart, & Lipton, 1998)
Prevalence for ETTH peaks between ages 30 and 39 years (Schwartz et al., 1998)
30–36% of the population has a tension-type headache at least once a month (Rasmussen et al., 1991; Schwartz et al., in press)
Prevalence of ETTH is directly related to educational level (Schwartz et al., 1998)
Caucasians have a higher prevalence of ETTH than African Americans (Schwartz et al., 1998)
Only about 18% of ETTH sufferers ever seek medical treatment for their headaches (Schwartz et al., 1998)
Most common precipitant for ETTH: Stress (Rasmussen, 1993)

Chronic tension-type headache

Prevalence of CTTH: 5% of women; 2% of men (Rasmussen, 1995)
Prevalence of CTTH is inversely related to educational level (Schwartz et al., 1998)
Caucasians have a higher prevalence of CTTH than African Americans (Schwartz et al., 1998)
Only about 50% of persons with CTTH seek medical treatment for their headaches (Schwartz et al., 1998)
Most common precipitant for CTTH: Stress (Rasmussen, 1993)

1991) (see Table 13.3 for review of highlights). Though typically associated with less individual burden than migraine, the high incidence of TTH probably creates a greater societal burden. Thus, a recent Danish population study found 820 work days lost per year per thousand employees due to TTH compared to 270 work days lost per year per thousand employees due to migraine (Rasmussen, Jensen, & Olesen, 1992). As with migraine, it appears that a small segment of the most disabled TTH sufferers account for the greatest proportion of the total costs to society (Schwartz, Stewart, & Lipton, 1998).

Episodic TTH is not typically associated with significant levels of impairment. However, frequent and severe TTH appear to have a significant impact on quality of life and daily functioning (Schwartz et al., 1998). In a recent clinical trial (Lipchik et al., 1998), 65% of chronic tension-type headache (CTTH) sufferers recorded 25 or more headache days per month, and the majority (55.2%) of the patients showed clinically significant levels of impairment on either the physical, role, or social functioning subscales of the Medical Outcomes Survey–Short Form. Compared to the Medical Outcomes Survey national population sample, CTTH sufferers were two to five times more likely to be identified as impaired (Ware, Sherbourne, & Davis, 1992). This suggests that CTTH is associated with significant impairment in activities of daily living. Affective distress (presence of clinically significant levels of anxiety or depression) was associated with elevated levels of impairment in quality of life, work performance, and number of disability days. It thus appears that CTTH has greater impact on individuals' lives than has generally been realized, with affective distress being an important correlate of impairment.

PSYCHOSOCIAL FACTORS

In recent years migraine and tension-type headache increasingly have been viewed as primary medical disorders caused by biochemical mechanisms in the brain, most likely dysregulation in serotonergic pathways (Silberstein, 1992). When noted, psychological factors are frequently considered to be incidentally associated with headaches. In part, this is a reaction to earlier psychosomatic formulations that emphasized the causal role of specific personality traits and psychiatric morbidity in headache disorders. These earlier formulations probably led

some clinicians to pay insufficient attention to the primary headache problem.

In light of recent advances in our understanding of the association between psychosocial factors and recurrent headaches disorders, we believe that neither extreme is correct. Although we agree that recurrent headache disorders result from biological mechanisms, we also believe there is evidence that psychosocial factors play a significant role in the exacerbation and maintenance of headache disorders and most likely in the transformation of episodic headaches into chronic headaches. Here we review advances in our understanding of (1) the association between headache disorders and personality traits, (2) the association between headache disorders and psychopathology, and (3) psychosocial factors that trigger, exacerbate, or maintain headaches.

Headache and Personality Traits

For most of this century, migraineurs have been characterized as tense, driven, obsessionally perfectionistic, rigid, resentful, hostile, angry, insecure, unable to adapt to novel circumstances, and liable to react excessively, often with a migraine (see Martin, 1993, for review). Similarly, TTH sufferers had been described as "sensitive, perfectionistic, worrisome, chronically tense and apprehensive" (Martin, 1966, p. 49). These descriptions, based largely on anecdotal observations, were widely accepted in the medical and psychological community (Silberstein, Lipton, & Breslau, 1995).

Most studies investigating the association between headache disorders and personality traits have been clinic-based, which limits their generalizability. We now know that fewer than 50% of headache sufferers ever seek medical treatment and only about 2% consult headache specialists, for example, at subspecialty centers. The association between headache disorders and personality traits has been investigated primarily with the Minnesota Multiphasic Personality Inventory (MMPI) and the Eysenck Personality Questionnaire (EPQ). Most investigators found that MMPI scores of most individuals with recurrent headache disorders fall within the normal range, but that headache sufferers exhibit slight elevations on the neurotic triad (hypochondriasis, depression, and hysteria) of the MMPI (Silberstein et al., 1995). The few community epidemiological studies investigating the association between personality traits and migraine have found similar elevations in neuroticism, suggesting that these findings are not simply a function of sample selection biases (Brandt, Celentano, Stewart, Linet, & Folstein, 1990; Breslau & Andreski, 1995; Rasmussen, 1992).

Unfortunately, investigators have generally failed to account for presence of headache at the time of assessment, headache frequency or disability, and drug use, all of which can influence responses to personality assessments. For example, higher levels of psychological symptoms are reported when psychological tests are completed during a headache episode than when completed between headache episodes (Holroyd & Penzien, 1990), and thus the presence of pain is likely to elevate the psychological symptom and neuroticism scores of individuals with recurrent headache disorders. Consistent with this possibility, at least one study found that elevations on the MMPI scales were normalized in headache sufferers following treatment (Ellerstein, 1992). We thus believe there is no convincing evidence of a migraine or headache personality.

Headache and Psychopathology

Population-based studies indicate that most headache sufferers do not experience concomitant psychopathology. However, associations between migraine, depression, and anxiety disorders have been noted in recent years. For example, 20 to 30% of migraineurs, compared to 10% of persons without migraine, have a lifetime prevalence of major depression; 10% of migraineurs, compared to 2% of nonmigraineurs, have a lifetime prevalence of panic disorder (Breslau & Davis, 1992). Recent longitudinal studies indicate not only that migraines increase the risk of subsequently developing major depression (relative risk = 4.8) but also that the presence of major depression increases the risk of subsequently developing migraine (relative risk = 3.8) (Breslau, Merikangas, & Bowden, 1994). This bidirectional effect suggests that major depression is not always simply a reaction to recurrent, disabling migraine episodes, as has sometimes been suggested. The bidirectional influence has been interpreted as suggesting a common genetic vulnerability for migraine and depression. However, patterns of cotransmission of migraine and anxiety/depression have failed to reveal evidence for a shared genetic predisposition to migraine and major affective disorders (Breslau et al., 1994). It

may be that a dysregulation in the brain neurochemical system, possibly the serotonergic system, increases an individual's vulnerability to both disorders (Silberstein et al., 1995). Alternatively, it may be that the presence of each disorder increases the risk for the other disorder. For example, anxiety and affective disorders may be risk factors for transforming episodic headache problems into more severe chronic problems. Longitudinal studies of migraineurs with comorbid affective or anxiety disorders might thus provide useful insights into the pathophysiology of migraine and chronic headache.

Psychosocial Factors Influencing Attacks

In the past 25 years we have learned that headache precipitants are not universal, do not necessarily precipitate an attack on every exposure, and are not necessarily specific to a particular type of headache. Precipitants may include a variety of psychosocial, hormonal, environmental, and dietary factors (Blau & Thavapalan, 1988; Radnitz, 1990; Rains, Penzien, & Hursey, 1996; Rasmussen, 1993). Recent general population studies indicate psychosocial factors such as stress and sleep difficulties, and hormonal factors are the most commonly identified triggers (Rasmussen, 1993). Significant headache improvement often results from teaching patients to avoid, modify, or cope more effectively with headache precipitants. For example, patients who identify sleep difficulties as headache precipitants should be instructed in sleep hygiene and should be advised to maintain regular sleep schedules.

Stress

Stress is the primary trigger for both tension and migraine headache identified by headache sufferers (Rasmussen, 1993). However, our understanding of the role that stress plays in triggering and maintaining headache problems is limited and rather nonspecific. Recurrent headache sufferers do not report a greater number of major life stressors than matched controls, although recurrent headache sufferers do report more minor daily stressors than controls (e.g., De Beneditiis & Lorenzetti, 1992; Holm, Holroyd, Hursey, & Penzien, 1986). Some findings also suggest that individuals with recurrent headache disorders use coping strategies of avoidance and self-blame more frequently and seek social support less frequently in response to stress than do controls (e.g., De Beneditiis &

Lorenzetti, 1992; Edhe & Holm, 1992; Holm et al., 1986). However, it is unclear whether the use of these coping strategies is a consequence of or a contributor to recurrent headache problems or both. Longitudinal studies of daily life stress, coping, and mood and affective disorders similar to those being conducted with other pain disorders may help untangle this relationship. In any case, stress-management interventions that teach patients to identify stressors that trigger or exacerbate their headaches and to modify their response to these stressors have the potential to play a role in headache management.

Sleep

The relationship between sleep and headaches remains unclear, but we do know that a large proportion of headache sufferers identify insufficient or unrefreshing sleep as a headache precipitant, especially for tension-type headache (Rasmussen, 1993). Prolonged or unusually deep sleep also may precipitate headaches in some individuals (Sahota & Dexter, 1995). There is recent evidence that for some, headaches may arise as a consequence of a sleep disorder, such as sleep apnea, suggesting that it is worthwhile to screen for the presence of a sleep disorder and to refer to a sleep specialist when this seems likely (Paiva, Batista, Martins, & Martins, 1995).

Hormonal Factors

In the past two decades, an association between fluctuations in reproductive hormones and headache disorders, particularly migraine, has been clarified (for reviews, see Holroyd & Lipchik, 1997; Silberstein et al., 1995). We know that for many women, headaches are exacerbated or triggered by menarche, menstruation, pregnancy, menopause, and hormone supplements (e.g., oral contraceptives, estrogen replacement therapy). For example, the majority of women with migraine (52 to 70%) and a significant percentage of women with tension-type headaches (39%) report that some of their headaches are associated with their menstrual cycle, with attacks occurring either before or during menstruation (e.g., Granella et al., 1993; Rasmussen, 1993). There is evidence to suggest that menstrual headaches are related to the abrupt fall of estrogens that occurs shortly before menstruation and are prevented by the premenstrual administration of estrogens but not of progesterone (Silberstein & Merriam, 1991; Somerville, 1972; Somerville,

1975). Fluctuations in estrogen levels induce a variety of biochemical changes that might trigger migraines, including changes in prostaglandins, prolactin release, and endogenous opioid regulation (see Bouser & Massiou, 1993, and Silberstein & Merriam, 1993, for reviews). However, the specific mechanism whereby the fluctuation of estrogen levels associated with menstruation induces migraine is unknown.

Dietary Factors

Close to 30% of headache sufferers report that dietary factors sometimes trigger their headaches (e.g., Robbins, 1994). However, most of the data on dietary factors comes from surveys and clinical reports. Few double-blind studies of dietary triggers have been conducted, and clinical opinions differ regarding the benefits to be expected from dietary alterations (e.g., Baumgartner, Wesseley, Bingol, Maly, & Holzner, 1989; Blau & Thavapalan, 1988; Medina & Diamond, 1978). Nonetheless, a diet that eliminates possible dietary precipitants can serve as a valuable assessment device (e.g., Rapoport & Sheftell, 1996).

BEHAVIORAL MANAGEMENT

Interest in the use of behavioral interventions for the management of recurrent headache disorders was stimulated 25 years ago, when promising outcomes were first reported with biofeedback training (e.g., Budzynski, Stoyva, Adler, & Mullaney, 1973) and, shortly thereafter, with cognitive-behavior therapy (e.g., Holroyd, Andrasik, & Westbrook, 1977). At that time it was widely expected that these developments would rapidly lead to new and even more powerful therapeutic technologies for controlling headaches. However, 25 years later it is clear that these high expectations were not realized: The very therapies that were the focus of attention 25 years ago—relaxation training, electromyograph (EMG) biofeedback training and cognitive therapy for tension headache, and relaxation training and thermal ("handwarming") biofeedback training for migraine—remain the primary nonpharmacologic therapies for recurrent headache disorders today. Contrary to expectations 25 years ago, no new behavioral technologies were able to supplant these early therapies in the following 2 decades.

Fortunately, our understanding of the benefits and limitations of these therapies has advanced considerably in the last 25 years. We will focus here on five questions that we have made progress in answering:

1. How effective is behavioral treatment?
2. Who benefits from behavioral treatment?
3. How long do improvements produced by behavioral treatments last?
4. Can behavioral treatments be administered cost effectively?
5. Should behavioral and drug treatments be combined?

Space did not permit us to discuss a number of current topics. These include the mechanisms whereby behavioral treatment produces improvements in headache activity (see Blanchard et al., 1997; Holroyd et al., 1984; Rokicki et al., 1997); developments in psychophysiology underlying self-regulatory therapies (see Lipchik, Holroyd, Talbot, & Greer, 1997, and Schoenen, 1997); other types of behavioral interventions, for example, those that focus primarily on improving medication compliance (cf. Holroyd et al., 1989); or topics of special interest to women, for example, the management of menstrual migraines or migraines during pregnancy (see Holroyd & Lipchik, 1997, for a review).

How Effective Is Behavioral Treatment?

Relaxation and biofeedback therapies have been evaluated in more than 100 studies in the last 25 years, so a substantial body of evidence is now available on the outcomes that are produced by these therapies. However, available studies have been conducted primarily in headache clinics or in specialized university or medical school settings and have generally been small, averaging 20 patients per treatment group in migraine studies and about 10 patients per treatment group in tension-type headache studies (Holroyd & Penzien, 1986; Holroyd & Penzien, 1990). Information about the benefits that can be expected when relaxation/biofeedback therapies are integrated into busy primary care or general neurology settings or when these therapies are administered conjointly with drug therapies thus remains limited.

Relaxation and Biofeedback Therapies

Average percentage reductions in headache activity with commonly used relaxation and biofeedback therapies reported in studies conducted over the last 25 years are summarized in Table 13.4. It can be seen that for tension-type headaches, relaxation and EMG biofeedback therapies have yielded about a 50% reduction in headache activity. However, for migraine, only the combination of relaxation and thermal biofeedback training has yielded a 50% reduction in migraine activity; somewhat smaller improvements have been reported with relaxation training alone or with thermal biofeedback training alone. Nonetheless, for both headache disorders, improvements reported with each of the relaxation and biofeedback therapies have been at least three times as large as the improvements reported with placebo control treatments (Table 13.4). Thus, 25 years after relaxation and biofeedback therapies were developed, considerable evidence has accumulated to indicate that these interventions can produce clinically significant improvements in headache activity.

Cognitive-Behavioral (Stress Management) Therapy

Although cognitive-behavioral therapy has received less attention than biofeedback training, the use of cognitive-behavioral interventions in the management of recurrent tension-type headaches has received relatively strong empirical support in the last 25 years. Cognitive-behavioral therapy not only effectively reduces tension headache activity but also appears to enhance the effectiveness of relaxation training for a significant number of patients (for reviews see Blanchard, 1992; Holroyd & French, 1995). Cognitive-behavior therapy may be particularly helpful when psychological or environmental problems (e.g., chronic work stress, depression, or other adjustment problems) that are not effectively addressed by relaxation/biofeedback therapies aggravate headaches or prevent patients from effectively using self-regulation skills. Thus, in one study, patients exhibiting high levels of daily life stress (as assessed by the Hassles Scale; DeLongis, Coyne, Dakof, Folkman, & Lazarus, 1982) were unlikely to improve with relaxation training alone but were likely to improve when cognitive-behavior therapy interventions were added to relaxation training (Tobin, Holroyd, Baker, Reynolds, & Holm, 1988).

Although migraines also may improve with cognitive-behavior therapy, cognitive-behavioral interventions have not been found to enhance the effectiveness of relaxation/thermal biofeedback therapy in reducing migraine activity (see Blanchard & Andrasik, 1982, for a review). However, studies with migraine to date have adopted cognitive-behavior therapy interventions largely unchanged

TABLE 13.4. Average Improvement by Type of Treatment and Type of Headache

Type of treatment	Average % improvement	Treatment groups (n)	Improvement range (%)
Tension-type headache			
Combined EMG biofeedback and relaxation training	57	9	29 to 88
EMG biofeedback training	46	26	13 to 87
Relaxation training	45	15	17 to 94
Placebo control (noncontingent biofeedback)	15	6	-14 to 40
Headache monitoring control	-4	10	-28 to 12
Migraine			
Combined relaxation training and thermal biofeedback	56	35	11 to 93
Relaxation training	37	38	5 to 81
Thermal biofeedback training	35	14	-8 to 80
Cephalic vasomotor biofeedback training	34	11	2 to 82
Placebo control (medication placebo)	12	20	-23 to 32
Headache monitoring control	3	15	-30 to 33

Note. All relaxation and biofeedback therapies produced significantly larger improvements than placebo and headache monitoring controls. Combined relaxation training and thermal biofeedback also produced larger improvements in migraine than relaxation or thermal biofeedback training alone. Data from Holroyd and Penzien (1986), Holroyd, Penzien, and Cordingley (1991), and Penzien et al. (1985).

from studies with tension-type headache. Interventions developed specifically for the management of migraine, with which, for example, daily life stresses and headache onset are typically less obviously associated than in tension headache, might thus prove more effective. At this point, however, there is no convincing evidence that the addition of cognitive-behavior therapy interventions can increase the effectiveness of relaxation/biofeedback therapies.

More detailed reviews of this literature and, in some instances, alternate interpretations of findings can be found in Blanchard (1992), Blanchard and Andrasik (1987), Holroyd (1986), and Holroyd and French (1995). Clinical issues that arise in administering behavioral treatments are discussed in Arena and Blanchard (1996), Blanchard and Andrasik (1985), Hatch (1993), Holroyd, Penzien, and Holm (1988), and Holroyd, Lipchik, and Penzien (1998).

Who Benefits from Behavioral Treatments?

The efficacy of relaxation and biofeedback therapies was relatively well established by the mid-1980s, when a series of meta-analyses appeared (Blanchard & Andrasik, 1982; Blanchard, Andrasik, Ahles, Teders, & O'Keefe, 1980; Holroyd & Penzien, 1986). However, it was evident that one-third to one-half of patients in the typical study

failed to show a clinically significant improvement with behavioral treatment. Investigators thus began to look for commonalities among these unimproved patients in the hopes that more effective treatments for these subgroups of nonresponsive patients could be developed.

Excessive Medication Use

In spite of the fact that the role that excessive analgesic use plays in aggravating headaches was recognized in Germany in the 1940s and that the deleterious effects of excessive abortive medication use was recognized in the 1950s in the United States (Isler, 1988), these problems were not generally recognized by physicians or psychologists until the mid-1980s. By the end of the decade, however, several clinical series (Baumgartner et al., 1989; Diener et al., 1989) had documented the benefits of analgesic and abortive medication withdrawal in patients who consumed high levels of these medications (patients averaged 35 to 40 doses per week). For example, when medication withdrawal was included in their treatment program, Baumgartner et al. (1989) judged that 61% of patients who had been excessively using medication significantly reduced both medication use and headache activity at follow-up (mean = 17 months). Although studies to date have not included comparison or control groups, reported improvement figures are encouraging because these patients typically are unresponsive to drug or behavioral therapies. Controlled trials of medication withdrawal programs in patients with clearly described medication overuse patterns are nonetheless needed.

Continuous Headaches

Headaches characterized by near-daily, sometimes disabling, pain, termed chronic daily headaches or transformed migraines by some clinicians, also may respond poorly to relaxation and biofeedback therapies, even when excessive medication use is not present. For example, Blanchard, Appelbaum, Radnitz, Jaccard, & Dentinger (1989) reported that patients who recorded nearly continuous (1 or 0 headache-free days during a 4-week baseline), at times intensely painful, headaches were unlikely to benefit from relaxation or EMG biofeedback training: Only 13% of these patients showed a 50% or greater improvement in headache activity, whereas more than half of patients with more episodic headaches (two or more headache-free days per week) showed this level of improvement. Because only about 10% of patients with continuous headaches met criteria for excessive medication use, headache problems in these patients, for the most part, could not be attributed to the overuse of medication. The conventional wisdom is that management of near-daily headaches often requires aggressive multimodal therapy, for example, conjoint prophylactic medication and behavior therapy; however, controlled trials of such multimodal therapies, or, for that matter, of intensive behavior therapies in this population have yet to be conducted.

Comorbid Psychiatric Symptoms

Elevated scores on psychological tests that assess depression or other psychiatric symptoms have identified patients who would respond poorly to behavioral treatment in some, but not in other, studies. Of course, elevated psychological test scores may simply co-occur with other, better established, predictors of a poor treatment response, such as excessive medication use or continuous headaches. However, little overlap in these three predictors of negative treatment response was observed in a sample of patients recruited into studies evaluating behavioral treatments: Patients with continuous headaches showed only small elevations in Beck Depression Inventory or MMPI scores (Blanchard et al., 1989), whereas patients who were identified as using medication excessively did

not differ from controls on these psychological tests (Michultka, Blanchard, Appelbaum, Jaccard, & Dentinger, 1989). In contrast, at a specialized headache treatment center, patients with continuous headaches, particularly those unresponsive to treatment, tended to exhibit both elevated MMPI profiles (100% of unresponsive patients) and problems with the overuse of medication (Mathew, Reuveni, & Perez, 1989). Unresponsive patients also tended to report a history of parental alcoholism and sexual or physical abuse, and one-third exhibited an abnormal response to the dexamethasone suppression test. Treatment protocols that incorporate elements of cognitive-behavioral or drug therapies for anxiety and mood disorders deserve evaluation in this population of patients. In primary care or general neurology settings, treatment outcomes might also be improved if patients receiving treatment for headaches were routinely screened for the most common anxiety and mood disorders and symptoms identified were appropriately addressed.

Children and Adolescents

Until the mid-1980s virtually no information was available concerning the effectiveness of behavioral interventions with children and adolescents; unfortunately, information remains quite limited today. However, the handful of, for the most part, small studies published to date suggest that some behavioral treatments are as effective or more effective with children and adolescents than with adults. Thermal biofeedback training and combined relaxation/thermal biofeedback training—but not necessarily relaxation training—may be particularly effective in controlling migraines in children and adolescents (see review by Hermann, Kim, & Blanchard, 1995). For example, in an illustrative study, Blanchard and Andrasik (1985) reported an 82% reduction in migraine activity with relaxation/thermal biofeedback training and a 45% reduction in migraine activity with relaxation training alone in children 8 to 16 years of age. The positive results that have been reported with relaxation/thermal biofeedback training and the reluctance of parents and many physicians to use drug therapies in young children raise the possibility that relaxation/thermal biofeedback training is the treatment of choice for pediatric migraine. In the only study (Olness, MacDonald, & Uden, 1987) to directly compare the effectiveness of behavioral and drug therapy in children (6 to 12 years of age), combined relaxation and self-hypnosis training (5 treatment sessions) yielded significantly better results than propranolol (3 mg per kg per day). In fact, although combined relaxation and self-hypnosis produced better results than placebo, results achieved with propranolol and a placebo did not differ.

Less is known about the treatment of tension-type headache than migraine in children and adolescents, though the data that is available is encouraging. For example, in a reanalysis of data from three controlled studies, Larsson and Melin (1988) concluded that therapist-administered relaxation training produced larger improvements (63% reduction in headache activity) in adolescents (aged 16 to 18) than a pseudotherapy control treatment designed to control for therapist contact and other nonspecific aspects of therapy. Clearly more information is needed about the effectiveness of behavioral treatments in this population.

Older Adults

It was first noted in the mid-1980s that relaxation and EMG biofeedback therapies, at least as administered in trials being conducted at that time, were ineffective for tension headache sufferers over the age of about 50 (Blanchard, Andrasik, Evans, & Hillhouse, 1985; Holroyd & Penzien, 1986). Investigators quickly generated complex explanations for this apparent age effect. However, in subsequent studies when relatively simple adjustments were made in treatment protocols, quite positive outcomes were reported, particularly with combined relaxation and cognitive-behavior therapy (e.g., Arena, Hannah, Bruno, & Meador, 1991; Arena, Hightower, & Chong, 1988; Mosley, Grotheus, & Meeks, 1995). For example, Mosley and colleagues (1995) treated patients who ranged in age from 60 to 78 years of age (mean = 68 years) and found that 64% of patients who received 12 sessions of combined relaxation and cognitive-behavior therapy showed clinically significant improvements in tension-type headache activity. In this study, audiotapes and written materials designed specifically to assist acquisition of self-regulatory skills were provided to patients, and weekly phone contacts following each session to answer questions and identify problems were included in treatment procedures. These recent findings suggest that the provision of more detailed verbal and written explanations of treatment procedures, the review of the material covered, and the allowance of more time to practice elementary skills before more advanced skills are introduced eliminates the age effect observed in earlier studies.

How Long Do Improvements Last?

In studies conducted over the last 25 years, improvements achieved with behavioral treatments have generally been maintained, at least for the 3- to 9-month follow-up periods that have most frequently been assessed. For example, improvements reported at such short-term follow-up evaluations were larger than improvements reported at immediate posttreatment evaluations in 65 patient samples included in two meta-analytic reviews (Holroyd & Penzien, 1986; Penzien, Holroyd, Holm, & Hursey, 1985).

Positive but much less definitive statements can be made about the long-term (greater than 1 year) maintenance of improvements. At least 45% reduction in headache activity has been reported in 14 of 15 studies that used daily headache recordings to assess improvement 1 to 3 years following behavioral treatment and in three studies that assessed improvement 5 to 7 years following treatment (see Blanchard, 1987; Blanchard, 1992; Holroyd & French, 1995, for reviews). However, a significant proportion of patients is typically lost to follow-up in these studies, and patients who do complete the follow-up evaluation may have received other treatment during the follow-up period, so these findings must be interpreted cautiously. If we could identify patients at high risk for relapse, it might help us prevent relapse in these patients. Booster sessions have not been found to enhance the maintenance of improvements, possibly because good maintenance has frequently been found without booster sessions (Andrasik, Blanchard, Neff, & Rodichok, 1984; Blanchard et al., 1988). It is possible, however, that patients at high risk for relapse would benefit from booster sessions. One 5-year retrospective follow-up of more than 400 patients reported relatively poor long-term results for patients over 30 years of age, for males, and for patients who had exhibited excessive medication use prior to treatment (Diamond, Mediana, Diamond-Falk, & DeVeno, 1979). Unfortunately, the possibility that patients who were doing poorly at follow-up actually were less improved at the end of treatment (as opposed to having relapsed following initial improvement) was not ruled out; nonetheless, these results raise the possibility that variables associated with initial treatment response also predict maintenance of treatment gains.

Can Behavioral Treatments Be Administered Cost Effectively?

For many patients treatment procedures can be effectively administered in limited-contact or group treatment formats. In a limited-contact or "home-based" treatment, headache management skills are introduced in periodic clinic sessions, but written materials and audiotapes are used to enable patients to acquire skills at home that would be typically taught in clinic sessions. As a result, only three to four (monthly) clinic sessions may be required to complete limited-contact behavioral treatment. This contrasts with the 10 to 20 (often weekly) clinic sessions required for completely therapist-administered "clinic-based" treatment. In the studies that have directly compared the effectiveness of the same behavioral intervention given in both therapist-administered and minimal-contact treatment formats, these two treatment formats have yielded similar outcomes both in adults and children, although improvements in children were possibly somewhat smaller (see reviews by Haddock et al., 1997; Hermann et al., 1995; Nash & Holroyd, 1992; Rowan & Andrasik, 1996). The limited available evidence also suggests that group treatment can be as effective as individual treatment, even with interventions such as biofeedback (Gauthier, Cote, Cote, & Drolet, in press). These alternate formats thus appear to be cost-effective methods for providing treatment. Some proportion of patients will, of course, continue to require more therapist-intensive treatment. Individuals who excessively use analgesic medication, are clinically depressed, or suffer from near-daily headache problems may require more intensive treatment. Other patients simply do not persist in efforts to learn or apply self-regulation skills without regular contact with a health professional.

Should Behavioral and Drug Therapy Be Combined?

The comparative effectiveness and combined effects of behavioral and drug therapies have rarely been directly assessed. Consequently, the effectiveness of these two treatment modalities can only be examined via meta-analysis of the separate drug therapy and behavior therapy literatures (see Holroyd, 1993, for a more detailed review). Average improvements in migraine with the most widely used preventive drug (propranolol hydrochloride; 25 clinical trials) and nondrug (relaxation/thermal biofeedback; 35

clinical trials) therapies reported in a meta-analysis of these two literatures suggested that two treatments produced almost identical improvements in migraine: Each yielded a 55% reduction in migraine activity in the typical patient, whereas the average patient treated with pill placebo showed only a 12% reduction in migraine activity. Less information is available concerning the effectiveness of prophylactic agents other than propranolol; however, in direct comparisons other agents have generally proven no more effective than propranolol (Holroyd, Penzien, & Cordingley, 1991). In many cases prophylactic drug and behavioral therapies may thus be equally viable treatment options.

Two of three studies that have evaluated conjoint propranolol and relaxation/thermal biofeedback training found this treatment highly effective in managing recurrent migraines (yielding more than a 70% headache reduction on average; Holroyd, Cordingley, France, Rokicki, & Kvaal, 1992; Mathew, 1981). In fact, this combination therapy proved significantly more effective than relaxation/biofeedback training alone in both studies. In developing a treatment algorithm (Holroyd et al., 1998), we have argued that if migraines are frequent or severe or if psychological problems complicate treatment, conjoint behavior and drug therapy should be considered. If migraines are less frequent and not complicated by psychological problems, behavioral and drug therapies may be equally viable treatment alternatives. In the latter case, patient preference, treatment costs, or presence of medication contraindications (e.g., possibility of pregnancy, breast-feeding) might then influence the treatment modality chosen.

In the only study that has examined the long-term effects of a combined drug and behavioral therapy, amitriptyline initially enhanced the effectiveness of biofeedback training in patients who appear likely to have had both migraine and tension-type headache diagnoses (Reich & Gottesman, 1993). However, beginning at month 8 and continuing through the 24-month observation period, results achieved with biofeedback training alone were superior to those obtained with the combination of amitriptyline and biofeedback training.

The comparative effectiveness of preventive drug and behavior therapies in the management of tension-type headache has been examined in only one study (Holroyd, Nash, Pingel, Cordingley, & Jerome, 1991). Patients with frequent (either episodic or chronic) tension-type headaches (mean = 5 headache days per week) received either cognitive-behavioral therapy (administered in a limited-therapist contact treatment format) or amitriptyline HCl (individualized dose of 25 to 75 mg per day). Cognitive-behavioral therapy and amitriptyline each yielded significant improvements in headache activity, both when improvement was assessed with patient daily recordings (56% and 27% reduction, respectively) and when improvement was assessed by neurologist ratings (94% and 69%, respectively, of patients rated as at least moderately improved). In instances in which differences in treatment effectiveness were observed, cognitive-behavioral therapy yielded somewhat more positive outcomes than did amitriptyline. It is unclear if brief cognitive-behavioral therapy would yield equally positive results if only patients with near-daily pain were treated, because patients who are rarely headache-free often are unable to make use of the skills for preventing headaches that are an important component of this treatment. In developing a treatment algorithm (Holroyd et al., 1998), we have suggested that both antidepressant medication and behavior therapy be considered when pain is unremitting or when a comorbid mood or anxiety disorder is present; when neither of these conditions is present, cognitive-behavioral therapy may be the treatment of choice.

PROSPECTS

Here we discuss three developments we believe will influence the behavioral management of headaches in the next decade: (1) the development of treatment programs tailored to empirically defined segments of the population of headache sufferers, (2) the development of new migraine medications, and (3) the growth of managed care. Although we discuss these three developments separately, they are not independent but interdependent developments.

Segmenting the Population

The epidemiologic research reviewed above suggests that the medical management of headache disorders might be improved if the population of headache sufferers could be segmented and well-defined management strategies systematically implemented to address the differing needs of each population segment. Here we draw upon epidemiologic findings to identify three population segments and note some of the ways behavioral intervention strat-

egies might contribute to the treatment of individuals within each population segment. The three population segments are (1) individuals not currently receiving treatment for their headaches, (2) individuals with severe disabling headaches, and (3) individuals exhibiting high levels of affective distress or comorbid psychiatric disorders. Other issues involved in changing health care delivery to systematically match treatments with patient characteristics are discussed in the subsequent section on managed care.

Most individuals with recurrent disorders either have never sought care or have lapsed from care (Stang et al., 1994). However, more than 80% of untreated headache sufferers report some disability associated with their headaches, and at least 25% experience severe impairment in work, daily life, and recreational activities, so failure to consult is not limited to individuals with minimally impairing headache problems (Lipton, Stewart, Celentano, & Reed, 1992). The factors that influence consultation have not been systematically studied. However, a significant proportion of individuals probably do not seek treatment because they are unaware that effective treatments are available (Lipton et al., 1992). In the United States (but not in western Europe) persons with migraines are less likely to be diagnosed as household income decreases, suggesting that access to health care may be an important factor in consultation, particularly for individuals with limited income (Stewart, Lipton, Celentano, & Reed, 1992). Over half of individuals who do consult and later lapse from care report that they were dissatisfied with the care they received from their physicians or that they experienced problems with prescribed medications that were not effectively addressed (Edmeads et al., 1993). This suggests that outcomes might be improved if the management of headaches, including physician–patient communication, were improved in the primary care setting.

Reaching individuals who are not currently receiving care will likely require public education campaigns to increase awareness about headaches and the availability of effective treatments. Screening programs also might be designed to identify headache problems that have a high individual and societal impact (e.g., Lipton, Amatniek, Ferrari, & Gross, 1994). For example, screening and providing treatment or referral at worksites where females between ages 25 and 55 are employed might be a cost-effective method of reaching untreated individuals and of reducing work-related disability costs (Cortelli et al., 1997). However, proposals that would bring more headache sufferers into the health care system highlight difficult cost–benefit choices. Although this may reduce headache-related disability and improve satisfaction with health care, it also is likely to dramatically increase health care costs.

Programs to facilitate effective self-management may be one way to address this problem. For example, patient education campaigns designed to help individuals with recurrent headache disorders identify patterns in headache activity and avoid or modify headache triggers might effectively reduce the frequency of attacks for a significant number of individuals (Blau & Thavapalan, 1988). It may also be possible to administer behavioral interventions, including relaxation and coping skills training for the prevention and management of headaches, via the mass media. In a novel public health effort in the Netherlands, 10 TV programs were used to teach headache management skills to more than 15,000 individuals. Participants were provided home-study materials that included a workbook and audiocassettes, and 10 accompanying call-in radio programs allowed them to address common difficulties encountered when learning or using these self-management skills. Although methodological limitations of the program evaluation component of the study limit conclusions that can be drawn about the effectiveness of this pioneering intervention, the subsample of participants who were evaluated reported a 50% average reduction in headache frequency (de Bruin-Kofman, van de Wiel, Groenman, Sorbi, & Klip, 1997). These promising results raise the possibility that the mass media might be used cost effectively to teach headache management skills. Similar programs might also be developed and administered through employee assistance or wellness programs.

Patients with severe disabling headaches incur the lion's share of medical and lost labor costs, and thus increasingly there are financial incentives to effectively manage severe headache problems. However, many of these individuals are currently ineffectively treated. For example, close to half of migraineurs who report sufficiently frequent and disabling headaches to justify a trial of prophylactic medication do not receive this type of medication (Celentano, Stewart, Lipton, & Reed, 1992). Similarly, the majority of migraineurs who appear to be good candidates for prescription abortive medications do not receive these medications (Celentano et al., 1992). We expect to see the development of programs targeted at reducing workplace absenteeism and increasing effectiveness at

work. These programs would emphasize a stepped-care approach utilizing self-management interventions and appropriate medication use (see the subsequent section on managed care).

Patients with clinically significant levels of anxiety or depression or with a comorbid psychiatric disorder are probably less likely to have their headaches effectively managed than individuals without these problems, though there is little hard evidence to support this contention. It has been suggested that patients with comorbid psychiatric conditions also account for a disproportionate share of direct and indirect costs associated with headache (Lipton et al., 1997). Thus we expect that treatment outcomes could be improved if patients receiving treatment for headaches in primary care or general neurology settings were routinely screened for the most common anxiety, mood, and substance abuse disorders and if problems identified were appropriately treated. Treatment protocols that incorporate empirically validated cognitive-behavioral interventions and/or drug therapies for anxiety and mood disorders deserve evaluation in this population of patients.

Impact of New Migraine Medications

The efficacy of the first 5-HT1 agonists or "triptans" is leading abortive medications to play an increasingly important role in migraine management. At the same time, the high cost of the "triptans" assures that methods of helping patients effectively use these costly medications will be in demand. Thus we expect to see a demand for psychosocial interventions that enhance the effectiveness of the new abortive medications or that reduce the number of doses that are required.

The triptans, which are potent vasoconstrictors, might be expected to override the physiological changes induced by hand warming or by relaxation exercises, attenuating the effects of some behavioral interventions, though no hard data evaluating this possibility is available. Thus behavioral interventions in the next decade may focus more on teaching headache management skills than on the modification of specific physiological responses through biofeedback procedures. For example, methods of deciding when to use analgesic, abortive, or other medications, as well as psychological and behavioral skills for managing headaches, are likely to be included in self-management interventions.

The Impact of Managed Care

Health maintenance organizations, pharmaceutical companies, and managed care companies have all begun to design disease management systems to help control the costs of common disorders such as headache in capitated health care systems. As these disease management systems are implemented, we believe there will be less need for health psychologists to provide direct clinical services—for example, administering behavior therapies—so professionals involved in headache management will need to carve out new professional roles.

The general outline of the headache management systems currently being developed is known, though the nature of the future systems that will actually be implemented will not be clear until pilot programs are evaluated and, if successful, further refined. However, an effective headache management system is likely to require improvements in patient education and changes in physician behavior, patient assessment procedures, medical information systems, and possibly other aspects of health care delivery (Wagner, Austin, & Von Korff, 1996). To illustrate both the challenges and the opportunities presented by the development of disease management systems, we will briefly outline likely characteristics of future systems.

First, a successful headache management system must improve the management of headaches in primary care, where most patients are seen. The components of current behavioral therapies most appropriate for the primary care setting, such as education about the self-management of headaches, including headache monitoring and the use of basic relaxation skills to prevent and manage headache episodes, will thus need to be modified for the primary care setting. Second, a successful system should incorporate cost-effective methods of facilitating self-management to reduce the future need for health care services. Automated telephone assessment and other communication technologies now make it possible and cost effective to offer brief screening evaluations to a large population of plan members; identified headache sufferers can then be provided with individualized home-based headache management materials, and individuals with frequent disabling headaches who are not currently receiving treatment could be encouraged to seek appropriate treatment. Third, medical information systems will need to be modified to support effective headache management. For example, computer systems that now typically serve medical record keeping and scheduling functions might flag patients likely to benefit from special attention, such as patients who are depressed, who use problematic levels of analgesic medication, or who have made emergency room visits for headache problems. Computer systems might also encourage clinicians to use empirically based treatments by displaying relevant clinical guidelines when a patient's record is displayed or updated. Fourth, brief, easily administered, standardized assessment procedures will be needed if treatments are to be reliably tailored to patients' clinical needs and outcomes reliably evaluated. For example, a brief measure of headache severity (e.g., Von Korff, Ormel, Keefe, & Dworkin, 1992) might be used to increase the likelihood that patients with headache problems of different severities are appropriaely treated. An algorithm might be developed that (1) initiates the treatment of mild uncomplicated headache problems with education, home-based self-management interventions, and over-the-counter medications, (2) initiates the treatment of moderately severe but uncomplicated headache problems with basic drug therapies, as well as the previous interventions, and (3) initiates the treatment of frequent and disabling headaches or complicated headache problems with more aggressive drug therapy and a headache management class in which behavioral interventions and the self-management of headaches are covered more intensively.

ACKNOWLEDGMENT

Support for preparation of this chapter was provided in part by Grant No. NS32374 from the National Institute of Neurological Disorders and Stroke.

REFERENCES

American Psychiatric Association. (1994). *Diagnostic and statistical manual of mental disorders* (4th ed.). Washington, DC: Author.

Andrasik, F., Blanchard, E. B., Neff, D. F., & Rodichok, L. D. (1984). Biofeedback and relaxation training for chronic headache: A controlled comparison of booster treatments and regular contacts for long-term maintenance. *Journal of Consulting and Clinical Psychology, 52*, 609–615.

Arena, J. G., & Blanchard, E. B. (1996). Biofeedback and relaxation therapy for chronic pain disorders. In R. J. Gatchel & D. C. Turk (Eds.), *Psychological approaches to pain management: A practitioner's handbook* (pp. 179–230). New York: Guilford Press.

Arena, J. G., Hannah, S. L., Bruno, G. M., & Meador, K. J. (1991). Electromyographic biofeedback training for tension headache in the elderly: A prospective study. *Biofeedback and Self-Regulation, 35*, 187–195.

Arena, J. G., Hightower, N. E., & Chong, G. C. (1988). Relaxation therapy for tension headache in the elderly: A prospective study. *Psychology and Aging, 1*, 96–98.

Baumgartner, C., Wesseley, P., Bingol, C., Maly, J., & Holzner, F. (1989). Long-term prognosis of analgesic withdrawal in patients with drug-induced headaches. *Headache, 29*, 510–514.

Blanchard, E. B. (1987). Long-term effects of behavioral treatment of chronic headache. *Behavior Therapy, 23*, 375–385.

Blanchard, E. B. (1992). Psychological treatment of benign headache disorders. *Journal of Consulting and Clinical Psychology, 60*, 537–551.

Blanchard, E. B., & Andrasik, F. (1982). Psychological assessment and treatment of headache: Recent developments and emerging issues. *Journal of Consulting and Clinical Psychology, 50*, 859–879.

Blanchard, E. B., & Andrasik, F. (1985). *Management of chronic headache: A psychological approach*. Elmsford, New York: Pergamon Press.

Blanchard, E. B., & Andrasik, F. (1987). Biofeedback treatment of vascular headache. In J. P. Hatch, J. D. Rugh, & J. G. Fisher (Eds.), *Biofeedback studies in clinical efficacy* (pp. 1–79). New York: Plenum.

Blanchard, E. B., Andrasik, F., Ahles, T. A., Teders, S. J., & O'Keefe, D. M. (1980). Migraine and tension headache: A meta-analytic review. *Behavior Therapy, 11*, 613–631.

Blanchard, E. B., Andrasik, F., Evans, D. D., & Hillhouse, J. (1985). Biofeedback and relaxation treatments for headache in the elderly: A caution and a challenge. *Biofeedback and Self-Regulation, 10*, 69–73.

Blanchard, E. B., Appelbaum, K. A., Guarnieri, P., Neff, D. F., Andrasik, F., Jaccard, J., & Barron, K. D. (1988). Two studies of the long-term follow-up of minimal-therapist contact treatments of vascular and tension headache. *Journal of Consulting and Clinical Psychology, 56*, 427–432.

Blanchard, E. B., Appelbaum, K. A., Radnitz, C. L., Jaccard, J., & Dentinger, M. P. (1989). The refractory headache patient: I. Chronic, daily, high-intensity headache. *Behaviour Research and Therapy, 27*, 403–410.

Blanchard, E. B., Peters, M. L., Herman, C., Turner, S. M., Buckley, T. C., & Barton, S. M. (1997). Direction of temperature control in the thermal biofeedback treatment of vascular headache. *Applied Psychophysiology and Biofeedback, 22*, 227–246.

Blau, J. N., & Thavapalan, M. (1988). Preventing migraine: A study of precipitating factors. *Headache, 28*, 481–483.

Bouser, M. G., & Massiou, H. (1993). Migraine in the reproductive cycle. In J. Olesen, P. Tfelt-Hansen, & K. M. A. Welch (Eds.), *The headaches* (pp. 413–419). New York: Raven Press.

Brandt, J., Celentano, D., Stewart, W., Linet, M., & Folstein, M. F. (1990). Personality and emotional disorder in a community sample of migraine headache sufferers. *American Journal of Psychiatry, 147*, 303–308.

Breslau, N., & Andreski, P. (1995). Migraine, personality, and psychiatric comorbidity. *Headache, 35*, 382–386.

Breslau, N., & Davis, G. C. (1992). Migraine, major depression and panic disorder: A prospective epidemiologic study of young adults. *Cephalalgia, 12*, 85–90.

Breslau, N., Merikangas, K., & Bowden, C. L. (1994). Comorbidity of migraine and major affective disorders. *Neurology, 44*(Suppl. 7), S17–S22.

Budzynski, T. H., Stoyva, J. M., Adler, C. S., & Mullaney, D. J. (1973). EMG biofeedback and tension headache: A controlled outcome study. *Psychosomatic Medicine, 6*, 509–514.

Celentano, D. D., Stewart, W. F., Lipton, R. B., & Reed, M. L. (1992). Medication use and disability among migraineurs: A national probability sample survey. *Headache, 32*, 223–228.

Cortelli, P., Dahlof, C., Bouchard, J., Heywood, J., Jansen, J. P., Pham, S., Hirsch, J., Adams, J., & Miller, J. W. (1997). A multinational investigation of the impact of subcutaneous sumatriptan: 3. Workplace productivity and non-workplace activity. *PharmacoEconomics, 11*, 35–42.

Davidoff, R. A. (1995). *Migraine: Manifestations, pathogenesis, and management*. Philadelphia: Davis.

De Benedittis, G., & Lorenzetti, A. (1992). Minor stressful life events (daily hassles) in chronic primary headache: Relationship with MMPI personality patterns. *Headache, 32*, 330–332.

de Bruin-Kofman, A. T., van de Wiel, H., Groenman, N. H., Sorbi, M. J., & Klip, E. (1997). Effects of a mass media behavioral treatment for chronic headache: A pilot study. *Headache, 37*, 415–420.

DeLongis, A., Coyne, J. C., Dakof, G., Folkman, S., & Lazarus, R. S. (1982). Relationship of daily hassles, uplifts, and major life events to health status. *Health Psychology, 1*, 119–136.

Diamond, S., Mediana, J., Diamond-Falk, J., & DeVeno, T. (1979). The value of biofeedback in the treatment of chronic headache: A five-year retrospective study. *Headache, 19*, 90–96.

Diener, H. C., Dichgans, J., Scholz, E., Geiselhart, S., Gerber, W. D., & Bille, A. (1989). Analgesic-induced chronic headache: Long-term results of withdrawal therapy. *Journal of Neurology, 236*, 9–14.

Diener, H. C., & Tfelt-Hansen, P. (1993). Headache associated with chronic use of substances. In J. Olesen, P. Tfelt-Hansen, & K. M. A. Welch (Ed.), *The headaches* (pp. 721–728). New York: Raven Press.

Diener, H. C., & Wilkinson, M. E. (1988). *Drug-induced headache*. New York: Springer-Verlag.

Edhe, D. M., & Holm, J. E. (1992). Stress and headache: Comparison of migraine, tension, and headache-free subjects. *Headache Quarterly, 1992*, 54–60.

Edmeads, J., Findlay, H., Tugwell, P., Pryse-Phillips, W., Nelson, R. F., & Murray, T. J. (1993). Impact of migraine and tension-type headaches on life-style, consulting behavior, and medication use: A Canadian population survey. *Canadian Journal of Neurological Science, 20*, 131–137.

Ellerstein, B. (1992). Personality factors in recurring and chronic pain. *Cephalalgia, 12*, 129–132.

Gauthier, J. G., Cote, G., Cote, A., & Drolet, M. (in press). Group versus individual thermal biofeedback in the treatment of migraine: A comparative outcome study. *Headache*.

Goadsby, P. J., & Silberstein, S. D. (Eds.). (1997). *Blue books of practical neurology: Headache* (Vol. 17). Boston: Butterworth-Heinemann.

Gobel, H. (1994). Objective headache classification on the computer according to the IHS classification. In J. Olesen (Ed.), *Headache classification and epidemiology* (Vol. 4, pp. 55–62). New York: Raven Press.

Granella, F., Sances, G., Zanferrari, C., Costa, A., Martignoni, E., & Manzoni, G. C. (1993). Migraine without aura and reproductive life events: A clinical epidemiological study in 1300 women. *Headache, 33,* 385–389.

Granella, R., Alessandro, R. D., Manzoni, G. C., Cerbo, R., Collucci D'Amato, C., Pini, L. A., Savi, L., Zanferrari, C., & Nappi, G. (1994). International Headache Society classification: Interobserver reliability in the diagnosis of primary headaches. *Cephalalgia, 14,* 16–20.

Haddock, C. K., Rowan, A. B., Andrasik, F., Wilson, P. G., Talcott, G. W., & Stein, R. J. (1997). Home-based behavioral treatments for chronic benign headache: A meta-analysis of controlled trials. *Cephalalgia, 17,* 113–118.

Hatch, J. P. (1993). Headache. In R. J. Gatchel & E. B. Blanchard (Eds.), *Psychophysiological disorders: Research and clinical applications* (pp. 111–150). Washington, DC: American Psychological Association.

Hermann, C., Kim, M., & Blanchard, E. B. (1995). Behavioral and pharmacological intervention studies of pediatric migraine: An exploratory meta-analysis. *Pain, 60,* 239–256.

Holm, J. E., Holroyd, K., Hursey, K. G., & Penzien, D. (1986). The role of stress in recurrent tension headaches. *Headache, 26,* 160–167.

Holroyd, K. (1993). Integrating pharmacologic and nonpharmacologic treatments. In C. D. Tolison & R. S. Kunkel (Eds.), *Headache diagnosis and interdisciplinary treatment* (pp. 309–320). Baltimore: Williams & Wilkins.

Holroyd, K. A. (1986). Recurrent headache. In K. A. Holroyd & T. L. Creer (Eds.), *Self management of chronic disease: Handbook of clinical interventions and research* (pp. 373–413). Orlando, FL: Academic Press.

Holroyd, K. A., Andrasik, F., & Westbrook, T. (1977). Cognitive control of tension headache. *Cognitive Therapy and Research, 1,* 121–133.

Holroyd, K. A., Cordingley, G. E., France, J. L., Rokicki, L., & Kvaal, S. (1992). Combining propranolol and biofeedback for treatment of migraine. *Headache, 32,* 254–255.

Holroyd, K. A., Cordingley, G. E., Pingel, J. D., Jerome, A., Theofanous, A. G., Jackson, D. K., & Leard, L. (1989). Enhancing the effectiveness of abortive therapy: A controlled evaluation of self-management training. *Headache, 29,* 148–153.

Holroyd, K. A., & French, D. (1995). Recent advances in the assessment and treatment of recurrent headaches. In A. J. Goreczny (Ed.), *Handbook of health and rehabilitation psychology* (pp. 3–30). New York: Plenum Press.

Holroyd, K. A., & Lipchik, G. L. (1997). Recurrent headache disorders. In S. J. Gallant, G. P. Keita, & R. Royak-Schaler (Eds.), *Psychosocial and behavioral factors in women's health care: A handbook for medical educators, practitioners, and psychologists* (pp. 365–384). Washington, DC: American Psychological Association.

Holroyd, K. A., Lipchik, G. L., & Penzien, D. B. (1998). Psychological management of recurrent headache disorders: Empirical basis for clinical practice. In K. S.

Dobson & K. D. Craig (Eds.), *Best practice: Developing and promoting empirically supported interventions* (pp. 187–236). Newbury Park, CA: Sage.

Holroyd, K. A., Nash, J. M., Pingel, J. D., Cordingley, G. E., & Jerome, A. (1991). A comparison of pharmacological (amitriptyline HCl) and nonpharmacological (cognitive-behavioral) therapies for chronic tension headaches. *Journal of Consulting and Clinical Psychology, 59,* 387–393.

Holroyd, K. A., & Penzien, D. B. (1986). Client variables in the behavioral treatment of recurrent tension headache: A meta-analytic review. *Journal of Behavioral Medicine, 9,* 515–536.

Holroyd, K. A., & Penzien, D. B. (1990). Pharmacological vs. nonpharmacological prophylaxis of recurrent migraine headache: A meta-analytic review of clinical trials. *Pain, 42,* 1–13.

Holroyd, K. A., Penzien, D. D., & Cordingley, G. (1991). Propronolol in the management of recurrent migraine: A meta-analytic review. *Headache, 31,* 333–340.

Holroyd, K. A., Penzien, D. D., & Holm, J. E. (1988). Clinical issues in the treatment of recurrent headache disorders. In P. A. Keller & L. G. Ritt (Eds.), *Innovations in clinical practice: A source book* (Vol. 7, pp. 433–458). Sarasota, FL: Professional Resource Exchange.

Holroyd, K. A., Penzien, D. B., Hursey, K. G., Tobin, D. L., Rogers, L., Holm, J. E., Marcille, P. J., Hall, J. R., & Chila, A. G. (1984). Change mechanisms in EMG biofeedback training: Cognitive changes underlying improvements in tension headache. *Journal of Consulting and Clinical Psychology, 52,* 1039–1053.

Isler, H. (1988). Headache drugs provoking chronic headache: Historical aspects and common misunderstandings. In H. C. Diener & M. E. Wilkinson (Eds.), *Drug-induced headache* (pp. 87–94). New York: Springer-Verlag.

Lance, J. W. (1993). *Mechanisms and management of headache* (5th ed.). Boston: Butterworth-Heinemann.

Larsson, B., & Melin, L. (1988). The psychological treatment of recurrent headache in adolescents—short-term outcome and its prediction. *Headache, 28,* 187–195.

Leone, M., Filippini, G., D'Amico, D., Farinotti, M., & Bussone, G. (1994). Assessment of IHS diagnostic criteria: A reliability study. *Cephalalgia, 14,* 280–284.

Lipchik, G. L., Holroyd, K. A., Pinnell, C., Stensland, M., Hill, K., Malinoski, P., & Boyer, D. (1998, March). *Chronic tension-type headaches: Clinical characteristics and impact on quality of life.* Paper presented at the annual meeting of the Society of Medicine, New Orleans, LA.

Lipchik, G. L., Holroyd, K. H., Talbot, F., & Greer, M. (1997). Pericranial muscle tenderness and exteroceptive suppression of temporalis muscle activity: A blind study of chronic tension-type headache. *Headache, 37*(6), 368–376.

Lipton, R. B., Amatniek, J. C., Ferrari, M. D., & Gross, M. (1994). Migraine: Identifying and removing barriers to care. *Neurology, 44*(Suppl. 4), S63–S68.

Lipton, R. B., Ottman, R. B., Ehrenberg, B. L., & Hauser, W. A. (1994). Comorbidity of migraine: The connection between migraine and epilepsy. *Neurology, 44* (Suppl. 7), S28–S32.

Lipton, R. B., & Stewart, W. F. (1993). Migraine in the United States: A review of epidemiology and health care use. *Neurology, 48*(Suppl. 3), S6–S10.

Lipton, R. B., Stewart, W. F., Celentano, D. D., & Reed, M. L. (1992). Undiagnosed migraine headaches: A comparison of symptom-based and reported physician diagnosis. *Archives of Internal Medicine, 152,* 1273–1278.

Lipton, R. B., Stewart, W. F., & Von Korff, M. (1997). Burden of migraine: Societal costs and therapeutic opportunities. *Neurology, 48*(Suppl. 3), S4–S9.

Manzoni, G. C., Granella, F., Sandrini, G., Cavallini, A., Zanferrari, C., & Nappi, G. (1995). Classification of chronic daily headache by IHS criteria: Limits and new proposals. *Cephalalgia, 15,* 37–43.

Martin, M. J. (1966). Tension headache, a psychiatric study. *Headache, 6,* 47–54.

Martin, P. R. (1993). *Psychological management of chronic headaches.* New York: Guilford Press.

Mathew, N. T. (1981). Prophylaxis of migraine and mixed headache: A randomized controlled study. *Headache, 21,* 105–109.

Mathew, N. T. (1990). Drug-induced headache. *Neurologic Clinics, 8,* 903–912.

Mathew, N. T. (1993). Transformed *migraine. Cephalalgia, 13*(Suppl. 12), 78–83.

Mathew, N. T., Reuveni, V., & Perez, F. (1987). Transformed or evolutive headache. *Headache, 27,* 102–106.

Mathew, N. T., Reuveni, V., & Perez, F. (1989). Intractable chronic daily headache: A persistent neurobehavioral disorder. *Cephalalgia, 9*(Suppl. 1a), 180–181.

Medina, J. L., & Diamond, S. (1978). The role of diet in migraine. *Headache, 5,* 1020–1026.

Michultka, D. M., Blanchard, E. B., Appelbaum, K. A., Jaccard, J., & Dentinger, M. P. (1989). The refractory headache patient: II. High medication consumption (analgesic rebound) headache. *Behaviour Research and Therapy, 27,* 411–420.

Mosley, T. H., Grotheus, C. A., & Meeks, W. M. (1995). Treatment of tension headache in the elderly: A controlled evaluation of relaxation training and relaxation combined with cognitive-behavior therapy. *Journal of Clinical Geropsychology, 1,* 175–188.

Nash, J., & Holroyd, K. (1992). Home-based behavioral treatment for recurrent headache: A cost-effective alternative. *American Pain Society Bulletin, 2,* 1–6.

O'Brien, B., Goeree, R., & Streiner, D. (1994). Prevalence of migraine headache in Canada: A population-based survey. *International Journal of Epidemiology, 25*(5), 1020–1026.

Olesen, J. (Chair). (1988). Classification and diagnostic criteria for headache disorders, cranial neuralgias, and facial pain: Headache Classification Committee of the International Headache Society [Special issue]. *Cephalalgia, 8*(Suppl. 7).

Olesen, J., & Rasmussen, B. K. (1996). The International Headache Society classification of chronic daily and near-daily headaches: A critique of the critique. *Cephalalgia, 16,* 407–411.

Olesen, J., Tfelt-Hansen, P., & Welch, K. M. A. (Eds.). (1993). *The headaches.* New York: Raven Press.

Olness, K., MacDonald, J. T., & Uden, D. L. (1987). Comparison of self-hypnosis and propranolol in the treatment of juvenile migraine. *Pediatrics, 79,* 593–597.

Ophoff, R. A., Terwindt, G. M., Vergouwe, M. N., Frants, R. R., & Ferrari, M. D. (1997). Involvement of a Ca2+ channel gene in familial hemiplegic migraine and migraine with and without aura. *Headache, 37,* 479–485.

Osterhaus, J. T., Gutterman, D. L., & Plachetka, J. R. (1992). Healthcare resource and lost labour costs of migraine headache in the United States. *Pharmaco-Economics, 2*(1), 67–76.

Osterhaus, J. T., Townsend, R. J., Gandek, B., & Ware, J. E. (1994). Measuring the functional status and well-being of patients with migraine headache. *Headache, 34,* 337–343.

Paiva, T., Batista, A., Martins, P., & Martins, A. (1995). The relationship between headaches and sleep disturbances. *Headache, 35,* 590–596.

Penzien, D. B., Andrew, M. E., Knowlton, G. E., McAnulty, R. D., Rains, J. C., Johnson, C. A., Hursey, K. G., & Jacks, S. D. (1991). Computer-aided system for headache diagnosis with the IHS headache diagnostic criteria: Development and validation. *Cephalalgia, 11*(Suppl. 11), 325–326.

Penzien, D. B., Holroyd, K. A., Holm, J. E., & Hursey, K. G. (1985). Behavioral management of migraine: Results from five dozen group outcome studies. *Headache, 25,* 162.

Pryse-Philips, W., Findlay, H., Tugwell, P., Edmeads, J., Murray, T. J., & Nelson, R. F. (1992). A Canadian population survey on the clinical, epidemiologic and societal impact of *migraine and* tension-type headache. *Canadian Journal of Neurological Sciences, 19,* 333–339.

Radnitz, C. L. (1990). Food-triggered migraine: A critical review. *Annals of Behavioral Medicine, 12,* 51–65.

Rains, J. C., Penzien, D. B., & Hursey, K. G. (1996). Precipitants of episodic migraine: Behavioral, environmental, hormonal, and dietary factors. *Headache, 36,* 247–275.

Rapoport, A. M., & Sheftell, F. D. (1993a). Headache associated with medication and substance withdrawal. In C. D. Tollison & R. S. Kunkel (Eds.), *Headache: Diagnosis and treatment* (pp. 227–231). Baltimore: Williams & Wilkins.

Rapoport, A. M., & Sheftell, F. D. (1993b). *Headache disorders: A management guide for practitioners.* Philadelphia: Saunders.

Rapoport, A. M., & Sheftell, F. D. (1996). *Headache disorders: A management guide for practitioners.* Philadelphia: Saunders.

Rasmussen, B. K. (1992). Migraine and tension-type headache in a general population: Psychosocial factors. *International Journal of Epidemiology, 21,* 1138–1143.

Rasmussen, B. K. (1993). Migraine and tension-type headache in a general population: Precipitating factors, female hormones, sleep pattern and relation to lifestyle. *Pain, 53,* 65–72.

Rasmussen, B. K. (1995). Epidemiology of headache. *Cephalalgia, 14,* 45–68.

Rasmussen, B. K., Jensen, R., & Olesen, J. (1992). Impact of headache on sickness absence and utilization of medical services: A Danish population study. *Journal of Epidemiology and Community Health, 46,* 443–446.

Rasmussen, B. K., Jensen, R., Schroll, M., & Olesen, J. (1991). Epidemiology of headache in a general population—a prevalence study. *Journal of Clinical Epidemiology, 44*(11), 1147–1157.

Reich, B. A., & Gottesman, M. (1993). Biofeedback and psychotherapy in the treatment of muscle contraction/tension-type headache. In C. D. Tollison & R. S. Kunkel (Eds.), *Headache diagnosis and inter-*

disciplinary treatment (pp. 167–180). New York: Urban & Schwartzenberg.

Robbins, L. (1994). Precipitating factors in migraine: A retrospective review of 494 patients. *Headache, 34,* 214–216.

Rokicki, L. A., Holroyd, K. A., France, C. R., Lipchik, G. L., France, J. L., & Kvaal, S. A. (1997). Change mechanisms associated with combined relaxation/EMG biofeedback training for chronic tension headache. *Applied Psychophysiology and Biofeedback, 22,* 21–41.

Rowan, A. B., & Andrasik, F. (1996). Efficacy and cost-effectiveness of minimal therapist contact treatments of chronic headache: A review. *Behavior Therapy, 27,* 207–234.

Sahota, P. K., & Dexter, J. D. (1995). Sleep and headache syndromes: A clinical review. *Headache, 35,* 80–84.

Sanin, L. C., Mathew, N. T., Belmeyer, L. R., & Ali, S. (1994). The International Headache Society (IHS) Headache Classification as applied to a headache clinic population. *Cephalalgia, 14,* 443–446.

Schoenen, J. (1997). Clinical neurophysiology of headache. *Neurologic Clinics, 15*(1), 85–105.

Schwartz, B. S., Stewart, W. F., & Lipton, R. B. (1998). A population-based study of the epidemiology of tension-type headache. *Journal of the American Medical Association, 279,* 381–383.

Silberstein, S. D. (1992). Advances in understanding the pathophysiology of headache. *Neurology, 42,* 6–10.

Silberstein, S. D., Lipton, R. B., & Breslau, N. (1995). Migraine: Association with personality characteristics and psychopathology. *Cephalalgia, 15,* 358–369.

Silberstein, S. D., Lipton, R. B., & Sliwinski, M. (1996). Classification of daily and near-daily headaches: Field trial of revised IHS criteria. *Neurology, 47*(4), 871–875.

Silberstein, S. D., Lipton, R. B., Solomon, S., & Mathew, N. T. (1994). Classification of daily and near-daily headaches: Proposed revisions to the IHS criteria. *Headache, 34,* 1–7.

Silberstein, S. D., & Merriam, G. R. (1991). Estrogens, progestins, and headache. *Neurology, 22,* 239–244.

Silberstein, S. D., & Merriam, G. R. (1993). Sex hormones and headache. *Journal of Pain and Symptom Management, 8,* 98–114.

Somerville, B. W. (1972). The role of estradiol withdrawal in the etiology of menstrual migraine. *Neurology, 22,* 355–365.

Somerville, B. W. (1975). Estrogen-withdrawal migraine: I. Duration of exposure required and attempted prophylaxis by premenstrual estrogen administration. *Neurology, 22,* 239–244.

Stang, P. E., Osterhaus, J. T., & Celentano, D. D. (1994). Migraine: Patterns of healthcare use. *Neurology, 44*(Suppl. 44), S47–S55.

Stewart, W. F., Lipton, R. B., Celentano, D. D., & Reed, M. L. (1992). Prevalence of migraine headache in the United States: Relationship to age, income, race and other sociodemographic factors. *Journal of the American Medical Association, 267,* 64–69.

Stewart, W. F., Schecter, A., & Lipton, R. B. (1994). Migraine heterogeneity, disability, pain intensity, attack frequency, and duration. *Neurology, 44,* S24–S39.

Tobin, D. L., Holroyd, K. A., Baker, A., Reynolds, R. V. C., & Holm, J. E. (1988). Development and clinical trial of a minimal contact, cognitive-behavioral treatment for tension headache. *Cognitive Therapy and Research, 12*(4), 325–339.

Von Korff, M., Ormel, J., Keefe, F. J., & Dworkin, S. F. (1992). Grading the severity of chronic pain. *Pain, 50,* 133–149.

Wagner, E. H., Austin, B. T., & Von Korff, M. (1996). Improving outcomes in chronic illness. *Managed Care Quarterly, 4,* 12–25.

Ware, J. E., Sherbourne, C. D., & Davis, A. R. (1992). Developing and testing the MOS 20-item short form health survey: A general population application. In A. L. Stewart & J. E. Ware (Eds.), *Measuring functioning and well-being: The Medical Outcomes Study approach* (pp. 277–290). Durham, NC: Duke University Press.

Chapter 14

Temporomandibular Disorders: A Problem in Dental Health

SAMUEL F. DWORKIN

Temporomandibular disorders (TMD) comprise a cluster of related musculoskeletal conditions that affect the hard and soft structures involved in movement of the mandible (lower jaw) and that are characterized principally by (1) the presence of pain typically in the preauricular area in front of the ear, the cheeks, and/or temporal area; (2) limitations in movement of the mandible, reflected largely as impairment of vertical range of mandibular motion or restricted ability to open the mouth; and (3) joint sounds detected in the temporomandibular joint (TMJ) during functional excursions of the jaw (Dworkin, Huggins et al., 1990).

The purpose of this chapter is (1) to summarize the scientifically based evolution of TMD assessment and management as a bio-psycho-socially determined chronic pain condition; (2) to present evidence-based methods for the psychosocial assessment of the TMD patient; and (3) to consider evidence-based management methods derived from the arenas of behavioral medicine and health psychology, the latter sharing many common features with biobehaviorally derived methods that constitute the standard of care for the most common chronic pain conditions.

The orofacial region affected houses several organs of special sense, notably taste, smell, and hearing, and, of course, is heavily vascularized. Not surprisingly, this relatively compact anatomical region is further characterized by an especially complex

network of central and autonomic nervous system pathways. The central nervous system pathways implicated in TMD derive mainly from the maxillary (second) and mandibular (third) divisions of the trigeminal (fifth) cranial nerve, carrying both sensory and motor innervation to the masticatory muscles and the TMJ. The TMJ, located immediately in front of the ear, articulates the mobile lower jaw with the fixed temporal bone of the skull. The trigeminal nerve is also the primary sensory innervation for major intraoral structures, including the teeth and their supporting hard and soft tissue components constituting the periodontium, as well as those masticatory muscle and joint components located intraorally.

The craniofacial and perioral structures involved in TMD and the stomatognathic system they subserve are responsible for several life-sustaining physiological processes, including eating, breathing, swallowing, and verbal and nonverbal communication. Inevitably, these physiological processes are also associated with psychological and psychosocial functions of tremendous significance to the individual, functions that underlie the development of singularly unique intrapersonal and psychosocial characteristics that contribute to distinguishing one individual from another, including, but not limited to, facial appearance and interpersonal behavior.

The scientific rationale for including TMD in the series of prevalent clinical conditions represented in various chapters in this book rests on confirmed observations from scientific studies, as well as abundant clinical experience, that adaptive behaviors, psychological status, and psychosocial functioning can all be affected by persistent TMD-related pain. Chronic pain arising in conjunction with impairment of the masticatory system, from whatever etiology, affects the lives of TMD pain sufferers—from mild alterations in eating behaviors to profoundly disabling depression and appreciable interference with activities of daily living. In other words, patterns of psychosocial disability appear that are similar to those associated with other common musculoskeletal conditions in which chronic pain is an important clinical feature, such as back pain, headache, and fibromyalgia. Indeed, as a review of *all* the chapters in Part II will reveal, all the chronic pain conditions discussed in Chapters 10 through 20 share common features from the psychosocial domain (e.g., depression, limitations in activities, increased health care utilization) while each retains those unique physical features from the biological (or physical) domain that are related to a specific body site (e.g., headache, back pain) or specific pathophysiological processes (e.g., postherpetic neuralgia, cancer).

Although a large number of pathological states and diseases affect the tissues of the face and jaws, the term temporomandibular disorders (TMD) is generally restricted to painful and dysfunctional conditions affecting the muscles of mastication and the TMJ. Multiple labels have been applied to the condition, including myofascial pain disorder (MPD), temporomandibular joint syndrome (TMJS), and craniomandibular disorder (CMD). I prefer the relatively neutral (with regard to etiology and presumed site of pathology) and all-inclusive term TMD, as recommended by the American Dental Association (1983). All the nosology systems are in agreement that the predominant clinical subtypes of TMD are classified as (1) masticatory muscle disorders, by far the most common form of TMD; (2) derangements (i.e., displacements) of the articular disk of the temporomandibular joint, which rarely occur alone; and (3) degenerative joint changes typically classified as arthralgia, arthritis, and arthroses of the joint. The latter two conditions are also rare, whereas arthralgia (representing a painful or inflamed TMJ) is common among those diagnosed with TMD. Many TMD patients carry more than one of these physical diagnoses.

TMD is a common disorder, and the 6-month prevalence of persistent TMD-related pain has been estimated at about 12% in the U.S. population (Von Korff, Dworkin, LeResche, & Kruger, 1988). Any one of the three major clinical indicators of TMD (i.e., pain, limitations in jaw opening, and joint noises) is estimated to be present in 5–50% of the population at any one time (Carlsson & LeResche, 1995; Locker & Slade, 1989). Treatment seeking, however, seems only poorly correlated with the presence of other TMD signs and symptoms than pain, while treatment is generally not recommended for self-reported TMJ sounds per se, such as joint clicking or popping, in the absence of pain. Intensity of TMD-related pain seems the most reliable predictor of treatment seeking. Modal TMD patients are women in the childbearing years. The rate at which women seek treatment for TMD is four to seven times greater than that for men, although the prevalence of TMD pain in the population is only about twice as high for women (Dworkin, Huggins, et al., 1990; Von Korff et al., 1988). The condition is most prevalent in women during the reproductive years and falls off sharply with advancing middle age. All epidemiological studies of TMD report these similar patterns, and, other than age and gender, there are no known risk factors for TMD that emerge with any reliability (Dworkin, Von Korff, & LeResche, 1992).

Since behavioral, psychological, and psychosocial factors often play important roles in shaping the behavior, thinking, and emotions of all chronic pain patients, attending to these personal and interpersonal factors is indicated when diagnosing and planning treatment for TMD patients. Characteristics of TMD found in common with other chronic pain conditions include the following:

- Poor correspondence between the nature or extent of pathophysiological change and global severity of pain and suffering.
- Dysfunctional behaviors that directly affect the pain condition, such as oral parafunctional habits.
- Transient psychological distress.
- The potential for clinically meaningful depression, anxiety, and somatization.
- Interference with ability to perform usual activities at home, work, or school.
- Frequent use of the health care system, with potential for excessive treatment seeking and abuse of medications.

PSYCHOSOCIAL ASSESSMENT OF THE TMD PATIENT: BEHAVIORAL, PSYCHOLOGICAL, AND PSYCHOSOCIAL APPROACHES

Observational Methods

Reliable and valid observational methods have been developed for assessing pain-related behaviors, especially back pain. These observational measures have gained widespread acceptance and are discussed in several chapters throughout this book. At this point, however, observational methods applied to TMD have been limited to recording facial expressions of TMD-related pain (Craig, 1989; LeResche & Dworkin, 1988; Prkachin & Mercer, 1990). LeResche (LeResche, Dworkin, Wilson, & Ehrlich, 1992) has shown that persons with recent-onset TMD emit few facial expressions of pain overall but that facial expressions increase in frequency as a function of chronicity of the disorder, implying that facial expressions become increasingly important to the more chronic TMD pain patient as a means for communicating pain and suffering. However, at present, the coding and analysis of facial expression data for pain and other emotions remains a relatively specialized and labor-intensive undertaking, limiting its clinical utility.

Self-Report Methods

Typically, these self-report methods include use of interview schedules, symptom checklists, and psychological and biobehavioral rating scales and psychological tests that assess mental and emotional status, psychosocial adaptation, coping behaviors, and health care utilization. It is beyond the scope of the chapter to review the many published measures that have received at least some attention from biobehaviorally oriented TMD clinical researchers. The following self-report measures are most commonly used for biobehavioral assessment of chronic pain conditions.

Minnesota Multiphasic Personality Inventory (MMPI)

Perhaps the best known and most widely used instrument for assessing psychological status, the MMPI is not intended as a diagnostic instrument but rather to give a personality profile of psychological function. The test is long and takes highly specialized training to interpret; hence, it is not deemed suitable for use by many clinicians. The clinical value of the MMPI to many non-mental-health and biomedical clinicians remains somewhat problematic. Standardization samples used for MMPI scale construction are reported as inappropriate for chronic pain patients in several independent studies. However, the use of clustering methods to identify MMPI scale profiles that characterize pain patients, including TMD patients, has proven somewhat more useful. Generally, whether using the MMPI or the more recently revised and restandardized MMPI-2, elevations on scales 1, 2, and 3—Hypochondriasis, Depression, and Hysteria—were associated with perceptions of severe pain, affective disturbance, and maladaptive patterns of psychosocial functioning. When elevations on the Psychopathic Deviate and Schizophrenia scales were found accompanying elevations in scales 1, 2, and 3, not surprisingly, higher levels of psychopathology and resistance to modification of pain behavior were observed (Bradley, McDonald Haile, & Jaworski, 1992).

Although it was originally anticipated that distinct MMPI profiles would be confirmed for chronic pain patients, these have not emerged clearly. Nevertheless, the MMPI has been used in many studies of TMD patients, and these studies support the conclusion that clinical psychopathology is present in an appreciable number of TMD patients presenting for treatment (Deardorff, 1995). Using the MMPI in a study predicting response to treatment for TMD, McCreary and colleagues (McCreary, Clark, Oakley, & Flack, 1992) found that somatization was related to jaw function problems at long-term follow-up but not at early follow-ups. They found that "somatization was a significant predictor of outcome" for chronic TMD patients and concluded, "if treatment does not address this somatization process, there is an increased risk there will be no improvement" (1992, p. 168). The MMPI may potentially be useful to oral and maxillofacial surgeons if the patient is referred to a psychologist for administration of the test and interpretation of results.

Research Diagnostic Criteria for TMD (RDC/TMD)

Consistent with the integrative concepts imbedded in a biopsychosocial model of chronic pain (Dworkin, Von Korff, & LeResche, 1992), a coordinated system has been developed for assessing physical findings and biomedical diagnosis with behavioral, psychological, and psychosocial assessment of the current level of functioning of the TMD patient.

This classificatory system, the RDC/TMD, uses a dual axis system for diagnosing and classifying TMD patients (Dworkin & LeResche, 1992). Axis I is reserved for physical diagnoses of the most commonly occurring masticatory muscle and/or TMJ disorders. Axis II is used to assess (1) clinically relevant pain status variables; (2) jaw disability; (3) psychological distress, specifically depression, anxiety, and the presence of nonspecific physical symptoms that reflect somatization tendencies based on use of Symptom Checklist 90–Revised (SCL-90-R) subscales (Derogatis, 1983); and (4) pain severity and related psychosocial interference using a graded scale of chronic pain.

The RDC/TMD criteria for both Axes I and II, operationally defined and empirically supported and with demonstrated reliability, have been used in numerous clinical research studies to characterize TMD (Dworkin & LeResche, 1992; List & Dworkin, 1996; Ohrbach & Dworkin, 1998; Rudy, Turk, Kubinski, & Zaki, 1995). Because the RDC/TMD represents a standardized method for assessing both physical and biobehavioral aspects of TMD, it allows comparison of TMD populations across diverse clinical settings. For example, use of the standardized RDC/TMD methods detected comparable prevalence rates for the most common types of TMD at both a major U.S. clinic and a regional TMD public health clinic in Sweden: Muscle disorders and joint pain conditions predominated, whereas disk derangements with limitations in mandibular opening were rare, as were the most advanced forms of degenerative joint disease (List & Dworkin, 1996). The RDC/TMD was initially offered as a research instrument to the clinical research community for further assessment of reliability and validity of its integrated biopsychosocial components, an assessment which has only been partially achieved to date. The RDC/TMD has gained acceptance as a basic clinical instrument for the integrated assessment of TMD patients at several U.S., Canadian, and European university-based TMD and orofacial pain centers. Independently, the RDC/TMD has been recommended by at least one team of non-TMD clinical pain researchers as a model system for approaching the diagnosis and assessment of all chronic pain conditions (Garofalo & Wesley, 1997).

Symptom Checklist 90–Revised SCL-90-R

The SCL-90-R is a 90-item symptom checklist that yields several scales, of which the most relevant for us are scales that assess depression, anxiety, and somatization. The SCL-90-R is much briefer than the MMPI; however, its overall usefulness with chronic pain patients has not been unequivocally established, and some problems have emerged with its use on chronic pain populations. For example, using the entire SCL-90-R, researchers have had difficulty in replicating the original 10-factor structure obtained by Derogatis (Bradley et al., 1992). Nevertheless, the SCL-90-R has been used extensively to study all types of chronic pain populations, including persons with TMD. When comparing responses of chronic pain and psychiatric populations, the chronic pain population was distinguished, in studies by Buckelew and colleagues (1986), by reports of psychological distress limited to somatic, as opposed to emotional or cognitive, symptoms of anxiety and depression.

My colleagues and I have used several of the SCL-90-R scales in our own longitudinal research, after having developed population norms derived from our own epidemiological, or population-based, studies for the scales in the assessment instrument we used clinically and in research. The scales include those that assess anxiety, depression, and somatization (Dworkin & LeResche, 1992; Dworkin, Von Korff, & LeResche, 1990; Dworkin, Wilson, & Massoth, 1994). Both depression and somatization have been heavily implicated in chronic pain, including TMD (Dworkin, Wilson, & Massoth, 1994; Wilson, Dworkin, Whitney, & LeResche, 1994). Findings comparable to ours have been reported using the SCL-90-R in a similar fashion (List & Dworkin, 1996) to relate levels of depression and somatization to clinical findings from a TMD physical examination, as well as to examine the relationship between clinical depression and the presence of chronic pain problems. Taken together, these studies find poor relationships between physical signs or extent of physical jaw impairment in TMD patients and extent of psychological distress.

Somatization, as implied earlier, has emerged as increasingly relevant to chronic pain and is currently understood as a dimension of personal functioning characterized by the tendency to report distress arising from multiple, nonspecific physical symptoms (e.g., night sweats, tremors, heart palpitation) accompanied by increased health care visits. A spectrum of severity has been described for somatization (Katon, Lin, Von Korff, Russo, Lipscomb, & Bush, 1991). One end of the spectrum is occupied by somatoform psychiatric disorders recognized in the *Diagnostic and Statistical Manual of Mental Disorders* (DSM-IV) of the American Psychiatric Association (1994) that require the presence of as many as eight physical symptoms distributed over multiple organ systems and not explained by a diagnosable medical condition. More relevant to clinicians working with chronic pain problems is the end of the somatization spectrum represented by four or five similarly nonspecific physical symptoms that are perceived as distressful (Escobar et al., 1987; Simon, 1993). Of related interest, it is very difficult to qualify for a formal (DSM-IV) affective psychiatric disorder (such as a major depressive disorder or anxiety disorder) without identifying a number of nonspecific physical symptoms as frequently present and distressing. In addition, somatization consistently emerges as a major predictor or correlate of such pain behaviors as treatment seeking and prevalence of physical symptoms (Wilson et al., 1994).

Multidimensional Pain Inventory (MPI)

Turk and colleagues (Rudy, Turk, Zaki, & Curtin, 1989; Turk & Rudy, 1988) have developed the MPI, perhaps the most widely used self-report measure, to assess the psychosocial and cognitive responses of patients with chronic pain. Unlike the IMPATH and TMJ scales, which will be discussed later, its use is not limited to patients with TMD, and it has been extensively investigated for its psychometric properties, demonstrating acceptable levels of reliability, validity, and predictability of pain response pattern. The measure was developed with pain clinic populations and has been found to yield three distinct patient clusters that appear consistently across diverse chronic pain conditions, including back pain, headache, and TMD.

The chronic pain groups distinguished by the triaxial MPI are labeled *adaptive copers, interpersonally stressed,* and *dysfunctional,* and the three types reflect a continuum of increasing disability and pain-related psychosocial dysfunction. Rudy and Turk (Rudy et al., 1989) have demonstrated that TMD patients characterized as dysfunctional show significantly elevated depression and report significantly more physical symptoms than those TMD patients the MPI categorizes as adaptive copers. By contrast, dysfunctional TMD patients and adaptive copers were not found to differ significantly along physical parameters (e.g., proportion of positive CT scan findings, objective findings from a TMD clinical exam). More recently, Rudy and colleagues (Rudy, Turk, Kubinski, & Zaki, 1994) have used the MPI to assess the relative efficacy of a cognitive-behavioral treatment intervention compared to a physical treatment that involved use of an intra-oral occlusal splint. They presented evidence indicating that dysfunctional patients, as opposed to adaptive copers and interpersonally stressed patients, responded differentially to these treatments, supporting their conclusion that clinical treatment decisions for TMD should include not only assessment of biobehavioral status but assignment of TMD patients to treatment interventions specifically designed according to the assessed level of psychosocial function. It seems fair to say that the MPI is one of the most carefully designed and well-studied self-report measures for assessing biobehavioral and psychosocial functioning in chronic pain patients.

Graded Chronic Pain Measure (GCP)

The RDC/TMD incorporates an easy-to-use Graded Chronic Pain measure (GCP), which grades chronic pain severity from Grade 0 through Grade IV. The development of the GCP and its psychometric properties have been described in detail elsewhere (Von Korff, Ormel, Keefe, & Dworkin, 1992). Because the GCP was derived from population-based studies of chronic pain in the community and not from a pain clinic population, it can be used for data collection under a variety of research designs, ranging from random sample surveys to clinical intervention studies, and it has proven a very useful clinical measure for assessing the impact of chronic TMD on our patients.

The GCP was created not only to provide a meaningful quantitative index of the extent to which pain is perceived as mild or severe in intensity but also to capture in a single quantitative index the extent to which pain is psychosocially disabling.

The GCP measures disability by assessing both pain intensity and the extent of pain-related interference with daily activities and number of lost activity days (e.g., days unable to go to work or school or to attend to household responsibilities) attributed to TMD pain. Grade I is defined as TMD pain of low intensity, averaging less than 5.0 on a 10-point scale and associated with little pain-related interference in daily living. Grade II is defined as high-intensity pain, above 5.0 on a 10-point scale, with moderate amounts of pain-related interference. Grades III and IV are associated with increasing levels of pain-related psychosocial disability regardless of pain level. Data are provided in Table 14.1 to show the relationship between the I–IV GCP and selected biobehavioral variables. For clinical purposes, functional TMD patients, that is, individuals not significantly disabled by their

TABLE 14.1. TMD Graded Chronic Pain Scale

Grade	TMD pain					Headache					Back pain				
	I	II	III	IV	Total	I	II	III	IV	Total	I	II	III	IV	Total
Graded pain variables															
Average pain intensity	3.4	5.9	5.8	7.4	5.0	4.3	6.3	7.1	7.5	6.0	3.1	5.5	5.4	6.0	4.7
Disability days	0.8	1.7	31.3	114.4	10.4	1.8	2.9	13.9	55.7	10.1	2.9	3.3	23.3	76.8	19.8
Percent high intensity	0.0	100.0	90.2	95.2	58.1	0.0	100.0	91.0	96.1	68.1	0.0	100.0	71.7	89.7	57.6
Selected variables															
Percent 90+ pain days	36.0	59.8	65.0	76.2	51.7	16.9	30.1	20.9	40.8	25.4	24.8	51.9	31.3	58.6	39.4
Number of days in pain	68.3	104.2	104.4	132.9	91.7	38.1	63.4	45.7	88.8	55.2	52.9	93.9	70.9	111.1	78.5
Number of years since onset	5.6	6.2	5.4	7.6	6.0	17.1	18.0	16.9	17.4	17.5	11.8	14.0	12.5	10.1	12.3
Percent elevated depression	16.4	29.4	29.3	57.1	25.6	13.5	30.7	35.9	48.1	28.4	12.1	20.3	24.5	41.7	22.0
Percent, health rated fair-poor	6.9	12.9	14.6	55.0	12.8	6.6	12.3	21.2	24.7	13.7	4.1	9.1	11.8	20.6	9.9
Percent, frequent opioid use	0.0	3.5	4.9	19.1	3.1	0.0	2.6	1.9	9.1	2.3	0.5	4.2	5.1	15.8	5.1
Percent, frequent pain visits	1.3	7.7	22.5	23.8	7.5	1.8	4.6	19.5	29.3	9.2	1.2	5.2	8.0	27.5	8.1
Percent, high pain impact	5.1	25.4	63.4	71.4	23.8	14.7	33.1	50.7	75.0	35.4	10.4	25.5	48.5	72.1	32.8
Percent, unemployed	3.9	7.3	12.5	28.6	7.4	1.7	2.4	8.3	21.8	5.2	1.4	0.8	6.3	26.6	6.1

Note. Relationship of chronic pain grade to biobehavioral variables: mean values for graded pain variables and distributions for selected pain, psychological, and behavioral variables by chronic pain grade (I–IV) and total sample for TMD, headache, and back pain.

TMD condition, are defined as Grades I and II. By contrast, we define dysfunctional chronic pain as Grades III and IV on the GCP.

It is important to point out that these demarcations of functional and dysfunctional grades of chronic pain, although having empirical support (Von Korff et al., 1992), have nevertheless not been subject to cross-validation of their clinical utility. Such studies, however, are now under way, involving randomized clinical trials of TMD treatments based on level of psychosocial functioning as determined by the GCP measure. Similarly, it is important to note that despite widespread agreement regarding its public health, research, and treatment implications, the concept of dysfunctional chronic pain has only minimally been extended to TMD research and clinical application.

In addition to the measures already discussed for assessing psychological and psychosocial status of TMD patients, several other measures, some of them well known and discussed more extensively elsewhere in this book, have also been applied to the assessment of TMD in research and clinical settings.

Illness Behavior and Sickness Impact Measures

The Illness Behavior Questionnaire (IBQ; Pilowsky, 1986) and the Sickness Impact Profile (SIP; Bergner, Bobbitt, Carter, & Gilson, 1981) have been used to assess the psychological and biobehavioral impact of illness and illness beliefs. These measures have provided useful information about biobehavioral adaptation to chronic pain, including disability associated with chronic pain conditions, notably back pain, and differences in beliefs and expectations between pain clinic populations and chronic pain patients seeking treatment elsewhere. Although results obtained with these measures have appeared in the TMD literature, again supporting the conclusion that for a significant minority of clinic cases TMD has an appreciable impact on personal functioning, neither the IBQ nor the SIP is in common use by TMD clinicians or researchers.

Pain Coping Measures

Two approaches to assessing how patients cope with chronic pain have received attention. A well-known measure of pain coping, developed by Keefe and colleagues (Keefe & Gil, 1986) and widely used, indicates that passive coping strategies, particularly catastrophizing and praying, seem to be common among those who respond less well biobehaviorally and emotionally to their chronic pain problem. Supporting data come from use of a measure developed by Brown and Nicassio (1987), which indicates that those who use active versus passive pain coping styles and those who perceive themselves as having some control over their pain condition remain better able to minimize its personal and psychological negative impact.

Numerous additional measures exist that assess diverse dimensions of the chronic pain experience. Some of the more interesting-appearing ones that seem to warrant attention from biobehavioral TMD researchers include: the Ways of Coping Checklist (Lazarus, 1986), which measures strategies for coping with stress not specific to chronic pain; measures of daily stress used by Dohrenwend, Marbach, and their colleagues (Lennon, Dohrenwend, Zautra, & Marbach, 1990) to study psychosocial adaptation of TMD patients; and the Millon Biobehavioral Health Inventory, the Chronic Illness Problem Inventory, the Psychosocial Pain Inventory, and the Pain Beliefs Questionnaire (Bradley et al., 1992; Gatchel & Baum, 1983). Reports using these measures, taken together, also confirm the extent to which TMD can be psychosocially disabling for an appreciable segment of TMD sufferers.

Finally, two measures specific to TMD are available to provide TMD clinicians with global assessments of the TMD patient.

TMJ Scale

The TMJ Scale (Levitt, 1990; Levitt, 1991; Levitt, Lundeen, & McKinney, 1988; Levitt, Lundeen, & McKinney, 1994) has been developed as a self-report measure for use in the home or office and assesses three domains: physical, psychosocial, and global. The physical domain includes assessment of pain, whereas the psychosocial domain assesses psychological factors and stress. The scale, which the developers report has been used quite extensively, requires scoring and interpretation by its developers. It yields information that may be useful to guide clinicians treating TMD, although some questions of its validity as a psychological assessment tool have been noted by Rugh (Rugh, Woods, & Dahlstrom, 1993) and by Deardorff (1995), as well as by others (Glaros & Glass, 1993). Findings from the TMJ Scale indicate that women with TMD report a higher level of severity of all physical and psychological symptoms than men, and a relationship between severity of psychological problems and chronicity of TMD is noted. It is important to note, as the authors readily acknowledge, that the TMJ Scale has not been the subject of longitudinal studies—that is, cohorts of patients have not been repeatedly assessed with the TMJ Scale over time—but substantial data are available as cross-sectional data collected over a number of years.

IMPATH Scale

The IMPATH Scale for TMD (Fricton & Schiffman, 1987) is an interactive computer-based assessment instrument developed at the University of Minnesota by Fricton and colleagues for use as a screening and personal history instrument. In contrast to the TMJ Scale, IMPATH does include a carefully constructed component allowing it to be used to derive physical diagnoses of TMD subtypes. It has the advantage of instantaneous feedback, but, unfortunately, the psychometric characteristics of its illness-behavior components have not yet been well established. It is mentioned here because, like the TMJ Scale, it may serve as a useful guide to clinicians wishing to obtain a clinical impression of how their patients are doing psychologically and biobehaviorally.

PSYCHOSOCIAL APPROACHES TO THE MANAGEMENT OF THE TMD PATIENT

The treatment of all chronic pain conditions, including TMD, emphasizes a rehabilitation approach to treatment rather than a cure model (Fordyce, 1990). Consistent with such an approach, reliance is placed on the patient's acquiring a useful set of self-management strategies that facilitate more adaptive pain coping behaviors, emotional responses, and thought patterns.

With a view to guiding more rational management decisions concerning behavioral, psychological, and psychosocial factors that may influence the clinical course of TMD, attention to four domains of biobehavioral assessment is recommended (LeResche et al., 1997). From a practical treatment perspective, it should be noted that the assessment of these biobehavioral domains is possible largely through routine history and examination methods and requires no special measuring instruments or questionnaires; where specialized measures may be useful, they are indicated.

Patient's Self-Assessment

Included here is the recording of *pain complaint* (with special attention to consistency of the subjective report with relevant anatomy and physiology); *treatment history* (with attention to the record of prior successful and unsuccessful treatments and/or experiences with health professionals); and the patient's *explanatory model* for his or her condition—the patient's perceived etiology, maintenance, and exacerbation of the condition (with attention to physical versus behavioral factors, such as stress). Patients with a rigidly held physical, or biomedical, model of their condition will be more resistant to consideration of behavioral change strategies that may help them cope more adequately with their chronic pain problem (Massoth et al., 1994).

Jaw Disability and Oral Parafunction

Included here is assessment of *oral parafunction* habits such as nocturnal and diurnal bruxism (tooth grinding) and jaw clenching. The major theories of TMD etiology include the possibility that such parafunctional oral behaviors may be stress-related and represent opportunities for masticatory muscle physical abuse and physiological impairment—the latter primarily manifested as prolonged and painful inflammatory reactions in response to muscle overuse (Fricton, Kroening, & Hathaway, 1987; Ohrbach & McCall, 1996). There is, in fact, little evidence for peripheral inflammation in the masticatory muscle (Lund, Dong, Widmer, & Stohler, 1991), but it is also widely accepted that tooth grinding and clenching represent a contributing factor to TMD-related pain for many patients. Because its principal treatment is, in effect, to change behavior, it is reasonable to include its assessment as part of the full psychosocial assessment of the TMD patient. Again, it seems fair to say that more attention has been directed by dentists and psychologists and other mental health workers to modifying maladaptive parafunctional oral behaviors than to any other clinical segment of the TMD condition.

Psychological Status

Included here is assessment of *depression, anxiety,* and *somatization*. Formal assessment of psychological status requires specialized measurement instruments and/or diagnostic interview schedules.

However, the inclusion of relatively straightforward measures in a clinical data base, such as the SCL-90-R, used routinely with all patients, minimizes resistance to the perception that attention is being unduly given to psychological factors when the patient feels a physical pain problem is being presented. Such measures are more appropriate as screening aids and allow clinical impressions to be formed concerning the need for more specialized psychological assessment, generally achieved through referral to a psychiatrist or clinical psychologist. Depression commonly co-occurs with chronic pain conditions and has been documented as present in TMD clinic populations. Similarly, somatization is present in a significant minority of TMD patients, and there is ample evidence that even moderately elevated levels of long-standing somatization represent an important obstacle to successful treatment outcome.

Psychosocial Status

Included here is assessment of current level of psychosocial functioning, generally reflected for chronic pain patients in extent of interference with activities of daily living attributed to TMD and extent of health care utilization. Prognosis is more guarded when self-reported activity limitations due to TMD are high and when pain interferes appreciably with ability to discharge responsibilities at home, school, or work and/or limits socializing activities. The assessment of both psychological status and level of psychosocial functioning is viewed as essential to allowing rational clinical decisions concerning management of TMD. Most useful for assessing level of psychosocial functioning are the MPI and the GCP contained in the RDC/TMD.

Biobehavioral Management

General agreement has emerged that cognitive-behavioral, behavioral, and educational modalities—here collectively labeled "biobehavioral" for convenience—are useful and effective in the management of chronic pain conditions (Keefe, Dunsmore, & Burnett, 1992), although gains achieved are often modest and factors contributing to the efficacy of such modalities remain to be more precisely defined. The efficacy of psychodynamic and psychoanalytic treatment approaches for management of chronic pain has not yet been scientifically validated. In any event, at present, biobehavioral treatment modalities constitute a component of virtually every reported chronic pain treatment program, as numerous chapters in this text readily attest. Although biobehavioral management methods for chronic pain have the virtual status of a standard of care for all the well-known chronic pain conditions, their incorporation into care for TMD patients is not yet as systematic.

With regard to these modalities as applied to TMD management, although the use of educational approaches to modifying TMD-related pain and dysfunction has not been extensively studied, there is evidence from a randomized clinical trial (Dworkin, Turner, et al., 1994) that a single psychoeducational group session early in treatment for TMD resulted in reduced TMD pain-related interference with psychosocial function compared to usual treatment and that the benefits gained continued to be present at 1-year follow-up. Educational methods have been demonstrated efficacious in the self-management of headache and back pain, using both group and individual approaches to deliver the educational interventions (Blanchard et al., 1985; Turner, LeResche, Von Korff, & Ehrlich, 1998).

By and large, when biobehavioral treatments are employed in the management of TMD, effects are positive and in the hypothesized beneficial direction, though often effects are moderate in size. However, these biobehavioral methods, especially those subsumed under the label "cognitive-behavioral," appear to have the potential for producing long-lasting benefits when compared to usual clinical treatment for TMD. Increasingly, as noted, conservative, noninvasive approaches to TMD management are being advocated as the preferred overall treatment approach for this hard-to-understand chronic pain problem. These so-called conservative treatments generally incorporate many of the same elements (e.g., relaxation, stress education, habit behavior modification) found in cognitive-behavioral and behavioral therapies for TMD. Thus both the usual clinical treatment for TMD and biobehavioral treatment employ multimodal approaches, and it does not yet appear possible to determine which of the multiple therapeutic components are most efficacious. If one method had to be singled out, relaxation seems to emerge consistently as an effective method for chronic pain management across a wide variety of pain conditions and over a wide variety of clinical settings (Dworkin, 1997). In any event, although the combined biobehavioral methods commonly used in clinical practice have as yet failed to establish one modality as superior to another, it is important to note that much the same situation obtains with regard to biomedical-based TMD treatments. Little is known about the superiority of any one of the multiple methods commonly employed to manage TMD biomedically—there is no strong scientific evidence to substantiate invasive versus noninvasive treatments or pharmacological treatments emphasizing analgesics versus those stressing antidepressants or muscle relaxants. It is the absence of compelling evidence to the contrary that has led many clinical researchers to advocate conservative, reversible therapies for the largest majority of TMD patients.

For most patients, the TMD experience is associated with fluctuations in symptoms. Recurrences of pain are fairly common, and exacerbations or "flare-ups" tend to be responded to with increasingly extensive and/or invasive and/or irreversible treatments, although there is no scientific evidence to warrant changes away from conservative and reversible management methods in the largest majority of cases. The eventual course of TMD pain seems to be remission without recurrence, as is evident from the extremely small number of TMD pain cases among those over 55 years old that can be identified in population-based studies.

The most common conservative forms of biomedical treatments for TMD are briefly presented here because, in almost all instances, it is self-evident that these treatments incorporate self-management behavioral components such as patient education, treatment compliance, relapse prevention, and maintenance of successful treatment outcomes. For the largest number of TMD cases, it is advocated that both the biomedical and biobehavioral aspects of treatment be integrated and delivered by dentists who are sensitive and knowledgeable as to the psychosocial implications of viewing TMD as a chronic pain condition. A brief cognitive-behavioral intervention study that incorporates a biopsychosocial model (Dworkin, Turner et al., 1994) and addresses aspects of TMD assessed by the RDC/TMD and that also incorporates integrated participation by dentist- and psychologist-clinicians confirmed the usefulness of the conceptual model system as a mechanism for guiding integrated treatment approaches. In any case, there is now appreciable evidence to confirm that issues of psychological distress and psychosocial disruption of activities at home, work, or school need to be addressed with the TMD patient to maximize likelihood of a positive outcome.

Initial biomedical management typically includes careful instructions for elimination of habitual jaw activities, including clenching, jaw posturing, bruxism, fingernail biting, and jaw tensing, which occurs when the teeth are held together even without actual clenching. TMD resulting from trauma or other events can be sustained through dysfunctional jaw function patterns. Stress often increases existing patterns of jaw parafunction; therefore, attention to physical reactions to stressors is essential. Application of ice or heat packs to tender muscles is very effective symptomatic therapy and often provides transient relief of pain. Passive jaw-opening exercises (once it is clear that a disc displacement without reduction is not present) are also of benefit and have been found to improve pain-free mandibular opening. Usually, the only opening exercise needed is passive vertical opening, and lateral or protrusive exercises are unnecessary. Professional physical therapy is not usually necessary in the treatment of TMD except after surgical treatment of the joint, and most patients can provide the needed physical therapy themselves at home (Dworkin & Truelove, 1997; Dworkin, Truelove, Bonica, & Sola, 1990). In the early stages, medications can be of value, but use of narcotic analgesics should be limited to 1 or 2 weeks except in cases of clear physical damage to the joint or capsule. Often nonsteroidal anti-inflammatory drugs (NSAIDs) are as effective as codeine while providing the added benefit of reducing joint inflammation if the joint is tender. Controversy exists as to the value of muscle relaxants in TMD, and care is needed in prescribing muscle relaxants for other than the acute phase of TMD since some potential for dependency exists. Use of muscle relaxants for periods greater than 3 to 4 weeks is not generally advised. When TMD is accompanied by significant anxiety or situational stress, transient use of an anxiolytic agent such as diazepam or similar agents can be of significant value. Long-term use is not advised for most patients unless the medication is being used to treat the anxiety state rather than the pain. Antidepressants have been used increasingly to provide relief in chronic TMD. They improve sleep, which is frequently disturbed in chronic TMD, and may offer analgesic effects.

A widespread common treatment for TMD involves the construction of jaw habit appliances, used in perhaps 40% of TMD cases. For most cases of TMD, a simple flat-plane night guard made of acrylic and designed to not reposition the jaw is reported as useful in assisting the patient to control jaw parafunction during times when conscious control is difficult (sleep, driving, concentration). Although this intraoral appliance is used quite extensively, its mechanism of action is far from clear. Several studies have shown it to have significant placebo (Greene, Olson, & Laskin, 1982) or otherwise nonspecific effects. In one well-done clinical trial, such an appliance was equally effective for pain relief when worn only during dental visits as when worn many hours of the day and night (Dao, Lavigne, Charbonneau, Feine, & Lund, 1994); in a second clinical trial, preliminary data comparing an inexpensive athletic mouth guard that could be fabricated by the patient to the conventional, and much more expensive, dentist-fabricated appliance could find no differences in pain reduction or any measure of jaw function (Huggins et al., 1998; Truelove et al., 1998).

A great deal more research is needed before it is possible to adequately evaluate how biobehavioral interventions achieve their desired effects and which components of the multimodal approaches now in common use are most potent. Perhaps of greatest interest is the need to develop treatment approaches tailored to both the physical and the behavioral status of the patient. There is little indication, either from the scientific clinical research literature or even from conventional clinical wisdom, that psychosocial considerations are addressed in any systematic fashion by most clinicians managing the condition. Typically, treatment of TMD currently seems driven largely by the physical diagnosis alone, without addressing the personal or psychosocial impact of TMD pain or the patterns of coping with TMD used by TMD patients. Although TMD is regarded by many as a condition in which psychosocial factors influence the course of the condition, in fact, little attention has been paid to assessing how psychological or psychosocial factors influence treatment outcome and whether successful clinical outcome is associated with improved psychosocial functioning. It seems fair to say that outcome assessment for TMD, except for self-report of pain, is focused almost exclusively on assessment of physical factors (range of jaw motion, joint sounds, etc.).

Most recently, biobehavioral treatment approaches have been advocated that differ according to the differing levels of psychosocial functioning and/or level of cognitive or emotional disturbance exhibited by specific TMD patients or by groups of TMD patients. Such approaches give at least equal emphasis to biobehavioral assessment (e.g., RDC/TMD Axis II components) as to biomedical assessment (e.g., RDC/TMD Axis I components) for deriving treatment modalities tailored not only to the individual patient's biomedical status but also to the patient's biobehavioral status. The available data from at least one well-done clinical trial (Rudy et al., 1995) confirm the utility of tailoring TMD treatments to the level of TMD-related psychosocial impairment, and this

approach to TMD management seems most promising. Future clinical research will determine whether such an approach is indeed effective in the management of TMD, in which chronic pain plays such a dominant role.

SUMMARY AND CONCLUSIONS

TMD is treated for the most part by either general practicing dentists or dental specialists—principally oral surgeons, prosthodontists, and orthodontists—as well as by an increasing number of dentists whose specialized practice is limited to the diagnosis and management of TMD. In all fairness, it must be acknowledged that not all segments of the practicing dental community endorse a biopsychosocial model for TMD. A significant (and often vocal) minority view the condition as arising from and being maintained by pathobiological processes affecting the TMJ and/or abnormal patterns of dental occlusion that influence how the teeth come together during eating, swallowing, and so forth, resulting in unhealthy patterns of masticatory function that yield pain. Advocates of this more biomedical model would probably view as revolutionary (read, radical) the adoption of a biopsychosocial explanatory model for TMD, since they minimize the necessity, indeed even the possibility, of assessing psychosocial aspects of the TMD patient's overall functioning. These latter remarks are intended to reflect the fact that the clinical arena of TMD remains a controversial one—including an unnecessary controversy over the legitimacy of psychosocial perspectives—so that workers from other health care disciplines, notably medicine, psychology, and social work, who are often involved in the diagnosis and assessment of TMD patients may be aware of the existence of such a controversy. However, it seems equally fair to say that the largest number of dentists seem to recognize and, in many cases, eagerly adopt the concepts and methods of the prevalent biopsychosocial model. Thus, although it may have revolutionary implications to those who continue to hold older, outmoded, and often scientifically unfounded views, the biopsychosocial perspective on pain has evolved as the dominant evidence-based model in health care for the assessment and management of all health conditions, including those in which pain is an imortant clinical feature. Hence this perspective serves as the unifying basis for this book, as well as the organizing concept for this chapter on TMD.

TMD is best understood as a recurrent, chronic musculoskeletal pain condition that is self-limiting and, from the available scientific data, seems only rarely associated with significant physical disease progression. Simultaneously, it has been repeatedly demonstrated that a significant minority of chronic TMD sufferers exhibit significant psychological disturbance, most frequently apparent as manifestation of depression and somatization, as well as a tendency to hold a heavily biomedical explanatory model for their condition. These findings in the psychosocial domain seem to be relatively independent of physical findings derived from clinical examination. Reversible and "conservative" (i.e., noninvasive) treatment approaches are almost universally recommended and are virtually the only treatments considered appropriate in early stages of the problem (Dworkin, 1997). The most common treatments available for TMD using largely reversible treatment approaches per force rely heavily on patient education and self-management methods—that is, methods that seek to change health behaviors and beliefs. Because it is now well accepted that TMD involves both physical disease and subjective illness processes, it is increasingly accepted that integrated biomedical and biobehavioral approaches to the entire spectrum of diagnosis, assessment, and management of TMD are required.

REFERENCES

American Dental Association. (1983). *The president's conference on the examination, diagnosis and management of temporomandibular disorders.* Chicago: Author.

American Psychiatric Association. (1994). *Diagnostic and statistical manual of mental disorders* (4th ed.). Washington, DC: Author.

Bergner, M., Bobbitt, R. A., Carter, W. B., & Gilson, B. S. (1981). The Sickness Impact Profile: Development and final revision of a health status model. *Medical Care, 19,* 787–805.

Blanchard, E. B., Andrasik, F., Appelbaum, K. A., Evans, D. D., Jurish, S. E., Teders, S. J., Rodichok, L. D., & Barron, K. D. (1985). The efficacy and cost-effectiveness of minimal-therapist-contact non-drug treatments of chronic migraine and tension headache. *Headache, 25*(4), 214–220.

Bradley, L. A., McDonald Haile, J., & Jaworski, T. M. (1992). Assessment of psychological status using interviews and self-report instruments. In D. C. Turk & R. Melzack (Eds.), *Handbook of pain assessment* (pp. 193–213). New York: Guilford Press.

Brown, G. K., & Nicassio, P. M. (1987). Development of a questionnaire for the assessment of active and passive coping strategies in chronic pain patients. *Pain, 31,* 53–64.

Buckelew, S. P., DeGood, D. E., Schwartz, D. P., & Kerler, R. M. (1986). Cognitive and somatic item response pattern of pain patients, psychiatric patients, and hospital employees. *Journal of Clinical Psychology, 42,* 852–860.

Carlsson, G. E., & LeResche, L. (1995). Epidemiology of temporomandibular disorders. In B. J. Sessle, P. S. Bryant, & R. A. Dionne (Eds.), *Progress in pain research and management* (pp. 211–226). Seattle, WA: IASP Press.

Craig, K. D. (1989). Emotional aspects of pain. In P. D. Wall & R. Melzack (Eds.), *Textbook of pain* (pp. 220–230). Edinburgh: Churchill Livingstone.

Dao, T. T. T., Lavigne, G. J., Charbonneau, A., Feine, J. S., & Lund, J. P. (1994). The efficacy of oral splints in the treatment of myofascial pain of the jaw muscles: A controlled clinical study. *Pain, 56,* 85–94.

Deardorff, W. H. (1995). TMJ scale. In J. C. Conoley & J. C. Impara (Eds.), *The twelfth mental measurements yearbook* (pp. 1070–1071). Lincoln: University of Nebraska, Buros Institute of Mental Measurements.

Derogatis, L. R. (1983). *SCL-90-R: Administration, Scoring and Procedures Manual–II for the Revised Version.* Towson, MD: Clinical Psychometric Research.

Dworkin, S. F. (1997). Behavioral and educational modalities. *Oral Surgery, Oral Medicine, Oral Pathology, Oral Radiology and Endodontics, 83*(1), 128–133.

Dworkin, S. F., Huggins, K. H., LeResche, L., Von Korff, M., Howard, J., Truelove, E., & Sommers, E. (1990). Epidemiology of signs and symptoms in temporomandibular disorders: Clinical signs in cases and controls. *Journal of the American Dental Association, 120,* 273– 281.

Dworkin, S. F., & LeResche, L. (1992). Research Diagnostic Criteria for Temporomandibular Disorders: Review, criteria, examinations and specifications, critique. *Journal of Craniomandibular Disorders: Facial and Oral Pain, 6*(4), 301–355.

Dworkin, S. F., & Truelove, E. L. (1997). Temporomandibular disorders. In R. E. Rakel (Ed.), *Conn's current therapy.* New York: Saunders.

Dworkin, S. F., Truelove, E. L., Bonica, J. J., & Sola, A. (1990). Facial and head pain caused by myofascial and temporomandibular disorders. In J. J. Bonica (Ed.), *The management of pain* (pp. 727–745). Philadelphia: Lea & Febiger.

Dworkin, S. F., Turner, J. A., Wilson, L., Massoth, D., Whitney, C., Huggins, K. H., Burgess, J., Sommers, E., & Truelove, E. (1994). Brief group cognitive-behavioral intervention for temporomandibular disorders. *Pain, 59,* 175–187.

Dworkin, S. F., Von Korff, M., & LeResche, L. (1992). Epidemiologic studies of chronic pain: A dynamic-ecologic perspective. *Annals of Behavioral Medicine, 14,* 3–11.

Dworkin, S. F., Von Korff, M. R., & LeResche, L. (1990). Multiple pains and psychiatric disturbance: An epidemiologic investigation. *Archives of General Psychiatry, 47,* 239–244.

Dworkin, S. F., Wilson, L., & Massoth, D. L. (1994). Somatizing as a risk factor for chronic pain. In R. C. Grzesiak & D. S. Ciccone (Eds.), *Psychologic vulnerability to chronic pain* (pp. 28–54). New York: Springer.

Escobar, J. I., Jacqueline, M. G., Hough, R. L., Karno, M., Burnam, M. A., & Wells, K. B. (1987). Somatization in the community: Relationship to disability and use of services. *American Journal of Public Health, 77*(7), 837–840.

Fordyce, W. E. (1990). Contingency management. In J. J. Bonica, C. R. Chapman, W. E. Fordyce, & J. D. Loeser (Eds.), *The management of pain in clinical practice* (pp. 1702–1710). Philadelphia: Lea & Febiger.

Fricton, J. R., Kroening, R. J., & Hathaway, K. M. (1987). *TMJ and craniofacial pain: Diagnosis and management.* St. Louis, MO: Ishiyaku EuroAmerica.

Fricton, J. R., & Schiffman, E. L. (1987). The craniomandibular index: Validity. *Journal of Prosthetic Dentistry, 58*(2), 222–228.

Garofalo, J. P., & Wesley, A. L. (1997, May/June). Research Diagnostic Criteria for Temporomandibular Disorders: Reflection of the physical–psychological interface. *American Pain Society Bulletin, 7,* 4–16.

Gatchel, R. J., & Baum, A. (1983). Pain and pain management techniques. In *An introduction to health psychology* (pp. 259–277). New York: Random House.

Glaros, A. G., & Glass, E. G. (1993). Temporomandibular disorders. In R. J. Gatchel & E. B. Blanchard (Eds.), *Psychophysiological disorders* (pp. 299–356). Washington DC: American Psychological Association.

Greene, C. S., Olson, R. E., & Laskin, D. M. (1982). Psychological factors in the etiology, progression, and treatment of MPD syndrome. *Journal of the American Dental Association, 105,* 443–448.

Huggins, K. H., Truelove, E. L., Dworkin, S. F., Mancl, L., Sommers, E., & LeResche, L. (1998). Initial outcomes in RCT of splint for TMD: Clinical findings [Abstract]. *Journal of Dental Research, 77,* 112.

Katon, W., Lin, E., Von Korff, M., Russo, J., Lipscomb, P., & Bush, T. (1991). Somatization: A spectrum of severity. *American Journal of Psychiatry, 148,* 34–40.

Keefe, F. J., Dunsmore, J., & Burnett, R. (1992). Behavioral and cognitive-behavioral approaches to chronic pain: Recent advances and future directions. *Journal of Consulting and Clinical Psychology, 60*(4), 528–536.

Keefe, F. J., & Gil, K. M. (1986). Behavioral concepts in the analysis of chronic pain syndromes. *Journal of Consulting and Clinical Psychology, 54,* 776–783.

Lazarus, R. S. (1986). Coping strategies. In S. McHugh & T. M. Vallis (Eds.), *Illness behavior: A multidisciplinary model* (pp. 303–308). New York: Plenum Press.

Lennon, M. C., Dohrenwend, B. P., Zautra, A. J., & Marbach, J. J. (1990). Coping and adaption to facial pain in contrast to other stressful life events. *Journal of Personality and Social Psychology, 59*(5), 1040–1050.

LeResche, L., & Dworkin, S. F. (1988). Facial expressions of pain and emotions in chronic TMD patients. *Pain, 35,* 71–78.

LeResche, L., Dworkin, S. F., Massoth, D., Wilson, L., Truelove, E., Burgess, J., & Sommers, E. (1997). *Comprehensive assessment and management of temporomandibular disorders: Dentist's handbook* (rev. ed.). Unpublished manual.

LeResche, L., Dworkin, S. F., Wilson, L., & Ehrlich, K. J. (1992). Effect of temporomandibular disorder pain duration on facial expressions and verbal report of pain. *Pain, 51,* 289–295.

Levitt, S. R. (1990). Predictive value of the TMJ Scale in detecting clinically significant symptoms of temporomandibular disorders. *Journal of Craniomandibular Disorders: Facial and Oral Pain, 4,* 177–185.

Levitt, S. R. (1991). Predictive value: A model for dentists to evaluate the accuracy of diagnostic tests for temporo-

mandibular disorders as applied to the TMJ scale. *Journal of Prosthetic Dentistry, 66,* 385–390.

Levitt, S. R., Lundeen, T. F., & McKinney, M. W. (1988). Initial studies of a new assessment method for temporomandibular joint disorders. *Journal of Prosthetic Dentistry, 59*(4), 490–495.

Levitt, S. R., Lundeen, T. F., & McKinney, M. W. (1994). *The TMJ Scale Manual.* Durham, NC: Pain Resource Center.

List, T., & Dworkin, S. F. (1996). Comparing TMD diagnoses and clinical findings at Swedish and U.S. TMD centers using research diagnostic criteria for temporomandibular disorders. *Journal of Orofacial Pain, 10*(3), 240–253.

Locker, D., & Slade, G. (1989). Association of symptoms and signs of TM disorders in an adult population. *Community Dentistry and Oral Epidemiology, 17,* 150–153.

Lund, J. P., Dong, R., Widmer, C. G., & Stohler, C. S. (1991). The pain-adaption model: A discussion of the relationship between chronic pain and musculoskeletal pain and motor activity. *Canadian Journal of Physiology and Pharmacology, 69,* 683–693.

Massoth, D. L., Dworkin, S. F., Whitney, C. W., Harrison, R. G., Wilson, L., & Turner, J. (1994). Patient explanatory models for temporomandibular disorders. In G. F. Gebhart, D. L. Hammond, & T. S. Jensen (Eds.), *Proceedings of the 7th World Congress on Pain* (pp. 187–200). Seattle: IASP Press.

McCreary, C. P., Clark, G. T., Oakley, M. E., & Flack, V. (1992). Predicting response to treatment for temporomandibular disorders. *Journal of Craniomandibular Disorders: Facial and Oral Pain, 6*(3), 161–169.

Ohrbach, R., & Dworkin, S. F. (1998). Five-year outcomes in TMD: Relationship of changes in pain to changes in physical and psychological variables. *Pain, 74,* 315–326.

Ohrbach, R., & McCall, W. D., Jr. (1996). The stress-hyperactivity-pain theory of myogenic pain: Proposal for a revised theory. *Pain Forum, 5*(1), 51–66.

Pilowsky, I. (1986). Abnormal illness behaviour: A review of the concept and its implications. In S. McHugh & T. M. Vallis (Eds.), *Illness behavior: A multidisciplinary model* (pp. 391–396). New York: Plenum Press.

Prkachin, K., & Mercer, S. R. (1990). Pain expression in patients with shoulder pathology: Validity, properties and relationship to sickness impact. *Pain, 39,* 257–265.

Rudy, T., Turk, D., Kubinski, J., & Zaki, H. (1994). Efficacy of tailoring treatment for dysfunctional TMD patients [Abstract]. *Journal of Dental Research, 73,* 439.

Rudy, T. E., Turk, D. C., Kubinski, J. A., & Zaki, H. S. (1995). Differential treatment responses of TMD patients as a function of psychological characteristics. *Pain, 61*(1), 103–112.

Rudy, T. E., Turk, D. C., Zaki, H. S., & Curtin, H. D. (1989). An empirical taxometric alternative to traditional classification of temporomandibular disorders. *Pain, 36,* 311–320.

Rugh, J. D., Woods, B. J., & Dahlstrom, L. (1993). Temporomandibular disorders: Assessment of psychosocial factors. *Advances in Dental Research, 7,* 127–136.

Simon, G. E. (1993). Somatization and psychiatric disorders. In L. J. Kirmayer & J. M. Robbins (Eds.), *Progress in psychiatry: Vol. 31. Current concepts of somatization: Research and clinical perspectives* (pp. 37–61). Washington DC: American Psychiatric Press.

Truelove, E. L., Huggins, K. H., Dworkin, S. F., Mancl, L., Sommers, E., & LeResche, L. (1998). RCT splint treatment outcomes in TMD: Initial self-report findings [Abstract]. *Journal of Dental Research, 77,* 112.

Turk, D. C., & Rudy, T. E. (1988). Toward an empirically derived taxonomy of chronic pain patients: Integration of psychological assessment data. *Journal of Consulting and Clinical Psychology, 56*(2), 233–238.

Turner, J. A., LeResche, L., Von Korff, M., & Ehrlich, K. (1998). Back pain in primary care: Patient characteristics, content of initial visit, and short-term outcomes. *Spine, 23,* 463–469.

Von Korff, M., Dworkin, S. F., LeResche, L., & Kruger, A. (1988). An epidemiologic comparison of pain complaints. *Pain, 32,* 173–183.

Von Korff, M., Ormel, J., Keefe, F. J., & Dworkin, S. F. (1992). Grading the severity of chronic pain. *Pain, 50,* 133–149.

Wilson, L., Dworkin, S. F., Whitney, C., & LeResche, L. (1994). Somatization and pain dispersion in chronic temporomandibular pain. *Pain, 57,* 55–61.

Chapter 15

Fibromyalgia: Search for Mechanisms and Effective Treatments

AKIKO OKIFUJI
DENNIS C. TURK

Fibromyalgia syndrome (FMS) is a chronic musculoskeletal pain disorder, often classified as a nonarticular rheumatologic condition. The cardinal features of FMS consist of generalized pain and hypersensitivity to palpation at specific body locations ("tender points" [TPs]; see Table 15.1 and Figure 15.1). In addition, patients with FMS typically report a range of functional limitations and psychological dysfunction, including chronic fatigue, sleep disturbance, feelings of stiffness, headaches, irritable bowel disorders, depression, and anxiety (Baumstark & Buckelew, 1992). The natural course of FMS symptoms seems to be chronic; however, FMS is neither progressive nor lethal. Radiographic and laboratory findings tend to be negative. Despite the absence of any definitive neurophysiological pathology, FMS patients report substantially compromised quality of life compared to patients with other rheumatologic and chronic diseases (Burckhardt, Clark, & Bennett, 1993).

In this chapter, we will review the classification of FMS and describe the etiological mechanisms and models that have been proposed to explain the syndrome. Based on the review, we will propose a dynamic process model that integrates predispositional neuroendocrine and psychosocial factors and physical and psychological precipitants ("stressors"). Thus our proposed model is a diathesis (biological and psychosocial)–stress model.

Following presentation of the dynamic process model, we will review and evaluate the efficacy of the various treatments (i.e., pharmacological, physical, psychological, and multicomponent) that have been used to treat FMS. We will enumerate some of the problems inherent in the treatment outcome research. Finally, we will emphasize variability of patients diagnosed with FMS and suggest that matching treatments to patient characteristics may be the most appropriate way to proceed.

CLASSIFICATION OF FIBROMYALGIA SYNDROME

Due to the absence of definitive neurophysiological markers in FMS, classification has relied on physical signs and patients' reports of symptoms. Historically, various diagnostic criteria have been used (Wolfe, 1986). The lack of a standard diagnostic system has contributed to the confusing impression of the disorder.

The set of symptoms associated with FMS has appeared in various forms and with different names (e.g., fibrositis, tension myalgia, psychogenic rheumatism) in the medical literature since the early 1900s. In addition to the problem of multiple labels, diverse criteria (e.g., pain reported on palpation of 11, 22, or 43 locations) and symptoms (e.g., sleep

227

TABLE 15.1. The 1990 ACR Criteria for the Classification of FMS

1. Presence of widespread pain for at least 3 months. Pain must be present in all of the body quadrants and axial skeletal area.

2. Presence of pain in at least 11 of 18 tender points on digital palpation with approximately 4-kg force. Tender points are located in nine bilateral sites as described below:

   Occiput: at the suboccipital muscle insertions.
   Low cervical: at the anterior aspects of the intertransverse spaces at C_5-C_7.
   Trapezius: at the midpoint of the upper border.
   Supraspinatus: at origins, above the scapula spine near the medial border.
   Second rib: at the second costochondral junctions, just lateral to the junctions on upper surfaces.
   Lateral epicondyle: at 2 cm distal to the epicondyles.
   Gluteal: in upper outer quadrants of buttocks in anterior fold of muscle.
   Greater trochanter: posterior to the trochanteric prominence.
   Knee: at the medial fat proximal to the joint line.

Note. Adapted from Wolfe et al. (1990). Copyright 1990 by Lippincott Williams & Wilkins. Adapted by permission.

disorders, diarrhea, headaches, fatigue) have been presented as core features of FMS. Given the inconsistencies in the literature, some have suggested that FMS is merely a vague set of associated symptoms that does not warrant a specific label and, furthermore, that any label such as FMS is detrimental to the patient as it reifies the individual's belief that he or she is ill (Hadler, 1997).

In 1990, the American College of Rheumatology (ACR) proposed a classification system for the diagnosis of FMS comprising two specific criteria to be used for the diagnosis of FMS (see Table 15.1 and Figure 15.1). These criteria were derived from a multicenter study (Wolfe et al., 1990) that demonstrated that of all symptoms and physical signs frequently reported, only these two criteria significantly discriminated between FMS patients and patients with other chronic pain problems. The ACR criteria have become accepted as the standard classification system for FMS.

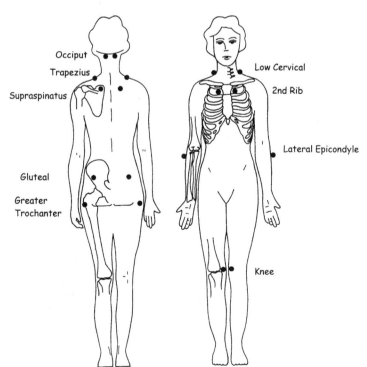

FIGURE 15.1. Locations of tender points.

The procedures proposed to evaluate the ACR criteria are relatively broad and imprecise. Several sets of investigators have attempted to increase the precision for assessing the ACR criteria. For example, a comprehensive, standardized protocol for examining tender points has been developed (Starz, Sinclair, Okifuji, & Turk, 1997). The protocol, Manual Tender Point Survey (MTPS), has been shown to be reliable with good sensitivity and specificity (Okifuji, Turk, Sinclair, Starz, & Marcus, 1997). The MTPS also yields tender points severity scores, in addition to the number of positive tender points, that can be used to evaluate changes over time or outcome of treatments. MacFarlane and colleagues (MacFarlane, Croft, Schollum, & Silman, 1996) have proposed a specific coding system to refine the definition of "widespread pain."

PREVALENCE

FMS is a prevalent condition, estimated to affect 3 to 6 million individuals in the United States (Goldenberg, 1987). In general populations the prevalence of FMS is estimated to range from .66% to 10.50% (Schochat, Croft, & Raspe, 1994). The variability may have resulted from differences in classification criteria, since not all of these studies used the 1990 ACR criteria. FMS is one of the most common disorders evaluated in outpatient rheumatologic clinics (White, Speechley, Harth, & Østbye, 1995). It is also worth noting that although FMS seems relatively common in the general population, severity of the symptoms in the "population-based" FMS tends to be less severe and disabling compared to those FMS patients who seek treatment (Prescott et al., 1993).

MECHANISMS

A number of attempts have been made to describe the underlying mechanisms that can explain the diverse set of symptoms reported by FMS patients. These can be grouped roughly into two groups, peripheral and central mechanisms.

Peripheral Hypotheses

The cardinal feature of FMS is diffuse musculoskeletal pain, although weakening of muscle strength is commonly observed in FMS patients (Mengshoel, Førre, & Komnæs, 1990). These observations have led to a hypothesis that FMS may result from abnormality in muscle structures and metabolisms. Although somewhat higher incidence of "ragged red fibers" was observed (Bengtsson, Henriksson, & Larsson, 1986), microscopic examinations of muscle tissues generally reveal no definitive pathology (Drewes, Andreasen, Schroder, Hogsaa, & Jennum, 1993). Similarly, FMS does not seem to be associated with spontaneous muscle denervation (Durette, Rodriquez, Agre, & Silverman, 1991) or an increased muscle sympathetic nerve discharge (Elam, Johansson, & Wallin, 1992).

Decreased levels of oxygen pressure in the trapezius muscles have been reported (Bengtsson & Henriksson, 1989), suggesting that FMS may be related to local hypoxia in muscles. The hypoxia hypothesis, however, has been criticized for the lack of specificity of the model and for its failure to account for a range of problems associated with FMS (Wolfe, 1996).

The critical weakness of the peripheral hypotheses is that they all fail to explain the diffused and generalized nature of the symptoms in FMS. The peripheral pathology may have been present at the beginning of FMS development, especially in those patients whose FMS symptoms began following musculoskeletal injuries. However, FMS seems to evolve such that the original pathology is no longer a factor in FMS. It is more likely that FMS involves the central mechanisms, both neurochemical and psychological factors.

Central Hypotheses

Several models based on hypothesized central mechanisms have been proposed. These include the hypervigilance model, the central modulation model, and the psychogenic model.

Hypervigilance Model

The diffused and generalized nature of FMS has led some investigators to consider impairment or dysfunction in information processing as a critical factor in FMS. Research investigating sensory processing of FMS patients has consistently demonstrated that FMS patients exhibit lower pain threshold than do age-matched and sex-matched healthy individuals (e.g., Kosek, Ekholm, & Hansson, 1996; McDermid, Rollman, & McCain, 1996). Lowered thresholds are noted not only at affected locations (i.e., TPs) but also in the non-FMS areas. Additionally, FMS patients seem to experience slower recovery from induced pain compared to healthy individuals (Kosek & Hansson, 1997). Based on these results, Rollman and Lautenbacher (1993) have proposed a "hypervigilance model" in which heightened sensory vigilance is considered to be a predisposing factor in FMS.

Vigilance to sensory information in FMS may not be limited to pain. For example, FMS patients tend to exhibit a lower threshold to perceiving fatigue. Research has shown that FMS patients are likely to rate exercise as more demanding than healthy controls, controlling for their aerobic capacity (VO_2 max) (Nørregaard, Bülow, Mehlsen, & Danneskiold-Samsøse, 1994). Similarly, FMS patients tend to terminate physical exercise more quickly than do healthy individuals, despite comparable heart rates under the same workload (van Denderen, Boersma, Zeinstra, Hollander, & van Neerbos, 1992). There is also some evidence that FMS patients are sensitive to non-noxious stimulation such as sound (McDermid et al., 1996). These results seem to suggest that FMS is related to a dysfunction of central processing of somatosensory input.

There are several possible pathways by which individuals develop hypervigilance. For example, there may be genetic or neuroendocrine predispositions that signal the brain to lower background sensory noise, thereby increasing the chance to perceive novel sensory information even at minimal input level. Cognitive processes may be a critical factor in determining vigilance (Chapman, 1986), with past experience with noxious stimulation having an accumulating impact on how one defines and responds to noxious sensory input. Moreover, focusing attention and responding to sensory events may encourage environmental reinforcement (e.g., solicitous reaction by others) or may act as a psychological defense against fear of acquiring serious illness. An excessive amount of orienting attention may further compromise adaptive cognitive, affective, and behavioral responses due to a deficiency of attentional resources to support the self-regulatory process (Wallace & Newman, 1997).

Central Modulation Model: Neuroendocrine Factors

Observation that FMS is associated with lowered thresholds in general suggests that hypervigilance in FMS may be accounted for by dysregulatory processes in the central nervous system (CNS). The central modulation model proposes that maladaptive mechanisms exist in the CNS that interact with peripheral pain modulation (Yunus, 1992). According to this model, the dysfunctional pain mechanisms in the CNS are caused by abnormality in the neuroendocrine system, and over time plasticity in the CNS may result in the adverse feedback from pain to the CNS pain modulation. There are several neuroendocrine factors that may be associated with the CNS pain modulation.

Hypothalamic–Pituitary–Adrenal Axis. Because FMS is often associated with a stressful event as a stimulating or exacerbating factor (Wolfe et al., 1990), disturbance in the hypothalamic–pituitary–adrenal (HPA) axis may be expected. In support of this hypothesis, FMS patients appear to have lower levels of basal cortisol than healthy individuals, as well as abnormal reactivity to stressors (Crofford et al., 1994; van Denderen et al., 1992).

A wide range of sequelae from dysfunction in the HPA axis, from peripheral effects such as muscle pain to central effects such as sleep disturbance, seem to strengthen further the validity of the dysfunctional HPA axis hypothesis (Crofford, Engleberg, & Demitrack, 1996). The dysfunction of the HPA, however, is not specific to FMS. Similar "blunted" stress reactions in the HPA axis have been shown to be associated with obesity and depression (Chrousos & Gold, 1992). Considering the common features among these disorders, dysfunctional HPA responses may be more related to decreased mobility and negative affect than to generalized pain.

Serotonin. Many other functions in the CNS are regulated by or interact with activities at the HPA axis. Several specific neurochemical factors have been investigated as potentially pathophysiological. In particular, the role of serotonin deficiency in the FMS pathophysiology has been of considerable interest, as serotonin is known to be associated with various symptoms related to FMS (e.g., headaches, depression, sleep problems) and nociceptive experience (Richardson, 1990). A series of studies have demonstrated that FMS does seem to be associated with lowered level of serotonin, on the bases of plasma concentration (Wolfe, Russell, Vipraio, Ross, & Anderson, 1997), transfer ratio of tryptophan (a precursor of serotonin; Yunus, Dailey, Aldag, Masi, & Jobe, 1992), cerebrospinal fluid (CFS) concentration (Russell, Vaeroy, Javors, & Nyberg, 1992), and reuptake site density (Russell, Michaleck, et al., 1992). Furthermore, significantly elevated level of substance P present in the cerebrospinal fluid in FMS patients (Russell et al., 1994; Vaeroy, Helle, Forre, Káss, & Terenius, 1988) suggests the presence of hyperalgesia, since the dampening effects on the nociceptive process by substance P cannot be exerted in low levels of serotonin (Murphy & Zemlan, 1987).

Sleep. FMS patients frequently complain of poor sleep and feeling unrefreshed on waking (Wolfe et al., 1990). In an attempt to clarify the relationship between FMS and sleep, Moldofsky and colleagues (Moldofsky & Scarisbrick, 1976; Moldofsky, Scarisbrick, England, & Smythe, 1975) have conducted a series of studies and found that (1) FMS patients tended to exhibit "alpha–delta sleep," characterized by the intrusion of fast-frequency alpha into the delta frequency of slow-wave sleep during non-rapid-eye-movement (NREM) sleep, and (2) artificial induction of alpha–delta sleep in healthy individuals during the Stage IV NREM sleep resulted in reports of symptoms similar to those of FMS. These results suggested that FMS might be considered as an arousal disorder during sleep and that the alpha–delta sleep may have a pathogenetic role in FMS.

The results from subsequent studies, however, have not been consistent. Although some studies (e.g., Drewes, Svendsen, Nielsen, Taagholt, & Bjerregad, 1994) demonstrated higher alpha–delta ratios in Stages II, III, and IV NREM sleep in FMS patients compared to healthy individuals, others (e.g., Shaver et al., 1997) failed to reveal the increased level of alpha activity in FMS patients. The inconsistency may be related to within-group variability. Carette, Oakson, Guimont, & Steriade (1995) found the incidence of alpha–delta sleep in FMS patients to be far from 100%; only 36% of FMS patients they tested showed abnormal alpha intrusion.

Insulin-Like Growth Factor-I (Somatomedin C). Attention has also been given to the level of somatomedin C in FMS. The somatomedin C deficiency hypothesis is derived from the findings that FMS is associated with disturbance in nonrestorative sleep, characterized by alpha-wave intrusion into the normal delta rhythm (Moldofsky et al., 1975). Stage IV sleep is essential in the secretion of the growth hormone that plays an important role in muscle homeostasis and repair. Thus it is possible that the levels of somatomedin C (growth-hormone-related peptide) are impaired in FMS. The research findings on somatomedin C are equivocal. Although Bennett, Clark, Campbell, and

Burckhardt (1992) demonstrated significantly lower levels of somatomedin C in FMS patients than in healthy individuals, a recent study (Buchwald, Umali, & Stene, 1996) failed to find significant differences among FMS patients, FMS patients with chronic fatigue syndrome (CFS), CFS patients, and healthy individuals.

Comments on the Central Hypotheses. We have described two models that are relevant to the central hypotheses of FMS: the hypervigilance model and the central pain modulation model. The two models have produced separate lines of research: the former with behaviorally measured psychophysical studies and the latter with biomedical assay studies. However, it should be noted that the two models are not mutually exclusive; both models define FMS as a disorder primarily characterized by maladaptive information processing.

What is most notable in the studies examining various neuroendocrine substances in FMS seems to be the large intragroup variability observed with any of the substances. Thus, although statistically FMS patients may be different from non-FMS individuals, the large individual differences within FMS patients may make it difficult to interpret the results.

Although most studies may indicate the presence of neuroendocrine dysfunction at the CNS in FMS patients as a whole, roles of the CNS dysfunction in the FMS symptoms are not well understood. Hypothesized mechanisms should be able to account at least partially for the variability in symptom severity. Negative relationships between pain thresholds and pain reports (e.g., present pain severity) are very modest and not observed consistently (Lautenbacher, Rollman, & McCain, 1994). Only a few studies have attempted to determine the roles of neuroendocrine dysfunctions; however, the results have been confusing. In attempting to examine the role of low levels of serotonin in FMS, for example, Wolfe et al. (1997) revealed correlations between serotonin levels and the number of painful TPs in the *opposite direction* from what was expected of the relationship.

The confusing results may be explained by the heterogeneity of FMS patients. This may be present in the biomedical, as well as the psychosocial, domains of chronic illness (Turk & Flor, 1989). For example, several distinctive nociceptive pathways (Sörensen et al., 1997) and cognitive-behavioral styles (Turk, Okifuji, Sinclair, & Starz, 1996; Turk, Okifuji, Starz, & Sinclair, 1996) have been suggested to be present in FMS patients. Identification of factors that define subgroups of FMS may be helpful in determining the associated pathophysiological mechanisms and may serve as a basis for prescribing treatments.

Psychogenic Model

As is so often the case in medicine, when the presence of persistent pain is not explained by organic pathology, pain is often considered as psychogenic (i.e., psychiatric disorder). The high prevalence rate of depression in FMS has led some to hypothesize that the affective disorder is the primary mechanism underlying FMS. For example, Alfici, Sigal, and Landau (1989) found that a significant proportion of FMS patients report past and present depression. They have proposed a model in which individuals with preexisting psychological vulnerability (i.e., personality) develop a depressive disorder that is expressed in a somatic format (e.g., pain).

In general, results from studies fail to support the psychogenic model of FMS. First, the model cannot explain the presence of large individual differences in the presence and degree of depression and other types of psychological distress in FMS patients (Ahles, Khan, Yunus, Spiegel, & Masi, 1991). Similarly, depression is not specific to FMS, nor do all FMS patients consistently report elevated levels of depression. Although some studies show FMS patients to be more distressed than other chronic pain, including arthritic, patients (e.g., Hawley & Wolfe, 1993; Payne et al., 1982), other studies failed to show significant group differences (e.g., Birnie, Knipping, van Rijswijk, de Blécourt, & de Voogd, 1991).

Affective Spectrum Disorder Model

Based on the observation that major depression was common in FMS patients and their first-degree relatives (Hudson, Hudson, Pliner, Goldenberg, & Pope, 1985), Hudson and Pope (1989) proposed the concept of affective spectrum disorder (ASD). Unlike the psychogenic model, the ASD model does not suggest a causal relationship between depression and FMS. Instead, the model proposes that there is a family of medical and psychiatric disorders that share common pathophysiology, such as FMS, irritable bowel syndrome, migraine headache, and major depression. These disorders tend to co-occur with FMS, and, according to the

model, the comorbidity is due to the common abnormality. Positive responses of the ASDs to antidepressants have been posed as supporting evidence for the ASD model.

At the present time, arguments and empirical evidence in support of the ASD model are inconsistent. In addition to the methodological problems in the studies noted, greater prevalence of depression is not always observed in FMS than in other pain conditions. The effectiveness of antidepressant medication on FMS seems to be overestimated in this model (see the later section on pharmacological treatment). Furthermore, the assumption that if one medication improves multiple disorders, then all of those disorders share a common pathology is not always warranted. Medications, such as tricyclics, may affect several aspects of the CNS and in turn have an impact on a range of symptoms.

Muscle Tension

The similarity between FMS and myofascial pain syndrome (MPS) led some investigators to suggest a uniform classification, tension myalgia (Thompson, 1990). The concept of tension myalgia implies that muscle tension, resulting from a variety of causes (e.g., spasms, overuse, poor posture), significantly contributes to the development and maintenance of chronic pain. Tension myalgia also implies that elevated tension levels are tonic and therefore present at all times. Thus patients with tension myalgia should exhibit elevated baseline levels of muscle tension in the pain-relevant areas (i.e., localized in MPS, widespread in FMS) compared to healthy individuals. The available data generally do not support the tension myalgia model. Two studies (Durette et al., 1991; Zidar, Backman, Bengtsson, & Henriksson, 1990) examining baseline level of muscle tension in FMS found no difference between FMS and healthy individuals or patients with non-FMS chronic pain.

An alternative model linking chronic pain and muscle tension considers the interaction of psychological and physiological factors. Hyperactivity of muscles, induced by stress, may lead to ischemia, spasms, and oxygen depletion of the area, thereby increasing individuals' susceptibility to pain. Individuals with a predisposition to tense their back muscles in reaction to stress or those who have learned to increase muscle tension, for example, may be at increased risk of developing chronic pain (Flor & Turk, 1989).

One study (Svebak, Anija, & Kårstad, 1993) reported that FMS patients did not differ from healthy individuals in EMG reactivity to a perceptual–motor task. However, there are methodological concerns that may have confounded the results, such as a small sample size ($n = 10$), inadequate baseline adaptation phase, and questionable validity of the stressor. Generic types of stressors, such as the one that was used in this study, may not be potent enough to elicit EMG reactivity in contrast to "personally relevant" stressors (Flor & Turk, 1989). At the present time, it is difficult to conclude whether elevated reactivity in muscle tension plays any significant role in FMS. Research is required to establish the relationships between FMS and elevated EMG reactivity to stress and to determine the role of EMG reactivity in the initiation, maintenance, and exacerbation of pain and other associated symptoms in FMS.

Physical Factors

Given the chronic and generalized nature of pain in FMS, it appears reasonable to assume that the activity levels of FMS patients would be limited, thereby facilitating and maintaining physical deconditioning. Despite the emphasis on aerobic conditioning as a treatment for FMS, research investigating the physical fitness in FMS patients has yielded inconsistent results. FMS patients' aerobic capacity has not been shown to be significantly different from that of age-matched healthy individuals (e.g., Mengshoel et al., 1990; Nørregaard et al., 1994), whereas a below-average level of aerobic fitness was observed in the majority of FMS patients (Jacobsen & Holm, 1992). The differences may be due to the methodological inconsistencies (e.g., sample sizes) or the predispositional factors (i.e., premorbid level of fitness).

When muscle strength and endurance are tested, however, FMS patients consistently exhibit a significantly lower level of muscle fitness than do healthy individuals (Mengshoel et al., 1990; Nørregaard et al., 1994) and non-FMS pain patients (Jacobsen & Danneskiold-Samsøe, 1992). It should be noted that muscle fitness tests generally depend on participants' voluntary muscle movement; thus results are subjected to the motivational and emotional factors. For example, anticipatory fear of producing pain by excessive muscle contraction may inhibit FMS patients from exerting their maximal muscle strength (Lindh, Johansson, Hedberg, & Grimby, 1994).

The current status of research on fitness in FMS suggests that large individual variation exists in the levels of aerobic and muscular fitness of FMS patients. Relevant factors include premorbid fitness levels, as well as emotional and cognitive factors associated with activities. The intimate relationships between physical functioning abilities and psychological factors have been demonstrated in chronic pain (Dolce et al., 1986). Thus special attention may be warranted for those FMS patients who maintain sedentary lifestyles with progressive deconditioning.

Cognitive Factors

Past research has repeatedly demonstrated that cognitive factors (e.g., beliefs, appraisals) play an important part in determining the adaptation of chronic pain patients to their symptoms (e.g., Turk & Rudy, 1986). Cognitive factors are not generally considered to be etiological. However, research examining the effects of maladaptive cognition on maintenance and aggravation of chronic pain suggests that physical pathology that may have initiated the symptoms play a diminished role over time. On the other hand, perception and interpretation of the symptoms contribute to an internal representation of chronic pain. The dysfunctional representation is likely to facilitate an environment that supports "sick behaviors" and reduction of activities; in turn, patients experience decreased levels of social reinforcement and sense of accomplishment, along with progressive physical deconditioning, all of which will facilitate further disability, distress, and pain.

Although the volume of research in this arena is relatively limited for FMS compared to other types of chronic pain syndromes, the results have consistently indicated that maladaptive thinking is commonly observed in FMS patients. For example, FMS patients, compared to patients with other rheumatological conditions, tend to feel that they have very little control over their pain (Burckhardt & Bjelle, 1996; Pastor et al., 1993). As has been observed in many chronic pain syndromes, maladaptive cognitions seem to be closely associated with functional limitations and affective distress in FMS. Perceptions of uncontrollability, belief that behaviors do not have significant impact on one's condition, and self-efficacy beliefs have been shown to be related to greater pain, disability, and depressive mood in FMS (Buckelew, Murray, Hewett, Johnson, & Huyser, 1995; Turk & Okifuji, 1997a).

It should be noted, however, that not all FMS patients appear to have numerous maladaptive cognitions. Approximately one-third of FMS patients seem to adapt well to their conditions despite unremitting pain and other associated disorders (Turk, Okifuji, Starz, & Sinclair, 1996). All patients were referred for evaluation to a specialized pain center with an average pain duration of 10 years; thus they would hardly qualify as the "healthier" group of individuals who would marginally meet the FMS classification criteria in the community samples. Again, we are struck by the heterogeneity of FMS patients. Although all patients actively create their own cognitive representations of their symptoms, the levels and nature of maladaptive thoughts varies greatly across patients.

TOWARD AN INTEGRATED MODEL

Based on past FMS research, it is reasonable to assume that both neuroendocrine dysfunction and maladaptive psychological responses are associated with FMS. The variable results in FMS research make it difficult to develop a model that is capable of explaining every FMS case. Yunus (1992) proposed a schematic representation of the biophysiological mechanisms of FMS in which FMS symptoms, environmental factors, behavioral factors, and neuroendocrine dysfunction interact with each other. The model was a first attempt to integrate multiple factors. It is primarily symptom-based in conceptualization. Although Yunus mentions the importance of those factors interacting at the CNS levels, the contribution of cognitive and behavioral factors is not specifically included in the model. In this section, we will describe a preliminary model that extends Yunus's. The model is designed to be heuristic, serving as a guide for a comprehensive conceptualization of FMS that incorporates our current understanding of the literature. We have labeled our model "dynamic process." We consider FMS to be a disorder of information processing due to the dysregulated stress-response system. Our model is a diathesis (predisposition)–stress model that integrates premorbid factors, precipitating factors, and stress responses in the development and maintenance of the symptoms associated with FMS.

Figure 15.2 describes a hypothesized process that places individuals at risk of developing FMS. A stressor (box A) triggers physiological (oval D) and psychosocial (oval E) responses, mediated by biological (e.g., genetic information; oval B) and experiential (e.g., prior learning history; oval C) predispositions. At this point, an individual may

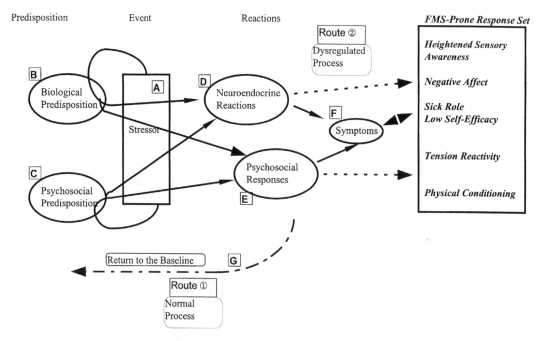

FIGURE 15.2. Dynamic process model of FMS: Evolving processes toward FMS-prone response set.

become aware of certain symptoms, such as mild aching and fatigue (oval F). Ordinarily, this process is self-corrective. Adaptive responses (e.g., relaxation, rehabilitative effort) are hypothesized to play a homeostatic role in returning both physiological and psychological reactions to the system baseline.

For some individuals, however, the system fails to exert the self-corrective process. The self-corrective process may be inhibited due to predispositional factors (e.g., CNS reactivity, dysfunctional thoughts) or environmental factors (e.g., potency and number of stressors in a given time, social supports) or possibly the interaction of these two factors. When the system fails to self-correct, dysregulations of the CNS (e.g., blunted HPA reaction; Crofford et al., 1994; van Denderen et al., 1992 or serotonin deficiency; Russell & Michaleck, 1992; Wolfe et al., 1997) and maladaptive cognitive-behavioral responses (e.g., cognitive errors; Buckelew et al., 1995; Turk & Okifuji, 1997a) are activated (Figure 15.2). Since the system fails to return to the baseline, a new baseline is set (i.e., modification of predispositional factors that will interact with future stressors), further reinforcing the dysregulation of the system. In this model, a response set that places individuals "at risk" for developing FMS ("FMS-prone response set"; see Figure 15.2) is hypothesized to emerge as a result of repeated activations of the dysregulated system. The FMS-prone response set should not be confused with personality traits. The response set is considered as a dominant biopsychological repertoire with which individuals respond to stressors, but it is modifiable.

The FMS-prone response set can be described in terms of several constructs that have been shown to be associated with FMS. The dysregulated stress reactions in the CNS and psychosocial adaptations result in increased attention to sensory information (lowered thresholds; e.g., Kosek et al., 1996; McDermid et al., 1996), negative mood (e.g., Hawley & Wolfe, 1993; Hudson et al., 1985), cognitions consistent with being chronically ill (e.g., lack of control, catastrophizing; Burckhardt & Bjelle, 1996), declined activities and increased deconditioning (e.g., Nørregaard et al., 1994), and muscle tension reactivity (Flor & Turk, 1989). The strength of the FMS-prone response set is determined by potency of each of the mediating factors.

It should be noted that the model presents an oversimplified view of FMS. As we reviewed various factors in this chapter, a set of factors can be included within each oval. Intra- and interoval interactions among factors are likely to occur. The strength of these interactions may vary. Some factors may be more influential than others with different individuals, with some having acute effects and with others having long-term (i.e., chronic) effects.

Over time, the FMS-prone response set and associated symptoms will be manifested as generalized hypervigilance and result in diffuse somatic complaints (see Figure 15.3). Presentations of diffuse symptoms may lead to inconclusive diagnostic results, which may contribute to frustration and anxiety in patients and families, possibly changing the dynamics of patients' interpersonal environments. Modification of the environment forms a new frame, in which patients undergo various experiences, and feeds back into the characteristics of the psychosocial predisposition, thereby affecting the subsequent processes.

Figure 15.4 presents the overall scheme of the evolution of the FMS-related factors as a function of predisposition, time, and stressors. During the acute stage, a precipitator, either physical injury or psychological trauma, that is sufficiently potent to trigger both physiological and psychosocial stress-defense responses, interacts with predispositional biological and psychological tendencies. The interactions elicit responses in the system (neuroendocrine as well as psychosocial). For the majority of individuals, the neuroendocrine and psychosocial systems return to the baseline once they adjust and adapt to a challenging event or situation. Alternative processes, as we described earlier, are hypothesized be in effect for some individuals—the process that eventually leads to FMS. As those individuals undergo multiple stressors, the predispositional factors themselves are modified and eventually evolve into a new predispositional state that guides the individuals in reacting to stressors with the FMS-prone response set (as symbolized in the darkened shade).

Time is central to our model, since time allows the FMS-prone response set eventually to evolve as a default mode of responding to stressors. Furthermore, as the FMS-prone response set becomes more dominant, thresholds for even minor stressors may be lowered. In other words, a whole set of physiological and psychosocial reactions can be triggered to relatively minor stressors that might not even be considered as "stressful" by many individuals.

The clinical implications of the model emphasize the importance of multifactorial assessment and treatment. Given the complex web of interactive

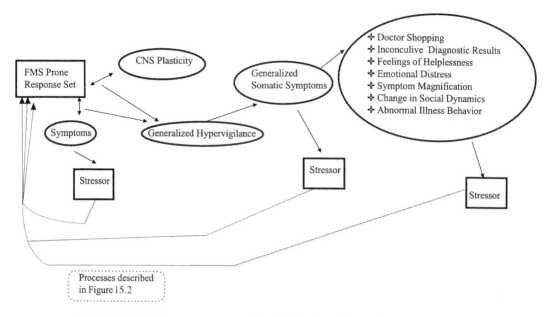

FIGURE 15.3. Dynamic process model of FMS: Toward generalized hypervigilance.

pathways, targeting any single factor (e.g., seroto-nin) will be inadequate and will not likely lead to a substantial change in the maladaptive process it-self or the FMS symptoms. The model also sug-gests that FMS is a disorder of biopsychosocial processes (Turk, 1996; see also Turk & Flor, Chap-ter 2, this volume). Assessment therefore should include identification of the predispositional factors that are likely to mediate the relationships between stressors and maladaptive stress responses, as well as current physical and psychological conditions.

We might set a goal for an FMS treatment to "normalize" the process, targeting the FMS-prone response set. The most reasonable course seems to be to manipulate the CNS and maladaptive psychosocial responses, thereby modifying the way stressors and predispositional factors interact with one another. A number of treatment modalities have been used in an attempt to alleviate the symp-toms of FMS. Many of the treatment modalities described subsequently can be used to modify the maladaptive responses and processes incorporated in the dynamic process model. However, because the FMS-prone response set is a result of complex interactions between the neuroendocrine and psy-chosocial factors, comprehensive interventions that target a range of variables will likely be most effec-tive in alleviating FMS symptoms.

Even though the model presents the evolving processes of the system for FMS as a whole, it is important to acknowledge that FMS patients are not a homogeneous group (Turk, Okifuji, Sinclair, & Starz, 1996). It is reasonable to assume that large individual differences existed prior to FMS onset in the neuroendocrine and psychosocial systems. Thus, although the evolving processes may be present in all FMS patients, the degrees to which the processes become dysregulated may vary across individuals due to differences in the predispositional factors. As we note later in this chapter, research suggests the pres-ence of distinctive subgroups of FMS patients on the basis of biomedical and psychosocial factors. These subgroups may respond to an identical inter-vention in different manners. In short, the "one-size-fits-all" approach of treating FMS patients is not likely to be effective. Identifying patients' character-istics and matching them to specific treatment may be the best way to maximize the clinical efficacy.

TREATMENT

FMS patients complain of a whole panoply of so-matic and psychological symptoms. Although no organic pathology has been identified, patients' quality of life is substantially compromised. In the past few decades, a number of approaches have been tested for the treatment of FMS. Despite ex-tensive research efforts, however, no treatment has proven to be universally effective. In the following

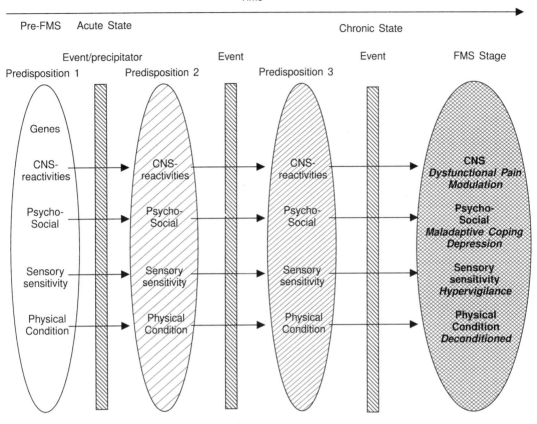

FIGURE 15.4. Dynamic process model of FMS: Time course.

section, we present an overview of research evaluating different types of treatment for FMS. Before we begin, however, there are several issues that need to be kept in mind.

Outcome Variables

Some of the difficulties in evaluating treatment outcome studies in FMS relate to inconsistency in outcome variables. The inconsistency reflects the diverse nature of the disorder and the particular interests and discipline of the investigators. Most studies, if not all, include some measure of pain, the cardinal feature of FMS, either in the form of TP assessment or self-report of pain severity. However, emotional distress, cognitive factors, perceived disability, functional limitation, and physical conditioning were not included in all studies. Studies evaluating psychological treatment, for example, tend to focus more on psychosocial variables, whereas studies testing the physical modality tend to collect more functional data.

The inconsistency of outcome variables across studies seems also to be related to the lack of a "gold standard" for treatment efficacy. Defining success in treating multifactorial chronic conditions with no identifiable pathology is not a simple task (Turk & Okifuji, 1997b). In an attempt to determine standard criteria for evaluating treatment efficacy in FMS, Simms, Felson, & Goldenberg (1991) delineated several criteria on the basis of the assumption that treatment response to amitriptyline is the gold standard for treatment efficacy. As can been seen in the following section, amitriptyline is one of the most effective pharmacological therapies; however, the estimated efficacy rate is only 36% (Carette et al., 1994), thereby making it difficult to assess the validity of the criteria presented by Simms et al. (1991).

In addition, many outcome variables are measured in an unstandardized format with questionable validity. An example of such items would be the widely used "physician's global assessment," in which a physician (often the one who provides the treatment) rates patient's improvement on an ordinal scale (e.g., "got worse," "no change," "mild improvement," "moderate improvement," "marked improvement"). Bias for or against the treatment and the patient may substantially influence such ratings, especially since physicians are commonly aware of the treatment patients are receiving even in a blind setting (Quimby, Gratwick, Whitney, & Block, 1989).

Designs and Analyses

Types and qualities of research designs and analytic approaches also vary across studies. Generally, evaluation of pharmacological treatment has used randomized, controlled trials. Many used a crossover design so that all participants received the same treatment by the end of the project. A large dropout rate (up to 57%; e.g., Wolfe, Cathey, & Hawley, 1994) is quite common in these studies, and statistical considerations such as "intention-to-treat" analyses are not generally included. In contrast, nonrandomized designs dominate in studies of multidisciplinary treatments in which randomization and placebo control are ethically and practically difficult to achieve.

UNIMODAL INTERVENTIONS

A wide variety of pharmacological, physical, and psychological interventions has been used in an attempt to treat FMS patients. As we shall see, the rationales for these different modalities seem reasonable in some, though not all, instances; yet the results are rather modest.

Pharmacological Therapies

Anti-Inflammatory Medications

Corticosteroids are often used to treat inflammatory conditions such as rheumatoid arthritis. They were one of the first classes of medications to be tested for the treatment of FMS. A double-blind, crossover trial of prednisone (Clark, Tindall, & Bennett, 1985) revealed no difference between the treatment and control conditions. Nonsteroidal anti-inflammatory drugs (NSAIDs) are another choice of anti-inflammatory therapy. NSAIDs are commonly used analgesics. Double-blind, placebo-controlled studies failed to show any significant effects of ibuprofen (Russell, Fletcher, Michaleck, McBroom, & Hester, 1991) or naproxen (Goldenberg, Felson, & Dinerman, 1986). Because inflammation typically is not involved in FMS, the failure of these medications to treat FMS is not surprising. Moreover, there is no good rationale for prescribing corticosteroids, especially given the potential adverse effects.

Benzodiazepines

Many FMS patients report chronic anxiety and sleep disturbances. The efficacy of benzodiazepines was tested on the basis of the assumption that improvement of sleep and mood regulation may help FMS patients. However, the results from the two studies (Hench, Cohen, & Mitler, 1989; Russell et al., 1991) seem to suggest that benzodiazepines are no better than a placebo and have minimal, if any, significant impact on the FMS symptomatology. Adverse effects, such as dependence, are serious concerns with benzodiazapines that should dissuade any long-term use.

Tricyclics

Since serotonin deficiency has been hypothesized to play an important role in modulation of pain and sleep, agents that were considered as serotonergic, such as imipramine, doxepin, amitriptyline, and cycrobenzaprine, have been used to treat FMS. Low-dose amitriptyline is probably the most frequently evaluated drug. The prescribed dose for FMS is usually too low to expect significant antidepressant effects as well as serious anticholinergic effects.

Variability in the methodologies and outcome variables makes it difficult to draw a definitive conclusion as to the clinical value of tricyclics. Some studies (e.g., Goldenberg et al., 1986) report significant decreases in pain responsiveness and other FMS symptoms. However, more modest results have also been reported by others. For example, Carette et al. (1994) observed that only 36% of FMS patients receiving low-dose amitriptyline showed clinical improvement in various FMS affected areas.

The research findings from the cyclobenzaprine trials are similar to those of the amitriptyline trials. Cyclobenzaprine is a tricyclic that is chemically very similar to amitriptyline, generally used as muscle relaxant with no expected antidepressant effect. Although some studies (e.g., Bennett et al.,

1988) have shown improvement in a range of areas (e.g., pain, fatigue, mood) with cyclobenzaprine, others (Reynolds, Moldofsky, Saskin, & Lue, 1991; Simms et al., 1991) did not. For example, of nine patients who completed the trial in the Reynolds et al.'s study (1991), only two patients reported the medication as "moderately helpful." Similarly, Simms et al. (1991) estimated 30% sensitivity and 96% specificity for the efficacy of cyclobenzaprine for improving sleep, decreasing TPs, and better clinical impression. Carette et al. (1994), in the same study referred to in the test of amitriptyline, tested cyclobenzaprine and estimated the efficacy rate as only 33%.

Selective Serotonin Reuptake Inhibitors

Research results demonstrating that a lowered level of serotonin may be associated with FMS (Wolfe et al., 1997) and that tricyclics may be beneficial, at least for some FMS patients (Carette et al., 1994), have led to a hypothesis that another type of antidepressant, the selective serotonin reuptake inhibitor (SSRI), may be helpful. The SSRI has increasingly become a treatment of choice for depression, probably due to the increased safety, decreased side effects, and wide publicity SSRIs (particularly fluoxetine) have received, and this excitement for SSRIs seems to have been taken up by those who investigate pharmacological treatments of FMS. In a 3-month open trial of fluoxetine with 23 FMS patients, Cortet, Houvenagel, Forzy, Vincent, and Delcambre (1992) found no improvement in pain or TPs but some improvement in sleep. Similarly, in a double-blind placebo-controlled trial, Wolfe et al. (1994) reported that patients who received fluoxetine reported modest but statistically significant improvement in mood and sleep, but not in the TP, pain, and fatigue variables. These findings should be reviewed cautiously, however, due to the high dropout rates (29% in the treatment group, 57% in the placebo group).

Recently, Goldenberg, Mayskiy, Mossey, Ruthazer, and Schmid (1996) reported the results from a randomized, double-blind crossover trial with amitriptyline and fluoxetine. Each patient in this study underwent 6-week trials of placebo, fluoxetine, amitriptyline, and combination of fluoxetine and amitriptyline. Comparisons with the baseline levels revealed that the use of fluoxetine and amitriptyline was associated with improvements in pain, sleep, fatigue, and moods. Furthermore, the combination of two drugs yielded even better outcome than the use of either medication alone. Again,

however, two factors that may have affected the outcome should be mentioned: high dropout rates (nearly 40% of the total sample) and the exclusion of patients with high levels of depression from the study. Because depression is a prevalent problem in FMS, the sample representativeness may have been skewed by the exclusion of depressed patients in addition to the high dropout rate. Moreover, the range of improvement in each group seemed to vary greatly, reflecting the various levels of response to the medications.

Nonpharmacological Therapies

Chiropractic Therapy

Although infrequently subjected to empirical research, chiropractic therapy is one of the most widely utilized treatment modalities for FMS. For example, approximately 40% of FMS patients referred for evaluation at a university-based pain program report to have had chiropractic services (Turk, Okifuji, Sinclair, & Starz, 1996). In attempt to evaluate the efficacy of chiropractic therapy for FMS, Blunt, Rajwani, and Cuerriero (1997) compared nine patients who received a session including soft tissue massage, soft tissue stretching, spinal manipulation, and education four to five times a week for 4 weeks to 10 waiting-list control participants. No statistically significant differences were found in the improvement in physical functions, pain, and perceived disability. The lack of improvement may be related to diminished statistical power due to the small sample size. Given the popularity of the therapy, it is important to test the efficacy of chiropractic therapy. It is imperative, however, that the research design include an attention-controlled group, since patients in the treatment group receive extensive "hands-on" care. Waiting-list controls, such as the ones used in this study, would not be adequate to rule out a possibility that the observed efficacy may be due to nonspecific effects of chiropractic intervention.

Exercise

Although the central feature of FMS is generalized pain, many FMS patients, after years of living with constant pain, are physically deconditioned. Thus it is generally thought that treatment of FMS should include a component that improves physical fitness. Several studies have examined the efficacy of exercise programs with various levels of rigorousness. McCain, Bell, Mai, and Halliday (1988) tested a cardiovascular training program in which patients underwent sustained heart rate elevation training for 60 minutes, three times a week, for 20 weeks. Patients receiving flexibility training for the same amounts of minutes served as controls. Results revealed that those who received the cardiovascular training exhibited significantly more improved aerobic capacity and pain sensitivity on TPs than the controls; however, no group differences were found in pain severity, sleep, mood, and fatigue. Similar results were obtained by Wigers, Stiles, and Vogel (1996), whose patients underwent a 14-week program of submaximal aerobic exercises for 45 minutes three times per week (aiming at 60–70% of maximum heart rate for 20 minutes). Wigers et al. (1996) also followed their patients for 4 years and concluded that the efficacy of the aerobic exercise program depended largely on adherence to the regimen.

Muscle strength, endurance, and flexibility are important aspects of overall fitness in addition to improved cardiovascular capacity. Martin et al. (1996) developed a 1-hour exercise program consisting of 20-minute submaximal fast walk, 20-minute flexibility, and 20-minute muscle-strengthening training. Patients underwent the training program three times per week for 6 weeks. Results were similar to those findings from the aerobic training alone. At posttreatment, the patients in this training program showed significant reduction in TP counts and pain sensitivity in the TP areas.

Long-term compliance with ergometric and muscle-endurance training tasks is not easy even for healthy individuals. In attempt to enhance the efficacy of fitness programs for FMS by making the exercise more "interesting," some researchers (Nørregaard, Lykkegaard, Mehlgen, & Danneskiold-Samsøe, 1997) evaluated the efficacy of low-impact aerobic dance programs. This study failed to show significant improvement in any of the FMS symptoms, suggesting low-impact aerobic exercise is not by itself effective for FMS.

Other Nonpharmacological, Single-Modality Interventions

Technique-driven treatments, such as meditation, hypnosis, relaxation, biofeedback, and other behavioral therapy techniques, generally aim at better management of stress and coping. They are widely available and utilized to treat various stress-related conditions despite limited guidance to ascertain quality and appropriateness of the care. Research

investigating the effectiveness of various single-modality stress management programs for FMS suggests that those modalities also seem to offer few therapeutic benefits.

Progressive muscle relaxation is commonly used to reduce tension and anxiety by manipulating the autonomic nervous system. When applied to treat FMS by itself, patients seem to exhibit only minor changes at posttreatment in comparison to baseline (Martin et al., 1996) or relative to patients receiving "bath therapy" (Gunther, Mur, Kinigadner, & Miller, 1994). Ferraccioli et al. (1987) evaluated the effectiveness of frontal electromyographic biofeedback training for FMS patients. A large proportion (56%) of the six patients who received "true" feedback reported improvement in various symptoms. However, several factors, including the small sample size, nonstandardized outcome measures, and unexplained inconsistency that only regional effects, but not generalized, are expected from frontal biofeedback, make the results difficult to interpret.

Haanen et al. (1991) evaluated the efficacy of hypnotherapy compared to a program consisting of massage and relaxation training. Statistically significant improvements in pain, fatigue, sleep, and emotional distress were observed in patients receiving hypnotherapy at posttreatment and at a 3-month follow-up. No changes in pain sensitivity on TPs were observed. Although the results seem promising, the clinical significance of the changes was not clear, especially with the posttreatment and follow-up levels of pain at 6.0 and 7.1 respectively, on a 0–10 scale in the hypnotherapy group. Furthermore, the ACR criteria (Wolfe et al., 1990) were not used for patient selection.

Several investigators have combined several treatment modalities. De Voogd and colleagues (1993) tested a program involving active visualization and relaxation in addition to other behavioral techniques to improve interpersonal communication (e.g., assertiveness training). Although patients' satisfaction with the program and their subjective feelings of better coping were high, those scores were not reflected on standardized measures of psychological distress and sleep. Kaplan, Goldenberg, and Galvin-Nadeau (1993) developed a meditation-based cognitive-behavioral therapy program aiming at modifying stress responses. Approximately 50% of their patients showed at least 50% improvement in various standardized measures of FMS symptoms. Unfortunately, the interpretation of their results is compromised by the lack of parametric statistics and control groups.

In a recent report, Nicassio et al. (1997) examined the efficacy of behavior therapy versus educational sessions. In the behavior therapy group, patients received education (e.g., gate control theory of pain) and relaxation training, were conducted goal setting, and were able to involve significant others in the therapy. The education group received general information about FMS and supportive discussions. Results showed significant decreases in pain sensitivity on TPs, depression, and pain behaviors in the behavior therapy group compared to the education group but not in overall pain and sense of well-being, although the same effects were found in the control group that received educational sessions. The authors further reported that the critical factor in improvement was change in perceived helplessness—when patients' levels of perceived helplessness declined substantially, patients' reports of pain and depression seemed to improve. Although there are several problems in this study, including a high dropout rate (25%) in the treatment group, lack of statistical control (i.e., intention-to-treat analyses), statistically significant but only modest changes, failure to consider physical functioning abilities, and unclear descriptions of pain severity index, the results from this study suggest that treatment efforts to modify how individuals psychologically adapt to FMS may be critical.

The results of the unimodal-treatment outcome studies have led some to pessimism and resignation about the ability to successfully treat FMS patients. Solomon and Liang (1997) have questioned the appropriateness of rheumatologists continuing to treat FMS patients, given the limited results. Although we are sympathetic to the concerns raised, as we note below, we believe that one of the major problems is that FMS patients are being treated as a homogeneous set. It is more likely that there are subgroups of FMS patients and that treatment will be more effective when it is matched to the unique characteristics of each group. Thus at this point it may be premature to rule out the potential value of the unimodal therapies described. Moreover, we will note that some of these individual therapies may be incorporated within comprehensive programs.

Multidisciplinary Treatments

In the past few decades, a growing number of investigators have emphasized the importance of addressing multiple factors associated with FMS (e.g., Bennett, 1996). Various types of multidisciplinary treatment programs have been developed for FMS, although programs tend to include some common components, such as physical exercise, education, and some type of cognitive treatment to improve coping.

Burckhardt, Mannerkorpi, Hedenberg, and Bjelle (1994) conducted a randomized clinical trial evaluating the efficacy of a program consisting of six 90-minute education and 1-hour physical exercise sessions. Education was designed to facilitate self-management of pain and symptoms, mostly providing information and instructions for cognitive-behavioral coping strategies. Patients who received these sessions, compared to patients on the waiting list or those receiving only education sessions, tended to report improved self-efficacy at posttreatment. Other functional and pain variables did not change, except for modest change in the mood and pain sensitivity scores on TPs in the education-only group. Similarly, Mengshoel, Forseth, Haugen, Walle-Hansen, and Førre (1995) reported modest reduction in pain (no cognitive-behavioral variables were measured) reports from their evaluation of twenty 2-hour sessions involving dietary adjustment, group discussion of coping, relaxation training, and strength and flexibility exercise.

The modest nature of the efficacy of the program reviewed here may be due to the lack of intensity of the education program. Patients may need to exercise and internalize new and adaptive cognitive-behavioral coping strategies during sessions. Nielson, Walker, and McCain (1992) developed a comprehensive inpatient program consisting of exercise, relaxation training, coping training, family education, and pacing and demonstrated that their program was effective in reducing pain, emotional distress, pain behaviors, and maladaptive cognitive set. A subsequent study (White & Nielson, 1995) demonstrated the maintenance of treatment benefit at 30-month follow-up in emotional distress and pain behaviors. Unfortunately, they did not assess typical FMS symptoms such as fatigue and sleep problems.

Other investigators (Bennett et al., 1996; Turk, Okifuji, Sinclair, & Starz, 1998) developed comprehensive outpatient programs consisting of cognitive-behavioral therapy, exercise, medication management, and pacing. Bennett et al. (1996) provided weekly 90-minute sessions over 6 months, and Turk et al. (1998) provided six half-day sessions over 4 weeks. In both programs, patients reported significant improvements in various FMS-related areas, including reduced pain, fatigue, and distressed mood and improved perceived functioning.

The demonstrated efficacy of multidisciplinary treatment programs suggests that the combination of medical, physical, and cognitive-behavioral treatment paradigms should be the treatment of choice for all FMS patients. Certainly, treatment effects on the average were statistically significant. However, large individual differences in treatment responses were also present. For example, using the empirically derived index of clinical significance (Jacobson, Follette, & Revenstorf, 1984), Turk et al. (1998) found approximately 40% of patients could be considered to have had meaningful changes in pain after treatment. The demonstrated variability in treatment responses suggests that matching treatment to clinical needs of subgroups of FMS patients may be critical in optimizing treatment efficacy.

Turk, Okifuji, Sinclair, and Starz (1996) reported that FMS patients could be classified into three groups based on their cognitive-behavioral responses to their symptoms as measured by the Multidimensional Pain Inventory (Kerns, Turk, & Rudy, 1985). On the basis of this psychosocial classification, a subsequent study (Turk, Okifuji, Starz, & Sinclair, 1998) demonstrated that treatment responses varied significantly across subgroups of FMS patients who were divided on the basis of their cognitive-behavioral responses to their pain conditions. Individuals who tended to have high levels of pain, poor coping, emotional distress, and perceived disability benefited most from the treatment, whereas those whose distress and disability were associated with their interpersonal problems did not improve, suggesting that an additional treatment component addressing the interpersonal issues may be needed for the latter group of patients. Furthermore, a group of patients who were coping relatively well showed minimal changes, probably due to the floor effect, raising the question of whether these patients would need the comprehensive treatment.

The research consistently indicates that FMS patients are not homogenous, and we need to pay attention to the individual differences of FMS in not only psychosocial but also biomedical factors. By matching treatment needs to treatment protocols, we should be able to optimize the clinical and the cost effectiveness of the treatments.

CONCLUDING COMMENTS

In this chapter we attempted to provide an overview of the current status of research on the mechanisms and treatment of FMS. Despite extensive research, the mechanisms of FMS are still not well understood. However, the accumulated research results seem to rule out some of the most prevalent hypotheses—namely, the cause–effect relationship between peripheral pathology and FMS and the linear relationships among various neuroendocrine abnormalities, psychological distress, and FMS. In order to integrate the current understanding of FMS, we described the dynamic process model of FMS, proposing FMS as a disorder of information processing due to impaired stress reactivity. Systematic research is needed to test hypotheses based on the model to establish its validity.

The review of clinical trials revealed mostly mediocre results. However, investigators are now recognizing the heterogeneity of FMS patients and the importance of taking individual differences into account when developing treatment protocols. So far, the heterogeneity of psychosocial factors has been empirically considered; however, other factors, such as neuroendocrine and demographic variables, may be critical in addressing clinical needs of patients. Attempts to customize treatments to patients' clinical needs should help us develop optimal therapy protocols for a larger number of FMS patients than is currently possible.

REFERENCES

Ahles, T. A., Khan, S. A., Yunus, M. B., Spiegel, D. A., & Masi, A. T. (1991). Psychiatric status of patients with primary fibromyalgia, patients with rheumatoid arthritis and subjects without pain: A blind comparison of DSM-III diagnoses. *American Journal of Psychiatry, 148,* 1721–1726.

Alfici, S., Sigal, M., & Landau, M. (1989). Primary fibromyalgia syndrome: A variant of depressive disorder. *Psychotherapy and Psychosomatics, 51,* 156–161.

Baumstark, K. E., & Buckelew, S. P. (1992). Fibromyalgia: Clinical signs, research findings, treatment implications, and future directions. *Annals of Behavioral Medicine, 14,* 282–291.

Bengtsson, A., & Henriksson, K. G. (1989). The muscle in fibromyalgia: A review of Swedish studies. *Journal of Rheumatology, 19,* 144–149.

Bengtsson, A., Henriksson, K. G., & Larsson, J. (1986). Muscle biopsy in primary fibromyalgia: Light-microscopical and histochemical findings. *Scandinavian Journal of Rheumatology, 15,* 1–6.

Bennett, R. M. (1996). Multidisciplinary group programs to treat fibromyalgia patients. *Rheumatic Diseases Clinics of North America, 22,* 351–367.

Bennett, R. M., Burckhardt, C. S., Clark, S. R., O'Reilly, C. A., Wiens, A. N., & Campbell, S. M. (1996). Group treatment of fibromyalgia: A 6-month outpatient program. *Journal of Rheumatology, 23,* 521–528.

Bennett, R. M., Clark, S. R., Campbell, S. M., & Burckhardt, C. S. (1992). Low levels of somatomedin C in patients with the fibromyalgia syndrome: A possible link between sleep and muscle pain. *Arthritis and Rheumatism, 35,* 1113-1116.

Bennett, R. M., Gatter, R. A., Campbell, S. M., Andrews, R. P., Clark, S. R., & Scarola, J. A. (1988). A comparison of cyclobenzaprine and placebo in the management of fibrositis: A double-blind controlled study. *Arthritis and Rheumatism, 32,* 1535-1542.

Birnie, D. J., Knipping, A. A., van Rijswijk, M. H., de Blécourt, A. C., & de Voogd, J. N. (1991). Psychological aspects of fibromyalgia compared with chronic and nonchronic pain. *Journal of Rheumatology, 18,* 1845-1848.

Blunt, K. L., Rajwani, M. H., & Cuerriero, R. (1997). The effectiveness of chiropractic management of fibromyalgia patients: A pilot study. *Journal of Manipulative and Physiological Therapeutics, 20,* 389-399.

Buchwald, D., Umali, J., & Stene, M. (1996). Insulin-like growth factor-I (somatomedin C) levels in chronic fatigue syndrome and fibromyalgia. *Journal of Rheumatology, 23,* 739-742.

Buckelew, S. P., Murray, S. E., Hewett, J. E., Johnson, J., & Huyser, B. (1995). Self-efficacy, pain, and physical activity among fibromyalgia subjects. *Arthritis Care Research, 8,* 43-50.

Burckhardt, C. S., & Bjelle, A. (1996). Perceived control: A comparison of women with fibromyalgia, rheumatoid arthritis, and systemic lupus erythematosus using a Swedish version of the Rheumatology Attitude Index. *Scandinavian Journal of Rheumatology, 25,* 300-306.

Burckhardt, C. S., Clark, S. R., & Bennett, R. M. (1993). Fibromyalgia and quality of life: A comparative analysis. *Journal of Rheumatology, 20,* 475-479.

Burckhardt, C. S., Mannerkorpi, K., Hedenberg, L., & Bjelle, A. (1994). A randomized, controlled trial of education and physical training for women with fibromyalgia. *Journal of Rheumatology, 21,* 714-720.

Carette, S., Bell, M. J., Reynolds, W. J., Haraoui, B., McCain, G., Bykerk, V. P., Edworthy, S. M., Baron, M., Koehler, B. E., Fam, A. G., Bellamy, N., & Guimont, C. (1994). Comparison of amitriptyline, cyclobenzaprine, and placebo in the treatment of fibromyalgia: A randomized, double-blind clinical trial. *Arthritis and Rheumatism, 37,* 32-40.

Carette, S., Oakson, G., Guimont, C., & Steriade, M. (1995). Sleep electroencephalography and the clinical response to amitriptyline in patients with fibromyalgia. *Arthritis and Rheumatism, 38,* 1211-1217.

Chapman, C. R. (1986). Pain, perception, and illness. In R. A. Sternbach (Ed.), *The psychology of pain* (2nd ed.). New York: Raven Press.

Chrousos, G. P., & Gold, P. W. (1992). The concepts of stress and stress system disorders: Overview of physical and behavioral homeostatis. *Journal of the American Medical Association, 267,* 1244-1252.

Clark, S., Tindall, E., & Bennett, R. M. (1985). A double blind crossover trial of prednisone versus placebo in the treatment of fibrositis. *Journal of Rheumatology, 12,* 980-983.

Cortet, B., Houvenagel, E., Forzy, G., Vincent, G., & Delcambre, B. (1992). Evaluation of the effectiveness of serotonin (flouxetine hydrochloride) treatment: Open study in fibromyalgia. *Revue du Rhumatisme et des Maladies Ostéo-Articulaires, 59,* 497-500.

Crofford, L. J., Engleberg, N. C., & Demitrack, M. A. (1996). Neurohormonal perturbations in fibromyalgia. *Baillieres Clinical Rheumatology, 10,* 365-378.

Crofford, L. J., Pillemer, S. R., Kalogeras, K. T., Cash, J. M., Michelson, D., Kling, M. A., Sternberg, E. M., Gold, P. W., Chrousos, G. P., & Wilder, R. L. (1994). Hypothalamic–pituitary–adrenal axis perturbations in patients with fibromyalgia. *Arthritis and Rheumatism, 37,* 1583-1592.

de Voogd, J. N., Knipping, A. A., de Blécourt, A. C. E., & van Rijswijk, M. H. (1993). Treatment of fibromyalgia syndrome with psychomotor therapy and marital counselling. *Journal of Musculoskeletal Pain, 3/4,* 273-281.

Dolce, J. J., Doleys, D. M., Racyznski, J. M., Lossie, J., Poole, L., & Smith, M. (1986). The role of self-efficacy expectancies in the prediction of pain tolerance. *Pain, 27,* 261-272.

Drewes, A. M., Andreasen, A., Schroder, H. D., Hogsaa, B., & Jennum, P. (1993). Pathology of skeletal muscle in fibromyalgia: A histo-immuno-chemical and ultrastructural study. *British Journal of Rheumatology, 32,* 479-483.

Drewes, A. M., Svendsen, L., Nielsen, K. D., Taagholt, S. J., & Bjerregad, K. (1994). Quantification of alpha-EEG activity during sleep in fibromyalgia: A study based on ambulatory sleep monitoring. *Journal of Musculoskeletal Pain, 2,* 33-53.

Durette, M. R., Rodriquez, A. A., Agre, J. C., & Silverman, J. L. (1991). Needle electromyographic evaluation of patients with myofascial or fibromyalgic pain. *American Journal of Physical Medicine and Rehabilitation, 70,* 154-156.

Elam, M., Johansson, G., & Wallin, B. G. (1992). Do patients with primary fibromyalgia have an altered muscle sympathetic nerve activity? *Pain, 48,* 371-375.

Ferraccioli, G., Ghirelli, L., Scita, F., Nolli, M., Mozzani, M., Fontana, S., Scorsonelli, M., Tridenti, A., & De Risio, C. (1987). EMG-biofeedback training in fibromyalgia syndrome. *Journal of Rheumatology, 14,* 820-825.

Flor, H., & Turk, D. C. (1989). Psychophysiology of chronic pain: Do chronic pain patients exhibit symptom-specific psychophysiological responses? *Psychological Bulletin, 105,* 215-259.

Goldenberg, D. L. (1987). Fibromyalgia syndrome: An emerging but controversial condition. *Journal of the American Medical Association, 257,* 2782-2787.

Goldenberg, D. L., Felson, D. T., & Dinerman, H. (1986). A randomized, controlled trial of amitriptyline and naproxen in the treatment of patients with fibromyalgia. *Arthritis and Rheumatism, 29,* 1371-1377.

Goldenberg, D., Mayskiy, M., Mossey, C., Ruthazer, R., & Schmid, C. (1996). A randomized, double-blind crossover trial of fluoxetine and amitriptyline in the treatment of fibromyalgia. *Arthritis and Rheumatism, 39,* 1852-1859.

Gunther, V., Mur, E., Kinigadner, U., & Miller, C. (1994). Fibromyalgia—the effect of relaxation and hydrogalvanic bath therapy on the subjective pain experience. *Clinical Rheumatology, 13,* 573-578.

Haanen, H. C., Hoenderdos, H. T., van Romunde, L. K., Hop, W. C., Mallee, C., Terwiel, J. P., & Hekster, G. B. (1991). Controlled trial of hypnotherapy in the treatment of refractory fibromyalgia. *Journal of Rheumatology, 18,* 72-75.

Hadler, N. M. (1997). Fibromyalgia, chronic fatigue, and other iatrogenic diagnostic algorithms: Do some labels escalate illness in vulnerable patients? *Postgradute Medicine, 102,* 161–172.

Hawley, D. J., & Wolfe, F. (1993). Depression is not more common in rheumatoid arthritis: A 10-year longitudinal study of 6,153 patients with rheumatic disease. *Journal of Rheumatology, 20,* 2025–2031.

Hench, P. K., Cohen, R., & Mitler, M. M. (1989). Fibromyalgia: Effects of amitriptyline, temazepam, and placebo on pain and sleep. *Arthritis and Rheumatism, 32,* S47.

Hudson, J. I., Hudson, M. S., Pliner, L. F., Goldenberg, D. L., & Pope, H. G. (1985). Fibromyalgia and major affective disorder: A controlled phenomenology and family history study. *American Journal of Psychiatry, 142,* 441–466.

Hudson, J. I., & Pope, H. G. (1989). Fibromyalgia and psychopathology: Is fibromyalgia a form of "affective spectrum disorder"? *Journal of Rheumatology, 19,* 15–22.

Jacobsen, S., & Danneskiold-Samsøe, B. (1992). Dynamic muscular endurance in primary fibromyalgia compared with chronic myofascial pain syndrome. *Archives of Physical Medicine and Rehabilitation, 73,* 170–173.

Jacobson, N. S., Follette, W. C., & Revenstorf, D. (1984). Psychotherapy outcome research: Methods for reporting variability and evaluating clinical significance. *Behavior Therapy, 15,* 336–352.

Jacobson, S., & Holm, B. (1992). Muscle strength and endurance compared to aerobic capacity in primary fibromyalgia syndrome. *Clinical and Experimental Rheumatology, 10,* 419–420.

Kaplan, K. H., Goldenberg, D. L., & Galvin-Nadeau, M. (1993). The impact of a meditation-based stress reduction program on fibromyalgia. *General Hospital Psychiatry, 15,* 284–289.

Kerns, R. D., Turk, D. C., & Rudy, T. E. (1985). The West Haven-Yale Multidimensional Pain Inventory (WHYMPI). *Pain, 23,* 345–356.

Kosek, E., Ekholm, J., & Hansson, P. (1996). Sensory dysfunction in fibromyalgia patients with implications for pathogenic mechanisms. *Pain, 68,* 375–383.

Kosek, E., & Hansson, P. (1997). Modulatory influence on somatosensory perception from vibration and heterotopic noxious conditioning stimulation (HNCS) in fibromyalgia patients and healthy subjects. *Pain, 70,* 41–51.

Lautenbacher, S., Rollman, G. B., & McCain, G. A. (1994). Multi-method assessment of experimental and clinical pain in patients with fibromyalgia. *Pain, 59,* 45–53.

Lindh, M. H., Johansson, L. G., Hedberg, M., & Grimby, G. L. (1994). Studies on maximal voluntary muscle contraction in patients with fibromyalgia. *Archives of Physical Medicine and Rehabilitation, 75,* 1217–1222.

MacFarlane, G. J., Croft, P. R., Schollum, J., & Silman, A. J. (1996). Widespread pain: Is an improved classification possible? *Journal of Rheumatology, 23,* 1628–1632.

Martin, L., Nutting, A., Macintosh, B. R., Edworthy, S. M., Butterwick, D., & Cook, J. (1996). An exercise program in the treatment of fibromyalgia. *Journal of Rheumatology, 23,* 1050–1053.

McCain, G. A., Bell, D. A., Mai, F. M., & Halliday, P. D. (1988). A controlled study of the effects of a supervised cardiovascular fitness training program on the manifestations of primary fibromyalgia. *Arthritis and Rheumatism, 31,* 1135–1141.

McDermid, A. J., Rollman, G. B., & McCain, G. A. (1996). Generalized hypervigilance in fibromyalgia: Evidence of perceptual amplification. *Pain, 66,* 133–144.

Mengshoel, A. M., Førre, O., & Komnæs, H. B. (1990). Muscle strength and aerobic capacity in primary fibromyalgia. *Clinical and Experimental Rheumatology, 8,* 475–479.

Mengshoel, A. M., Forseth, K. O., Haugen, M., Walle-Hansen, R., & Førre, O. (1995). Multidisciplinary approach to fibromyalgia: A pilot study. *Clinical Rheumatology, 14,* 165–170.

Moldofsky, H., & Scarisbrick, P. (1976). Induction of neurasthenic musculoskeletal pain syndrome by selective sleep stage deprivation. *Psychosomatic Medicine, 38,* 35–44.

Moldofsky, H., Scarisbrick, P., England, R., & Smythe, H. (1975). Musculosketal symptoms and non-REM sleep disturbance in patients with "fibrositis syndrome" and healthy subjects. *Psychosomatic Medicine, 37,* 341–351.

Murphy, R. M., & Zemlan, F. P. (1987). Differential effects of substance P on serotonin-modulated spinal nociceptive reflexes. *Psychopharmacology, 93,* 118–121.

Nicassio, P. M., Radojevic, V., Weisman, M. H., Schuman, C., Kim, J., Schoenfeld-Smith, K., & Krall, T. (1997). A comparison of behavioral and educational interventions for fibromyalgia. *Journal of Rheumatology, 24,* 2000–2007.

Nielson, W. R., Walker, C., & McCain, G. A. (1992). Cognitive behavioral treatment of fibromyalgia syndrome: Preliminary findings. *Journal of Rheumatology, 19,* 98–103.

Nørregaard, J., Bülow, P. M., Mehlsen, J., & Danneskiold-Samsøe, B. (1994). Biochemical changes in relation to a maximal exercise test in patients with fibromyalgia. *Clinical Physiology, 14,* 159–167.

Nørregaard, J., Lykkegaard, J. J., Mehlgen, J., & Danneskiold-Samsøe, B. (1997). Exercise training in treatment of fibromyalgia. *Journal of Musculoskeletal Pain, 5,* 71–79.

Okifuji, A., Turk, D. C., Sinclair, J. D., Starz, T. W., & Marcus, D. A. (1997). A standardized Manual Tender Point Survey: I. Development and determination of a threshold point for the identification of positive tender points in fibromyalgia syndrome. *Journal of Rheumatology, 24,* 377–383.

Pastor, M. A., Salas, E., Løpez, S., Rodriguez, Sanchez, S., & Pascual, E. (1993). Patients' beliefs about their lack of pain control in primary fibromyalgia syndrome. *British Journal of Rheumatology, 32,* 484–489.

Payne, T. C., Leavitt, F., Garron, D. C., Katz, R. S., Golden, H. E., Glickman, P. B., & Vanderplate, C. (1982). Fibrositis and psychologic disturbance. *Arthritis and Rheumatism, 25,* 213–217.

Prescott, E., Jacobsen, S., Kjoller, M., Bulow, P. M., Danneskiold-Samsøe, B., & Kamper-Jorgesen, J. (1993). Fibromyalgia in the adult Danish population: I. Prevalent study. *Scandinavian Journal of Rheumatology, 22,* 238–242.

Quimby, L. G., Gratwick, G. M., Whitney, C. D., & Block, S. R. (1989). A randomized trial of cyclobenzaprine for the treatment of fibromyalgia. *Journal of Rheumatology, 16,* 140–143.

Reynolds, W. J., Moldofsky, H., Saskin, P., & Lue, F. A.

(1991). The effects of cyclobenzaprine on sleep physiology and symptoms in patients with fibromyalgia. *Journal of Rheumatology, 18,* 452–454.

Richardson, B. P. (1990). Serotonin and nociception. *Annals of the New York Academy of Sciences, 600,* 511–519.

Rollman, G. B., & Lautenbacher, S. (1993). Hypervigilance effects in fibromyalgia: Pain experience and pain perception. In H. Vaeroy & H. Merskey (Eds.), *Progress in fibromyalgia and myofascial pain.* Amsterdam: Elsevier.

Russell, I. J., Fletcher, E. M., Michaleck, J. E., McBroom, P. C., & Hester, G. G. (1991). Treatment of primary fibrositis/fibromyalgia syndrome with ibuprofen and alprazolam: A double-blind, placebo-controlled study. *Arthritis and Rheumatism, 34,* 552–560.

Russell, I. J., Michaleck, J. E., Vipraio, G. A., Fletcher, E. M., Javors, M. A., & Bowden, C. A. (1992). Platelet ^{3}H-imipramine uptake receptor density and serum serotonin levels in patients with fibromyalgia/fibrositis syndrome. *Journal of Rheumatology, 19,* 104–109.

Russell, I. J., Orr, M. D., Littman, B., Ipraio, G. A., Alboukrek, D., Michaleck, J. E., Lopez, Y., MacKillip, F. (1994). Elevated cerebrospinal fluid levels of substance P in patients with the fibromyalgia syndrome. *Arthritis and Rheumatism, 37,* 1593–1601.

Russell, I. J., Vaeroy, H., Javors, M., & Nyberg, F. (1992). Cerebrospinal fluid biogenic amine metabolites in fibromyalgia/fibrositis syndrome and rheumatoid arthritis. *Arthritis and Rheumatism, 35,* 550–556.

Schochat, T., Croft, P., & Raspe, H. (1994). The epidemiology of fibromyalgia. *British Journal of Rheumatology, 33,* 783–786.

Shaver, J. L., Lentz, M., Landis, C. A., Heitkemper, M. M., Buchwald, D. S., & Woods, N. F. (1997). Sleep, psychological distress, and stress arousal in women with fibromyalgia. *Research in Nursing and Health, 20,* 247–257.

Simms, R. W., Felson, D. T., & Goldenberg, D. L. (1991). Development of preliminary criteria for response to treatment in fibromyalgia syndrome. *Journal of Rheumatology, 18,* 1558–1563.

Solomon, D. H., & Liang, M. H. (1997). Fibromyalgia: Scourge of humankind or bane of a rheumatologist's existence? *Arthritis and Rheumatism, 40,* 1553–1555.

Sörensen, J., Bengtsson, A., Ahlner, J., Henriksson, K. G., Ekselius, L., & Bengtsson, M. (1997). Fibromyalgia— are there different mechanisms in the processing of pain? A double blind crossover comparison of analgesic drugs. *Journal of Rheumatology, 24,* 1615–1621.

Starz, T. W., Sinclair, J. D., Okifuji, A., & Turk, D. C. (1997). Putting the finger on fibromyalgia: The Manual Tender Point Survey. *Journal of Musculoskeletal Medicine, 14,* 61–67.

Svebak, S., Anija, R., & Kårstad, S. I. (1993). Task-induced electromyographic activation in fibromyalgia subjects and controls. *Scandinavian Journal of Rheumatology, 22,* 124–130.

Thompson, J. M. (1990). Tension myalgia as a diagnosis at the Mayo Clinic and its relationship to fibrositis, fibromyalgia, and myofascial pain syndrome. *Mayo Clinic Procedures, 65,* 1237–1247.

Turk, D. C. (1996). Biopsychosocial perspective on chronic pain. In R. J. Gatchel & D. C. Turk (Eds.), *Psychological approaches to pain management: A practitioner's handbook.* New York: Guilford Press.

Turk, D. C., & Flor, H. (1989). Primary fibromyalgia is more than tender points: Toward a multiaxial taxonomy. *Journal of Rheumatology, 16,* 80–86.

Turk, D. C., & Okifuji, A. (1997a). Evaluating the role of physical, operant, cognitive, and affective factors in the pain behaviors of chronic pain patients. *Behavior Modification, 21,* 259–280.

Turk, D. C., & Okifuji, A. (1997b). Multidisciplinary approach to pain management: Philosophy, operations, and efficacy. In M. A. Ashburn and L. J. Rice (Eds.), *The management of pain.* Baltimore: Churchill Livingstone.

Turk, D. C., Okifuji, A., Sinclair, J. D., & Starz, T. W. (1996). Pain, disability, and physical functioning in subgroups of patients with fibromyalgia. *Journal of Rheumatology, 23,* 1255–1262.

Turk, D. C., Okifuji, A., Sinclair, J. D., & Starz, T. W. (1998). Interdisciplinary treatment for fibromyalgia syndrome: Clinical and statistical significance. *Arthritis Care and Research, 11,* 186–195.

Turk, D. C., Okifuji, A., Starz, T. W., & Sinclair, J. D. (1996). Effects of type of symptom onset on psychological distress and disability in fibromyalgia syndrome patients. *Pain, 68,* 423–430.

Turk, D. C., Okifuji, A., Starz, T. W., & Sinclair, J. D. (1998). Differential responses by psychosocial subgroups of fibromyalgia syndrome patients to an interdisciplinary treatment. *Arthritis Care and Research, 11,* 397–404.

Turk, D. C., & Rudy, T. E. (1986). Assessment of cognitive factors in chronic pain: A worthwhile enterprise? *Journal of Consulting and Clinical Psychology, 54,* 760–768.

Vaeroy, H., Helle, R., Førre, O., Káss, E., & Terenius, L. (1988). Elevated CSF levels of substance P and high incidence of Raynaud's phenomenon in patients with fibromyalgia: New features for diagnosis. *Pain, 32,* 21–26.

van Denderen, J. C., Boersma, J. W., Zeinstra, P., Hollander, A. P., & van Neerbos, B. R. (1992). Physiological effects of exhaustive physical exercise in primary fibromyalgia syndrome (PFS): Is PFS a disorder of neuroendocrine reactivity? *Scandinavian Journal of Rheumatology, 21,* 35–37.

Wallace, J. F., & Newman, J. P. (1997). Neuroticism and the attentional mediation of dysregulatory psychopathology. *Cognitive Therapy and Research, 21,* 135–156.

White, K. P., & Nielson, W. R. (1995). Cognitive behavioral treatment of fibromyalgia syndrome: A follow-up assessment. *Journal of Rheumatology, 22,* 717–721.

White, K. P., Speechley, M., Harth, M., & Østbye, T. (1995). Fibromyalgia in rheumatology practice: A survey of Canadian rheumatologists. *Journal of Rheumatology, 22,* 722–726.

Wigers, S. H., Stiles, T. C., & Vogel, P. A. (1996). Effects of aerobic exercise versus stress management treatment in fibromyalgia: A 4.5-year prospective study. *Scandinavian Journal of Rheumatology, 25,* 77–86.

Wolfe, F. (1986). Development of criteria for the diagnosis of fibrositis. *American Journal of Medicine, 81,* 99–104.

Wolfe, F. (1996). Fibromyalgia and myofascial pain syndrome. In W. N. Kelley, E. D. Harris, S. S. Ruddy, & B. Clement (Eds.), *Textbook of rheumatology* (5th ed.). Philadelphia: Saunders.

Wolfe, F., Cathey, M. A., & Hawley, D. J. (1994). A double-blind placebo controlled trial of fluoxetine in fibromyalgia. *Scandinavian Journal of Rheumatology, 23,* 255–259.

Wolfe, F., Russell, I. J., Vipraio, G., Ross, K., & Anderson, J. (1997). Serotonin levels, pain threshold, and fibromyalgia symptoms in the general population. *Journal of Rheumatology, 24,* 555–559.

Wolfe, F., Smythe, J. A., Yunus, M. B., Bennett, R. M., Bombardier, C., Goldenberg, D. J., Tugwell, P., Campbell, S. M., Abeles, M., Clark, P., Fam, A. G., Farber, S. J., Fiechtner, J. J., Franklin, C. M., Gatter, R. A., Hamaty, D., Lessard, J., Lichtbroun, A. S., Masi, A. T., McCain, G. A., Reynolds, W. J., Romano, T. J., Russell, I. J., & Sheon, R. P. (1990). The American College of Rheumatology 1990 criteria for the classification of fibromyalgia: Report of the multicenter criteria committee. *Arthritis and Rheumatism, 36,* 160–172.

Yunus, M. B. (1992). Towards a model of pathophysiology of fibromyalgia: Aberrant central pain mechanisms with peripheral modulation. *Journal of Rheumatology, 19,* 846–850.

Yunus, M. B., Dailey, J. W., Aldag, J. C., Masi, A. T., & Jobe, P. C. (1992). Plasma tryptophan and other amino acids in primary fibromyalgia: A controlled study. *Journal of Rheumatology, 19,* 90–94.

Zidar, J., Backman, B., Bengtsson, A., & Henriksson, K. G. (1990). Quantitative EMG and muscle tension in painful muscle in fibromyalgia. *Pain, 40,* 249–254.

Chapter 16

A Vulnerability–Diathesis–Stress Model of Chronic Pain: Herpes Zoster and the Development of Postherpetic Neuralgia

ROBERT H. DWORKIN

SARA M. BANKS

> For that which is but a flea-biting to one, causeth insufferable
> torment to another; and which one by his singular moderation
> and well-imposed carriage can happily overcome, a second is
> no whit able to sustain. . . .
> —ROBERT BURTON, *The Anatomy of Melancholy*, 1621
> (cited in Kendler et al., 1995, p. 833)

The natural history, pathophysiology, and treatment of pain in herpes zoster ("shingles") and postherpetic neuralgia (PHN) have been reviewed in a number of publications (Dworkin & Johnson, 1998; Dworkin & Portenoy, 1996; Kost & Straus, 1996; Loeser, 1990; Portenoy, Duma, & Foley, 1986; Rowbotham, 1994; Watson, 1993; Watson & Evans, 1986), and we therefore do not review this material again in this chapter. Rather, our aim is to present a model of the pathogenesis of chronic pain in patients with herpes zoster. We begin by reviewing representative multifactorial models of the development of chronic pain and then compare these with diathesis–stress models of psychopathology. We then present a vulnerability–diathesis–stress model of chronic pain. Following the description of this model, we review studies of risk factors for chronic pain in herpes zoster patients. The

results of these studies are then used as a basis for applying our model of the pathogenesis of chronic pain to the development of PHN.

MULTIFACTORIAL MODELS OF THE PATHOGENESIS OF CHRONIC PAIN

Despite the long-standing recognition that chronic pain develops from and is maintained by a combination of neurobiological, psychological, and social factors, surprisingly few comprehensive models have been proposed that explain the pathogenesis of chronic pain in terms of an interaction between biological and psychosocial factors. Those models that have done so remain at the conceptual and descriptive stages of model development and have yet to progress to the predictive stage. Although these

247

models have been comprehensive, including multiple factors and suggesting that there are interactive relationships among them, they have not specified how these factors interact nor have they proposed specific testable predictions about these factors and their relationships. We briefly describe three recent and representative biopsychosocial models of chronic pain to illustrate these limitations and the need for additional models of the pathogenesis of chronic pain.

S. F. Dworkin, Von Korff, and LeResche (1992) presented a comprehensive ecological model of chronic pain that synthesizes biopsychosocial components with three perspectives of epidemiology—the population perspective, the developmental perspective, and the ecological perspective. In keeping with the biopsychosocial perspective, these authors proposed an interaction between physiological factors that influence nociception, psychological factors that affect pain perception and appraisal, and social factors that shape pain behaviors and social roles. However, the model went beyond traditional biopsychosocial models in suggesting that the nature of the interactions between the biopsychosocial variables is dynamic rather than static—that these factors are in a dynamic flux and interact differently at different points in time. Consequently, the model introduced the construct of time and operationalized it along two dimensions: life span development and natural history of pain.

Kerns and colleagues (Kerns & Jacob, 1995; Kerns & Payne, 1996) presented a model for the development of persistent pain, disability, and distress in chronic pain patients. They proposed that an individual may have preexisting vulnerabilities in any one or a combination of cognitive, affective, behavioral, social, and biological domains that place that individual at risk for developing chronic pain following the experience of acute pain. In addition, they suggested that the experience of acute pain may create challenges or stressors for the individual across these same domains. Kerns and colleagues hypothesized that individuals in whom there is a match between a vulnerability and a specific challenge or stressor may go on to develop chronic pain and its associated disability and distress. In other words, the stressors associated with acute nociception were hypothesized to activate preexisting vulnerabilities to produce the clinical manifestations of the chronic pain syndrome. Akin to S. F. Dworkin et al.'s (1992) ecological model, the model proposed by Kerns and colleagues emphasized a temporal context in which biopsychosocial variables interact. It also emphasized the social and family context of the pain experience, within which interpersonal interactions exert change

and maintenance effects on the chronic pain patient's functioning primarily by way of operant learning.

Flor and colleagues (Flor & Birbaumer, 1994; Flor, Birbaumer, & Turk, 1990; Turk & Flor, 1984) proposed a psychobiological model of chronic musculoskeletal pain that highlights the dynamic interaction among psychological and biomedical variables. Specifically, these authors suggested several interacting preconditions for the development and maintenance of chronic pain syndromes:

1. *Predisposing factors*—physiological predispositions that consist of a reduced threshold for nociceptive activation that may be related to genetic variables, previous trauma, or social learning experiences and that result in a physiological response stereotypy of a specific body system.
2. *Precipitating stimuli*—persistent aversive external or internal stimuli with negative meaning that activate the sympathetic nervous system and/or various muscular processes and also motivate avoidance responses.
3. *Precipitating responses*—maladaptive information processing of and coping with pain-related social and/or physiological stimuli.
4. *Maintaining processes*—operant, respondent, and observational learning processes that serve to maintain pain.

Similar to the model of Kerns and colleagues (Kerns & Jacob, 1995; Kerns & Payne, 1996), the model proposed by Flor and colleagues emphasized not only that premorbid vulnerabilities interact with stressors but also that learning processes contribute to the maintenance of chronic pain; both models were described by their authors as diathesis–stress models of chronic pain.

Each of these three models proposes that biological, psychological, and social factors are essential in understanding the pathogenesis of chronic pain. Two of the models even conceptualized the development of chronic pain in terms of preexisting vulnerabilities and stressors that combine in some way to produce the clinical manifestations of the chronic pain syndrome. However, none of the models specified which factors are necessary and which are sufficient for the emergence of chronic pain, and none included hypotheses about how the various factors may combine to produce chronic pain (e.g., whether in an additive fashion or through an interaction). Neither the descriptions of the models nor the illustrative figures that accompanied them offered specific predictions that could be subjected to statistical testing.

For example, S. F. Dworkin et al. (1992) suggested that "chronic pain and chronic pain behavior result from the dynamic interaction of nociception, pain perception, pain appraisal, behavioral response to pain, and social roles for persons in pain" (p. 4), but went no further in defining what is meant by dynamic interaction. The authors' suggestion that the biopsychosocial variables coexist in a dynamic flux over two dimensions of time may actually defy generation of testable hypotheses. In fact, the authors state that "the large number of possibilities for the interaction of these biologic, psychologic, and social factors through the different stages of development of pain dysfunction allows for highly varied individual expression of subjective pain experience and overt pain behaviors" (p. 5). Kerns and Jacob (1995) proposed "a congruence between a preexisting vulnerability to develop chronic pain and a specific challenge or stress represented by the pain problem" (p. 330), but again they did not describe precisely what is meant by congruence and whether this congruence must occur within the biological or psychosocial domains or between these domains of functioning. That is, there was little discussion of how or if the vulnerabilities and challenges within the psychosocial domains interact with the vulnerabilities and challenges within the biological domain. Finally, although Flor and colleagues (Flor & Birbaumer, 1994; Flor et al., 1990) described potential mechanisms for how predisposing factors, precipitating stimuli, precipitating responses, and maintaining processes may lead to chronic pain, their descriptions were again largely conceptual and lacked specific testable predictions.

These three models and much current theory and research on chronic pain are based, at least nominally, on a biopsychosocial approach in which the interaction of biological, psychological, and social factors is thought to account for the development of chronic pain (Turk, 1996). Surprisingly, however, in the recently published *Curriculum on Pain for Students in Psychology* (International Association for the Study of Pain, 1997), little attention is paid to the role of psychosocial factors in the etiology of chronic pain, and no mention at all appears of the interaction between biological and psychosocial factors. Perhaps this neglect is a result of the failure of most existing biopsychosocial models of chronic pain to provide an adequate basis for specifying testable hypotheses. In the next section, we briefly review major diathesis–stress models of psychopathology from the perspective of providing a framework for our model of the pathogenesis of chronic pain.

DIATHESIS–STRESS MODELS OF PSYCHOPATHOLOGY

Thirty years ago, Mednick and McNeil (1968) published a now classic article titled "Current methodology in research on the etiology of schizophrenia: Serious difficulties which suggest the use of the high-risk method." They argued that identifying etiological factors had been the goal of much schizophrenia research but that studies of individuals with schizophrenia could not satisfactorily identify such factors because the characteristics of patients may be a consequence either of their disorder or of its treatment. This observation provided the impetus for their proposal that future research on the etiology of schizophrenia could identify causal factors by examining individuals at "high risk" for the later development of the disorder using prospective methods.

This attention to distinguishing causal antecedents of a disorder from abnormalities that may be concomitants or consequences of the disorder remains an important focus of research on psychopathology (e.g., Haynes, 1992; Kraemer et al., 1997). One important result has been the development of diathesis–stress models in which it is hypothesized that psychopathology is caused by specific interactions between biological and psychosocial processes. These models of psychopathology have had enormous heuristic value and are central components of theory and research on diverse psychiatric disorders. Unfortunately, such attempts to specify the nature of the interactions between biological and psychosocial processes have not been characteristic of theory and research on the etiology of chronic pain. When compared to the biopsychosocial approaches discussed in the previous section, the most important advantage of diathesis–stress models of psychopathology is their greater emphasis on the investigation and identification of specific interactions between biological and psychosocial causal factors.

We believe such models are very valuable, not only in understanding psychopathology but also as a guide to future theory and research on the pathogenesis of chronic pain. In this section, we therefore briefly review several diathesis–stress models of the etiology of schizophrenia and depression that can provide a basis for a diathesis–stress model of the pathogenesis of chronic pain. In these models, an interaction between an organic predisposition (the diathesis) and psychosocial stress is hypothesized to account for the development of a disorder. The diathesis may be a genetic vulnerability, a disease, an injury, or another predisposing condition of the organism. The psychosocial stress components of these models have included stressful life events, diminished social support, and various aspects of personality and psychopathology.

Current diathesis–stress models of psychopathology originated in theories of the etiology of schizophrenia (Meehl, 1962; Rosenthal, 1963). Two diathesis–stress models of schizophrenia that have had great influence are Zubin and Spring's (1977) vulnerability model and Nuechterlein and Dawson's (1984) vulnerability-stress model. Zubin and Spring proposed that vulnerability to schizophrenia is a relatively permanent, enduring trait and that "each of us is endowed with a degree of vulnerability that under suitable circumstances will express itself in an episode of schizophrenic illness" (p. 109). They suggested that there are numerous factors contributing to an individual's degree of vulnerability, including not only genetic influences but also acquired components of vulnerability resulting from, for example, perinatal complications, family experiences, and "other life events that either enhance or inhibit the development of subsequent disorder" (p. 109). The essence of Zubin and Spring's model was the proposition that an individual's vulnerability to schizophrenia determines how readily an episode of illness occurs in response to "challenges," which include endogenous biochemical or neurophysiological events as well as exogenous challenges, such as stressful life events. The hypothesized relationship between the degree of vulnerability and the degree of stress needed for illness to occur is illustrated in Figure 16.1. As can be seen from the figure, a highly vulnerable individual will cross the threshold into an episode of illness in response to a minimal

challenge, whereas the individual with a low level of vulnerability requires a considerable degree of stress to become ill.

Nuechterlein and Dawson (1984) proposed a vulnerability–stress model of schizophrenia that was based on the results of longitudinal studies of psychological and psychophysiological abnormalities, stressful life experiences, and outcome in individuals with schizophrenia. Their model included both the vulnerability factors and the environmental challenges that had been discussed by Zubin and Spring (1977). In addition, the model identified specific sets of vulnerability factors and environmental factors that were hypothesized to interact with each other. Importantly, Nuechterlein and Dawson's model also included feedback loops between these factors and transient intermediate states that might or might not progress to a full episode of illness.

The transient intermediate states in this model provide a point at which the vicious cycle between vulnerability and stress and progressively increasing dysfunction can be interrupted. This attention to the possibility of prevention was one of the most important contributions of Nuechterlein and Dawson's (1984) model. Before prevention can be attempted, it is first necessary to identify those individuals who require preventive efforts and to specify the point at which prevention becomes needed. Nuechterlein and Dawson distinguished stable vulnerability indicators, mediating vulnerability factors, and episode indicators. Stable vulnerability indicators are present before, during, and after episodes of illness and, as can be seen from the top panel of Figure 16.2, are independent of changes in symptoms. Nuechterlein and Dawson noted that stable vulnerability indicators could be used to identify individuals at risk for the development of schizophrenia but that their accuracy will be incomplete because the indicators may be present in individuals who never develop the disorder. Mediating vulnerability factors are also deviant during the disorder and when the individual is asymptomatic, but they differ from stable vulnerability indicators because they covary with symptomatology, as the middle panel of Figure 16.2 shows. Mediating vulnerability factors were hypothesized to play a role in the causal chain of events leading to schizophrenia and to become more deviant during the transient intermediate states preceding an episode of the disorder. Changes in mediating vulnerability factors therefore have the potential to predict an impending episode of disorder. Nuechterlein and Dawson distinguished these two types of

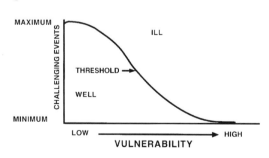

FIGURE 16.1. Relation between vulnerability and challenging events. From Zubin and Spring (1977). Copyright 1977 by the American Psychological Association. Reprinted by permission.

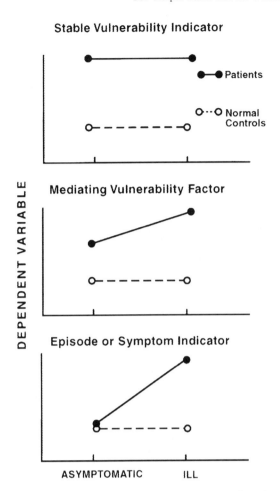

FIGURE 16.2. Characteristic patterns across clinical states for stable vulnerability indicators, mediating vulnerability factors, and episode or symptom indicators. Adapted from Nuechterlein and Dawson (1984).

1992). Similar diathesis–stress models of depression have also been proposed. In an important series of studies, Kendler and colleagues have presented and tested an "integrated etiologic model" of depression (Kendler, Kessler, Neale, Heath, & Eaves, 1993, p. 139; Kendler et al., 1995). This model proposes that at least four major interacting risk factor domains play a role in the etiology of major depression—genetic factors, traumatic experiences, temperament, and interpersonal relations. The model includes the vulnerability factors (e.g., genetic factors, parental loss) and stressful life events that have been the central components of diathesis-stress models of schizophrenia. The results of a recent study provided evidence of a statistically significant interaction between genetic vulnerability and stress in which the increased risk of depression following a stressful life event was significantly greater for individuals with high levels of genetic vulnerability than for those with lower levels of genetic vulnerability (Kendler et al., 1995).

As researchers in schizophrenia and depression have recognized, interactions between diathesis (or vulnerability) and stress may take many forms (e.g., Kendler & Eaves, 1986; Monroe & Simons, 1991). For some disorders, the diathesis may not interact at all with stress, and the development of illness may be a result of additive effects of these factors, as illustrated in the top panel of Figure 16.3. For other disorders, diathesis and stress may interact. For example, stress may have a greater effect in individuals with a more severe diathesis than in individuals with little or no vulnerability, the interaction found by Kendler et al. (1995) and shown in the middle panel of Figure 16.3. It is also possible that stress may have a greater effect in individuals with a moderate diathesis than in those whose diathesis is either high or low in severity, as the bottom panel of Figure 16.3 shows. Other models of the interaction between diathesis and stress are possible, including those with threshold effects for either the diathesis or stress components of the model and those in which diathesis and stress are not independent (e.g., the diathesis may influence the individual's exposure to stress; Kendler & Eaves, 1986; Monroe & Simons, 1991). It is this emphasis on specifying testable hypotheses about interactions between risk factors that we believe is the most valuable feature of diathesis–stress models of psychopathology. Indeed, the strength of these models is in their "in-depth probing of associations between the components of the model, often multidirectional and transpiring over time" (Monroe & Simons, 1991, p. 422).

vulnerability factors from episode or symptom indicators. As can be seen from the bottom panel of Figure 16.2, episode indicators are normal when the individual is asymptomatic—that is, before and after episodes of illness—but are deviant when the individual is ill. Such indicators have little value in distinguishing causal antecedents from consequences of a disorder and no value in predicting onset, but they can be used to evaluate clinical improvement and treatment efficacy (see Kraemer, Gullion, Rush, Frank, & Kupfer, 1994, for another approach to distinguishing the state and trait components of measures used in psychopathology research).

These two models of schizophrenia have been very influential and continue to be revised and refined (e.g., Green, 1998; Nuechterlein et al.,

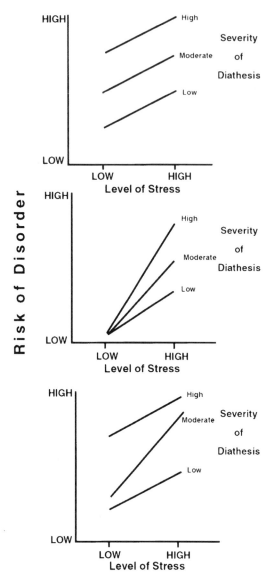

FIGURE 16.3. Hypothetical relationships between diathesis and stress.

A VULNERABILITY–DIATHESIS–STRESS MODEL OF CHRONIC PAIN

In this section, we propose a vulnerability–diathesis–stress model of the pathogenesis of chronic pain that not only includes biological, psychological, and social factors but that also makes it possible to examine hypothesized interactions among these causal factors. In this model, the pathogenesis of chronic pain originates in neurobiological and psychosocial predisposing factors that precede the

onset of pain. The neurobiological factors that predispose individuals to develop chronic pain are undoubtedly diverse. They include the genetic factors that underlie individual differences in physiology or structure that make an individual more likely to develop chronic pain (e.g., sympathetic reactivity, scoliosis). These neurobiological factors also include physiological and structural abnormalities resulting from prior disease or injury or their treatment (e.g., diabetic neuropathy, musculoskeletal pathology). Although it is beyond the scope of this chapter to review these neurobiological predisposing factors, few prospective studies have been conducted that directly address such factors in the development of chronic pain. Accordingly, much of our very limited understanding of neurobiological predispositions for chronic pain is indirect and consists of informed hypotheses that are based on animal models, clinical observations, and studies of patients already suffering from chronic pain.

The psychosocial factors that predispose individuals to develop chronic pain are also likely to be diverse. Such factors probably include pain-relevant personality traits (e.g., somatization, somatic amplification, hypervigilance; Dworkin, 1997a; Gamsa, 1994a, 1994b; McDermid, Rollman, & McCain, 1996) and psychopathology, perhaps especially mood, anxiety, and substance abuse disorders (e.g., Atkinson, Slater, Patterson, Grant, & Garfin, 1991; Banks & Kerns, 1996; Dworkin, 1997a; Dworkin & Gitlin, 1991; Walker, Keegan, Gardner, Sullivan, Katon, et al., 1997). Physical and sexual abuse and other traumatic events (e.g., emotional abuse and neglect) occurring before the onset of pain, perhaps especially during childhood, also appear to be risk factors for the development of chronic pain (e.g., Linton, 1997; Schofferman, Anderson, Hines, Smith, & Keane, 1993; Schofferman, Anderson, Hines, Smith, & White, 1992; Walker, Keegan, Gardner, Sullivan, Bernstein, et al., 1997). In addition, the individual's prior experiences with pain may also be a psychosocial predisposing (or protective) factor (Bachiocco, Scesi, Morselli, & Carli, 1993; Dar, Ariely, & Frenk, 1995), although it is also possible that such experiences result in, for example, central sensitization or increased descending inhibition and could therefore be considered neurobiological predisposing factors. Other pain-relevant attitudes, beliefs, and behaviors that are a consequence of the individual's socialization experiences and that develop during childhood and adolescence are very likely to be psychosocial predisposing factors (e.g., Grunau, Whitfield, Petrie, & Fryer, 1994). For example, modeling of responses to pain and illness by significant others in childhood and adolescence is commonly thought to be an important influence on how an adult responds to a painful injury or illness (e.g., Chaturvedi, 1987; Violon & Giurgea, 1984). Unfortunately, however, virtually all existing studies of this question make it impossible to distinguish the relative effects of shared genetic and environmental influences (but see the adoption study of somatoform disorders conducted by Bohman, Cloninger, von Knorring, & Sigvardsson, 1984).

In our proposed vulnerability–diathesis–stress model of chronic pain, the neurobiological and psychosocial predisposing factors that precede the onset of pain constitute the vulnerability component of the model. This vulnerability is conceptualized as a continuum to which both the neurobiological and psychosocial predisposing factors contribute. Individuals therefore range from low to high in their vulnerability to the development of chronic pain. The neurobiological and psychosocial predisposing factors may contribute to this continuum of vulnerability in an additive fashion, or interactions within and between these two domains of risk factors may occur.

D. Cohen (1974) proposed that the etiology of neurosis is based on two sequential interactions—the first between organismic factors and socialization, which results in the individual having a "disposition" to develop a neurosis, and the second between this disposition and the environmental "condition," which results in the neurosis. As in Cohen's model and the vulnerability models of schizophrenia discussed previously, we propose that the individual's combined neurobiological and psychosocial predisposing factors constitute an enduring vulnerability to chronic pain that interacts with subsequent events. Our model differs from these, however, in proposing that this second interaction occurs between the individual's vulnerability and *two* other antecedents of chronic pain, a diathesis and stress. In our model, the diathesis for chronic pain is not the premorbid neurobiological and psychosocial vulnerability but rather is an illness or injury that causes an episode of acute pain. Because the distinction between acute and chronic pain is based on pain duration (e.g., 3 months; Merskey & Bogduk, 1994), all chronic pain patients, by definition, have suffered from acute pain that did not resolve. The presence of acute pain, therefore, places a person at risk for the subsequent development of chronic pain.

We have therefore proposed that an illness or injury that causes an episode of acute pain is a necessary but not sufficient diathesis for the development of chronic pain (Dworkin, 1991; R. H. Dworkin et al., 1992; Dworkin & Portenoy, 1996). There are many examples of such diatheses: the diathesis for chronic low back pain is an acute back injury; the diathesis for reflex sympathetic dystrophy (complex regional pain syndrome, Type I) is trauma from a surgical procedure or a typically mild injury; the diathesis for phantom limb pain is amputation; and the diathesis for postherpetic neuralgia is acute herpes zoster. Although these diatheses are either present or absent in an individual, when present the diathesis should be considered a continuum of severity. Individuals therefore vary from low to high with respect to how severe their diathesis is, that is, the degree to which their diathesis places them at risk for the development of chronic pain. For most diatheses, this continuum of severity is probably reflected in the severity of the acute pain that accompanies the diathesis. This acute pain, at least in part, reflects the pathophysiological process or processes that not only contribute to acute pain but also increase an individual's risk for the development of chronic pain (Dworkin, 1997a). Strictly speaking, it is these pathophysiological processes that are the diatheses for chronic pain; unfortunately, however, current knowledge of the pathophysiology of chronic pain is limited, and our ability to directly measure the severity of the damage or dysfunction underlying acute and chronic pain is minimal.

As in the diathesis–stress models of psychopathology discussed above, we hypothesize that the diathesis for chronic pain interacts with the degree of psychosocial stress being experienced by the individual during the months directly preceding the injury or illness. A valuable guide to choosing the types of variables to be examined in this domain has been provided by the Dohrenwends and their colleagues (B. S. Dohrenwend & Dohrenwend, 1981; B. P. Dohrenwend, Shrout, Link, Martin, & Skodol, 1986), who propose that the "life-stress process" includes recent stressful life events and the relative absence of ongoing social supports. They suggest that these variables can be antecedents of both physical and psychological disorder—a hypothesis clearly applicable to chronic pain, a disorder which almost always involves both physical and psychological processes.

Relationships between stressful life events and the onset and course of physical illness have been reported frequently, and a number of studies have examined the relationship between stressful life events and various chronic pain syndromes (e.g.,

Affleck, Tennen, Urrows, & Higgins, 1994; Arena, Sherman, Bruno, & Smith, 1990; De Benedittis, Lorenzetti, & Pieri, 1990; Feuerstein, Sult, & Houle, 1985; Gervais et al., 1991; Marbach, Lennon, & Dohrenwend, 1988). Numerous associations between social support and susceptibility to and recovery from physical illness have also been found (S. Cohen, 1988; S. Cohen & Williamson, 1991), and the relationship between social support and chronic pain has been examined in several studies. The results of this research suggest that social support may have detrimental as well as beneficial effects in chronic pain patients (e.g., Gervais et al., 1991; Gil, Keefe, Crisson, & Van Dalfsen, 1987; Kerns, Haythornthwaite, Southwick, & Giller, 1990; Kerns, Southwick, Giller, Haythornthwaite, & Rosenberg, 1991; Kerns & Turk, 1984; Klapow et al., 1995; Marbach et al., 1988; Paulsen & Altmaier, 1995; Turk, Kerns, & Rosenberg, 1992).

There are complex conceptual and methodological issues involved in examining the relationships between social support and stressful life events and the development of a disorder such as chronic pain. Among these are the different models of the relationship between social support and health (e.g., direct effect vs. buffering models; S. Cohen, 1988) and the confounding of social support with preexisting psychological or physical disorder (e.g., psychologically distressed or physically disabled individuals may be less able to establish supportive relationships; Monroe & Steiner, 1986). There are a variety of methods that have been used to measure social support, and numerous distinctions have been made regarding different types, sources, and dimensions of social support (e.g., Dunkel-Schetter & Bennett, 1990; House, Umberson, & Landis, 1988; Smith, Fernengel, Holcroft, Gerald, & Marien, 1994; Wethington & Kessler, 1986).

Not surprisingly, a variety of different models of the relationship between life events and physical illness has also been proposed (S. Cohen & Williamson, 1991), and various suggestions have been made regarding the types of life events that have the greatest impact on health (e.g., Shrout et al., 1989). It has been recognized that the methods used to assess stressful life events have often led to a confounding with the consequences of physical and psychological disorder (e.g., marital difficulties can be a stressful event but they may also reflect psychopathology; B. S. Dohrenwend, Dohrenwend, Dodson, & Shrout, 1984; Schroeder & Costa, 1984); this problem, however, can be addressed by examining separately those life events that do not reflect such consequences. It has also been noted that although most existing measures of life events have focused on temporally discrete events, many physical and psychological disorders may be more closely associated with ongoing chronic stressors (e.g., Monroe & Roberts, 1990; Moos, 1992).

Many life events involve important changes in an individual's relationships, and so stressful life events often involve decreases in an individual's level of social support (Thoits, 1982). Indeed, Moos (1992) has argued that life events and social supports are closely interrelated and tend to influence each other over time and that an integrated approach to their assessment is therefore necessary. It is for this reason that the stress component of our vulnerability–diathesis–stress model of chronic pain comprises both stressful life events and the relative absence of social support (and any detrimental effects of its presence). We propose that this psychosocial stress interacts with the diathesis for chronic pain and that the relationships between diathesis and stress and the development of chronic pain vary depending on the individual's level of vulnerability.

An illustration of our model of the relationships between the individual's vulnerability, diathesis, and psychosocial stress and his or her probability of developing chronic pain is presented in Figure 16.4. As can be seen from the figure, individuals with low levels of neurobiological and psychosocial vulnerability have an overall lower risk of chronic pain than those with greater vulnerability (for clarity, we have chosen to represent vulnerability in this figure as dichotomous even though we believe, as discussed previously, that it is a continuum). Within these levels of vulnerability, diathesis and stress interact, with psychosocial stress having a more pronounced impact when the individual's diathesis is severe (of course, it is also possible that the diathesis and stress interact in a manner different from that depicted here, as illustrated in Figure 16.3). In this model, individuals with low levels of psychosocial and neurobiological vulnerability, little psychosocial stress at the time of their illness or injury, and a diathesis that is minimal in severity are not likely to develop chronic pain. However, those with high vulnerability, considerable stress, and a severe diathesis are at great risk of chronic pain. It is important to note that in this model low levels of vulnerability and stress can be thought of as serving to protect the individual from the development of chronic pain even when the diathesis is severe and that such effects

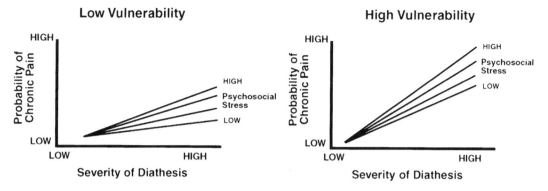

FIGURE 16.4. A vulnerability–diathesis–stress model of the pathogenesis of chronic pain.

have implications for the prevention of chronic pain (Dworkin, 1997a).

To this point, we have discussed chronic pain as something that is either present or absent. However, the nature of the chronic pain outcomes examined in the vulnerability–diathesis–stress model must be clearly specified. The outcome explained in a model of the pathogenesis of chronic pain is, of course, its central feature, and it would not be at all surprising if different risk factors were ultimately identified for different chronic pain outcomes (Dworkin, 1997b). Chronic pain has been defined differently in different studies, with 3 months and 6 months being the minimum durations most often used to identify samples of chronic pain patients. It has also been suggested that a combined measure of pain intensity and duration be used; this measure provides a continuous measure of chronic pain severity and reflects the total "burden" of pain experienced by the patient (Dworkin, Carrington, et al., 1997; Lydick, Epstein, Himmelberger, & White, 1995; Oxman et al., 1994).

But duration and intensity of pain are not the only variables that must be considered in defining chronic pain outcomes. Distinctions can be made between the presence of any pain, however mild; pain of moderate or greater intensity with minimal disability; and pain accompanied by significant disability and psychosocial distress (e.g., Klapow et al., 1993; Turk & Rudy, 1992; Von Korff, Ormel, Keefe, & Dworkin, 1992). Indeed, prospective studies designed to test the vulnerability–diathesis–stress model would make it possible to determine whether patients who are coping well with relatively low levels of chronic pain (so-called adaptive copers; Turk & Rudy, 1992) have, over time, developed effective coping strategies for minimizing pain and disability or whether these are individuals who

from the outset experienced minimal disability because their pain was never more than mild.

The selection of the specific chronic pain outcome to be examined in testing the vulnerability–diathesis–stress model of chronic pain will depend, in part, on the primary goal of the research program. If this goal is understanding the pathogenesis of chronic pain, then any pain—regardless of its intensity and whether or not it is accompanied by disability—may be the outcome of greatest interest. If the primary goal, however, is to design preventive interventions and identify those most in need of such efforts, then outcomes characterized by greater personal suffering and social costs must be examined. This is because screening and prevention programs are costly, especially with prevalent conditions such as acute back pain. Of course, with a large sample and with enough measures administered at baseline and follow-up assessments, it would be possible to examine different chronic pain outcomes within a single study.

The vulnerability–diathesis–stress model is a model of the pathogenesis of chronic pain. Many of the factors included in the model may also be relevant to the maintenance of chronic pain once it is established and may contribute to an explanation of why, for example, chronic pain resolves considerably more quickly in some individuals than in others. Diverse factors have been implicated in the maintenance of chronic pain (e.g., Banks & Kerns, 1996; Feuerstein, Papciak, & Hoon, 1987; Gatchel, 1996; Rohling, Binder, & Langhinrichsen-Rohling, 1995; Waddell, Newton, Henderson, Somerville, & Main 1993), and such maintaining factors would need to be included in any comprehensive model intended to address the duration of chronic pain as well as its origins.

The mechanisms by which chronic pain develops are largely unknown, and it is almost certainly true that these mechanisms are at least partially different for different pain syndromes. Our aim in proposing a vulnerability–diathesis–stress model of chronic pain is to provide a general framework for future research on the pathogenesis of chronic pain. It has been argued that research on psychosocial aspects of physical and psychological disorders has been hindered by a neglect of the possibility that the influence of psychosocial factors may be syndrome-specific (S. Cohen, 1988; S. Cohen & Williamson, 1991). If future prospective studies succeed in identifying antecedents of chronic pain and in distinguishing them from its concomitants and consequences, it will become possible to examine the applicability of our model to the wide variety of chronic pain syndromes that have been described (Merskey & Bogduk, 1994). Indeed, the results of recent studies suggest that our vulnerability–diathesis–stress model of chronic pain may also be applicable to acute pain (e.g., Bélanger, Melzack, & Lauzon, 1989; Syrjala & Chapko, 1995).

HERPES ZOSTER AND POSTHERPETIC NEURALGIA

The varicella-zoster virus (VZV) causes two different diseases: varicella (chicken pox), which typically occurs in children, and herpes zoster, which typically occurs in elderly individuals (Hope-Simpson, 1954; Weller, Witton, & Bell, 1958). The virus establishes latency in sensory ganglia following the varicella infection, and herpes zoster is the reactivation of the virus and its spread from a sensory ganglion to the corresponding dermatome (Hope-Simpson, 1965; Straus et al., 1984). Although the presentation of herpes zoster is variable, a prodrome of dermatomal pain typically precedes the appearance of the rash, which becomes pustular after several days and then forms a crust; thoracic dermatomes are the most commonly affected sites (Hope-Simpson, 1965; Portenoy et al., 1986). The nature and duration of pain in herpes zoster varies greatly among patients, and in a percentage of cases pain in the affected dermatome persists following the acute infection and healing of the rash (Dworkin & Johnson, 1998; Dworkin & Portenoy, 1996). Persisting herpes zoster pain is termed postherpetic neuralgia (PHN), a chronic pain syndrome that can last for years and cause substantial suffering.

As Weller (1992, p. S4) has noted, herpes zoster "will increase as the mean age of our population increases, reflecting both the age-related decay of cellular immunity and the enhanced propensity for malignancy in the elderly." PHN can therefore be expected to increase substantially in the next several decades (Donohue, Choo, Manson, & Platt, 1995; Schmader, 1995), not only because more individuals will develop herpes zoster but also because these elderly individuals will have an increased risk of PHN, as discussed subsequently. Unfortunately, even though numerous approaches are available for the treatment of PHN (Dworkin & Johnson, 1998; Watson, 1993), many patients either fail to respond or derive only limited benefit. Because PHN patients suffer from increased health care utilization, psychological distress, and physical and occupational disability (Davies, Cossins, Bowsher, & Drummond, 1994; Graff-Radford, Kames, & Naliboff, 1986), a substantial increase in the prevalence of PHN would be a major public health concern.

A greater understanding of the pathogenesis of PHN has the potential to contribute to the development of improved treatments and methods for reducing or even eliminating the risk that patients with acute herpes zoster will develop PHN. In the next section, we will review the results of research on risk factors for chronic pain in herpes zoster patients. The identification of individuals with acute herpes zoster who are at increased risk for the development of chronic pain has the potential to guide research on the pathogenesis of PHN. As we will discuss, the results of these studies provide support for a vulnerability–diathesis–stress model of PHN. In addition, knowledge of risk factors could be used in the design of interventions to prevent the development of PHN and to identify those individuals who most need such preventive efforts because of their increased risk of chronic pain (Dworkin, 1997a; see also Kraemer et al., 1997).

RISK FACTORS FOR CHRONIC PAIN IN HERPES ZOSTER PATIENTS

An increasing number of studies are being conducted in which the characteristics of acute herpes zoster patients who develop prolonged herpes zoster pain are being examined. The impetus for these studies has come from two sources. One is the examination of covariates in clinical trials that evaluate the impact of antiviral agents and other drugs on the persistence of pain in herpes zoster patients

(Dworkin, Carrington, et al., 1997). The second is research that seeks to increase understanding of the natural history and pathogenesis of PHN. Before reviewing these studies, we will discuss the different approaches that have been used to assess prolonged pain in herpes zoster—that is, to define the specific outcome for which some patients have an increased risk.

Assessing Prolonged Pain in Herpes Zoster

As discussed elsewhere (Dworkin, 1997c; Dworkin, Carrington, et al., 1997; Dworkin & Portenoy, 1996), a variety of approaches has been used to define PHN and to examine prolonged pain in herpes zoster patients. PHN has been defined as pain persisting after the herpes zoster rash has healed and as pain persisting beyond a specified interval after rash onset or after rash healing; for example, 3 months. The number of patients with persisting herpes zoster pain declines with time, and estimates of the prevalence of PHN—which range from 9% to 34%—vary with the criteria used to define it.

Because of the existence of different definitions of PHN, the use of a diagnosis of PHN in research on herpes zoster pain has recently become controversial. It has been suggested that pain in herpes zoster be considered "as a continuum, rather than distinguishing acute pain from an arbitrary definition of postherpetic neuralgia" (Huff et al., 1993, p. 93). Several recent studies have used this approach to examine the efficacy of various medications in reducing the duration of herpes zoster pain (e.g., Beutner, Friedman, Forszpaniak, Andersen, & Wood, 1995; Degreef, 1994; Whitley et al., 1996; Wood, Kay, Dworkin, Soong, & Whitley, 1996). In these trials, the primary endpoint used in evaluating treatment efficacy is the time from enrollment in the trial to complete cessation of all zoster-associated pain; no distinction is made between acute pain and PHN when herpes zoster pain is examined in this manner (Wood, 1995).

Such analyses of herpes zoster pain considered as a continuum can provide a worthwhile overview of factors associated with pain duration, not only in studies of the efficacy of treatments for reducing pain duration but also in research on risk factors for prolonged herpes zoster pain. One important advantage of examining herpes zoster pain as a continuum is that no assumption is required regarding the point at which PHN begins. However, to the extent that acute herpes zoster pain and PHN differ clinically and have different pathophysiologies, examining pain only as a continuum would be misleading and could impede progress in understanding herpes zoster.

The available data provide considerable support for the validity and importance of examining acute herpes zoster pain and PHN separately (Dworkin, 1997c; Dworkin, Carrington, et al., 1997; Dworkin & Portenoy, 1996). However, the two different approaches to the persistence of pain in herpes zoster are not mutually exclusive; data on herpes zoster pain collected on multiple occasions beginning during the acute infection and continuing for several months thereafter can be examined by using a continuum of pain duration as well as by analyzing the incidence and duration of PHN. Accordingly, in the following discussion of risk factors for chronic pain in patients with herpes zoster, findings based on a diagnosis of PHN, however defined, will be considered together with findings based on analyses in which herpes zoster pain is examined as a continuum of overall pain duration.

Greater Age

Until recently, the only factor that had been associated consistently with an increased risk of PHN was age (Brown, 1976; Burgoon, Burgoon, & Baldridge, 1957; Choo et al., 1997; De Moragas & Kierland, 1957; Guess, Broughton, Melton, & Kurland, 1985; Harding, Lipton, & Wells, 1987; Hope-Simpson, 1975; Raggozzino, Melton, Kurland, Chu, & Perry, 1982; Rogers & Tindall, 1971). PHN is infrequent in patients under 40, but as many as 65% of patients over 60 and 75% of those over 70 have pain at 1 month following healing; the proportion of patients with pain at 1 year approaches 50% in those over 70 (De Moragas & Kierland, 1957).

Greater Acute Pain Severity

The possibility that "there may be a correlation between the duration of pain and the severity of pain on presentation" in herpes zoster was proposed only several years ago as a hypothesis in need of further investigation (Wood et al., 1994, p. 900). However, there are now a considerable number of independent studies that have reported that patients with more severe acute pain are at greater risk for both prolonged herpes zoster pain (assessed as a continuum) and for PHN (Bamford & Boundy, 1968; Beutner et al., 1995; Bruxelle, 1995; Dworkin, Boon, Griffin, & Phung, 1998; Dworkin, Cooper, Walther, & Sweeney, 1997; R. H. Dworkin et al., 1992; Fiddian, 1995; Haanpää & Nurmikko, 1997; Harding et al., 1987; Leijon, Boivie, Roberg, & Forsberg, 1993; McKendrick, Care, Ogan, & Wood, 1994; Molin, 1969; Riopelle, Naraghi, & Grush, 1984; Whitley et al., 1996; Wood et al., 1996). In addition, acute pain severe enough to interfere with activities of daily living has also been reported to be a risk factor for PHN (Choo et al., 1997; Galil, Choo, Donahue, & Platt, 1997). The majority of these studies examined the persistence of pain using a 6–month follow-up period; however, greater acute pain severity has also been reported to predict greater duration of pain in patients with pain resolving before rash healing (Bamford & Boundy, 1968), as well as presence of PHN 9 years after an acute herpes zoster infection (McKendrick et al., 1994).

A variety of research designs, pain measures, and approaches to examining prolonged pain have been used in these studies, and several have serious methodological shortcomings, including small sample sizes and the use of retrospective methods. Nevertheless, given that a relationship between greater acute pain severity and prolonged herpes zoster pain has been found in all of these studies, this relationship can now be considered an established finding. The focus of future research should therefore become the identification of mechanisms accounting for this relationship. In pursuing this task, a priority should be to conduct a careful examination of the specific aspects of acute herpes zoster pain that predict the development of chronic pain (Dworkin, 1997a, 1997b).

Few of the studies that have reported a relationship between the severity of acute herpes zoster pain and PHN have examined the different types of pain associated with herpes zoster. For example, is the predominant quality of patients' acute herpes zoster pain—whether allodynia, burning, throbbing, or stabbing (Dworkin & Portenoy, 1996)—associated with their risk of developing PHN? Burning pain is more common in PHN patients than in acute herpes zoster patients, who are more likely to report sharp, stabbing pain (Bhala, Ramamoorthy, Bowsher, & Yelnoorker, 1988; Bowsher, 1993). In addition, burning pain was much *less* likely to be reported by PHN patients who had been treated with acyclovir during their acute infection compared to PHN patients who had not received acyclovir

(Bowsher, 1992, 1993). Acyclovir is an antiviral agent that inhibits VZV replication and may thereby limit the neural damage contributing to the development of PHN. Considered together, the greater prevalence of burning pain in PHN compared to acute herpes zoster and the reduced burning pain in PHN patients treated with acyclovir suggest that burning pain may reflect an important pathophysiological mechanism in the development of prolonged herpes zoster pain. It could therefore be hypothesized that acute herpes zoster patients with prominent burning pain are at greater risk for the development of PHN (Dworkin, 1997a). Preliminary reports of the results of two recent studies, however, suggested that patients who described their acute herpes zoster pain as sharp (Johnson, Shukla, & Fletcher, 1995) and who had mechanical allodynia (Haanpää & Nurmikko, 1997) were more likely to have pain that persisted 3 months after rash onset. Additional prospective studies are therefore needed to resolve the relationship between pain quality in herpes zoster and the development of PHN.

Greater Rash Severity

Several studies have reported that greater severity of the cutaneous manifestation of the acute herpes zoster infection is associated with prolonged herpes zoster pain and the development of PHN (Choo et al., 1997; Dworkin et al., 1998; Higa, Dan, Manabe, & Noda, 1988; Higa, Noda, Manabe, Sato, & Dan, 1992; Higa et al., 1997; Whitley et al., 1996; Wildenhoff et al., 1981; Wildenhoff, Ipsen, Esmann, Ingemann-Jensen, & Poulsen, 1979; Wilson, 1986). Rash severity has been assessed using a variety of methods in these studies. The duration of time until the occurrence of various aspects of rash healing has been examined, including assessments of time to cessation of new vesicle formation and time to complete crusting. In addition, assessments of rash severity have been conducted, including counts of the number of vesicles and ratings of the proportion of the dermatome affected. Few studies, however, have reported assessments of rash severity on multiple occasions, which would allow rash progression from onset to healing to be examined. Even fewer studies have evaluated the interrater reliability of their ratings of rash severity, ratings which often involve judgments with a subjective component.

Although scarring in the affected dermatome is common in patients following healing of the acute herpes zoster rash, there are no studies that have examined the relationship between the severity of the acute zoster rash and the development of scarring. Two studies, however, have examined the relationship between scarring and PHN; it has been reported that the presence (Battock, Finn, & Barnes, 1990; Nurmikko & Bowsher, 1990) and extent (Battock et al., 1990) of scarring distinguished patients with PHN from herpes zoster patients whose pain did not persist. Because it is likely that scarring is a consequence of a more severe rash during the acute infection, these findings are consistent with the data suggesting that greater rash severity is a risk factor for prolonged pain. It has also been reported that scarring is less severe in PHN patients with predominantly allodynic pain (Rowbotham & Fields, 1989), which suggests that scarring, and perhaps the more severe rash this implies, may be differentially associated with pain quality in herpes zoster and PHN.

Greater Sensory Dysfunction

A fourth risk factor that has been identified by several groups of investigators is the presence of greater sensory deficits in the affected dermatome during acute herpes zoster. Evaluations of sensory dysfunction in the affected dermatome have included clinical assessments of hypesthesia, as well as quantitative sensory testing. Acute herpes zoster patients with greater sensory abnormalities (e.g., hypesthesia, elevated thermal and vibration thresholds) in the affected dermatome, compared to the contralateral unaffected dermatome, were found to be at greater risk for PHN in most (Bruxelle, 1995; Leijon et al., 1993; Noda, Dan, Manabe, & Higa, 1987; Nurmikko, Rasanen, & Hakkinen, 1990) but not all (Haanpää & Nurmikko, 1997) of these studies.

Elevated vibration thresholds *outside* the affected dermatome (i.e., in the hands and feet) have also been found to distinguish herpes zoster patients who developed PHN from those who did not (Baron, Haendler, & Shulte, 1997). It was concluded that these results suggest that a generalized subclinical impairment of A-beta afferent fiber function (i.e., large fiber polyneuropathy) contributes to the development of PHN. Indirect support for this conclusion is provided by the report of an almost twofold greater risk of PHN in patients who developed herpes zoster after the onset of diabetes compared to patients who developed zoster before

they developed diabetes (McCulloch, Fraser, & Duncan, 1982); as the authors suggest, diabetic polyneuropathy may render the nerves more susceptible to damage from VZV.

It has also been reported that there is greater sensory dysfunction in the affected dermatome in patients with PHN than in herpes zoster patients whose pain did not persist (Leijon et al., 1993; Nurmikko & Bowsher, 1990; Wildenhoff et al., 1979, 1981). The results of these studies indicate that sensory dysfunction can persist well beyond the acute phase of herpes zoster and that it is a frequent concomitant of prolonged pain.

More Pronounced Immune Response

Greater magnitude and duration of humoral and cell-mediated immune responses in acute herpes zoster patients have been reported to predict prolonged pain (Dan, Higa, Tanaka, & Mori, 1983; Higa et al., 1988, 1992). It is possible that immune responses during acute herpes zoster predict prolonged pain because a more pronounced immune response reflects a more severe acute infection.

Several findings are consistent with this hypothesis. VZV-specific cell-mediated immune responses reach their maximum 1 to 2 weeks after the onset of herpes zoster, which is usually the time of maximal infection (Arvin, Pollard, Rasmussen, & Merigan, 1978). In addition, measures of both humoral and cell-mediated immunity were found to be lower in acyclovir-treated compared to placebo-treated acute zoster patients (Mitchell, Gehrz, & Balfour, 1986); although the group differences were not statistically significant, the dose of acyclovir used (400 mg, five times daily) in this study was only half of what is now accepted as adequate antiviral treatment for herpes zoster. In discussing their results, the investigators suggested that the lower values of the immune response measures may have reflected a reduced "antigenic burden" resulting from the inhibition of viral replication associated with acyclovir treatment (Mitchell et al., 1986). Similarly, antibody titers were found to be significantly lower in children with varicella treated with acyclovir compared to those treated with placebo (Balfour et al., 1990). And in research on two other herpes viruses—herpes simplex virus and Epstein–Barr virus—it has been noted that elevated antibody titers "are thought to reflect the increased production of viral antigens after reactivation" (Glaser & Kiecolt-Glaser, 1994, p. 251).

Presence of a Prodrome

In 70–90% of herpes zoster patients, a prodrome of dermatomal pain begins several days before the appearance of the characteristic rash (Beutner et al., 1995; Dworkin et al., 1998; Rogers & Tindall, 1971). The herpes zoster prodrome is often accompanied by other symptoms—including fatigue, dysesthesias, and headache—and some patients may have these prodromal symptoms in the absence of pain. In three recent studies, the presence of prodromal pain and symptoms was found to be associated with prolonged pain and the development of PHN (Beutner et al., 1995; Choo et al., 1997; Dworkin, Boon, & Griffin, 1995). In future studies of risk factors for PHN, it will be necessary to carefully distinguish prodromal pain from other prodromal symptoms. A series of patients in whom prodromal pain preceded the rash by 7 to more than 100 days has been described (Gilden et al., 1991), and so it will also be important to examine prodrome duration in future research.

Antiviral Therapy

It is well beyond the scope of this chapter to review the literature on the efficacy of antiviral therapy (and other treatments) in acute herpes zoster patients on the development of PHN and on prolonged herpes zoster pain assessed as a continuum. Recent studies have demonstrated that treatment of acute herpes zoster patients with the antiviral agents acyclovir, famciclovir, and valacyclovir reduces both the risk of developing PHN and the overall duration of pain (Beutner et al., 1995; Dworkin et al., 1998; Jackson, Gibbons, Meyer, & Inouye, 1997; Tyring et al., 1995; Wood et al., 1996). In the context of identifying risk factors, the *absence* of antiviral therapy in acute herpes zoster patients may therefore be considered a risk factor for PHN.

Fever

In one study, fever greater than 38°C during acute herpes zoster was reported to predict the development of PHN (Wildenhoff et al., 1981).

Sex

Several investigators have examined whether there is a relationship between the patient's sex and the risk of prolonged pain, and the majority of these studies have found that men and women are equally likely to develop PHN (Beutner et al., 1995; Brown, 1976; Choo et al., 1997; Dworkin et al., 1995, 1998; Fiddian, 1995; Harding et al., 1987; Hope-Simpson, 1975; Wildenhoff et al., 1979, 1981; Wood et al., 1996).

Dermatome

Several investigators have examined the relationship between the specific dermatome affected in acute herpes zoster and the risk of prolonged pain (Burgoon et al., 1957; Choo et al., 1997; De Moragas & Kierland, 1957; Fiddian, 1995; Higa et al., 1997; Hope-Simpson, 1975; Wildenhoff et al., 1979, 1981). Although the results of several of these studies have suggested that the likelihood of prolonged pain is greater in patients with ophthalmic or trigeminal zoster, this relationship has not been found consistently. The results of a recent preliminary analysis of the first 476 herpes zoster patients out of an anticipated total of 2000 suggested that pain was present in a higher proportion of patients with ophthalmic zoster than in patients with zoster in other dermatomes at 6 months after rash onset; the difference between these two groups, however, was not statistically significant (Stillman, 1997). Considered together with the results of previous research, these data suggest that even if future studies demonstrate that PHN is more likely to occur in patients with ophthalmic zoster, it is unlikely that this will be a risk factor with substantial potency (Kraemer et al., 1997).

Psychosocial Risk Factors

The risk factors for PHN discussed to this point have consisted of demographic and biomedical characteristics of patients with acute herpes zoster. It has also been suggested that psychosocial factors might play a role in determining which patients with acute herpes zoster will develop PHN. Pilowsky (1977) proposed that patients who develop PHN are characterized by a constellation of certain premorbid personality traits and stressful life events. Although this hypothesis was based on psychiatric interviews with patients who had suffered from PHN for as long as 15 years, several recent studies have provided data that are consistent with the hypothesis that psychosocial factors play a role in the development of both acute herpes zoster and PHN. In two studies of risk factors for acute herpes zoster, Schmader and colleagues reported that herpes zoster patients reported increased stressful life events and decreased social support preceding the onset of their infection compared to matched controls who had not had herpes zoster (Schmader, George, Burchett, & Pieper, 1998; Schmader, Studenski, Macmillan, Grufferman, & Cohen, 1990).

The results of other studies have suggested that greater levels of psychological distress (e.g., depression, anxiety) in herpes zoster patients may be risk factors for the development of PHN. In one cross-sectional study, PHN patients had more symptoms of anxiety and rated their past experiences of pain as more intense than herpes zoster patients whose pain had not persisted (Rose, Klenerman, Atchison, & Slade, 1992). In this study, PHN patients had also experienced *fewer* stressful life events in the preceding year, a finding that the authors attributed to the withdrawal from activities that characterizes chronic pain patients. The results of a second cross-sectional study that attempted to identify predictors of PHN "showed a higher frequency of psychopathological impairment" in patients with PHN than in patients with a history of herpes zoster who did not develop chronic pain (Leplow, Lamparter, Risse, & Wassilev, 1990, p. 46). In a recent retrospective study of patients with a history of herpes zoster, those who reported having other diseases and/or psychosocial stress at the onset of their infection were significantly more likely to have PHN, changed daily activities, and lower levels of well-being than patients who reported no other diseases or psychosocial stress at the onset of their infection (Bergbom Engberg, Gröndahl, & Thibom, 1995).

The results of these three studies are consistent with the existence of psychosocial risk factors for PHN. However, the use of cross-sectional and retrospective methods makes it impossible to determine whether psychosocial distress is a risk factor for PHN or whether the *recollection* of such distress being present at the time of the acute herpes zoster infection is simply one of the consequences of PHN. Prospective studies are necessary to determine whether variables that may plausibly be either antecedents or consequences of chronic pain are risk factors (Dworkin, 1991; Kraemer et al., 1997). In a prospective study of a small sample of herpes zoster patients, patients who developed PHN had greater depression, anxiety, and disease conviction and lower life satisfaction during their acute infection than patients who did not develop PHN (R. H. Dworkin et al., 1992). Preliminary analyses of the data from a recent prospective study of a larger sample of acute herpes zoster patients have provided additional evidence that psychosocial factors, including disease conviction and somatosensory amplification, are associated with an increased risk of PHN independently of age and acute pain severity (Dworkin, Cooper, et al., 1997). Two chronic stressors—poor physical health and financial resources—also predicted PHN in this study, but these did not remain significant when age and acute pain severity were controlled (Dworkin, Cooper, et al., 1997). Considered together, the results of the research on the role of psychosocial factors in the natural history of herpes zoster suggest that these factors may play a role in the onset of acute herpes zoster as well as in the development of PHN; this conclusion is consistent with the evidence suggesting that psychosocial factors contribute to the onset and course of other herpes virus infections (Glaser & Kiecolt-Glaser, 1994).

Associations among Risk Factors

There are important unanswered questions about risk factors for PHN that must be addressed in future research. One involves the nature of the associations among the risk factors that have been identified for PHN. For example, it would be valuable to know whether greater acute pain severity and greater rash severity are associated in acute herpes zoster patients. This relationship, however, has been examined in only two studies: In one of these, greater acute pain severity and greater rash duration were associated (Molin, 1969), whereas in the other, acute pain severity and rash severity (assessed by the number of vesicles) were uncorrelated (Bruxelle, 1995). A second important question is whether there are interactions among the risk factors for PHN. For example, is greater acute pain severity a risk factor for PHN in both younger and older patients, or is this relationship limited to only one age group? Similarly, few studies have examined treatment–covariate interactions in the development of PHN. Such analyses have the potential to reveal whether certain herpes zoster patients benefit more from treatment than others. For example, although it has been suggested that intravenous acyclovir has a greater effect on acute pain in older herpes zoster patients than in younger patients (Peterslund et al., 1981), the available data do not directly address whether antiviral treatment has a significantly greater effect on the risk of PHN in older patients.

Future Directions for Research on Risk Factors for Postherpetic Neuralgia

The most interesting unanswered question about risk factors for PHN is also the one with the longest history—that is, why is older age a risk factor for PHN (Wall, 1993)? It has been hypothesized that age is associated with the development of PHN because older patients have more severe acute herpes zoster infections (Higa et al., 1988, 1997). The results of several studies, however, are not entirely consistent with this hypothesis. Although significant associations between older age and greater rash duration have been reported (Harding et al., 1987; Wildenhoff et al., 1979, 1981), older age is inconsistently associated with greater lesion severity (Higa et al., 1988, 1997) and is not associated with greater acute pain severity (Bamford & Boundy, 1968; Dworkin, Cooper, et al., 1997; Harding et al., 1987). Moreover, the results of several recent studies suggest that age and acute pain severity make independent contributions to predicting which herpes zoster patients develop PHN (Beutner et al., 1995; Dworkin et al., 1998; Dworkin, Cooper, et al., 1997; Wood et al., 1996). To the extent that acute pain severity reflects a more severe acute infection, these findings suggest that the increased risk of PHN in the elderly is not completely accounted for by more severe acute infections and that this increased risk reflects an additional pathophysiological process. Indeed, Hope-Simpson (1967) recognized that although severe acute infections are frequently associated with PHN, even mild cases of zoster are sometimes followed by PHN.

One pathophysiological process that might contribute to an increased risk of PHN in the elderly involves nervous system senescence. The recent report, discussed previously, that large fiber polyneuropathy in acute herpes zoster patients predicts the development of PHN is consistent with this hypothesis and merits continued investigation (Baron et al., 1997). A second process that might explain the increased risk of PHN in the elderly involves immunopathogenesis. It has been hypothesized that autoimmune phenomena and age-associated disturbances in cytokine production, possibly involving cytokine neurotoxicity, may result in nerve damage and contribute to the development of prolonged pain in patients with herpes zoster (Dworkin &

Portenoy, 1996; Weksler, 1994). The contribution of immunopathological processes to the development of PHN has not been examined directly; however, this hypothesis is consistent not only with the greater risk of PHN in the elderly but also with several other recent findings, including the existence of pain-free intervals in PHN, evidence of inflammation in patients with well-established PHN, and possibly equivalent risks of PHN in immunocompromised and immunocompetent patients (Dworkin & Johnson, 1998; Dworkin & Portenoy, 1996).

A VULNERABILITY-DIATHESIS-STRESS MODEL OF POSTHERPETIC NEURALGIA

In this section, we will apply the vulnerability-diathesis–stress model of chronic pain presented above to the development of PHN.[1] As discussed previously, the vulnerability component of the model comprises neurobiological and psychosocial predisposing factors. Two of the risk factors for PHN—age and generalized large fiber impairment—can be considered neurobiological predisposing factors. Although older age may reflect psychosocial predisposing factors, as well as neurobiological predisposing factors, the results of a recent study suggested that the effect of age could not be accounted for by increased psychosocial distress in older patients (Dworkin, Cooper, et al., 1997). It is therefore likely that older age reflects neurobiological predisposing factors, and it is possible that subclinical large fiber polyneuropathy explains the greater risk of PHN in the elderly (Baron et al., 1997). Immunopathological processes may also account for the increased risk of PHN in older patients. It is important to note, however, that nervous system senescence and the autoimmune phenomena discussed previously are not mutually exclusive explanations of the relationship between age and PHN.

Several psychosocial risk factors for PHN have been identified and can be considered psychosocial predisposing factors contributing to an individual's vulnerability for PHN. As reviewed previously, symptoms of psychological distress—for example, depression and anxiety—have been found to distinguish patients with PHN from herpes zoster patients whose pain did not persist and to predict

---

[1] This is a revised and expanded version of a diathesis–stress model of PHN that was proposed recently (Dworkin & Portenoy, 1996).

the development of PHN in several recent cross-sectional and prospective studies. The results of these studies also suggest that somatosensory amplification, disease conviction, and increased pain sensitivity are associated with the development of PHN. Because these variables and acute pain severity have been found to make independent contributions to predicting PHN, they presumably reflect premorbid personality traits and not just the severity of the acute herpes zoster infection.

The diathesis component of the vulnerability-diathesis–stress model of PHN is the severity of the acute herpes zoster infection, and, more precisely, the neural damage that accompanies it. Except for age and the psychosocial variables, the risk factors for PHN that have been identified—acute pain severity, rash severity, sensory dysfunction, more pronounced immune responses, presence of a prodrome, fever, and the absence of antiviral therapy during acute zoster—can all be considered concomitants of a more severe acute herpes zoster infection. Several of these risk factors have been identified by independent groups of investigators, and they provide appreciable support for the conclusion that there is a greater risk of PHN in patients with more severe acute herpes zoster infections. Indeed, over 30 years ago, Hope-Simpson (1967) proposed that patients with more severe acute herpes zoster infections are more likely to develop PHN. More severe acute herpes zoster infections are accompanied by greater neural damage, and it has been proposed that this neural damage contributes prominently to the development of PHN in patients with herpes zoster (Bennett, 1994; Dworkin & Portenoy, 1996; for recent reviews of the pathophysiology of PHN, see Dworkin & Johnson, 1998; Rowbotham & Fields, 1996).

The stress component of our vulnerability-diathesis–stress model comprises stressful life events and social support and is hypothesized to interact with the diathesis in accounting for the development of PHN. As discussed previously, certain chronic stressors may be risk factors for PHN (Dworkin, Cooper, et al., 1997), and Schmader and colleagues (Schmader et al., 1990, 1998) have reported that various aspects of stress and social support appear to be risk factors for an acute herpes zoster infection. The risk of PHN is hypothesized to increase as both the severity of the neural damage and the severity of the psychosocial stress increase. As illustrated in Figure 16.3, the interaction between the diathesis and stress may have different forms. Preliminary analyses of the data from a prospective study of risk factors for PHN were consistent with the model illustrated in Figure 16.5 in suggesting that psychosocial factors may have a more pronounced effect on the risk of PHN in patients with more severe herpes zoster infections (Dworkin, Cooper, et al., 1997). Note that vulnerability is represented in this figure as a function of age and psychological distress—two risk factors for PHN that reflect putative neurobiological and psychosocial predisposing factors that must be examined in much greater detail in future prospective studies of patients with herpes zoster.

Although it has often been assumed that the diathesis and stress components of diathesis–stress models are independent, individuals with a more severe diathesis may be more likely to incur stressful life events, putting them at even greater risk of developing a disorder (Kendler & Eaves, 1986; Monroe & Simons, 1991; see also Walker, Downey, & Nightingale's [1989] discussion of the conceptual and statistical implications of correlations among

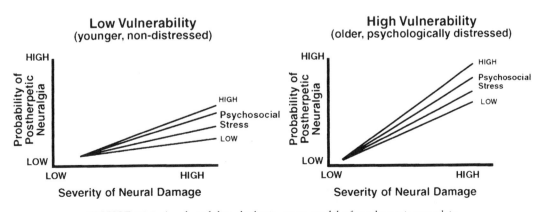

FIGURE 16.5. A vulnerability–diathesis–stress model of postherpetic neuralgia.

risk factors). The model of PHN presented here makes the assumptions that not only are the diathesis for PHN and the psychosocial stress with which it interacts independent, but also that the individual's neurobiological and psychosocial vulnerability is independent of the severity of the diathesis and the level of stress. However, a variety of bidirectional relationships between infectious and behavioral processes have been reported (e.g., Maier, Watkins, & Fleshner, 1994), and it is possible that individuals with more severe acute zoster infections experience increased psychosocial stress as a result of their infections, putting them at even greater risk of prolonged pain. Furthermore, although there is compelling evidence that a decrease in cell-mediated immunity plays an important role in the onset of herpes zoster (Gershon, 1993), the factors accounting for the severity of the acute infection have not been well studied. It is possible that those individuals who have high premorbid psychosocial vulnerability or who are experiencing stressful life events at the onset of their acute herpes zoster have more severe infections, which would put them at even greater risk of PHN. Although such relationships between vulnerability factors, diathesis, and stress do not invalidate the vulnerability–diathesis–stress model, they should be taken into account in future research.

CONCLUSIONS

We suggested previously that current research on chronic pain is characterized by the very same "serious difficulties which suggest the use of the high-risk method" identified by Mednick and McNeil (1968, p. 681)—that is, the difficulties associated with attempting to identify factors that contribute to the development of a disorder in patients who already have the disorder. Prospective studies of acute pain patients and other high-risk groups (e.g., the offspring of chronic pain patients), although requiring a major commitment of time and resources, are needed to address these difficulties. We believe that the goals of research on chronic pain are to understand its pathogenesis, improve its treatment, and prevent its development. To achieve these goals, prospective multivariate studies with testable hypotheses about the interactions among biological, psychological, and social risk factors are needed, and it is our hope that the vulnerability–diathesis–stress model presented in this chapter is a step in this direction.

ACKNOWLEDGMENT

Preparation of this chapter was supported in part by a research grant from the National Institute of Neurological Disorders and Stroke (No. NS-30714).

REFERENCES

Affleck, G., Tennen, H., Urrows, S., & Higgins, P. (1994). Person and contextual features of daily stress reactivity: Individual differences in relations of undesirable daily events with mood disturbance and chronic pain intensity. *Journal of Personality and Social Psychology, 66,* 329–340.

Arena, J. G., Sherman, R. A., Bruno, G. M., & Smith, J. D. (1990). The relationship between situational stress and phantom limb pain: Cross-lagged correlational data from six month pain logs. *Journal of Psychosomatic Research, 34,* 71–77.

Arvin, A. M., Pollard, R. B., Rasmussen, L. E., & Merigan, T. C. (1978). Selective impairment of lymphocyte reactivity to varicella-zoster virus antigen among untreated patients with lymphoma. *Journal of Infectious Diseases, 137,* 531–540.

Atkinson, J. H., Slater, M. A., Patterson, T. L., Grant, I., & Garfin, S. R. (1991). Prevalence, onset, and risk of psychiatric disorders in men with chronic low back pain: A controlled study. *Pain, 45,* 111–121.

Bachiocco, V., Scesi, M., Morselli, A. M., & Carli, G. (1993). Individual pain history and familial pain tolerance models: Relationships to post-surgical pain. *Clinical Journal of Pain, 9,* 266–271.

Balfour, H. H., Jr., Kelly, J. M., Suarez, C. S., Heussner, R. C., Englund, J. A., Crane, D. D., McGuirt, P. V., Clemmer, A. F., & Aeppli, D. M. (1990). Acyclovir treatment of varicella in otherwise healthy children. *Journal of Pediatrics, 116,* 633–639.

Bamford, J. A. C., & Boundy, C. A. P. (1968). The natural history of herpes zoster (shingles). *Medical Journal of Australia, No. 13,* 524–528.

Banks, S. M., & Kerns, R. D. (1996). Explaining high rates of depression in chronic pain: A diathesis–stress framework. *Psychological Bulletin, 119,* 95–110.

Baron, R., Haendler, G., & Schulte, H. (1997). Afferent large fiber polyneuropathy predicts the development of postherpetic neuralgia. *Pain, 73,* 231–238.

Battock, T. M., Finn, R., & Barnes, R. M. R. (1990). Observations on herpes zoster: 1. Residual scarring and postherpetic neuralgia; 2. Handedness and the risk of infection. *British Journal of Clinical Practice, 44,* 596–598.

Bélanger, E., Melzack, R., & Lauzon, P. (1989). Pain of first-trimester abortion: A study of psychosocial and medical predictors. *Pain, 36,* 339–350.

Bennett, G. J. (1994). Hypotheses on the pathogenesis of herpes zoster-associated pain. *Annals of Neurology, 35* (Suppl.), S38–S41.

Bergbom Engberg, I., Gröndahl, G.-B., & Thibom, K. (1995). Patients' experiences of herpes zoster and postherpetic neuralgia. *Journal of Advanced Nursing, 21,* 427–433.

Beutner, K. R., Friedman, D. J., Forszpaniak, C., Andersen, P. L., & Wood, M. J. (1995). Valaciclovir compared with acyclovir for improved therapy for herpes zoster in immunocompetent adults. *Antimicrobial Agents and Chemotherapy, 39*, 1546–1553.

Bhala, B. B., Ramamoorthy, C., Bowsher, D., & Yelnoorker, K. N. (1988). Shingles and postherpetic neuralgia. *Clinical Journal of Pain, 4*, 169–174.

Bohman, M., Cloninger, C. R., von Knorring, A.-L., & Sigvardsson, S. (1984). An adoption study of somatoform disorders: III. Cross-fostering analysis and genetic relationship to alcoholism and criminality. *Archives of General Psychiatry, 41*, 872–878.

Bowsher, D. (1992). Acute herpes zoster and postherpetic neuralgia: Effects of acyclovir and outcome of treatment with amitriptyline. *British Journal of General Practice, 42*, 244–246.

Bowsher, D. (1993). Sensory change in postherpetic neuralgia. In C. P. N. Watson (Ed.), *Herpes zoster and postherpetic neuralgia* (pp. 97–107). Amsterdam: Elsevier.

Brown, G. R. (1976). Herpes zoster: Correlation of age, sex, distribution, neuralgia, and associated disorders. *Southern Medical Journal, 69*, 576–578.

Bruxelle, J. (1995). Prospective epidemiologic study of painful and neurologic sequelae induced by herpes zoster in patients treated early with oral acyclovir. *Neurology, 45*(Suppl. 8), S78–S79.

Burgoon, C. F., Burgoon, J. S., & Baldridge, G. D. (1957). The natural history of herpes zoster. *Journal of the American Medical Association, 164*, 265–269.

Chaturvedi, S. K. (1987). Family morbidity in chronic pain patients. *Pain, 30*, 159–168.

Choo, P. W., Galil, K., Donahue, J. G., Walker, A. M., Spiegelman, D., & Platt, R. (1997). Risk factors for postherpetic neuralgia. *Archives of Internal Medicine, 157*, 1217–1224.

Cohen, D. B. (1974). On the etiology of neurosis. *Journal of Abnormal Psychology, 83*, 473–479.

Cohen, S. (1988). Psychosocial models of the role of social support in the etiology of physical disease. *Health Psychology, 7*, 269–297.

Cohen, S., & Williamson, G. M. (1991). Stress and infectious disease in humans. *Psychological Bulletin, 109*, 5–24.

Dan, K., Higa, K., Tanaka, K., & Mori, R. (1983). Herpetic pain and cellular immunity. In T. Yokota & R. Dubner (Eds.), *Current topics in pain research and therapy* (pp. 293–305). Amsterdam: Excerpta Medica.

Dar, R., Ariely, D., & Frenk, H. (1995). The effect of past-injury on pain threshold and tolerance. *Pain, 60*, 189–193.

Davies, L., Cossins, L., Bowsher, D., & Drummond, M. (1994). The cost of treatment for post-herpetic neuralgia in the UK. *PharmacoEconomics, 6*, 142–148.

De Benedittis, G., Lorenzetti, A., & Pieri, A. (1990). The role of stressful life events in the onset of chronic primary headache. *Pain, 40*, 65–75.

De Moragas, J. M., & Kierland, R. R. (1957). The outcome of patients with herpes zoster. *AMA Archives of Dermatology, 75*, 193–196.

Degreef, H. (1994). Famciclovir, a new oral antiherpes drug: Results of the first controlled clinical study demonstrating its efficacy and safety in the treatment of uncomplicated herpes zoster in immunocompetent patients. *International Journal of Antimicrobial Agents, 4*, 241–246.

Dohrenwend, B. P., Shrout, P. E., Link, B. G., Martin, J. L., & Skodol, A. E. (1986). Overview and initial results from a risk-factor study of depression and schizophrenia. In J. E. Barrett & R. M. Rose (Eds.), *Mental disorders in the community: Progress and challenge* (pp. 184–212). New York: Guilford Press.

Dohrenwend, B. S., & Dohrenwend, B. P. (1981). Life stress and illness: Formulation of the issues. In B. S. Dohrenwend & B. P. Dohrenwend (Eds.), *Stressful life events and their context* (pp. 1–27). New York: Prodist.

Dohrenwend, B. S., Dohrenwend, B. P., Dodson, M., & Shrout, P. E. (1984). Symptoms, hassles, social supports, and life events: Problem of confounded measures. *Journal of Abnormal Psychology, 93*, 222–230.

Donohue, J. G., Choo, P. W., Manson, J. E., & Platt, R. (1995). The incidence of herpes zoster. *Archives of Internal Medicine, 155*, 1605–1609.

Dunkel-Schetter, C., & Bennett, T. L. (1990). Differentiating the cognitive and behavioral aspects of social support. In B. R. Sarason, I. G. Sarason, & G. R. Pierce (Eds.), *Social support: An interactional view* (pp. 267–296). New York: Wiley.

Dworkin, R. H. (1991). What do we really know about the psychological origins of chronic pain? *American Pain Society Bulletin, 1* (5), 7–11.

Dworkin, R. H. (1997a). Which individuals with acute pain are most likely to develop a chronic pain syndrome? *Pain Forum, 6*, 127–136.

Dworkin, R. H. (1997b). Toward a clearer specification of acute pain risk factors and chronic pain outcomes. *Pain Forum, 6*, 148–150.

Dworkin, R. H. (1997c). Pain and its assessment in herpes zoster. *Antiviral Chemistry and Chemotherapy, 8* (Suppl. 1), 31–36.

Dworkin, R. H., Boon, R. J., & Griffin, D. R. G. (1995). Covariates in herpes zoster and interpretation of clinical trial data. *Antiviral Research, 26*, A344.

Dworkin, R. H., Boon, R. J., Griffin, D. R. G., & Phung, D. (1998). Postherpetic neuralgia: Impact of famciclovir, age, rash severity, and acute pain in herpes zoster patients. *Journal of Infectious Diseases, 178*(Suppl. 1), S76–S80.

Dworkin, R. H., Carrington, D., Cunningham, A., Kost, R., Levin, M., McKendrick, M., Oxman, M., Rentier, B., Schmader, K. E., Tappeiner, G., Wassilew, S. W., & Whitley, R. J. (1997). Assessment of pain in herpes zoster: Lessons learned from antiviral trials. *Antiviral Research, 33*, 73–85.

Dworkin, R. H., Cooper, E. M., Walther, R. R., & Sweeney, E. W. (1997, March). *Risk factors for postherpetic neuralgia: A prospective study of acute herpes zoster patients.* Paper presented at the Third International Conference on the Varicella-Zoster Virus, Palm Beach, FL.

Dworkin, R. H., & Gitlin, M. J. (1991). Clinical aspects of depression in chronic pain patients. *Clinical Journal of Pain, 7*, 79–94.

Dworkin, R. H., Hartstein, G., Rosner, H. L., Walther, R. R., Sweeney, E. W., & Brand, L. (1992). A high-risk method for studying psychosocial antecedents of chronic pain: The prospective investigation of herpes zoster. *Journal of Abnormal Psychology, 101*, 200–205.

Dworkin, R. H., & Johnson, R. W. (1998). A belt of roses from hell: Pain in herpes zoster and postherpetic neuralgia. In A. R. Block, E. F. Kremer, & E. Fernandez (Eds.), *Handbook of pain syndromes: Biopsychosocial perspectives* (pp. 371–402). Hillsdale, NJ: Erlbaum.

Dworkin, R. H., & Portenoy, R. K. (1996). Pain and its persistence in herpes zoster. *Pain, 67,* 241–251.

Dworkin, S. F., Von Korff, M. R., & LeResche, L. (1992). Epidemiologic studies of chronic pain: A dynamic-ecologic perspective. *Annals of Behavioral Medicine, 14,* 3–11.

Feuerstein, M., Papciak, A. S., & Hoon, P. E. (1987). Biobehavioral mechanisms of chronic low back pain. *Clinical Psychology Review, 7,* 243–273.

Feuerstein, M., Sult, S., & Houle, M. (1985). Environmental stressors and chronic low back pain: Life events, family and work environment. *Pain, 22,* 295–307.

Fiddian, A. P. (1995). A randomized, controlled trial of Zovirax (acyclovir, ACV) versus netivudine for the treatment of herpes zoster. *Antiviral Research, 26,* A297.

Flor, H., & Birbaumer, N. (1994). Acquisition of chronic pain: Psychophysiological mechanisms. *American Pain Society Journal, 3,* 119–127.

Flor, H., Birbaumer, N., & Turk, D. C. (1990). The psychobiology of chronic pain. *Advances in Behavior Research and Therapy, 12,* 47–84.

Galil, K., Choo, P. W., Donahue, J. G., & Platt, R. (1997). The sequelae of herpes zoster. *Archives of Internal Medicine, 157,* 1209–1213.

Gamsa, A. (1994a). The role of psychological factors in chronic pain: I. A half century of study. *Pain, 57,* 5–15.

Gamsa, A. (1994b). The role of psychological factors in chronic pain: II. A critical appraisal. *Pain, 57,* 17–29.

Gatchel, R. J. (1996). Psychological disorders and chronic pain: Cause-and-effect relationships. In R. J. Gatchel & D. C. Turk (Eds.), *Psychological approaches to pain management: A practitioner's handbook* (pp. 33–52). New York: Guilford Press.

Gershon, A. A. (1993). Zoster in immunosuppressed patients. In C. P. N. Watson (Ed.), *Herpes zoster and postherpetic neuralgia* (pp. 73–86). Amsterdam: Elsevier.

Gervais, S., Dupuis, G., Véronneau, F., Bergeron, Y., Millette, D., & Avard, J. (1991). Predictive model to determine cost/benefit of early detection and intervention in occupational low back pain. *Journal of Occupational Rehabilitation, 1,* 113–131.

Gil, K. M., Keefe, F. J., Crisson, J. E., & Van Dalfsen, P. J. (1987). Social support and pain behavior. *Pain, 29,* 209–217.

Gilden, D. H., Dueland, A. N., Cohrs, R., Martin, J. R., Kleinschmidt-DeMasters, B. K., & Mahalingam, R. (1991). Preherpetic neuralgia. *Neurology, 41,* 1215–1218.

Glaser, R., & Kiecolt-Glaser, J. K. (1994). Stress-associated immune modulation and its implications for reactivation of latent herpesviruses. In R. Glaser & J. F. Jones (Eds.), *Herpesvirus infections* (pp. 245–270). New York: Dekker.

Graff-Radford, S. B., Kames, L. D., & Naliboff, B. D. (1986). Measures of psychological adjustment and perception of pain in postherpetic neuralgia and trigeminal neuralgia. *Clinical Journal of Pain, 2,* 55–58.

Green, M. F. (1998). *Schizophrenia from a neurocognitive perspective: Probing the impenetrable darkness.* Boston: Allyn & Bacon.

Grunau, R. V. E., Whitfield, M. F., Petrie, J. H., & Fryer, E. L. (1994). Early pain experience, child and family factors, as precursors of somatization: A propsective study of extremely premature and fullterm children. *Pain, 56,* 353–359.

Guess, H. A., Broughton, D. D., Melton, L. J., III, & Kurland, L. T. (1985). Epidemiology of herpes zoster in children and adolescents: A population-based study. *Pediatrics, 76,* 512–517.

Haanpää, M., & Nurmikko, T. (1997, March). *Sensory thresholds, allodynia and pain in acute herpes zoster and their association with postherpetic neuralgia.* Paper presented at the Third International Conference on the Varicella-Zoster Virus, Palm Beach, FL.

Harding, S. P., Lipton, J. R., & Wells, J. C. D. (1987). Natural history of herpes zoster ophthalmicus: Predictors of postherpetic neuralgia and ocular involvement. *British Journal of Opthalmology, 71,* 353–358.

Haynes, S. N. (1992). *Models of causality in psychopathology: Toward dynamic, synthetic and nonlinear models of behavior disorders.* New York: Macmillan.

Higa, K., Dan, K., Manabe, H., & Noda, B. (1988). Factors influencing the duration of treatment of acute herpetic pain with sympathetic nerve block: Importance of severity of herpes zoster assessed by the maximum antibody titers to varicella-zoster virus in otherwise healthy patients. *Pain, 32,* 147–157.

Higa, K., Mori, M., Hirata, K., Hori, K., Manabe, H., & Dan, K. (1997). Severity of skin lesions of herpes zoster at the worst phase rather than age and involved region most influences the duration of acute herpetic pain. *Pain, 69,* 245–253.

Higa, K., Noda, B., Manabe, H., Sato, S., & Dan, K. (1992). T-lymphocyte subsets in otherwise healthy patients with herpes zoster and relationships to the duration of acute herpetic pain. *Pain, 51,* 111–118.

Hope-Simpson, R. E. (1954). Studies on shingles: Is the virus ordinary chicken pox virus? *Lancet, ii,* 1299–1302.

Hope-Simpson, R. E. (1965). The nature of herpes zoster: A long-term study and a new hypothesis. *Proceedings of the Royal Society of Medicine, 58,* 9–20.

Hope-Simpson, R. E. (1967). Herpes zoster in the elderly. *Geriatrics, 22,* 151–159.

Hope-Simpson, R. E. (1975). Postherpetic neuralgia. *Journal of the Royal College of General Practitioners, 25,* 571–575.

House, J. S., Umberson, D., & Landis, K. R. (1988). Structures and processes of social support. *Annual Review of Sociology, 14,* 293–318.

Huff, J. C., Drucker, J. L., Clemmer, A., Laskin, O. L., Connor, J. D., Bryson, Y. J., & Balfour, H. H., Jr. (1993). Effect of oral acyclovir on pain resolution in herpes zoster: A reanalysis. *Journal of Medical Virology*(Suppl. 1), 93–96.

International Association for the Study of Pain. (1997). *Curriculum on pain for students in psychology.* Seattle, WA: Author.

Jackson, J. L., Gibbons, R., Meyer, G., & Inouye, L. (1997). The effect of treating herpes zoster with oral acyclovir in preventing postherpetic neuralgia: A meta-analysis. *Archives of Internal Medicine, 157,* 909–912.

Johnson, R., Shukla, S., & Fletcher, P. (1995). *Qualitative aspects of zoster-associated pain: Evaluation of a new approach.* Paper presented at the Scientific Meeting of the European Federation of IASP Chapters, Verona, Italy.

Kendler, K. S., & Eaves, L. J. (1986). Models for the joint effect of genotype and environment on liability to psychiatric illness. *American Journal of Psychiatry, 143,* 279–289.

Kendler, K. S., Kessler, R. C., Neale, M. C., Heath, A. C., & Eaves, L. J. (1993). The prediction of major depression in women: Toward an integrated ecologic model. *American Journal of Psychiatry, 150,* 1139–1148.

Kendler, K. S., Kessler, R. C., Walters, E. E., MacLean, C., Neale, M. C., Heath, A. C., & Eaves, L. J. (1995). Stressful life events, genetic liability, and onset of an episode of major depression in women. *American Journal of Psychiatry, 152,* 833–842.

Kerns, R. D., Haythornthwaite, J., Southwick, S., & Giller, E. L. (1990). The role of marital interaction in chronic pain and depressive symptom severity. *Journal of Psychosomatic Research, 34,* 401–408.

Kerns, R. D., & Jacob, M. C. (1995). Toward an integrative diathesis–stress model of chronic pain. In A. J. Goreczny (Ed.), *Handbook of health and rehabilitation psychology* (pp. 325–340). New York: Plenum Press.

Kerns, R. D., & Payne, A. (1996). Treating families of chronic pain patients. In R. J. Gatchel & D. C. Turk (Eds.), *Psychological approaches to pain management: A practitioner's handbook* (pp. 283–304). New York: Guilford Press.

Kerns, R. D., Southwick, S., Giller, E. L., Haythornthwaite, J., & Rosenberg, R. (1991). The relationship between reports of pain-related social interactions and expressions of pain and affective distress. *Behavior Therapy, 22,* 101–111.

Kerns, R. D., & Turk, D. C. (1984). Depression and chronic pain: The mediating role of the spouse. *Journal of Marriage and the Family, 46,* 845–852.

Klapow, J. C., Slater, M. A., Patterson, T. L., Atkinson, J. H., Weickgenant, A. L., Grant, I., & Garfin, S. R. (1995). Psychosocial factors discriminate multidimensional clinical groups of chronic low back pain patients. *Pain, 62,* 349–355.

Klapow, J. C., Slater, M. A., Patterson, T. L., Doctor, J. N., Atkinson, J. H., & Garfin, S. R. (1993). An empirical evaluation of multidimensional clinical outcome in chronic low back pain patients. *Pain, 55,* 107–118.

Kost, R. G., & Straus, S. E. (1996). Postherpetic neuralgia: Pathogenesis, treatment, and prevention. *New England Journal of Medicine, 335,* 32–42.

Kraemer, H. C., Kazdin, A. E., Offord, D. R., Kessler, R. C., Jensen, P. S., & Kupfer, D. J. (1997). Coming to terms with the terms of risk. *Archives of General Psychiatry, 54,* 337–343.

Kraemer, H. C., Gullion, C. M., Rush, A. J., Frank, E., & Kupfer, D. J. (1994). Can state and trait variables be distinguished?: A methodological framework for psychiatric disorders. *Psychiatry Research, 52,* 55–69.

Leijon, G., Boivie, J., Roberg, M., & Forsberg, P. (1993). Sensory abnormalities accompanying herpes zoster and post-herpetic neuralgia. *Abstracts of the 7th World Congress on Pain* (pp. 184–185). Seattle, WA: IASP.

Leplow, B., Lamparter, U., Risse, A., & Wassilev, S. W. (1990). Die postherpetische Neuralgie: Klinische Prädiktoren und psychopathologischer Befund. *Nervenarzt, 61,* 46–51.

Linton, S. J. (1997). A population-based study of the relationship between sexual abuse and back pain: Establishing a link. *Pain, 73,* 147–153.

Loeser, J. D. (1990). Herpes zoster and postherpetic neuralgia. In J. J. Bonica (Ed.), *The management of pain* (2nd ed., pp. 257–263). Philadelphia: Lea & Febiger.

Lydick, E., Epstein, R. S., Himmelberger, D., & White, C. J. (1995). Area under the curve: A metric for patient subjective responses in episodic diseases. *Quality of Life Research, 4,* 41–45.

Maier, S. F., Watkins, L. R., & Fleshner, M. (1994). Psychoneuroimmunology: The interface between behavior, brain, and immunity. *American Psychologist, 49,* 1004–1017.

Marbach, J. J., Lennon, M. C., & Dohrenwend, B. P. (1988). Candidate risk factors for temporomandibular pain and dysfunction syndrome: Psychosocial, health behavior, physical illness and injury. *Pain, 34,* 139–151.

McCulloch, D. K., Fraser, D. M., & Duncan, L. P. J. (1982). Shingles in diabetes mellitus. *Practitioner, 226,* 531–532.

McDermid, A. J., Rollman, G. B., & McCain, G. A. (1996). Generalized hypervigilance in fibromyalgia: Evidence of perceptual amplification. *Pain, 66,* 133–144.

McKendrick, M. W., Care, C. D., Ogan, P., & Wood, M. J. (1994, July). *A retrospective study of the epidemiology of zoster with particular reference to factors pertinent to the development of chronic pain.* Paper presented at the Second International Conference on the Varicella-Zoster Virus, Paris.

Mednick, S. A., & McNeil, T. F. (1968). Current methodology in research on the etiology of schizophrenia: Serious difficulties which suggest the use of the high-risk method. *Psychological Bulletin, 70,* 681–693.

Meehl, P. E. (1962). Schizotaxia, schizotypy, schizophrenia. *American Psychologist, 17,* 827–838.

Merskey, H., & Bogduk, N. (Eds.). (1994). *Classification of chronic pain: Descriptions of chronic pain syndromes and definitions of pain terms* (2nd ed.). Seattle, WA: IASP.

Mitchell, C. D., Gehrz, R. C., & Balfour, H. H., Jr. (1986). Varicella-zoster-specific immune responses in acute herpes zoster during a placebo-controlled trial of oral acyclovir therapy. *Diagnostic Microbiology and Infectious Diseases, 5,* 113–126.

Molin, L. (1969). Aspects of the natural history of herpes zoster. *Acta Dermato-Venereologica, 49,* 569–583.

Monroe, S. M., & Roberts, J. E. (1990). Conceptualizing and measuring life stress: Problems, principles, procedures, progress. *Stress Medicine, 6,* 209–216.

Monroe, S. M., & Simons, A. D. (1991). Diathesis–stress theories in the context of life stress research: Implications for the depressive disorders. *Psychological Bulletin, 110,* 406–425.

Monroe, S. M., & Steiner, S. C. (1986). Social support and psychopathology: Interrelations with preexisting disorder, stress, and personality. *Journal of Abnormal Psychology, 95,* 29–39.

Moos, R. H. (1992). Understanding individuals' life contexts: Implications for stress reduction and prevention. In M. Kessler, S. E. Goldston, & J. M. Joffe (Eds), *The present and future of prevention* (pp. 196–213). Newbury Park, CA: Sage.

Noda, B., Dan, K., Manabe, H., & Higa, K. (1987). Prognostic clinical signs in herpes zoster pain. *Pain*(Suppl. 4), S382.

Nuechterlein, K. H., & Dawson, M. E. (1984). A heuristic vulnerability/stress model of schizophrenic episodes. *Schizophrenia Bulletin, 10,* 300–312.

Nuechterlein, K. H., Dawson, M. E., Gitlin, M., Ventura, J., Goldstein, M. J., Snyder, K. S., Yee, C. M., & Mintz, J. (1992). Developmental processes in schizophrenic disorders: Longitudinal studies of vulnerability and stress. *Schizophrenia Bulletin, 18,* 387-425.

Nurmikko, T. J., & Bowsher, D. (1990). Somatosensory findings in postherpetic neuralgia. *Journal of Neurology, Neurosurgery, and Psychiatry, 53,* 135-141.

Nurmikko, T. J., Rasanen, A., & Hakkinen, V. (1990). Clinical and neurophysiological observations on acute herpes zoster. *Clinical Journal of Pain, 6,* 284-290.

Oxman, M. N., Levin, M., Johnson, G. R., Arbeit, R., Barry, P., Gershon, A., Schmader, K., Straus, S. E., White, C. J., Collins, D., & Colling, C. L. (1994). *Trial of varicella vaccine for the prevention of herpes zoster and its complications: Vol. 1. Protocol* (VA Cooperative Study No. 403). San Diego, CA: Veterans Affairs Medical Center, Infectious Diseases Section.

Paulsen, J. S., & Altmaier, E. M. (1995). The effects of perceived versus enacted social support on the discriminative cue function of spouses for pain behaviors. *Pain, 60,* 103-110.

Peterslund, N. A., Seyer-Hansen, K., Ipsen, J., Esmann, V., Schonheyder, H., & Juhl, H. (1981). Acyclovir in herpes zoster. *Lancet, 2,* 827-830.

Pilowsky, I. (1977). Psychological aspects of post-herpetic neuralgia: Some clinical observations. *British Journal of Medical Psychology, 50,* 283-288.

Portenoy, R. K., Duma, C., & Foley, K. M. (1986). Acute herpetic and postherpetic neuralgia: Clinical review and current management. *Annals of Neurology, 20,* 651-664.

Raggozzino, M. W., Melton, L. J., III, Kurland, L. T., Chu, C. P., & Perry, H. O. (1982). Population-based study of herpes zoster and its sequelae. *Medicine, 61,* 310-316.

Riopelle, J. M., Naraghi, M., & Grush, K. P. (1984). Chronic neuralgia incidence following local anesthetic therapy for herpes zoster. *Archives of Dermatology, 120,* 747-750.

Rogers, R. S., III, & Tindall, J. P. (1971). Geriatric herpes zoster. *Journal of the American Geriatrics Society, 19,* 495-504.

Rohling, M. L., Binder, L. M., & Langhinrichsen-Rohling, J. L. (1995). Money matters: A meta-analytic review of the association between financial compensation and the experience and treatment of chronic pain. *Health Psychology, 14,* 537-547.

Rose, M. J., Klenerman, L., Atchison, L., & Slade, P. D. (1992). An application of the fear avoidance model to three chronic pain conditions. *Behaviour Research and Therapy, 30,* 359-365.

Rosenthal, D. (1963). A suggested conceptual framework. In D. Rosenthal (Ed.), *The Genain quadruplets* (pp. 505-516). New York: Basic Books.

Rowbotham, M. C. (1994). Postherpetic neuralgia. *Seminars in Neurology, 14,* 247-254.

Rowbotham, M. C., & Fields, H. L. (1989). Post-herpetic neuralgia: The relation of pain complaint, sensory disturbance, and skin temperature. *Pain, 39,* 129-144.

Rowbotham, M. C., & Fields, H. L. (1996). The relationship of pain, allodynia and thermal sensation in postherpetic neuralgia. *Brain, 119,* 347-354.

Schmader, K. (1995). Management of herpes zoster in elderly patients. *Infectious Diseases in Clinical Practice, 4,* 293-299.

Schmader, K., George, L. K., Burchett, B. M., & Pieper, C. F. (1998). Racial and psychosocial risk factors for herpes zoster in the elderly. *Journal of Infectious Diseases, 178*(Suppl. 1), S67-S70.

Schmader, K., Studenski, S., Macmillan, J., Grufferman, S., & Cohen, H. J. (1990). Are stressful life events risk factors for herpes zoster? *Journal of the American Geriatrics Society, 38,* 1188-1194.

Schofferman, J., Anderson, D., Hines, R., Smith, G., & Keane, G. (1993). Childhood psychological trauma and chronic refractory low-back pain. *Clinical Journal of Pain, 9,* 260-265.

Schofferman, J., Anderson, D., Hines, R., Smith, G., & White, A. (1992). Childhood psychological trauma correlates with unsuccessful lumbar spine surgery. *Spine, 17*(Suppl.), S138-S144.

Schroeder, D. H., & Costa, P. T., Jr. (1984). Influence of life event stress on physical illness: Substantive effects or methodological flaws? *Journal of Personality and Social Psychology, 46,* 853-863.

Shrout, P. E., Link, B. G., Dohrenwend, B. P., Skodol, A. E., Stueve, A., & Mirotznik, J. (1989). Characterizing life events as risk factors for depression: The role of fateful loss events. *Journal of Abnormal Psychology, 98,* 460-467.

Smith, C. E., Fernengel, K., Holcroft, C., Gerald, K., & Marien, L. (1994). Meta-analysis of the associations between social support and health outcomes. *Annals of Behavioral Medicine, 16,* 352-362.

Stillman, P. (1997, March). *Valaciclovir for the treatment of herpes zoster: A large-scale study assessing influence of age and dermatome on patient outcome.* Paper presented at the Third International Conference on the Varicella-Zoster Virus, Palm Beach, FL.

Straus, S. E., Reinhold, W., Smith, H. A., Ruyechan, W. T., Henderson, D. K., Blaese, R. M., & Hay, J. (1984). Endonuclease analysis of viral DNA from varicella and subsequent zoster infections in the same patient. *New England Journal of Medicine, 311,* 1362-1364.

Syrjala, K. L., & Chapko, M. E. (1995). Evidence for a biopsychosocial model of cancer treatment-related pain. *Pain, 61,* 69-79.

Thoits, P. A. (1982). Conceptual, methodological, and theoretical problems in studying social support as a buffer against life stress. *Journal of Health and Social Behavior, 23,* 145-159.

Tyring, S., Barbarash, R.A., Nahlik, J.E., Cunningham, A., Marley, J., Heng, M., Jones, T., Rea, T., Boon, R., Saltzman, R., & the Collaborative Famciclovir Herpes Zoster Study Group. (1995). Famciclovir for the treatment of acute herpes zoster: Effects on acute disease and postherpetic neuralgia: A randomized, double-blind, placebo-controlled trial. *Annals of Internal Medicine, 123,* 89-96.

Turk, D. C. (1996). Biopsychosocial perspective on chronic pain. In R. J. Gatchel & D. C. Turk (Eds.), *Psychological approaches to pain management: A practitioner's handbook* (pp. 3-32). New York: Guilford Press.

Turk, D. C., & Flor, H. (1984). Etiological theories and treatments for chronic back pain: II. Psychological models and interventions. *Pain, 19,* 209-233.

Turk, D. C., Kerns, R. D., & Rosenberg, R. (1992). Effects of marital interaction on chronic pain and disability: Examining the down side of social support. *Rehabilitation Psychology, 37,* 259-274.

Turk, D. C., & Rudy, T. E. (1992). Classification logic and strategies in chronic pain. In D. C. Turk & R. Melzack (Eds.), *Handbook of pain assessment* (pp. 409–428). New York: Guilford Press.

Violon, V., & Giurgea, D. (1984). Familial models for chronic pain. *Pain, 18,* 199–203.

Von Korff, M., Ormel, J., Keefe, F. J., & Dworkin, S. F. (1992). Grading the severity of chronic pain. *Pain, 50,* 133–149.

Waddell, G., Newton, M., Henderson, I., Somerville, D., & Main, C. J (1993). A Fear-Avoidance Beliefs Questionnaire (FABQ) and the role of fear-avoidance beliefs in chronic low back pain and disability. *Pain, 52,* 157–168.

Walker, E., Downey, G., & Nightingale, N. (1989). The nonorthogonal nature of risk factors: Implications for research on the causes of maladjustment. *Journal of Primary Prevention, 9,* 143–163.

Walker, E. A., Keegan, D., Gardner, G., Sullivan, M., Bernstein, D., & Katon, W. J. (1997). Psychosocial factors in fibromyalgia compared with rheumatoid arthritis: II. Sexual, physical, and emotional abuse and neglect. *Psychosomatic Medicine, 59,* 572–577.

Walker, E. A., Keegan, D., Gardner, G., Sullivan, M., Katon, W. J., & Bernstein, D. (1997). Psychosocial factors in fibromyalgia compared with rheumatoid arthritis: I. Psychiatric diagnoses and functional disability. *Psychosomatic Medicine, 59,* 565–571.

Wall, P. D. (1993). An essay on the mechanisms which may contribute to the state of postherpetic neuralgia. In C. P. N. Watson (Ed.), *Herpes zoster and postherpetic neuralgia* (pp. 123–138). Amsterdam: Elsevier.

Watson, C. P. N. (Ed.). (1993). *Herpes zoster and postherpetic neuralgia.* Amsterdam: Elsevier.

Watson, P. N., & Evans, R. J. (1986). Postherpetic neuralgia: A review. *Archives of Neurology, 43,* 836–840.

Weksler, M. E. (1994). Immune senescence. *Annals of Neurology, 35,* S35–S37.

Weller, T. H. (1992). Varicella and herpes zoster: A perspective and overview. *Journal of Infectious Diseases, 166*(Suppl. 1), S1–S6.

Weller, T. H., Witton, H. M., & Bell, E. J. (1958). The etiologic agents of varicella and herpes zoster: Isola-tion, propagation, and cultural characteristics in vitro. *Journal of Experimental Medicine, 108,* 843–868.

Wethington, E., & Kessler, R. C. (1986). Perceived support, received support, and adjustment to stressful life events. *Journal of Health and Social Behavior 27,* 78–89.

Whitley, R. J., Weiss, H., Gnann, J. W., Jr., Tyring, S., Mertz, G. J., Pappas, P. G., Schleupner, C. J., Hayden, F., Wolf, J., Soong, S-J., & the National Institute of Allergy and Infectious Diseases Collaborative Antiviral Study Group. (1996). Acyclovir with and without prednisone for the treatment of herpes zoster: A randomized, placebo-controlled trial. *Annals of Internal Medicine, 125,* 376–383.

Wildenhoff, K. E., Esmann, V., Ipsen, J., Harving, H., Peterslund, N. A., & Schonheyder, H. (1981). Treatment of trigeminal and thoracic zoster with idoxuridine. *Scandinavian Journal of Infectious Diseases, 13,* 257–262.

Wildenhoff, K. E., Ipsen, J., Esmann, V., Ingemann-Jensen, J., & Poulsen, J. H. (1979). Treatment of herpes zoster with idoxuridine ointment, including a multivariate analysis of symptoms and signs. *Scandinavian Journal of Infectious Diseases, 11,* 1–9.

Wilson, J. B. (1986). Thirty one years of herpes zoster in a rural practice. *British Medical Journal, 293,* 1349–1351.

Wood, M. J. (1995). For debate: How should zoster trials be conducted? *Journal of Antimicrobial Chemotherapy, 36,* 1089–1101.

Wood, M. J., Johnson, R. W., McKendrick, M. W., Taylor, J., Mandal, B. K., & Crooks, J. (1994). A randomized trial of acyclovir for 7 days or 21 days with and without prednisolone for treatment of acute herpes zoster. *New England Journal of Medicine, 330,* 896–900.

Wood, M. J., Kay, R., Dworkin, R. H., Soong, S-J., & Whitley, R. J. (1996). Oral acyclovir therapy accelerates pain resolution in patients with herpes zoster: A meta-analysis of placebo-controlled trials. *Clinical Infectious Diseases, 22,* 341–347.

Zubin, J., & Spring, B. (1977). Vulnerability: A new view of schizophrenia. *Journal of Abnormal Psychology, 86,* 103–126.

Chapter 17

Irritable Bowel Syndrome

EDWARD B. BLANCHARD
TARA GALOVSKI

IRRITABLE BOWEL SYNDROME AS A CHRONIC PAIN PROBLEM

Irritable bowel syndrome (IBS) is a widespread functional disorder of the lower gastrointestinal (GI) tract. Epidemiological studies indicate that it may affect 10-20% of adults in the United States. The most precise recent estimate by Talley, Zinsmeister, Van Dyke, and Melton (1991) showed that 17% of adults aged 30-64 met the criteria for IBS. Only about 14% of those who met the criteria had sought medical assistance for the problem in the past year, a point to which we will return later. It may be the second leading pain-related cause of lost work days in the United States (Sternbach, 1985).

Although IBS is a disorder characterized by many symptoms, in this chapter, consistent with the theme of this book, we will emphasize the pain aspects of the disorder, with attention paid to how IBS can be conceptualized as a chronic pain problem and what this might mean in terms of psychosocial assessment and psychosocial treatments. We will also summarize the psychosocial treatment literature, especially as it pertains to pain.

Definitions or Diagnostic Criteria for IBS

The older diagnostic criteria for IBS, also known as the clinical criteria (Latimer, 1983), are as follows:

1. Cramping abdominal pain and/or severe abdominal tenderness.
2. Altered bowel habits, either diarrhea or constipation or alternating diarrhea and constipation.
3. Symptoms present for most days over a 3-month or longer time span.
4. Ruling out by appropriate tests of the following medical disorders with similar symptoms:
   a. Inflammatory bowel disease (Crohn's disease or ulcerative colitis).
   b. Parasites.
   c. Lactose intolerance or lactose malabsorption syndrome.
   d. Other lower GI tract diseases.

Although these criteria have been widely used in research and probably form the basis for most clinical diagnoses, they have been criticized because they relegate IBS to the status of a residual category, that is, once all of the "real" diseases have been ruled out, patients with these symptoms are diagnosed with IBS.

An international group of GI specialists (primarily gastroenterologists but also at least one psychologist and one psychiatrist) have put forth a new definition of IBS, which emerged from a consensus conference in Rome, Italy; hence the criteria have come to be known as the Rome criteria:

At least three months continuous or recurrent symptoms of:

1. Abdominal pain or discomfort which is:
   (a) relieved with defecation,

(b) and/or associated with change in frequency of stool,

(c) and/or associated with change in consistency of stool;

2. Two or more of the following, at least a quarter of occasions or days:
   (a) altered stool frequency (> 3 bowel movements/day or < 3 bowel movements/week),
   (b) altered stool form (lumpy/hard or loose/watery stool),
   (c) altered stool passage (straining, urgency or feeling of incomplete evacuation),
   (d) passage of mucus,
   (e) bloating or feeling of abdominal distension. (Thompson, Creed, Drossman, Heaton, & Mazzacca, 1992, p. 77)

The Rome criteria thus represent an effort to change diagnostic practices so that the diagnosis of IBS is made *positively*, on the basis of the presence of specific symptoms, rather than as a residual diagnosis after other possible causes of the symptom picture have been ruled out.

The Rome criteria owe their intellectual heritage to work of Manning and others (Manning, Thompson, Heaton, & Morris, 1978), who compared the GI symptoms of 32 patients with IBS to those of 33 patients with various organic GI diseases. Seven symptoms (looser stools at onset of pain, more frequent bowel movements at onset of pain, pain eased after bowel movement [often]), visible distension, feeling of distension, mucus per rectum, and feeling of incomplete emptying [often], discriminated between the two groups at the .05 level or better. However, no single symptom discriminated perfectly. The best single-symptom discriminator correctly identified 45 of 61 patients (73.8%). Manning et al. (1978) did note that all but 3 IBS patients (91%) had two or more symptoms, whereas only 10 patients with organic disease (30%) had that many symptoms or more. They also noted that 30 of 33 patients with organic disease and 31 of 32 with IBS complained of pain. Clearly, abdominal pain per se does not identify IBS or functional GI disorders.

Talley, Phillips, Melton, Mulvihill, Wiltgen, and Zinsmeister (1990) conducted an expanded replication study of the Manning et al. (1978) criteria involving 82 IBS patients, 33 patients with nonulcer dyspepsia, 101 with organic GI disease, and 145 healthy controls. They found that the Manning criteria discriminated IBS from organic GI disease with a sensitivity of 58% and specificity of 74%. Thus, although abdominal pain and its relief is a major motivator for the IBS patients, it is not very specific to the disorder.

Functional Bowel Disorder Severity Index

Recently, Drossman et al. (1995) has developed a composite measure of functional bowel disorder (FBD) severity for research purposes (such as matching patients before randomization) and termed it the "FBD Severity Index" (FBDSI). Because IBS is the predominant functional bowel disorder, the index could be known as the IBS Severity Index. It was derived through having treating physicians initially rate the overall severity of the presenting problems for their patients with FBDs on a 0-to-5 scale. Then, through multiple regression analyses, a large number of potential predictors were reduced to 3, and the FBDSI derived: FBDSI = Pain severity (0–100 visual analogue scale rating by patient of current pain intensity) + 106 × (diagnosis of chronic functional abdominal pain [chronic pain complaints for 6 months or more plus disability] or not) + 11 × number of physician visits for abdominal pain in the last 6 months.

Scores of less than 36 are termed "mild," 36–110 "moderate," and greater than 110 "severe." It seems clear that a patient usually would need to be diagnosed with chronic functional abdominal pain to be labeled severe. The point from this work most pertinent to this chapter is the dominating role of abdominal pain in determining the severity of IBS.

Epidemiology, or the Size of the Problem

There have been two good epidemiological studies on the prevalence of IBS over the past few years. In the first (Drossman et al., 1993), termed the "U.S. Householder Survey of Functional Gastrointestinal Disorders," 5,430 households out of 8,250 approached and selected to represent the United States responded to a detailed questionnaire. From the responses, the survey revealed that 11.6% (n = 629) met diagnostic criteria for IBS (11.2% after excluding self-reported structural diagnoses); of these only 45.8% (n = 288) had ever seen a physician for the problem. Women outnumbered men about 2 to 1 (14.5% of women vs. 7.7% of men), and younger individuals (15–44) outnumbered older (45 years or greater) about 3 to 2 (13.3% vs. 9.4%). Those with IBS reported missing an average of 13.4 days of school or work in the past year.

Talley et al. (1991) surveyed 1,021 adult residents (age 30–64) in an upper midwestern county and received an 82% response. Abdominal pain more than six times in the prior year was present in 26.2% of respondents. IBS was diagnosed (using Manning criteria) in 17.0%, with women outnumbering men 18.2% to 15.8%. Only 14% of those with IBS or chronic diarrhea or constipation had seen a physician for the GI problems over the past year. Predictors of seeking medical attention were pain described as severe or very severe (affecting one's life), pain once a week or more, and pain interrupting daily activities.

Thus these data again demonstrate that among the wide array of symptoms present in IBS it is the pain, especially severe, interfering pain, that brings the patient to the attention of the health care system.

Psychological/Psychiatric Factors in IBS

It is reasonably well established that, as a group, IBS patients show a noticeable level of psychological distress or disturbance on standardized psychological tests and also show a high frequency of psychiatric diagnoses. For example, in a study from our center, we (Blanchard et al., 1986) compared IBS patients to two other chronic pain populations, patients with tension-type headache and patients with migraine headaches, and to nonpatient normal controls. The groups were matched for age and gender and the three patient groups had comparable lengths of illness. When we compared the groups on the Beck Depression Inventory (BDI; Beck et al., 1961) and the State–Trait Anxiety Inventory (STAI; Spielberger, Gorsuch, & Lushene, 1970) for both state and trait anxiety, we found significantly higher BDI scores for those with IBS ($\bar{X}$ = 13.4) than for the tension-type headache sufferers ($\bar{X}$ = 9.6), who in turn scored higher than those with migraine headache ($\bar{X}$ = 7.6). The latter group was not different from the nonpatient controls ($\bar{X}$ = 4.3). On both state and trait anxiety, those with IBS ($\bar{X}$ State = 41.9, $\bar{X}$ Trait = 47.7) were significantly more anxious than those with migraine headache ($\bar{X}$ State = 34.3, $\bar{X}$ Trait = 40.0). The IBS patients also were arithmetically higher than those with tension-type headache ($\bar{X}$ State = 37.9, $\bar{X}$ Trait = 44.1).

Whitehead et al. (1990) reported similar data on IBS patients compared to normal controls: BDI scores for the IBS group were 14.5 versus 2.2 for nonpatient controls, and STAI-Trait scores were 42.9 for IBS and 32.9 for controls. Interestingly, in the Whitehead et al. (1990) study, patients diagnosed with functional bowel disorder (essentially patients who meet the clinical criteria for IBS, but not the more precise Manning symptom [2+] criteria) were even more distressed, with BDI scores of 16.1 and STAI-Trait scores of 49.1.

We (Blanchard et al., 1987) have also found that successful psychosocial treatment of IBS, in which primary GI symptoms were reduced by 50% or more, led to a significant reduction in the psychological test scores, whereas treated patients whose GI symptoms did not improve significantly with treatment and GI symptom monitoring controls (who received no treatment) did not change appreciably. For example, BDI scores in successfully treated patients were reduced from 14.3 to 7.1 (this latter mean value is the normal range) and STAI-Trait scores were reduced from 45.4 to 38.7, whereas STAI-State scores went from 41.7 to 31.3. For the IBS patients whose treatments were not successful, BDI scores before and after treatment were 13.6 and 12.8, respectively, whereas STAI-Trait scores were 52.9 and 46.6 and STAI-State scores were 48.3 and 49.2, respectively. The symptom monitoring controls had BDI scores of 14.3 and 13.2, respectively, before and after the treatment interval. It thus appears that IBS might be construed as a "somatopsychic" disorder, with the psychological distress resulting from the somatic symptoms (and disappearing, relatively, when the somatic symptoms are reduced).

Psychiatric Diagnoses among IBS Patients

Beginning with the pioneering work of Young, Alpers, Norlend, and Woodruff (1976), a series of studies has found high prevalence of diagnosable psychiatric disorders among samples of IBS patients. Young et al. (1976), operating in the pre-DSM-III era, found that 72% of IBS patients attending a gastroenterology clinic met research criteria for psychiatric diagnoses (using Feighner et al., 1972, criteria), with the majority being mood disorders (mostly primary affective disorder). Walker et al. (1990), using structured psychiatric interviews and DSM-III-R criteria (American Psychiatric Association, 1987), found that 90% of IBS patients met current or lifetime criteria for at least one Axis I disorder. The vast majority of these diagnoses were among the anxiety or mood disorders.

Work from our center (Blanchard, Scharff, Schwarz, Suls, & Barlow, 1990) similarly shows a high prevalence of psychiatric disorders based on structured interviews utilizing the ADIS (Anxiety Disorders Interview Schedule; DiNardo & Barlow,

1988). We examined 68 IBS patients, 44 patients with inflammatory bowel disease (IBD), that is, lower-GI-tract diseases with some similar symptoms but with readily identifiable pathophysiology, and 38 age- and gender-matched non-ill controls. Overall, we found that 56% of IBS patients with lifetime prevalence met criteria for at least one Axis I disorder, as contrasted with 25% for those with IBD and 18% of the non-ill controls. The prevalence did not differ significantly between the latter two groups but was significantly ($p = .002$) higher for those with IBS.

Interestingly, 40% of the total IBS sample had primary diagnoses among the anxiety disorders, with 12% having a mood disorder diagnosis. Among the anxiety disorders, by far the most prevalent was generalized anxiety disorders (GAD): 20.5% of the total sample (and thus 37% of those with any Axis I diagnosis) met the DSM-III-R criteria for GAD. Thus worry, or apprehensive expectation, seems to play a major role in IBS. In this respect, IBS is different from many chronic pain syndromes, in which one expects to find primarily depression and mood disorders as the major psychiatric consequences of living with chronic pain.

A point that is not clear in these data is whether the GAD preceded or followed the IBS. (GAD is known to be an extremely chronic condition and is often present for much of the sufferer's adult life.) If the GAD developed before the IBS, it could be that the worry-prone or anxiety-prone individual is more susceptible to developing IBS, a point consistent with Paul Latimer's (1983) early theorizing that IBS develops in individuals who are fundamentally neurotic and who begin at some point to focus on bowel sensations and bowel symptoms. More research is obviously needed on this point of whether the IBS or the Axis I disorder is primary from a historical view.

IBS Sufferers and IBS Patients

About 10 years ago, two reports appeared independently from two laboratories that have been very prominent in the study of IBS. William Whitehead at Johns Hopkins University and Douglas Drossman at the University of North Carolina addressed the issue of whether everyone who suffers from the symptoms of IBS shows the characteristic psychological distress described previously. Thus both studies included individuals with IBS symptoms who had sought medical attention for the GI symptoms (whom we term IBS patients) and individuals with IBS symptoms who had not sought medical attention (whom we term IBS nonpatients). In the first study (Whitehead, Bosmajian, Zonderman, Costa, & Schuster, 1988), 149 middle-class women, average age 47, were examined by questionnaire and H_2 breath test to distinguish those with IBS, FBD (a group who met clinical criteria for IBS), lactose malabsorption and non-ill controls. They also completed the Hopkins Symptom Checklist. From the Johns Hopkins GI clinics, 121 women with diagnoses of IBS, FBD, or lactose malabsorption were also tested. Results showed higher levels of psychological distress on almost all measures, including the Global Severity Index, for clinic attendees versus diagnosable individuals not seeking care.

Of particular relevance were much higher scores on scales measuring somatization, depression, anxiety, and hostility among IBS clinic attendees versus IBS nonpatients and non-ill controls, who tended not to differ. Whitehead et al. (1988) also noted "robust correlations of abdominal pain with measures of psychological distress" (p. 712). Whitehead et al. (1988) concluded, however, "that symptoms of psychological distress are unrelated to the bowel symptoms that define IBS, but they do influence who will come to the medical clinic for treatment" (p. 713).

In the second study, Drossman et al. (1988) examined 72 IBS patients, 82 individuals with IBS who had not sought medical attention, and 84 normal non-ill controls. The average age was 28, and 89% were female. On the MMPI, the IBS patients scored higher than the IBS nonpatients on Hypochondriasis, Depression, and Ego Strength. On the McGill Pain Questionnaire (Melzack, 1975), which was taken daily for 2 weeks by all participants, the IBS patients had a significantly higher mean total pain score than the IBS patients or non-ill controls. Interestingly, the IBS patients reported abdominal pain 8.2 out of 14 days, whereas the IBS nonpatients reported it on only 3.0 days. Thus the diary was consistent with initial symptom questionnaires that found that 94% of patients but only 56% of IBS nonpatients reported more than six episodes of pain per year ($p < .001$).

Although it is clear that IBS sufferers who seek medical care (perhaps a majority) are more psychologically distressed along a number of dimensions than IBS sufferers who do not seek medical care, it is not clear whether the psychological distress (or neuroticism) causes the care seeking. It also may well be that the abdominal pain symptoms are most likely to lead the individual with IBS symptoms to seek medical care. Drossman et al.'s (1988) data seem to indicate more pain episodes and more severe pain when it occurs among IBS patients than IBS nonpatients. Perhaps the greater psychological distress among the help-seeking patients is a consequence of living with more chronic pain.

It should also be kept in mind that all of the treatment research and almost all of the other research on IBS has been done with IBS *patients*. One only treats those individuals who seek care for their ailments. It is also the case, as pointed out earlier, that successful alleviation of GI symptoms leads to significant improvement in psychological state. Thus it may be that the years of living with abdominal pain and the other symptoms of IBS exacts a psychological toll that is then detected when the patient seeks treatment.

Objective Measures of Pain Tolerance in IBS Patients

One possible basis for the pain complaints of the IBS patients is that they as a group are more sensitive to distension of the lower colon and rectum caused by normal filling with stool than normal individuals and thus are more likely to complain of abdominal pain. Gastroenterologists have developed a method of studying this phenomenon by inserting a deflated balloon into the rectum and sigmoid colon and then progressively inflating the balloon with known volumes of water or air while simultaneously recording resistant pressure from the rectocolonic tissue and self-report of sensations from fullness to discomfort to pain.

Ritchie (1973) initially reported 25 years ago that patients with IBS had a lower tolerance (because of pain) for distension of the colon through external inflation. Latimer et al. (1979), however, reported no difference in pain or discomfort reports between IBS patients and a comparison group of "neurotics." Cook, van Eeden, and Collins (1987) reported that IBS patients did not differ from normal controls in terms of pain threshold and pain tolerance when the painful stimulus was electric shock to the hand. Thus the picture was fairly muddled on this issue of possible physiological differences in colonic pain sensitivity among IBS sufferers.

A landmark study resolving some of these issues was published by Whitehead and colleagues (Whitehead et al., 1990). In this study participants' pain tolerance for a cold pressor test (the hand submerged in ice and water at 0°C for up to 4 minutes) and pain tolerance for inflation of a rectosigmoid balloon inserted through the rectum into the sigmoid colon were determined. In the latter procedure the balloon was filled stepwise in 20 ml increments of air up to the pain tolerance point or to a maximum of 200 ml. Participants were 16 IBS patients, 10 patients with functional bowel disorder (who met clinical criteria for IBS but not Rome criteria [see previous discussion]), 25 patients with lactose malabsorption, and 18 normal controls.

Results showed significantly lower tolerance among the IBS group (120 ml) than the normal controls (180 ml), with the other two groups intermediate and not different. There were no significant differences in cold pressor tolerance, although those with IBS (160 s) and FBD (165 s) were lower than the normal controls (220 s). Interestingly, both the IBS and FBD groups show noticeable bimodal distributions on the latter measure: About half of each group reached the 240 s limit of the test, and the other half clustered under 150 s. Whitehead et al. thus conclude that "reduced tolerance for distension of the bowel may contribute to the abdominal pain complaints of the IBS group" (1990, p. 1191).

Prior, Maxton, and Whorwell (1990) partially replicated this finding in that their diarrhea-predominant IBS patients show less tolerance for distension than normal controls, whereas the constipation-predominate subset of IBS patients showed greater tolerance.

Thus far we have focused on several psychosocial aspects of IBS, with particular attention to the role pain may play in determining the diagnosis of IBS, the severity of the IBS, and whether the IBS sufferer seeks medical attention and thus becomes an IBS patient. It is very clear that IBS patients, on average, have notable psychological distress and that many meet the criteria for Axis I psychiatric disorders. It also appears that psychosocial treatments that lead to substantial relief of GI symptoms also lead to reductions in psychosocial distress.

In the next section we summarize research on treatment of IBS, with most attention given to psychosocial treatments. Regarding the latter, we pay particular attention to the series of psychosocial treatment studies conducted at the Center for Stress and Anxiety Disorders of the University at Albany over the past 14 years. In all of these summaries, we focus on both the effect of the treatment on pain reduction and on reduction of the total symptom complex that makes up IBS.

TREATMENT OF IBS

Pharmacological Treatments

Although there have been many studies on the pharmacological treatment of IBS, for the most part this literature has not led to promising results. Klein (1988), in a widely heralded review, noted numerous methodological problems with almost all of the IBS drug treatment trials. He concluded that "not a single study offers convincing evidence that any (drug) therapy is effective in treating the IBS symptom complex" (p. 232).

This situation has not markedly improved over the 10 years since his review. One possible exception is a study by Greenbaum et al. (1987) evaluating desipramine. Both diarrhea-predominant ($n = 19$) and constipation-predominant ($n = 9$) IBS patients underwent three 6-week trials of either desipramine, atropine (as an active placebo), or placebo in a double-blind crossover design with evaluation both by patient symptom diary and by periodic structured interview evaluations.

Results from the symptom diaries showed greater reduction in stool frequency, in self-reports of diarrhea, and in pain index for the entire sample and for the diarrhea-predominant subsample when comparing desipramine to placebo. Importantly, the entire sample showed a reduction in pain index when comparing desipramine to atropine. None of the other desipramine-versus-atropine comparisons were significant: No analyses were reported for the constipation-predominant subsample because of small sample size. The total sample also showed more reduction in symptoms on the Brief Psychiatric Rating Scale for desipramine versus placebo and for desipramine versus atropine. Finally, 15 of 28 patients reported global improvement in all GI symptoms during desipramine treatment. It thus appears that desipramine, in doses of 50 to 150 mg per day, can be therapeutic with IBS, especially in diarrhea-predominant IBS patients.

Psychosocial Treatments: The Albany Studies

We have published seven controlled and one quasi-controlled treatment trials of IBS over the past 12 years. In all of these studies, the dependent variables and measurement procedures have been the same, as have patient selection criteria. Thus we believe the results are comparable from one study to the next.

Our chief measurement operation has been a daily GI-symptom diary in which patients rated the following GI symptoms on a scale of 0 = absent, 1 = mild severity and interference, 2 = moderate, 3 = severe, 4 = excruciating or debilitating severity and interference: abdominal pain, abdominal tenderness, diarrhea, constipation, flatulence, belching, nausea, and bloating. From the diary ratings of the primary clinical symptoms of IBS, pain and tenderness, diarrhea, and constipation, we calculated individual symptom reduction scores by averaging the ratings from 2 to 4 weeks of pretreatment monitoring and 2 weeks of posttreatment monitoring:

$$\text{Diarrhea reduction score} = 100 \times \frac{\text{Pre-tx. avg. diarrhea rating} - \text{Post-Tx. avg. diarrhea rating}}{\text{Pre-tx. avg. diarrhea rating}}$$

Next, we calculate a composite primary symptom reduction score (CPSR score) by combining the three symptom reduction scores.

$$\text{Composite primary symptom reduction (CPSR) score} = \frac{\text{Diarrhea reduc. score} + \text{constip. reduc. score} + \text{abdom. pain reduc. score}}{2 \text{ or } 3 \text{ (depending on number of symptoms present)}}$$

Thus the CPSR score represents the average degree of reduction in the primary symptoms of IBS; as such, it equates a reduction in diarrhea with a reduction in pain, and so forth. Whether this is justified is not known.

Table 17.1 summarizes the treatment conditions, sample sizes, CPSR scores, percent of sample who reached our criteria for clinically meaningful improvement (a CPSR score of 0.50 or greater), and the percent reduction in abdominal pain and tenderness for the sample.

Our early studies compared a multicomponent cognitive-behavioral treatment package (comprising brief education, training in progressive muscle relaxation, training in thermal biofeedback, and brief cognitive stress coping therapy) administered in 12 sessions over 8 weeks. Although the early studies (Neff & Blanchard, 1987; Blanchard & Schwarz, 1987) found treatment better than symptom monitoring, two later studies (Blanchard et al., 1992) failed to find an advantage for the cognitive-behavioral treatment over an attention placebo condition comprising biofeedback to suppress alpha in the EEG and pseudo-meditation.

TABLE 17.1. Summary of Albany Studies of IBS Treatment

Authors	Treatment conditions	Sample size	CPSR score	% of sample improved	% reduction in pain and tenderness
Neff & Blanchard (1987)	Multicomponent CBT	10	50.4	60%	62.8%
	Symptom monitoring	9	15.4	11%	6.0%
	Treatment of symptom monitoring (multicomponent CBT)	7	N/R	43%	38.3%
Blanchard & Schwarz (1987)	12 weeks symptom monitoring	14	N/R	0%	6.1%
	Group multicomponent CBT	14	47.5	64%	36.1%
Blanchard, Schwarz, et al. (1992)					
Study 1	Multicomponent CBT	10	45.2	60%	36.9%
	Attention placebo	10	38.0	50%	29.2%
	Symptom monitoring	10	9.5	20%	0%
Study 2	Multicomponent CBT	31	32.4	52%	22.9%
	Attention placebo	30	30.4	47%	34.4%
	Symptom monitoring	31	6.4	32%	-1.9%
	Treatment of symptom monitoring (multicomponent CBT)	29	N/R	41%	N/R
Blanchard et al. (1993)	Progressive muscle relaxation	8	51.6	50%	43.3%
	Symptom monitoring	8	-1.4	13%	14.3%
Greene & Blanchard (1994)	Cognitive therapy	10	66.2	80%	53.9%
	Symptom monitoring	10	2.1	10%	-2.9%
	Treatment of symptom monitoring	6	63.8	67%	N/R
Payne & Blanchard (1995)	Cognitive therapy	12	66.8	75%	63.5%
	Support groups	12	31.0	25%	9.7%
	Symptom monitoring	10	10.1	10%	-1.9%
Vollmer & Blanchard (1998)	Individual cognitive therapy	11	46.0	55%	50.0%
	Group cognitive therapy	11	51.6	64%	46.4%
	Symptom monitoring	10	-4.0	10%	26.5%

Note. CPSR, composite primary symptom reduction; CBT, cognitive-behavioral treatments; N/R, not reported. Negative values represent worsening symptoms.

Presence of an Axis I disorder predicted relatively poorer treatment response in the large sample.

We then switched to single-component treatments. We found progressive muscle relaxation alone was superior to symptom monitoring (however, it had a high dropout rate of almost 40%; Blanchard, Greene, Scharff, & Schwarz-McMorris, 1993).

Our best and most consistent results have come from a treatment utilizing purely cognitive therapy (an amalgam of ideas from Aaron Beck, Donald Meichenbaum, and Jacqueline Persons). Greene and Blanchard (1994) found cognitive therapy superior to symptom monitoring. Payne and Blanchard (1995) replicated the positive results from individual cognitive therapy for IBS and showed it to be superior to a self-help support group control and to a symptom monitoring control. Finally, Vollmer and Blanchard (1998) have shown equivalent positive

results for cognitive therapy delivered individually or in small groups in comparison to a symptom monitoring control.

In the last three studies, over 80% of IBS sufferers had at least one Axis I disorder. Thus the presence of the comorbid psychiatric disorders no longer predicted outcome.

It seems clear to us that a relatively brief treatment with purely cognitive therapy is very beneficial for IBS and that it replicates strongly across differing therapists with different cohorts of IBS patients.

Returning to Table 17.1, one can see that the various treatments have had noticeable impact on pain, as well as on the other GI symptoms. The average percent reduction in abdominal pain and tenderness for the multicomponent cognitive-behavioral therapy (CBT) treatment was 40% across four studies on a total of 65 IBS sufferers. For relaxation alone, the percent decrease in pain was 43%. For the trials of cognitive therapy alone, the average decrease in pain and tenderness was 54% across four separate sets of a total of 44 IBS patients. Clearly, no treatment procedure is effective with 100% of IBS patients, but the various treatments are having noticeable effects on abdominal pain.

We should note that the results for the cognitive-behavioral treatment of IBS have held up well at follow-ups of 1 year (Schwarz, Blanchard, & Neff, 1986), 2 years (Blanchard, Schwarz, & Neff, 1988) and even 4 years (Schwarz, Taylor, Scharff, & Blanchard, 1990), as documented by GI symptom diaries.

Psychosocial Treatments: The Rest of the World

Three different psychosocial treatments have been tested in two or more controlled trials over the past 15 years: hypnotherapy, brief psychodynamic psychotherapy, and combinations of cognitive and behavioral procedures. From the point of view of the psychosocial treatment of other chronic pain problems, two of the three—cognitive-behavioral treatment packages and hypnotherapy—are not unexpected and have certainly been found to be useful with other pain problems. In Tables 17.2, 17.3, and 17.4, these studies are summarized, again with an emphasis on total outcome and on pain reduction.

Hypnotherapy

Several years ago Whorwell and colleagues (Whorwell, Prior, & Faragher, 1984), working in the United Kingdom, described dramatic improvement in a group of 15 refractory IBS patients treated with seven sessions of hypnotherapy that focused on relaxation, control of bowel motility, and ego strengthening. Participants practiced autohypnosis with the aid of a tape on a daily basis. A control group received placebo medication and supportive psychotherapy. The hypnotherapy group had very large reductions in bowel dysfunction and about 85% reduction in abdominal pain. A follow-up at about 18 months showed excellent maintenance, with two patients suffering brief relapses that were treated with a single booster session (Whorwell, Prior, & Colgan, 1987).

As shown in Table 17.2, Whorwell and colleagues have published two replications of their results, all of which showed very positive effects of hypnotherapy on abdominal pain.

Also as noted in Table 17.2, Harvey, Hinton, Gunary and Barry (1989) have reported replicating Whorwell's results with hypnotherapy administered either individually or in small groups. The form of administration did not matter. Their overall results were a bit lower than Whorwell's in terms of percent of sample improved, but treatment was also briefer (4 sessions vs. 10 to 12 sessions). It seems clear that hypnotherapy reliably leads to improvement in IBS, specifically in the pain component.

Brief Psychodynamic Psychotherapy

There have been two large controlled trials of brief psychodynamic psychotherapy for IBS. Both utilized large samples and routine medical care as a control condition. Both also included 1-year follow-up data. They are summarized in Table 17.3.

Svedlund, Sjodin, Ottosson, and Dotevall (1983) found psychotherapy superior to conventional medical care in terms of physician ratings of improvement in patient's abdominal pain at end of treatment and at the 1-year follow-up (in fact, the degree of improvement is greater at follow-up [68%] than at end of treatment [50%]). At the follow-up, but not at the end of treatment, the treated group also had greater relief of bowel dysfunction than the controls.

Guthrie, Creed, Dawson, and Tonenson (1991) combined brief psychodynamic psychotherapy with regular home practice of relaxation (by means of an audiotape) and compared it to routine medical care for the first 3 months of the study. Then 33 of the controls were crossed over to receive the psychotherapy and relaxation. Treatment was superior to the control condition on both patient ratings and physician ratings of abdominal pain and diarrhea at the end of treatment. Overall improvement held up well at the 1-year follow-up.

Thus, brief psychodynamic psychotherapy has certainly been shown to be effective for IBS in both the short term and the long term. It is not possible to gain a good sense of what was done from the synoptic descriptions in the journal reports; thus we cannot know how similar the two treatments were. We do know that the patients in the Guthrie et al. study also received regular home practice in relaxation, an element also present in Whorwell's hypnotherapy studies and in many CBT treatments. These results are somewhat at odds with the general literature on psychosocial

TABLE 17.2. Treatment of IBS with Hypnotherapy

Authors	Conditions	No. of visits and treatment duration	Sample size	Overall results	% of sample improved	% reduction in pain
Whorwell et al. (1984)	Hypnotherapy for relaxation and control of bowel motility; ego-strengthening exercises; daily autohypnosis at home with tape	7 30-minute visits over 3 months	15	Hypnotherapy group improved more than controls on abdominal pain, abdominal distension, bowel habit dysfunction, and general well-being.	N/R	Hypnotherapy, 85%; placebo, 5%
	Placebo medication plus supportive psychotherapy with attention to life issues and symptoms	Same	15	Controls improved significantly on pain, distension, well-being.		
Whorwell et al. (1987)	Hypnotherapy	7–10 30-minute visits over 3 months	15 original + 35	95% of 38 classical cases improved; 43% of 7 atypical cases improved; 60% of 5 cases with severe psychopathology improved.	84%	69% reduction for whole sample
Houghton, Jeyman, & Whorwell (1996)	Hypnotherapy Assessment-only controls	12 30-minute visits over 3 months	25 25	Hypnotherapy group improved more than controls on overall, pain, bloating, bowel dysfunction, psychic well-being, and mood.	N/R	Hypnotherapy, 81%; controls, 0%
Harvey et al. (1989)	Hypnotherapy, similar to Whorwell Individual Small groups	4 40-minute visits over 7 weeks	16 17	No difference between individual and group treatment; 33% symptom-free, 27% improved, 40% unimproved.	60%	N/R

Note. N/R, not reported.

278

TABLE 17.3. Treatment of IBS with Brief Psychodynamic Psychotherapy

Authors	Conditions	No. of visits and treatment duration	Sample size	Overall results	% of sample improved	% reduction in pain
Svedlund et al. (1983)	Brief dynamically oriented and supportive psychotherapy plus conventional medical care	10 1-hour visits over 3 months	50	Both groups improved on somatic and mental symptoms. Psychotherapy group superior to controls on abdominal pain reduction at 3 months and 15 months.	N/R	50% reduction in pain at 3 months; 68% reduction in pain at 15 months (physician ratings); 18% reduction in pain at 3 months in controls
	Conventional medical care		51	Psychotherapy group superior to controls on bowel dysfunction at 15 months		
Guthrie et al. (1991)	Brief dynamically oriented psychotherapy plus routine medical care; regular home practice with relaxation tape	7 1-hour sessions over 3 months	46	Treatment group superior to controls at 3 months: patient ratings—pain, distension, diarrhea; physician ratings—abdominal discomfort, diarrhea. No data on crossover patients	Treatment, 72%	67% reduction in pain for treatment at 3 months
	Routine medical care; at 3 months, 33 were crossed over to receive brief psychotherapy + relaxation tape	Treated after 3-month assessment	43		Control, 23%	19% reduction in pain for controls at 3 months

Note. N/R, not reported.

279

TABLE 17.4. Treatment of IBS with Cognitive-Behavioral Therapies

Authors	Conditions	Sample size	No. of visits and treatment duration	Overall results	% of sample improved	% reduction in pain
Bennett & Wilkinson (1983)	Education; PMR; cognitive therapy; homework	12	8 1-hour visits over 8 weeks	Both conditions had reduced abdominal pain and discomfort, and reduced abnormal bowel movements	N/R	Pain and discomfort significantly ($p = .01$) reduced in both conditions.
	Combination of three drugs: bulking agent, smooth muscle relaxant, antidepressant or anxiolytic	12	Once per month medical checks	CBT group had reduction in STAI, but medical group did not.		
Lunch & Zambie (1989)	PMR; cognitive therapy; analysis of stressful situations; assertiveness training; homework	11	8 2-hour visits over 8 weeks	Treatment superior to wait-list on reduction of abdominal discomfort and constipation and on symptom composite.	64%	31% reduction in pain for combined (n = 21) treated patients; 39% reduction in pain at 6-month follow-up.
	Symptom monitoring wait-list; later crossed over to treatment	10			52% of total treated group	
Corney et al. (1991)	Education and correction of mistaken ideas; rehearsal to overcome avoidance; bowel retraining; operant pain management	21	6–15 1-hour visits + follow-up visits	No differences between conditions except treated group reduced avoidance behaviors more than controls. Both groups reduced stomach pain significantly ($p = .018$) and constipation ($p = .047$).	52%	11 of 21 patients said stomach pain was improved; 48% reduction in pain ratings at 9 months
	Routine medical care plus support	20	1–4 visits		25%	5 of 20 patients had reduced stomach pain; 20% reduction in pain ratings at 9 months.
Shaw et al. (1991)	Education: taught relation of stress to GI symptoms; breathing exercises for relaxation and to counter daily tensions	18	4–10 40-minute visits over 6 months	The treated group had significantly fewer IBS attacks and they were of less severity than the drug treatment control.	67%	3 out of 18 patients (17%) had noticeable improvement in abdominal pain.
	Antispasmodic medication plus education and relation of stress to Gi symptoms	17	Not specified		18%	
van Dulmen, Fennis, & Bleijenberg (1996)	Group treatment: education, cognitive therapy, PMR, homework; group support	27	8 2-hour visits over 3 months	Treatment was superior to wait-list on reduction of abdominal pain intensity and duration of pain, with trend ($p = .09$) for other GI symptoms.	44%	35% reduction in pain scores for treatment; –6% (worsening) in controls.
	Symptom monitoring wait-list	20			11%	

Note. PMR, progressive muscle relaxation; CBT, cognitive-behavioral treatments; STAI, State–Trait Anxiety Inventory; N/R, not reported.

treatment of pain in that brief psychodynamic psychotherapy has not been shown in that literature to be helpful in chronic pain problems.

Cognitive-Behavioral Treatments

In addition to our work, summarized previously and in Table 17.1, there have been a number of reports of the use of various combinations of behavioral (usually relaxation) and cognitive (based on Meichenbaum, Beck, etc.) treatments compared to various control conditions. These studies are summarized in Table 17.4.

Several things are obvious from the work summarized in Table 17.4 and our work shown in Table 17.1: (1) there have been more controlled trials of cognitive-behavioral therapy (CBT) for IBS (eight) than for any other form of psychosocial treatment; (2) strong results have been obtained when CBT was compared to a symptom monitoring and/or waiting-list control; (3) when CBT has been compared to active drug treatment (Bennett & Wilkinson, 1985; Shaw et al., 1991) or psychological placebo (Blanchard et al., 1992, Studies 1 and 2), the results are less impressive; (4) the sample sizes have tended to be on the low side, with only one study (Blanchard et al., 1992, Study 2) having samples of 30 or more and two others (Corney, Stanton, Newell, Clare, & Fairclough, 1991; van Dulmen, Fennis, & Bleijenberg, 1996) having samples of 20 or more. The latter is in contrast to the brief psychotherapy trials with samples of between 40 and 50. Nevertheless, the systematic replication available in the CBT work is impressive and the level of control conditions generally more rigorous than has been utilized with other treatments.

The pain relief from CBT has been substantial but not outstanding. The overall level of GI symptom relief is adequate. Long-term follow-ups by Blanchard and colleagues (Blanchard et al., 1988; Schwarz et al., 1990) have shown good maintenance of symptom relief over 2 and 4 years, respectively.

All but one CBT condition contained explicit training in, and regular home practice of, some form of relaxation (Blanchard et al., 1993, tested relaxation alone as a treatment), and all contained both some form of cognitive therapy to help individuals identify stressful circumstances and explicitly change their thoughts and attributions about them and methods of behavioral coping. Regular home practice of relaxation was an element in all of the hypnotherapy studies and in one of the two brief psychotherapy trials (Guthrie et al., 1991).

Conclusions on Psychosocial Treatment for IBS

From the material summarized in Tables 17.1–17.4 and reviewed in the preceding pages, two forms of treatment stand out. *Hypnotherapy* has been shown to be superior to a combination of placebo medication and supportive psychotherapy, and it has received independent replication (Harvey et al., 1989). Purely *cognitive therapy*, not the CBT combinations, has been shown to be superior to symptom monitoring in three separate trials and also to be superior to self-help support groups. The replications have all taken place within the same laboratory but with different therapists. Of special relevance to his book, both treatments are effective in reducing the abdominal pain of IBS.

We should also add that various forms of CBT and brief psychodynamic psychotherapy also show strong evidence of efficacy in the treatment of IBS. Thus, to some extent, we have a situation wherein any systematic treatment delivered with enthusiasm seems to be helpful in alleviating the symptoms of IBS. This situation makes one suspect a placebo effect except that the results hold up for a year or more.

A major research question with important clinical implications is, What are the mechanisms by which these treatments work? Research has only begun to address these questions. We know from Greene and Blanchard (1994) that cognitive therapy probably leads to changes in attributions and self-talk and also to a reduction in depression. However, we do not yet know how these cognitive changes relate to GI symptom changes or to changes in the gut itself. Likewise, there is some evidence that hypnotherapy leads to changes in the hyperalgesia of the colon and rectum (Prior, Colgan, & Whorwell, 1990). This could account for some of the improvement in abdominal pain but not for changes in bowel dysfunction or bloating. Even here, the mechanism by which this change occurs is not clear.

There is clearly much more to learn about the nature, the physiological substrate, and the treatment of this widespread pain problem.

REFERENCES

American Psychiatric Association. (1987). *Diagnostic and statistical manual of mental disorders* (3rd ed., rev.). Washington, DC: Author.

Beck, A. T., Ward, C. H., Mendelson, M., Mock, J., & Erbaugh, J. (1961). An inventory for measuring depression. *Archives of General Psychiatry, 5,* 561–571.

Bennett, P., & Wilkinson, S. (1985). Comparison of psychological and medical treatment of the irritable bowel syndrome. *British Journal of Clinical Psychology, 24,* 215–216.

Blanchard, E. B., Greene, B., Scharff, L., & Schwarz-McMorris, S. P. (1993). Relaxation training as a treatment for irritable bowel syndrome. *Biofeedback and Self-Regulation, 18,* 125–132.

Blanchard, E. B., Radnitz, C., Evans, D. D., Schwarz, S. P., Neff, D. F., & Gerardi, M. A. (1986). Psychological comparisons of irritable bowel syndrome to chronic tension and migraine headache and non-patient controls. *Biofeedback and Self-Regulation, 11,* 221–230.

Blanchard, E. B., Radnitz, C., Schwarz, S. P., Neff, D. F., & Gerardi, M. A. (1987). Psychological changes associated with self-regulatory treatments of irritable bowel syndrome. *Biofeedback and Self-Regulation, 12,* 31–38.

Blanchard, E. B., Scharff, L., Schwarz, S. P., Suls, J. M., & Barlow, D. H. (1990). The role of anxiety and depression in the irritable bowel syndrome. *Behaviour Research and Therapy, 28,* 401–405.

Blanchard, E. B., & Schwarz, S. P. (1987). Adaptation of a multi-component treatment program for irritable bowel syndrome to a small group format. *Biofeedback and Self-Regulation, 12,* 63–69.

Blanchard, E. B., Schwarz, S. P., & Neff, D. F. (1988). Two-year follow-up of behavioral treatment of irritable bowel syndrome. *Behavior Therapy, 19,* 67–73.

Blanchard, E. B., Schwarz, S. P., Suls, J. M., Gerardi, M. A., Scharff, L., Greene, B., Taylor, A. E., Berreman, C., & Malamood, H. S. (1992). Two controlled evaluations of multicomponent psychological treatment of irritable bowel syndrome. *Behaviour Research and Therapy, 30,* 175–189.

Cook, I. J., van Eeden, A., & Collins, S. N. (1987). Patients with irritable bowel syndrome have greater pain tolerance than normal subjects. *Gastroenterology, 93,* 727–733.

Corney, R. H., Stanton, R., Newell, R., Clare, A., & Fairclough, P. (1991). Behavioural psychotherapy in the treatment of irritable bowel syndrome. *Journal of Psychosomatic Research, 35,* 461–469.

DiNardo, P. A., & Barlow, D. H. (1988). *Anxiety Disorders Interview Schedule–Revised (ADIS-R).* (Available from the Phobia and Anxiety Disorders Clinic, Center for Stress and Anxiety Disorders Clinic, State University of New York, Albany, NY.)

Drossman, D. A., Li, Z., Andruzzi, E., Temple, R. D., Talley, N. J., Thompson, W. G., Whitehead, W. E., Janssens, J., Funch-Jensen, P., Corazziari, E., Richter, J. E., & Koch, G. G. (1993). U.S. Householder Survey of Functional Gastrointestinal Disorders: Prevalence, sociodemography and health impact. *Digestive Diseases and Sciences, 38,* 1569–1580.

Drossman, D. A., Li, Z., Toner, B. B., Diamant, N. E., Creed, F. H., Thompson, D., Read, N. W., Babbs, C., Barreiro, M., Bank, L., Whitehead, W. E., Schuster, M. M., & Guthrie, E. A. (1995). Functional bowel disorders: A multicenter comparison of health status and development of illness severity index. *Digestive Diseases and Sciences, 40,* 986–995.

Drossman, D. A., McKee, D. C., Sandler, R. S., Mitchell, C. M., Cramer, E. B., Lowman, B. C., & Burger,
A. L. (1988). Psychosocial factors in the irritable bowel syndrome: A multivariate study of patients and nonpatients with irritable bowel syndrome. *Gastroenterology, 95,* 701–708.

Feighner, J. P., Robins, E., Guze, S. B., Woodruff, R. A., Winokur, G., & Munoz, R. (1972). Diagnostic criteria for use in psychiatric research. *Archives of General Psychiatry, 26,* 57–63.

Greenbaum, D. S., Mayle, J. E., Vanegeren, L. E., Jerome, J. A., Mayor, J. W., Greenbaum, R. B., Matson, R. W., Stein, G. E., Dean, H. A., Halvorsen, N. A., & Rosen, L. W. (1987). Effects of desipramine on irritable bowel syndrome compared with atropine and placebo. *Digestive Diseases and Sciences, 32,* 257–266.

Greene, B., & Blanchard, E. B. (1994). Cognitive therapy for irritable bowel syndrome. *Journal of Consulting and Clinical Psychology, 62,* 576–582.

Guthrie, E., Creed, F., Dawson, D., & Tonenson, B. (1991). A controlled trial of psychological treatment for the irritable bowel syndrome. *Gastroenterology, 100,* 450–457.

Harvey, R. F., Hinton, R. A., Gunary, R. M., & Barry, R. E. (1989). Individual and group hypnotherapy in treatment of refractory irritable bowel syndrome. *Lancet, 1,* 424–425.

Houghton, L. A., Jeyman, D. J., & Whorwell, P. J. (1996). Symptomatology, quality of life and economic features of irritable bowel syndrome: The effect of hypnotherapy. *Alimentary Pharmacology and Therapeutics, 10,* 91–95.

Klein, K. B. (1988). Controlled treatment trials in the irritable bowel syndrome: A critique. *Gastroenterology, 95,* 232–241.

Latimer, P. R. (1983). *Functional gastrointestinal disorders: A behavioral medicine approach.* New York: Springer.

Latimer, P., Campbell, D., Latimer, M., Sarna, S., Danie, E., & Waterfall, W. (1979). Irritable bowel syndrome: A test of the colonic hyperalgesia hypothesis. *Journal of Behavioral Medicine, 2,* 285–295.

Lynch, P. N., & Zamble, E. (1989). A controlled behavioral treatment study of irritable bowel syndrome. *Behavior Therapy, 20,* 509–523.

Manning, A. P., Thompson, W. G., Heaton, K. W., & Morris, A. F. (1978). Towards positive diagnosis of the irritable bowel. *British Medical Journal, 2,* 653–654.

Melzack, R. (1975). The McGill Pain Questionnaire: Major properties and scoring methods. *Pain, 7,* 277–299.

Neff, D. F., & Blanchard, E. B. (1987). A multi-component treatment for irritable bowel syndrome. *Behavior Therapy, 18,* 70–83.

Payne, A., & Blanchard, E. B. (1995). A controlled comparison of cognitive therapy and self-help support groups in the treatment of irritable bowel syndrome. *Journal of Consulting and Clinical Psychology, 63,* 779–786.

Prior, A., Colgan, S. N., & Whorwell, P. J. (1990). Changes in rectal sensitivity after hypnotherapy in patients with irritable bowel syndrome. *Gut, 31,* 896–898.

Prior, A., Maxton, D. G., & Whorwell, P. J. (1990). Anorectal manometry and irritable bowel syndrome: Differences between diarrhea and constipation predominant subjects. *Gut, 31,* 458–462.

Ritchie, J. (1973). Pain from distention of the pelvic colon by inflating a balloon in the irritable colon syndrome. *Gut, 14,* 125–132.

Schwarz, S. P., Blanchard, E. B., & Neff, D. F. (1986). Behavioral treatment of irritable bowel syndrome: A 1-year follow-up study. *Biofeedback and Self-Regulation, 11,* 189–198.

Schwarz, S. P., Taylor, A. E., Scharff, L., & Blanchard, E. B. (1990). A four-year follow-up of behaviorally treated irritable bowel syndrome patients. *Behaviour Research and Therapy, 28,* 331–335.

Shaw, G., Srivastava, E. D., Sadlier, M., Swann, P., James, J. Y., & Rhodes, J. (1991). Stress management for irritable bowel syndrome: A controlled trial. *Digestion, 50,* 36–42.

Spielberger, C. D., Gorsuch, R. L., & Lushene, R. E. (1970). *STAI Manual for the State–Trait Anxiety Inventory.* Palo Alto, CA: Consulting Psychologists Press.

Sternbach, R. A. (1985). *Survey of pain in the United States: The Nuprin Pain Report,* New York: Louis Harris.

Svedlund, J., Sjodin, I., Ottosson, J-O., & Dotevall, G. (1983). Controlled study of psychotherapy in irritable bowel syndrome. *Lancet,* 589–592.

Talley, N. J., Phillips, S. F., Melton, L. J., Mulvihill, C., Wiltgen, C., & Zinsmeister, A. R. (1990). Diagnostic value of the Manning criteria in irritable bowel syndrome. *Gut, 31,* 77–81.

Talley, N. J., Zinsmeister, A. R., Van Dyke, C., & Melton, L. J. (1991). Epidemiology of colonic symptoms and the irritable bowel syndrome. *Gastroenterology, 101,* 927–934.

Thompson, W. G., Creed, F., Drossman, D. A., Heaton, K. W., & Mazzacca, G. (1992). Functional bowel disease and functional abdominal pain. *Gastroenterology International, 5,* 75–91.

van Dulmen, A. M., Fennis, J. F. M., & Bleijenberg, G. (1996). Cognitive-behavioral group therapy for irritable bowel syndrome: Effects and long-term follow-up. *Psychosomatic Medicine, 58,* 508–514.

Vollmer, A., & Blanchard, E. B. (1998). Controlled comparison of individual versus group cognitive therapy for irritable bowel syndrome. *Behavior Therapy, 29,* 19–33.

Walker, E. A., Roy-Byrne, P. P., Katon, W. J., Li, L., Amos, D., & Jiranek, G. (1990). Psychiatric illness and irritable bowel syndrome: A comparison with inflammatory bowel disease. *American Journal of Psychiatry, 147,* 1656–1661.

Whitehead, W. E., Bosmajian, L., Zonderman, A. B., Costa, P. T., & Schuster, M. M. (1988). Symptoms of psychologic distress associated with irritable bowel syndrome: Comparison of community and medical clinic samples. *Gastroenterology, 95,* 709–714.

Whitehead, W. E., Holtkotter, B., Enck, P., Hoelzl, R., Holmes, K. D., Anthony, J., Shabsin, H. S., & Schuster, M. M. (1990). Tolerance for rectosigmoid distention in irritable bowel syndrome. *Gastroenterology, 98,* 1187–1192.

Whorwell, P. J., Prior, A., & Colgan, S. M. (1987). Hypnotherapy in severe irritable bowel syndrome: Further experience. *Gut, 28,* 423–425.

Whorwell, P. J., Prior, A., & Faragher, E. B. (1984). Controlled trial of hypnotherapy in the treatment of severe refractory irritable bowel syndrome. *Lancet,* 1232–1234.

Young, S. J., Alpers, D. H., Norlend, C. C., & Woodruff, R. A. (1976). Psychiatric illness and the irritable bowel syndrome: Practical implications for the primary physician. *Gastroenterology, 20,* 162–166.

Chapter 18

Phantom Limb Pain: A Continuing Puzzle

JOEL KATZ
LUCIA GAGLIESE

Many patients awake from the anesthetic after an amputation feeling certain that the operation has not been performed. They feel the lost limb so vividly that only when they reach out to touch it or peer under the bedsheets to see it do they realize it has been cut off. This phenomenon has been termed the "phantom limb" and is usually described as having a tingling or numb quality. The nonpainful phantom is reported to develop within a day of amputation in approximately one-third of patients, and by 8 days the incidence is near 85% (T. Jensen, Krebs, Nielsen, & Rasmussen, 1984). The percentage of amputees that experience a phantom limb 6 months or 2 years later does not change appreciably, although with time there is a significant decrease both in the frequency with which the phantom limb occurs and in the duration of episodes.

For many amputees, however, a distressing problem is phantom limb pain (PLP; Sherman, 1989). The pain may be an intensification of the tingling sensation that defines the nonpainful phantom limb or it may consist of paroxysmal shooting pains that travel up and down the limb. The phantom limb may be reported to be in a cramped or unnatural posture that gives rise to excruciating pain. For many amputees, the phantom is the seat of an intense burning pain, as if the hand or foot were being held too close to an open flame. In still others, the pain in the phan-

tom limb is indistinguishable from the pain experienced in the limb prior to amputation (Katz & Melzack, 1990). Frequently, amputees suffer from several types of pain (T. Jensen & Rasmussen, 1994).

The variability in time course of PLP is much greater than that of the nonpainful phantom. According to recent prospective studies (T. Jensen, Krebs, Nielsen, & Rasmussen, 1985; Nikolajsen, Ilkjaer, Krøner, Christensen, & Jensen, 1997), the incidence of PLP ranges between 50% and 71% over a 2-year period, with a reduction in the frequency and duration of attacks over time (T. Jensen et al., 1985). The prevalence of PLP is equally grim when the time frame is extended beyond the 2-year mark (Houghton, Saadah, Nicholls, McColl, & Houghton, 1994). More than 70% of amputees continue to experience PLP of considerable intensity as long as 25 years after amputation (Sherman, Sherman, & Parker, 1984). Equally striking is the low success rate of treatments for PLP: In the long term only 7% of patients are helped by the more than 50 types of therapy used to treat PLP (Sherman, 1989).

Psychological and emotional factors have long been thought to play a role in the etiology and maintenance of PLP. In this chapter we review the evidence for the role of these factors in PLP. In the first section, we deal primarily with the problem of PLP in children and adolescents. We address the controversial psychological question of whether the body image is innate or develops as a consequence of experience through the assessment of children born missing limbs or those who experienced amputation at a young age. In the second section, we review evidence for and against psychodynamic and characterological theories that have been advanced as evidence for the amputee's difficulty adapting to the loss of a limb. The relationship between psychological distress and PLP is then explored in the third section, followed by a section covering the literature on coping with PLP. The fifth section deals with various psychological treatments that have been found useful in the treatment of PLP. In the final section, a model is presented that involves a sympathetic efferent–somatic afferent cycle of activity, initiated by higher brain centers involved in cognitive and affective processes. The model attempts to explain psychologically and emotionally triggered phantom limb sensations and pain.

PHANTOM LIMB PAIN IN CHILDREN AND ADOLESCENTS

There has been a considerable amount of research focused on whether phantom limbs occur in children born without limbs (congenital aplasia), in child and adolescent amputees, and in adults who underwent amputation in childhood or adolescence. These studies are usually carried out to support one of two opposing theories concerning the origins of the body schema or body image. Until recently, a frequently cited paper (Riese & Bruck, 1950) that found no evidence for phantoms in children under the age of 6 years has been used to support the view that the body image is a use-dependent phenomenon requiring years of sensory and motor experience to develop (Simmel, 1961, 1962).

More recent studies have presented conflicting data and point to the alternate view that the body image experience may result from processing within genetically determined, hardwired neural structures (Lacroix, Melzack, Smith, & Mitchell, 1992; Melzack, 1989). Phantom limbs do occur in young children, as well as in older individuals who underwent amputation in infancy or early childhood (Easson, 1961; Lacroix et al., 1992; Poeck, 1964; Sohn, 1914). The evidence that phantom limbs are reported by individuals with congenital absence of limbs (Melzack, Israel, Lacroix, & Schultz, 1997;

Vetter & Weinstein, 1967; Weinstein & Sersen, 1961; Weinstein, Sersen, & Vetter, 1964) provides some of the strongest data to support the suggestion that the phantom limb represents the perceptual correlate of an innate, neural substrate of the body experience (Melzack, 1989). Notwithstanding the absence of an intact limb from birth, as well as years of subsequent sensorimotor experience with the residual appendage, which arguably might lead to a reorganization of brain regions subserving the absent limb (Skoyles, 1990), the phantom limb is perceived to be remarkably similar to an intact limb.

In contrast to the relatively large literature on the origins of the body schema, the problem of PLP in children and adolescents has not received the clinical and research attention it deserves. Case studies of PLP in children (Bradley, 1955; Roger, 1989) and adolescents (Frazier & Kolb, 1970; McGrath & Hillier, 1992; Riddoch, 1941; Solomon & Schmidt, 1978) with congenital absence of limbs (Sohn, 1914) are rare, but this rarity does not seem to accurately reflect the scope of the problem. Up to 20% of these individuals report phantom sensations (Melzack et al., 1997; Wilkins, McGrath, Finley, & Katz, 1998). Fewer studies have measured PLP in these samples, although the preliminary data suggest that 3–4% experience PLP. The phantom limb sensations (PLS) were described as cold, tingling, itchy, numb, and pins-and-needles (Melzack et al., 1997). A detailed description of the qualitative characteristics of PLP experienced by this group is not available.

Phantom sensations and pain following childhood amputation are much more common, especially if amputation takes place after the age of 6 years (Melzack et al., 1997; Simmel, 1962; Wilkins et al., 1998). For example, Boyle, Tebbi, Mindell, and Mettlin (1982) reported that approximately 7 years after amputation performed in childhood or adolescence, 70–75% of individuals continue to experience PLP, although none reported the pain to be severe. Miser and Miser (1989) reported that PLP is more common if the child suffered preamputation pain, and they contend that the pain does not persist beyond several months after amputation, but they do not include data to support these claims. More recently, a retrospective survey of PLP in children found a prevalence of 83%, with pain persisting for years in some children (Krane & Heller, 1995).

The characteristics of PLP appear to be similar in children and adult amputees. PLP in children is more likely following preoperative limb pain

(Krane & Heller, 1995). The pain begins soon after or within weeks of amputation in the majority of children (Krane & Heller, 1995) although delayed onset of several years has also been reported (Krane & Heller, 1995; Melzack et al., 1997). The most common descriptors of this pain are sharp, tingling, stabbing, uncomfortable, throbbing, pins and needles, and aching (Krane & Heller, 1995; Melzack et al., 1997; Wilkins et al., 1998).

Although the characteristics of PLP in individuals with congenital limb deficiency have not been described, the time to phantom onset appears to be greater in these individuals than in those with early childhood amputations (9.0 vs. 2.3 years; Melzack et al., 1997).

These data suggest that PLP in children is not unusual and may even be a significant problem in a proportion of children. It is unclear whether the paucity of data represents an undetected problem, because a child's response to pain may differ from that of an adult depending, in part, on the child's age, cognitive level, and emotional maturity (McGrath, 1990). Supporting this idea is the discrepancy between the incidence of PLP as reported by the child and the relative lack of physician/nurse documentation of the problem (Krane & Heller, 1995). It is also possible that the absence of information in the literature reflects the lower priority assigned to PLP when compared with other obstacles the child or adolescent must contend with in coping with life after amputation (Boyle et al., 1982; Lasoff, 1985; Tebbi & Mallon, 1987; Tebbi, Petrilli, & Richards, 1989). Self-esteem, depression, social support, and family functioning have recently been assessed in child amputees (Varni, Rubenfeld, Talbot, & Setoguchi, 1989a; Varni, Rubenfeld, Talbot, & Setoguchi, 1989b; Varni, Rubenfeld, Talbot, & Setoguchi, 1989c; Varni, Setoguchi, Talbot, & Rubenfeld Rappaport, 1991), and strategies have been designed for them to cope directly with social and interpersonal situations that arise as a consequence of the amputation (Varni & Setoguchi, 1991).

With the exception of a recent study by Wilkins et al. (1998), there is a conspicuous absence of information regarding the impact of PLP on the psychosocial functioning of child and adolescent amputees. Wilkins et al. (1998) found that several physical and social/cognitive factors can affect phantom limb sensations (PLS) and pain. The physical factors included touching the stump, prosthesis use, and the weather. The social/cognitive factors included the perception of objects approaching the stump and certain negative cognitions (e.g., "bad memories") and negative emotional states (e.g., embarrassment, fright, shock, discouragement). The majority (76%) of these childhood amputees reported being able to decrease the pain by ignoring it. This suggests that they are using adaptive cognitive coping strategies and may be amenable to cognitive-behavioral interventions for pain management.

PSYCHODYNAMIC EXPLANATIONS OF PHANTOM LIMB PAIN

Psychodynamic explanations of phantom limb phenomena have been advanced as evidence of the amputee's difficulty in adapting to the mutilated state (Frazier & Kolb, 1970; Parkes, 1973; Parkes & Napier, 1975; Szasz, 1975). Denial (of the loss or the associated affect) and repression are the most common defense mechanisms proposed to explain the presence of a painless phantom (Szasz, 1975), painful phantom (Parkes, 1973; Parkes & Napier, 1975; Stengel, 1965; Szasz, 1975) and various alterations in the form of the phantom limb (Abramson & Feibel, 1981; Weiss, 1958).

Though often elegantly formulated, psychodynamic explanations are not consistent with the accumulation of physiological and psychological data. For example, many amputees become profoundly depressed after surgery, yet phantom pain and other sensations persist. The co-occurrence of depression and pain is inconsistent with the role of denial since the intense negative affect implies awareness, if not acceptance, of the loss (Caplan & Hackett, 1963). In fact, for many amputees, the affect associated with the loss is so overwhelming that it cannot be contained and seems to "spill over" into the phantom thereby increasing the intensity of the tingling sensations or paresthesias that define the normal phantom (Simmel, 1959).

There are other inconsistencies between psychodynamic theory and empirical evidence.

1. Apparently healthy individuals who, by all objective measures, have adjusted to the amputation continue to report the presence of a phantom years after amputation (Simmel, 1959).
2. Phantoms do not develop if the process of sensory loss is gradual, as in leprosy (Simmel, 1956b), yet there should be as great a need for denial in these cases.
3. Phantoms that occur after CNS lesions (e.g., root avulsions or spinal cord transection) are similar to amputation phantoms in quality of

sensation, even though the real limb(s) is still present but totally anesthetic and paralyzed. One would not expect denial of the loss of function to produce a phantom defined by paresthesias (Weinstein, 1962).

4. In refuting the view of the phantom limb as a wish fulfillment, Weinstein (1962) argues that an orphaned child would be in greater need of a parent than a child amputee would be of a limb, yet very few orphans hallucinate parents in an attempt to cope with their loss. As outlined earlier, a recent study found that 100% of children experienced PLS after amputation (Krane & Heller, 1995).

5. Procedures that temporarily block the supply of afferent impulses from reaching the CNS (e.g., anesthetic nerve blocks, blood pressure cuff occlusion) reliably result in the perception of a phantom limb that persists until the flow of afferent input has been restored (Melzack & Bromage, 1973; Wall, 1981). Under these circumstances, it is difficult to see the need of a phantom limb to fulfill the putative ego-protective function of defending the individual from a loss.

Although denial is more commonly associated with diseases that have no visual evidence of infirmity (Caplan & Hackett, 1963), the foregoing does not imply that denial of the loss, affect, illness, or future implications plays no part in the overall adaptation to amputation. Patients may demonstrate their denial of the importance of these realities in a variety of ways (Bradway, Malone, Racy, Leal, & Poole, 1984; Rosen, 1950; Turgay & Sonuvar, 1983), but these do not include having a phantom. For the vast majority of amputees, the presence of a phantom limb—painful or painless—is not a symptom of a psychological disorder.

Characterological Disturbances

In addition to the role of specific defense mechanisms in the genesis of PLP, it is postulated that PLP may be psychologically determined by characterological disturbances such as "compulsive self-reliance" and "rigidity" (Parkes, 1973). Parkes and Napier (1975) describe the "denier" or "defiant type" of amputee by the "obstinate refusal to admit defeat even against better advice . . . who never accepts that he has lost anything at all. He appears to have a compulsive need to do everything at least as well as he could before operation and if possible, better, as if to convince himself and everyone else that he is not incapacitated at all" (p. 442). With the exception of a recent review (Sherman, Sherman, & Bruno, 1987), this excessively negative depiction of patients with persisting PLP as rigid and compulsively self-reliant has been uncritically accepted by researchers and clinicians working in the field of PLP (see, e.g., Dawson & Arnold, 1981; Dernham, 1986; Lundberg & Guggenheim, 1986; Shukla, Sahu, Tripathi, & Gupta, 1982) despite the absence of empirical evidence to support this view.

Several studies have attempted to describe the personality structure of individuals with PLP. Parkes (1973) assessed rigidity and compulsive self-reliance in a group of 46 amputees. He found that self-assessed rigidity levels at 3–4 weeks postamputation were predictive of persistent pain at 13 months. Compulsive self-reliance measured at 13 months was associated with pain intensity at 13 months. Morgenstern (1970) administered the Eysenck Personality Inventory (EPI; Eysenck & Eysenck, 1968) and the Cornell Medical Index (CMI; Brodman, Erdmann, Lordge, Wolff, & Broadbent, 1951) to three groups of amputees: pain-free, high pain, and low pain in the stump or phantom limb at least 2 years following amputation. He found that patients reporting high levels of pain obtained significantly higher scores on the Neuroticism scales of the EPI and CMI and on the Psychosomatic and Symptoms scales of the CMI than patients reporting no pain. This latter scale is a measure of the number of symptoms endorsed. The pattern of scores on each scale across the three groups is not reported, making it impossible to draw conclusions regarding patients reporting low levels of pain. Steigerwald, Brass, and Krainick (1981) compared the personality profiles of male amputees with and without PLP but do not report the average length of time from amputation to participation in the study. They found that the group with PLP showed higher levels of conformity and rigidity and lower levels of flexibility and self-confidence than the amputees without PLP. The groups did not differ in levels of hypochrondriasis. The patients in the above studies were individuals seen in clinics that specialize in the treatment of amputees. It is not clear if the results from these samples are representative of amputees in the community. Katz and Melzack (1990, 1991) compared the personality structures using the EPI and levels of rigidity using the Wesley Rigidity Questionnaire (Wesley, 1953) in amputees with no phantom sensations, with painless phantom sensations, and with PLP. These subjects had undergone amputation on average 4.9 years prior to assessment and were recruited from the community so that their participation was in no way connected to their medical care. In these groups, there were no differences on any of the EPI subscales. More to the point, there were no significant between-group differences in scores on the measure of psychological "rigidity" as defined by a tendency to persist in behaviors that were effective at one time or in a particular situation but no longer are adequate to accomplish current goals. The inconsistency of these results with those described previously may be due to differences in the sample; subjects in the studies by Katz and Melzack (1990, 1991) were not assessed or recruited as part of a treatment program. This interpretation is consistent with the hypothesis that the "compulsive self-reliance" and "rigidity" of the amputees with PLP may be specific to those who continue to seek treatment.

In many instances an association between the presence of pain and psychological distress (e.g., depression and anxiety) or particular personality traits or styles (e.g., rigidity and compulsive self-reliance) is influenced by biased sampling procedures, so that the characteristics of a select group of patients (e.g., those referred to a pain center) come to define the population at large (Merskey, 1989; Sherman et al., 1987). The low success rate of most treatments for PLP serves as a deterrent to all but the most persistent or self-reliant individuals. Long after less assertive patients have given up actively seeking help, these sufferers of PLP continue to search for relief despite repeated failures. This self-selection bias has been advanced to explain the tendency for individuals with both "compulsively self-reliant" personality characteristics and PLP to dominate the clinical picture of the typical patient with PLP (Sherman et al., 1987).

One danger in attributing such negative traits to patients suffering from pain is the tendency for researchers and clinicians who are less careful to overgeneralize from a select group of individuals to all patients with PLP. Some health professionals adopt working definitions of terms such as "compulsively self-reliant" and "rigid" that are consistent with their role as helper. Patients who do not heed their advice, who try to rely on themselves, who attempt to make the best of a bad situation, and who persist in trying to overcome adversity may acquire these harmful labels because they do not behave in a way that conforms to the helper's expectations. Similar patients have been described as "oppositional individuals" (Ascher & Turner, 1980), "therapist killers" and "therapy addicts" (Weeks & L'Abate, 1982), and "help-rejecting complainers" (Tennen, Rohrbaugh, Press, & White,

1981). They resist most direct attempts at change. They fight the helper's moves to help (Katz, 1984). It is true that certain individuals are exceedingly difficult to treat, but we as clinicians and researchers must be mindful of our choice of words when attempting to "help." These terms have connotations that cast the behaviors and attitudes they describe in a negative light. They impede the already difficult processes of psychological and physical rehabilitation that confront the patient after the amputation of a limb. It is not too difficult to also see the positive traits possessed by these highly motivated and independent individuals.

As such, individuals with chronic PLP who continue to seek treatment may be similar to individuals with other forms of chronic pain who are seen in specialized pain clinics. Comparisons of the personality profiles of amputees with those of patients with chronic musculoskeletal pain seen in a pain clinic have shown that these groups do not differ on measures of histrionic or compulsive/conforming personality disorders (Marshall, Helmes, & Deathe, 1992). These data support the conclusion that the levels of characterological disturbance reported in the population of individuals with PLP may be due to the biased samples studied. In addition, none of the studies described above assessed personality structure prior to amputation, making it impossible to draw any conclusions regarding causality. Interpretation of these results is also limited by the variety of personality assessment instruments used.

PHANTOM LIMB PAIN AND PSYCHOLOGICAL DISTURBANCE

The co-occurrence of PLP and psychological disturbance has led to three conclusions: (1) pain is a symptom of a psychological disorder (Parkes, 1973; Szasz, 1975), (2) psychological disturbance is a consequence of pain (Sherman et al., 1987), or (3) the two are causally unrelated (Caplan & Hackett, 1963). At present, the consensus is that there is no difference in the prevalence rates of pain of psychological origin among amputees and the general population. There is no evidence to suggest that surgical amputation predisposes an individual to develop pain of psychological origin, nor that patients who undergo amputation are at greater risk for developing such pain. However, it should be noted that a prospective study has yet to be conducted in which preoperative measures of psychological and emotional functioning are obtained sufficiently prior to amputation so as to avoid the confounding effects of preamputation pain and hospitalization.

Anxiety and Depression

Given the intractability of PLP among the adult population, it should come as no surprise to find that amputees suffering with PLP exhibit higher than normal levels of psychological and emotional distress. The co-occurrence of chronic pain and psychological distress, especially symptoms of anxiety and depression, has been well documented (Caplan & Hackett, 1963; Lindesay, 1985; Parkes, 1973; Sherman et al., 1987; Shukla et al., 1982).

Depression has received the most empirical attention. Within samples of amputees with PLP seen in a clinical setting, up to 20% may meet the criteria for an ICD-8 diagnosis of depression (Lindesay, 1986). In addition, those who experience high levels of PLP are more likely to have elevated scores on the Beck Depression Inventory (BDI) than those who report low levels of PLP. However, Parkes (1973) reported that the intensity of PLP 13 months postamputation was not correlated with levels of depression. These inconsistent results may be due to methodological differences between the studies, especially in the psychometric instruments used to assess depression and pain. The majority of the studies suggests that depression may be a significant problem among those amputees with the most intense PLP seen in clinical settings. The evidence from samples of amputees recruited from the community, independent of treatment for PLP or amputation-related problems, suggests that levels of depressive symptomatology as assessed with the BDI do not discriminate between amputees with and without PLP (Katz & Melzack, 1990, 1991). The finding that individuals with chronic, intense PLP exhibit significant depressive symptomatology (Lindesay, 1986) may only be applicable to those amputees who are seen in the clinical setting and may not generalize to the larger population of amputees with PLP. In fact, comparisons between PLP patients and chronic musculoskeletal pain patients suggest that those with chronic musculoskeletal pain experience more intense dysthymia and somatoform symptoms, as measured on the Millon Clinical Multiaxial Inventory (MCMI), than amputees with chronic stump pain or PLP (Marshall et al., 1992).

The assessment of anxiety has received less empirical attention. In a group of amputees with significant PLP, not one reached the criteria for anxiety disorders using the General Health Questionnaire and ICD-8 (Lindesay, 1986). Consistent with this, several studies have shown that anxiety and PLP intensity are not correlated in clinical (Parkes, 1973; Steigerwald et al., 1981) or community samples (Katz & Melzack, 1990, 1991). In addition, amputees with stump pain or PLP receive lower MCMI anxiety scores than patients with chronic musculoskeletal pain (Marshall et al., 1992). Taken together, these data suggest that amputees with intense PLP may experience more depressive symptomatology than amputees without PLP. However, these groups do not differ on levels of anxiety. Of interest are the findings of Marshall et al. (1992). In this sample, amputees with stump pain or PLP reported less psychological distress but more impairment performing activities of daily life than other chronic pain patients. Therefore, the psychological distress associated with PLP does not appear to be greater than that usually associated with chronic pain and may, in fact, more accurately reflect distress associated with amputation rather than pain per se.

Pain "Memories" in Phantom Limbs

Recent studies show that the central nervous system is capable of long-term change in response to noxious somatosensory inputs. These long-term, injury-induced "plastic" changes may contribute to the experience of pain long after the offending stimulus has been removed or the injury has healed (Coderre & Katz, 1997; Katz et al., 1992, 1994). The most striking clinical evidence of injury-induced neuroplasticity comes from studies of amputees who report PLP resembling a pain experienced in the limb before amputation (Katz & Melzack, 1990). Amputees may experience the sensation of a painful ingrown toenail digging into the phantom toe or the steady, gnawing pain of a diabetic foot ulcer that was present at the time of amputation. These "somatosensory pain memories" are replicas of distressing preamputation lesions and pains that were experienced at or near the time of amputation. They are described as having the same qualities of sensation as the preamputation pain and are referred to the same location of the phantom limb. Patients who report these pains emphasize that they are suffering real pain and insist that the experience is not merely a cognitive recollection of an earlier pain.

It is not uncommon for proponents of theories of PLP to discount pain that could not be explained on the basis of current physiological and anatomical knowledge as psychological in origin (see e.g., Bailey & Moersch, 1941; Henderson & Smyth, 1948; Lakoff, 1990). The practice of relegating certain inexplicable phenomena to the psychological or emotional realm may free the theorist from considering them further, but it changes how the amputee is viewed and treated and implicitly blames him or her for the pain.

This reasoning has also been applied to the experience of pain memories in phantom limbs as well. It has been argued that the similarity of pain before and after amputation represents a psychopathological response to amputation in which the psychological or emotional importance of the preamputation pain determines the likelihood of its reexperience in the phantom limb. Bailey and Moersh (1941) provide an example of such a shift in theoretical orientation and level of analysis from biological to psychological when confronted with the otherwise inexplicable phenomenon of a patient whose phantom included the sensation of a wood sliver that had been under the nail of his index finger at the time of amputation. They write that the development of such phantom pains depends on the experience of "both psychical and physical trauma at the time of, or just prior to, the surgical amputation" (p. 41) and go on to equate "cerebral" with "psychical" and "psychical" with "obsession neurosis" without offering an explanation for their shift in orientation and leap in logic. The study by Bailey and Moersch is interesting from more than just a historical perspective, since the article has recently been reprinted in its entirety (Bailey & Moersch, 1992) without appropriate editorial commentary that would have addressed the issue of psychopathology and PLP based on empirical findings (Katz, 1992a).

Arguments that attempt to explain pain memories as a psychopathological response to amputation are untenable in the light of two lines of recent evidence. First, amputees who reported that their PLP was the same before and after amputation could not be differentiated on personality, depression, or anxiety inventories from those who did not have PLP or from subjects who had PLP that bore no resemblance to their preamputation pain (Katz & Melzack, 1990).

The second line of evidence comes from experiments that model the phantom limb in animals (Katz, Vaccarino, Coderre, & Melzack, 1991). Sectioning the sciatic and saphenous nerves in the rat is followed by self-mutilation (autotomy) of the

denervated hindpaw. It is well established that autotomy is a response to pain or dysesthesias (painful paresthesias or tingling) referred to the anesthetic limb and represents a model of the phantom limb. A brief thermal injury of a specific region of the hindpaw just prior to nerve sections changes the usual pattern of autotomy over the following days. Animals injured before but not after nerve sections direct autotomy to the site of prior injury. Because the nerve sections produce a deafferentation of the entire hindpaw, the central effects of the injury are sustained in the absence of further inputs from the hindpaw, implying that painful or dysesthetic sensations are referred specifically to the region of the denervated limb that had received the injury. The correspondence between the sites of prior injury and subsequent autotomy parallels descriptions of human amputees who report the persistence of a preamputation pain or lesion referred to the same location of the phantom limb.

In these experiments (Katz et al., 1991), the injury was always induced while the rats were under a general anesthetic, and they were maintained under the general anesthetic until well after the sciatic and saphenous nerve transections had been performed. Thus, although the rats never experienced the thermal injury in an awake state, their behavior in the days after the nerve sections revealed that the effects of the injury were still capable of influencing perception and behavior (in the absence of further inputs from the injured region). These findings imply that somatosensory pain memories reported by human amputees need not represent psychologically important pains and provide empirical support for the hypothesis that the unified experience of a pain memory involves two potentially dissociable forms of memory, one of which (the somatosensory component) is independent of the conscious experience of pain (Katz & Melzack, 1990).

Lacroix et al. (1992) have recently provided the most compelling clinical evidence to date of a dissociation between the cognitive and somatosensory memory components underlying the unified experience of a pain memory. They report the case of a 16-year-old girl who was born with a congenital deformity of the right foot, which was amputated when she was just 6 years old. At the time of the interview 10 years after amputation, the patient reported a flat phantom foot that was stuck in a forward position. This description corresponded to information subsequently obtained from her medical records verifying a right flatfoot that was locked in an equinovalgus position and incapable of movement. Interestingly, the patient was not aware that her foot had been deformed as a child, for she mistakenly described her foot as she remembered it prior to amputation as being normal and freely mobile. This case report demonstrates the remarkable capacity of the central nervous system to retain, for years after amputation, a complete representation of the cut-off part, including its somatosensory qualities, proprioceptive sensibility, and associated motor program. Moreover, the case demonstrates that the neural circuitry underlying the somatosensory component is capable of being activated and of influencing conscious awareness independent of the cognitive component, which usually suffuses the experience of the phantom limb with personal history and meaning tied to the original event.

COPING WITH PHANTOM LIMB PAIN

The experience of PLP and associated psychological distress may be directly related to the amputees' coping skills. Coping with pain may be defined as the thoughts and actions in which people engage in their efforts to manage pain on a daily basis (Katz, Ritvo, Irvine, & Jackson, 1996). These diverse efforts include interventions as global as cognitive-behavior therapy and other self-management programs developed to help patients cope with a multitude of problems associated with pain and specific strategies designed to manage the sensory intensity of a discrete episode of pain. In addition to the burden of pain, patients must contend with many secondary lifestyle changes that inevitably arise when pain becomes chronic. Among these downstream effects are loss of employment and income, mood disturbances such as depression and anxiety, changes in the marital relationship and family dynamics, and a reduction in social and leisure activities (Hitchcock, Ferrell, & McCaffery, 1994).

The literature on PLP spans more than 100 years, yet we know very little about the coping efforts and outcomes of amputees with PLP. To date, only two studies have evaluated use of coping strategies in patients with PLP (Hill, 1993; Hill, Niven, & Knussen, 1995). Amputees with PLP who made use of coping strategies indicative of helplessness, such as catastrophizing, reported more pain and psychological distress than patients who did not use these coping strategies (Hill, 1993; Hill et al.,

1995). In addition, catastrophizing was related to increased levels of physical and psychosocial distress (Hill et al., 1995).

These results are consistent with what is known about pain coping in other chronic pain populations; namely, patients who catastrophize fare worse than those who do not (M. Jensen, Turner, Romano, & Karoly, 1991). Factor analytic or principal component techniques often yield a factor that invariably includes the negative thinking characteristic of catastrophizing (e.g., helplessness, pain control and rational thinking, self-control and rational thinking). In general, these factors tend to be strongly correlated with depression, measures of physical impairment, and poor psychosocial adjustment. A reduction in catastrophizing, for example, was associated with less pain and improved psychosocial functioning following either cognitive-behavioral or operant behavioral therapy for low back pain (Turner & Clancy, 1986). In another study (Flor, Behle, & Birbaumer, 1993), the degree of catastrophizing was reduced significantly from pre- to posttreatment among patients who improved but not among patients who did not. In contrast, improvement was not accompanied by a strengthening of adaptive self-statements and beliefs. The association between reduced pain and a reduction in the use of catastrophizing without a strengthening of adaptive self-statements and beliefs suggests that maladaptive cognitions may have a stronger influence on negative outcomes than the utilization of adaptive coping strategies. In other words, it may be more important not to catastrophize than to engage in positive self-statements. This is a challenging area for future research and treatment development given the tendency for certain qualities of PLP to occur episodically and unpredictably (see, e.g., Hill, 1993; Hill et al., 1995). These parameters are likely to contribute to a sense of helplessness and lack of personal control.

Primary pain prevention and early detection of individuals at risk for developing chronic pain is of paramount importance. Keefe, Salley, and Lefebvre (1992) advocate use of longitudinal designs in which subjects are identified and assessed in terms of coping strategies prior to the development of chronic pain. Following these individuals over time would clarify the relationship between pain coping strategies and the development of persistent pain. Future research might best accomplish this objective by targeting patient populations, such as amputees, at relatively high risk for developing long-term pain problems.

TREATMENTS FOR PHANTOM LIMB PAIN

The psychological management of PLP has received very little empirical attention, although it has long been thought that psychological manipulations such as distraction might alleviate PLP (Morgenstern, 1964; Parkes, 1973). Specific interventions for PLP have not been developed, and the efficacy of standard psychological treatments for other chronic pain disorders has not been assessed in samples with PLP. Most of the available studies are retrospective and uncontrolled and lack appropriate comparison groups. This makes it very difficult to draw conclusions about the treatments that are most appropriate for these patients.

Preamputation Psychoeducation

Given that cognitive and affective processes may trigger or exacerbate PLP, it is of the utmost importance that patients be prepared prior to amputation for the presence of a phantom limb. Patient education programs and treatment of stress prior to and after amputation have become standard practice in some institutions (Butler, Turkal, & Seidl, 1992; McGrath & Hillier, 1992; Sherman, 1989). Patients who are ill prepared psychologically for amputation suffer needlessly with PLP and concern about their sanity (Solomon & Schmidt, 1978). This is equally true of children and adolescents, who may not fully comprehend the medical necessity and urgency of amputation and may all too often believe they are being punished (Turgay & Sonuvar, 1983). Misconceptions about methods of limb disposal after amputation have been reported to interfere with recovery and to be responsible for maintaining PLP in adolescents (Frazier & Kolb, 1970; Solomon & Schmidt, 1978). McGrath and Hillier (1992) recently outlined a supportive and collaborative approach to the assessment and management of phantom limb phenomena for adolescents that has significant potential for increasing patient control and decreasing fear and anxiety.

Psychotherapy

There have been reports of the usefulness of psychotherapy in the treatment of chronic PLP. Case reports suggest that psychodynamic and supportive approaches may be helpful (Blood, 1956; Rosen,

1950). It has also been suggested that amputees with PLP may benefit from psychoeducational group therapy with other amputees (Howard, 1983). Empirical studies to support the effectiveness of these treatments are not available.

Biofeedback and Relaxation Training

Relaxation training involves the use of standardized techniques to elicit the "relaxation response" (Jessup & Gallegos, 1994). Biofeedback training uses sensory stimuli to signal levels of a biological variable such as skin temperature or electromyographic (EMG) activity. The patient is guided by this signal or feedback to change the level of this variable, such as reducing EMG levels (Jessup & Gallegos, 1994). Biofeedback often includes relaxation training, and therefore studies using both or either of these strategies will be considered together. The effectiveness of these treatments in the management of chronic pain has been demonstrated in a number of empirical studies (see review by Jessup & Gallegos, 1994). There are case reports (Dougherty, 1980; Sherman, 1976; Sherman, Gall, & Gormly, 1979) of favorable outcomes with this treatment, but only one study has assessed the appropriateness of this treatment for patients with PLP. Unfortunately, the sample size is small, and appropriate controls are not included. Nonetheless, the majority of patients (14 of 16 or 87.5%) benefited from this treatment. These benefits were maintained from 6 months to 3 years following treatment (Sherman et al., 1979).

Hypnosis

The use of hypnosis for the management of PLP has received limited attention. Although hypnosis may reduce pain to a greater extent than no-treatment control conditions, hypnosis is not more effective than other forms of psychological management (Spanos, Carmanico, & Ellis, 1994). Several case reports (Baker, 1984; Muraoka, Komiyama, Hosoi, Mine, & Kubo, 1996; Seigel, 1979) and case series (Cedercreutz, 1954; Cedercreutz & Uusitalo, 1967) have been published of patients treated with hypnosis for PLP. Among the case series, the results suggest that over 50% of patients obtain complete relief and approximately 25% obtain at least partial relief immediately following treatment; however, neither of these studies (Cedercreutz, 1954; Cedercreutz & Uusitalo, 1967) included a comparison or placebo group. Unfortunately, these results are generally short-lived, with 49% reporting at least partial improvement at follow-up 1 to 8 years posttreatment (Cedercreutz & Uusitalo, 1967).

Virtual Reality/Mirror Box Intervention for Phantom Paralysis

Although this treatment is not among the traditional psychotherapies, it is indeed "psychological" in that it uses basic elements of perception to alleviate a specific quality of PLP, namely, painful phantom paralysis. In this condition, amputees report that their phantom is "frozen" in a fixed posture, incapable of voluntary movement. For some of these individuals, the problem of "phantom paralysis" is associated with pain (Ramachandran, 1994). For example, a common report is that the amputee's fingernails are felt to be digging into the palm of the phantom hand (Mitchell, 1872; Ramachandran, 1994; Ramachandran & Rogers-Ramachandran, 1996). In some cases this may be related to the position of the limb before amputation (i.e., a postural pain memory; Browder & Gallagher, 1948; Frederiks, 1963; T. Jensen et al., 1984; Katz & Melzack, 1990; Mitchell, 1872). In others, the inability to move the phantom limb may develop progressively after amputation (Ramachandran, 1994; Ramachandran & Rogers-Ramachandran, 1996). Until recently, there has been nothing in the way of treatment for this painful problem.

A clever solution has been devised that promises to restore, at least temporarily, a sense of voluntary movement to the paralyzed phantom limb (Ramachandran, 1994; Ramachandran & Rogers-Ramachandran, 1996). The solution is based on the assumption that the brain has "learned" that the phantom is paralyzed. The learning occurs either as a function of past experience with a paralyzed limb before amputation or subsequent to amputation due to the absence of visual feedback from the limb following attempts to move the phantom. The experiments involve a "virtual reality box" that makes use of mirrors to trick the brain into thinking that the phantom is moving. The amputee looks into a mirror at his or her contralateral intact hand while it is positioned to coincide spatially with the felt position of the phantom hand. The amputee is then instructed to carry out the same movement with both hands while looking at the phantom (i.e., the reflection of the intact hand). In the majority of cases, the sight of

the hand moving determines the ultimate perception, and the amputee feels as if the once paralyzed hand is now moving freely. These findings support the idea that vision dominates over other sensory modalities in determining the phantom limb percept (Katz, 1993). When there is a discrepancy or contradiction between incoming information from different modalities, or when a state of uncertainty exists based on somatosensory input alone, additional information is sought via the visual sense, which usually determines the perceptual experience.

The initial experiments carried out by Ramachandran and colleagues (Ramachandran, 1994; Ramachandran & Rogers-Ramachandran, 1996) suggest that in most cases the initiation of movement in the phantom is also associated with pain relief. From a clinical standpoint, controlled studies are needed to assess the duration of the analgesic effect, the percentage of patients in whom it is effective, and the possibility that a permanent effect can be achieved with repeated use of the mirrors.

These very preliminary data suggest that psychological interventions may play an important role in the management of PLP. However, this conclusion must remain tentative until data from randomized treatment studies with appropriate comparison groups and follow-up assessments are available. It is nonetheless interesting to speculate on one of the mechanisms by which the more traditional treatments may influence the experience of PLP.

COGNITIVE AND AFFECTIVE TRIGGERS ALTER PHANTOM LIMB EXPERIENCE BY A CYCLE OF SYMPATHETIC EFFERENT–SOMATIC AFFERENT ACTIVITY

As described in the previous sections, the idea that cognitive and affective processes can cause pain traditionally has been tied to the notion of psychopathology. However, it is becoming increasingly clear that under certain circumstances pain may be triggered by these processes in psychologically healthy individuals as well. Although instances of cognitively or affectively triggered pain and psychopathology may be present in the same amputee, their co-occurrence should not be taken as prima facie evidence of a causal link.

It is commonly accepted that anxiety or stress influence pain perception and subsequent behavior (Merskey, 1989). The aggravation or alleviation of pain referred to phantom body parts may also be mediated in part by psychological processes that alter anxiety levels (Kolb, 1954). Phantom breast pain after mastectomy is provoked by emotional distress in 6% of women 3 weeks after surgery and in 29% 1 year later (Krøner, Krebs, Skov, & Jørgensen, 1989). Half of all lower-limb amputees report that attacks of PLP can be brought on by emotional distress (T. Jensen et al., 1985) as long as 7 years after amputation (Krebs, Jensen, Krøner, Nielsen, & Jørgensen, 1985). A combination of progressive relaxation training and EMG biofeedback of stump and forehead muscles produces significant reductions in PLP and anxiety that are sustained for up to 3 years (Sherman, 1976; Sherman et al., 1979). Finally, stress levels and pain intensity ratings sampled over a 180-day observation period correlate significantly for most amputees (Arena, Sherman, & Bruno, 1990).

The literature contains many examples of cognitive or affective processes precipitating transient but profound alterations in the quality and intensity of PLS. These processes include hypnosis (Schilder, 1950), concentration (Morgenstern, 1964; Riddoch, 1941), distraction (Parkes, 1973), relaxation (Sherman, 1976; Sherman et al., 1979), fright (Henderson & Smyth, 1948), forceful reminders of the events that led to amputation (Simmel, 1956a), the sight of other amputees (Simmel, 1956a), and witnessing cruel and violent acts (Pilowsky & Kaufman, 1965; Stengel, 1965). One amputee interviewed by Katz described his reaction to an accident involving his wife by reporting "goose bumps and cold shivering down the phantom [leg]. It went through me. Everything emotional will get you that." Another amputee stated, "It's like everything I feel goes there—the good and the bad."

The material presented here indicates that cognitive and affective processes reliably trigger transient pains or sensations referred to the phantom limb. The model schematically represented in Figure 18.1 outlines a mechanism through which cognitive and affective processes associated with higher cortical and limbic centers may alter PLS. The reciprocal connections between cortical, limbic, and lateral hypothalamic structures are well documented (Brodal, 1981; Smith & DeVito, 1984). The lateral hypothalamus is involved in the control and integration of neural activity associated with affectively charged behavior (Brodal, 1981; Melzack & Casey, 1968; Smith & DeVito, 1984) and has direct projections to the lateral horn of the spinal cord. The intensity of phantom limb paresthesias and dysesthesias may thus be modulated by higher brain centers involved in cognitive

and affective processes via a multisynaptic network of descending inputs that impinges on preganglionic sympathetic neurons producing diffuse peripheral autonomic discharge and activation of primary afferent fibers located in stump neuromas.

Changes in the intensity of phantom limb paresthesias may thus reflect the joint activity of cholinergic (sudomotor) and noradrenergic (vasomotor) postganglionic sympathetic fibers on primary afferents located in the stump and stump neuromas (Katz, 1992b; Katz, France, & Melzack, 1989). As shown in Figure 18.1, release of acetylcholine and noradrenaline from postganglionic sympathetic fibers produces transient vasoconstriction and heightened skin conductance responses. Also, neurotransmitter release onto apposing peripheral fibers trapped in stump neuromas increases primary afferent discharge. This information is transmitted rostrally, where it gives rise to referred phantom sensations on reaching central structures subserving the amputated parts of the limb. The moment-to-moment fluctuations in the intensity of phantom limb paresthesias reported by many amputees may, in part, reflect a cycle of sympathetic efferent–somatic afferent activity. Increases in the intensity of phantom limb paresthesias would follow bursts of sympathetic activity, and decreases would correspond to periods of relative sympathetic inactivity.

Occasionally, the effects of intense affect (e.g., fright, horror) are experienced diffusely over the entire body as cutis anserina associated with pilomotor contraction (i.e., "goose bumps" or a tingling sensation). Among amputees, however, a more frequent occurrence is that the perception of less salient events and emotions precipitates these sensations throughout only the phantom limb. The tendency for affectively charged and psychologically meaningful experiences to be referred to the phantom limb but not to other parts of the body is consistent with two lines of evidence suggesting that the threshold for impulse generation is lower both in regenerating primary afferents in the stump and in deafferented central cells subserving the phantom limb than it is in the intact nervous system. First, regenerating sprouts, which are trapped in a neuroma, are exceedingly sensitive to the postganglionic sympathetic neurotransmitters noradrenaline (Wall & Gutnick, 1974) and acetylcholine (Diamond, 1959) and discharge rapidly when these substances are present. In contrast, intact peripheral fibers do not show this chemosensitivity and thus have a higher threshold compared with regenerating sprouts. Second, deafferentation results in

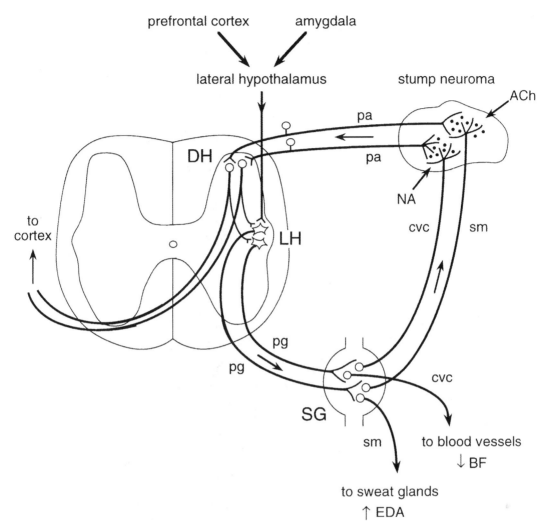

FIGURE 18.1. Schematic diagram illustrating a mechanism of sympathetically generated phantom limb paresthesias. Spontaneous activity or excitatory inputs descending from cortex (e.g., due to the perception of a salient event, loud noise, thought, feeling, etc.) increase the discharge rate of preganglionic (pg) sympathetic neurons with cell bodies in the lateral horn (LH) of the spinal cord and terminals in the sympathetic ganglion (SG). These neurons excite postganglionic noradrenergic (NA) cutaneous vasoconstrictor (cvc) and cholinergic (ACh) sudomotor (sm) fibers that impinge on effector organs (vascular smooth muscle and sweat glands) in the stump and on sprouts from large diameter primary afferent (pa) fibers that have been trapped in a neuroma. The release of ACh and NA on effector organs results in increased electrodermal activity (EDA) and decreased blood flow (BF) to the stump. Release of these chemicals in the neuroma activates primary afferents that project to spinal cord dorsal horn (DH) cells subserving the amputated parts of the limb. These neurons, in turn, feed back to the preganglionic sympathetic neurons and project rostrally where the impulses contribute to the perception of phantom limb paresthesias. If DH cells have been sensitized due to injury or if nociceptive primary afferents are activated, then the perception may be dysesthetic.

a loss of inhibitory control over cells in the dorsal horn and more rostral sensory structures, giving rise to the perception of a phantom limb (Melzack & Loeser, 1978; Wall, 1981). This consequence of deafferentation implies that the threshold for detecting sympathetically triggered afferent impulses

arising from stump neuromas should be lower than at other, intact body sites, since stump impulses would be subject to less inhibition on reaching the spinal cord. This fits well with the observation that the threshold for detecting sensations in the phantom limb during stimulation of the stump is lower than at the site of stimulation itself (Carlen, Wall, Nadvorna, & Steinbach, 1978).

Another possibility is that amputation leads to increased expression of alpha-1 adrenergic receptors located on mechanoreceptors or nociceptors (Campbell, Meyer, Davis, & Raja, 1992) in stump neuromas. This hypothesis would explain the perception of phantom limb paresthesias or dysesthesias in the absence of regional sympathetic hyperactivity. Taken together, these observations may explain the puzzling finding that only after amputation does the (phantom) limb become the site of affectively or cognitively triggered sensations.

The suggestion that the perception of PLS may reflect the activity of postganglionic sympathetic fibers on stump primary afferents is obviously not meant to imply that paresthesias arise only from a peripheral source. Blocking the afferent supply to a body region is sufficient to produce the experience of a painless phantom defined by paresthesias (Melzack & Bromage, 1973; Wall, 1981), and electrical stimulation of the medial lemniscal pathway gives rise to the sensation of paresthesias referred to the territory subserved by the cells being stimulated (Tasker, Organ, & Hawrylyshyn, 1982). Moreover, it is likely that through repeated activation neural circuitry is strengthened among brain regions subserving cognitive, affective, and sensory processes so that PLS and pain may be triggered by thoughts and feelings in the absence of primary afferent feedback from peripheral structures (LeDoux, 1989; Leventhal, 1982).

In summary, mental stress and anxiety not only provoke transient increases in the intensity of PLS and pain (Arena et al., 1990; Sherman, 1976; Sherman et al., 1979) but also induce reflex bursting activity in cutaneous sudomotor and vasomotor sympathetic fibers (Delius, Hagbarth, Hongell, & Wallin, 1972; Hagbarth, Hallin, Hongell, Torebjörk, & Wallin, 1972). Moreover, distraction or attention diversion that reduces PLP (Morgenstern, 1964; Parkes, 1973) also diminishes peripheral sympathetic nervous system activity (Hagbarth et al., 1972). These findings provide support for the model shown in Figure 18.1 and suggest that biofeedback, relaxation training, and other cognitive strategies directed at reducing anxiety and increasing self-control may be effective in reducing PLP in certain amputees.

SUMMARY AND CONCLUSIONS

A significant proportion of adult and child amputees experience PLS and PLP. This pain may continue for many years following amputation. Interestingly, up to 20% of individuals born missing a limb also report phantom sensations, although, fortunately, in only a small minority are these sensations painful.

There has been considerable interest in the role of psychosocial factors in the etiology and maintenance of PLS and PLP. In this chapter, we have shown that there is very little evidence that PLP or pain memories are psychogenic or the result of a character disturbance. In fact, the personality structure of individuals with PLP may not be different from that of other chronic pain patients. Therefore, the "rigid, compulsively self-reliant personality" invoked to explain PLP may more accurately reflect a stigmatization of individuals who are persistent in their efforts to obtain pain relief.

Similar to other chronic pain patients, many amputees who seek treatment for PLP report significant psychological distress, especially anxiety and depression. Furthermore, amputees have the added stress of adapting to the loss of the limb and the functional impairments that this involves. These factors may further contribute to the development of psychological distress. Prospective studies of the association of psychological variables and the development of PLP are urgently needed before firm conclusions can be drawn. Fortunately, there is some preliminary evidence to suggest that PLP can be alleviated with psychotherapeutic interventions such as biofeedback, relaxation, or group therapy. Although studies of the efficacy of cognitive-behavioral therapies for this type of pain are not available, the data regarding the coping strategies employed by both adult and child amputees suggest that this treatment may be appropriate for this group. Randomized, controlled studies of the outcome of psychological treatment strategies for PLP are lacking but would add significantly to our knowledge.

The data presented throughout this chapter suggest that PLP and PLS can be modified by both affective and cognitive triggers such as anxiety, stress, and relaxation training. The sympathetic nervous system may provide an important link between higher brain centers involved in cognitive and affective processes and PLS through its peripheral actions on primary afferents located in stump neuromas. A model has been proposed outlining a mechanism through which cognitive and affective processes associated with higher cortical and limbic centers may alter phantom limb sensations. It is hoped that this model will stimulate further research into the psychological factors associated with the experience of phantom limb sensations and pain.

ACKNOWLEDGMENT

This work was supported by grants from the Medical Research Council of Canada and the National Institute of Neurological Disorders and Stroke.

REFERENCES

Abramson, A. S., & Feibel, A. F. (1981). The phantom phenomenon: Its use and disuse. *Bulletin of the New York Academy of Medicine, 57,* 99–112.

Arena, J. G., Sherman, R. H., & Bruno, G. M. (1990). The relationship between situational stress and phantom limb pain: Cross-lagged correlational data from six-month pain logs. *Journal of Psychosomatic Research, 34,* 71–77.

Ascher, L. M., & Turner, R. M. (1980). A comparison of two methods for the administration of paradoxical intention. *Behaviour Research and Therapy, 18,* 121–126.

Bailey, A. A., & Moersch, F. P. (1941). Phantom limb. *Canadian Medical Association Journal, 45,* 37–42.

Bailey, A. A., & Moersch, F. P. (1992). Phantom limb. *Canadian Medical Association Journal, 146,* 1959–1965. (Original work published 1941)

Baker, S. R. (1984). Amelioration of phantom-organ pain with hypnosis and behavior modification: Brief case report. *Psychological Reports, 55,* 847–850.

Blood, A. M. (1956). Psychotherapy of phantom limb pain in two patients. *Psychiatry Quarterly, 30,* 114–122.

Boyle, M., Tebbi, C. K., Mindell, E. R., & Mettlin, C. J. (1982). Adolescent adjustment to amputation. *Medical and Pediatric Oncology, 10,* 301–312.

Bradley, K. C. (1955). *The sequelae of amputation.* Canberra, Australia: Trustees of the Services Canteens Trust Fund.

Bradway, J. K., Malone, J. M., Racy, J., Leal, J. M., & Poole, J. (1984). Psychological adaptation to amputation: An overview. *Orthotics and Prosthetics, 38,* 46–50.

Brodal, A. (1981). *Neurological anatomy in relation to clinical medicine* (3rd ed.). New York: Oxford University Press.

Brodman, K., Erdmann, A. J., Lordge, I., Wolff, H. G., & Broadbent, T. H. (1951). The CMI-Health Questionnaire. *Journal of the American Medical Association, 145,* 152–157.

Browder, J. G., & Gallagher, J. P. (1948). Dorsal cordotomy for painful phantom limbs. *Annals of Surgery, 128,* 456–459.

Butler, D. J., Turkal, N. W., & Seidl, J. J. (1992). Amputation: Preoperative psychological preparation. *Journal of the American Board of Family Practice, 5,* 69–73.

Campbell, J. N., Meyer, R. A., Davis, K. D., & Raja, S. N. (1992). Sympathetically maintained pain: A unifying hypothesis. In W. D. Willis (Ed.), *Hyperalgesia and allodynia* (pp. 141–150). New York: Raven Press.

Caplan, L. M., & Hackett, T. P. (1963). Emotional effects of lower-limb amputation in the aged. *New England Journal of Medicine, 269,* 1166–1171.

Carlen, P. L., Wall, P. D., Nadvorna, H., & Steinbach, T. (1978). Phantom limbs and related phenomena in recent traumatic amputations. *Neurology, 28,* 211–217.

Cedercreutz, C. (1954). Hypnotic treatment of phantom sensations in 100 amputees. *Acta Chirurgica Scandinavica, 107,* 158–162.

Cedercreutz, C., & Uusitalo, E. (1967). Hypnotic treatment of phantom sensations in 37 amputees. In J. Lassner (Ed.), *Hypnosis and psychosomatic medicine* (pp. 65–66). Berlin: Springer-Verlag.

Coderre, T. J., & Katz, J. (1997). Peripheral and central hyperexcitability: Differential signs and symptoms in persistent pain. *Behavioral and Brain Sciences, 20,* 404–419.

Dawson, L., & Arnold, P. (1981). Persistent phantom limb pain. *Perceptual and Motor Skills, 53,* 135–138.

Delius, W., Hagbarth, K. E., Hongell, A., & Wallin, B. G. (1972). Manoeuvres affecting sympathetic outflow in human skin nerves. *Acta Physiologica Scandinavica, 84,* 177–186.

Dernham, P. (1986). Phantom limb pain. *Geriatric Nursing (New York), 7,* 34–37.

Diamond, J. (1959). The effect of injecting acetylcholine into normal and regenerating nerves. *Journal of Physiology (London), 145,* 611–629.

Dougherty, J. (1980). Relief of phantom limb pain after EMG biofeedback-assisted relaxation: A case report. *Behaviour Research and Therapy, 18,* 355–357.

Easson, W. M. (1961). Body image and self-image in children. *Archives of General Psychiatry, 4,* 619–621.

Eysenck, H. L., & Eysenck, S. B. G. (1968). *Manual for the Eysenck Personality Inventory.* San Diego, CA: Educational and Industrial Testing Service.

Flor, H., Behle, D. J., & Birbaumer, N. (1993). Assessment of pain-related cognitions in chronic pain patients. *Behaviour Research and Therapy, 31,* 63–73.

Frazier, S. H., & Kolb, L. C. (1970). Psychiatric aspects of pain and the phantom limb. *Orthopedic Clinics of North America, 1,* 481–495.

Frederiks, J. A. M. (1963). Occurrence of phantom limb phenomena following amputation of body parts and following lesions of the central and peripheral nervous system. *Psychiatrica, Neurologica, Neurochirurgia, 66,* 73–97.

Hagbarth, K. E., Hallin, R. G., Hongell, A., Torebjörk, H. E., & Wallin, B. G. (1972). General characteristics of sympathetic activity in human skin nerves. *Acta Physiologica Scandinavica, 84,* 164–176.

Henderson, W. R., & Smyth, G. E. (1948). Phantom limbs. *Journal of Neurology, Neurosurgery and Psychiatry, 2,* 88–112.

Hill, A. (1993). The use of pain coping strategies by patients with phantom limb pain. *Pain, 55,* 347–353.

Hill, A., Niven, C. A., & Knussen, C. (1995). The role of coping in adjustment to phantom limb pain. *Pain, 62,* 79–86.

Hitchcock, L. S., Ferrell, B. R., & McCaffery, M. (1994). The experience of chronic nonmalignant pain. *Journal of Pain and Symptom Management, 9,* 312–318.

Houghton, A. D., Saadah, E., Nicholls, G., McColl, L., & Houghton, A. L. (1994). Phantom pain: Natural history and association with rehabilitation. *Annals of the Royal College of Surgeons of England, 76,* 22–25.

Howard, D. L. (1983). Group therapy for amputees in a ward setting. *Military Medicine, 148*, 678-680.

Jensen, M. P., Turner, J. A., Romano, J. M., & Karoly, P. (1991). Coping with chronic pain: A critical review of the literature. *Pain, 47*, 249-283.

Jensen, T. S., Krebs, B., Nielsen, J., & Rasmussen, P. (1984). Non-painful phantom limb phenomena in amputees: Incidence, clinical characteristics and temporal course. *Acta Neurologica Scandinavica, 70*, 407- 414.

Jensen, T. S., Krebs, B., Nielsen, J., & Rasmussen, P. (1985). Immediate and long-term phantom pain in amputees: Incidence, clinical characteristics and relationship to pre-amputation pain. *Pain, 21*, 268-278.

Jensen, T. S., & Rasmussen, P. (1994). Phantom pain and other phenomena after amputation. In P. D. Wall & R. Melzack (Eds.), *Textbook of pain* (3rd ed., pp. 651-665). Edinburgh: Churchill Livingstone.

Jessup, B. A., & Gallegos, X. (1994). Relaxation and biofeedback. In P. D. Wall & R. Melzack (Eds.), *Textbook of pain* (3rd ed., pp. 1321-1336). Edinburgh: Churchill Livingstone.

Katz, J. (1984). Symptom prescription: A review of the clinical outcome literature. *Clinical Psychology Review, 4*, 703-717.

Katz, J. (1992a). Phantom limbs still a ghostly phenomenon. *Canadian Medical Association Journal, 147*, 1632, 1636.

Katz, J. (1992b). Psychophysical correlates of phantom limb experience. *Journal of Neurology, Neurosurgery and Psychiatry, 55*, 811-821.

Katz, J. (1993). The reality of phantom limbs. *Motivation and Emotion, 17*, 147-179.

Katz, J., Clairoux, M., Kavanagh, B. P., Roger, S., Nierenberg, H., Redahan, C., & Sandler, A. N. (1994). Pre-emptive lumbar epidural anaesthesia reduces postoperative pain and patient-controlled morphine consumption after lower abdominal surgery. *Pain, 59*, 395- 403.

Katz, J., France, C., & Melzack, R. (1989). An association between phantom limb sensations and stump skin conductance during transcutaneous electrical nerve stimulation (TENS) applied to the contralateral leg: A case study. *Pain, 36*, 367-377.

Katz, J., Kavanagh, B. P., Sandler, A. N., Nierenberg, H., Boylan, J. F., Friedlander, M., & Shaw, B. F. (1992). Preemptive analgesia: Clinical evidence of neuroplasticity contributing to post-operative pain. *Anesthesiology, 77*, 439-446.

Katz, J., & Melzack, R. (1990). Pain "memories" in phantom limbs: Review and clinical observations. *Pain, 43*, 319-336.

Katz, J., & Melzack, R. (1991). Auricular TENS reduces phantom limb pain. *Journal of Pain and Symptom Management, 6*, 73-83.

Katz, J., Ritvo, P., Irvine, M. J., & Jackson, M. (1996). Coping with chronic pain. In M. Zeidner & N. S. Endler (Eds.), *Handbook of coping: Theory, research, applications* (pp. 252-278). New York: Wiley.

Katz, J., Vaccarino, A. L., Coderre, T. J., & Melzack, R. (1991). Injury prior to neurectomy alters the pattern of autotomy in rats. *Anesthesiology, 75*, 876-883.

Keefe, F. J., Salley, A. N. J., & Lefebvre, J. C. (1992). Coping with pain: Conceptual concerns and future directions. *Pain, 51*, 131-134.

Kolb, L. C. (1954). *The painful phantom: Psychology, physiology and treatment.* Springfield, IL: Thomas.

Krane, E. J., & Heller, L. B. (1995). The prevalence of phantom sensation and pain in pediatric amputees. *Journal of Pain and Symptom Management, 10*, 21-29.

Krebs, B., Jensen, T. S., Krøner, K., Nielsen, J., & Jørgensen, H. S. (1985). Phantom limb phenomena in amputees 7 years after limb amputation. In H. L. Fields, R. Dubner, & F. Cervero (Eds.), *Advances in pain research and therapy* (Vol. 9, pp. 425-429). New York: Raven Press.

Krøner, K., Krebs, B., Skov, J., & Jørgensen, H. S. (1989). Immediate and long-term phantom breast syndrome after mastectomy: Incidence, clinical characteristics and relationship to pre-mastectomy breast pain. *Pain, 36*, 327-334.

Lacroix, R., Melzack, R., Smith, D., & Mitchell, N. (1992). Multiple phantom limbs in a child. *Cortex, 28*, 503- 507.

Lakoff, R. (1990). The psychology and psychotherapy of the chronic pain patient. In T. W. Miller (Ed.), *Chronic pain* (Vol. 2, pp. 499-524). Madison, CT: International Universities Press.

Lasoff, E. M. (1985). When a teenager faces amputation. *RN, 48*, 44-45.

LeDoux, J. E. (1989). Cognitive-emotional interactions in the brain. *Cognition and Emotion, 3*, 267-289.

Leventhal, H. (1982). The integration of emotion and cognition: A view from the perceptual-motor theory of emotion. In M. Clark & S. Fiske (Eds.), *Affect and cognition: The 17th annual Carnegie Symposium on cognition* (pp. 122-156). Hillsdale, NJ: Erlbaum.

Lindesay, J. (1985). Multiple pain complaints in amputees. *Journal of the Royal Society of Medicine, 78*, 452-455.

Lindesay, J. (1986). Validity of the General Health Questionnaire (GHQ) in detecting psychiatric disturbance in amputees with phantom pain. *Journal of Psychosomatic Research, 30*, 277-281.

Lundberg, S. G., & Guggenheim, F. G. (1986). Sequelae of limb amputation. *Advances in Psychosomatic Medicine, 15*, 199-210.

Marshall, M., Helmes, E., & Deathe, B. (1992). A comparison of psychosocial functioning and personality in amputee and chronic pain populations. *The Clinical Journal of Pain, 8*, 351-357.

McGrath, P. A. (1990). *Pain in children: Nature, assessment, and treatment.* New York: Guilford Press.

McGrath, P. A., & Hillier, L. M. (1992). Phantom limb sensations in adolescents: A case study to illustrate the utility of sensation and pain logs in pediatric clinical practice. *Journal of Pain and Symptom Management, 7*, 46-53.

Melzack, R. (1989). Phantom limbs, the self, and the brain. *Canadian Psychology, 30*, 1-16.

Melzack, R., & Bromage, P. R. (1973). Experimental phantom limbs. *Experimental Neurology, 39*, 261-269.

Melzack, R., & Casey, K. L. (1968). Sensory, motivational, and central control determinants of pain. In D. Kenshalo (Ed.), *The skin senses* (pp. 423-439). Springfield, IL: Thomas.

Melzack, R., Israel, R., Lacroix, R., & Schultz, G. (1997). Phantom limbs in people with congenital limb deficiency or amputation in early childhood. *Brain, 120*, 1603-1620.

Melzack, R., & Loeser, J. D. (1978). Phantom body pain in paraplegics: Evidence for a central 'pattern generating mechanism' for pain. *Pain, 4*, 195-210.

Merskey, H. (1989). Psychiatry and chronic pain. *Canadian Journal of Psychiatry, 34*, 329-336.

Miser, A. W., & Miser, J. S. (1989). The treatment of cancer pain in children. *Pediatric Clinics of North America, 36,* 979-999.

Mitchell, S. W. (1872). *Injuries of nerves and their consequences.* Philadelphia: Lippincott.

Morgenstern, F. S. (1964). The effects of sensory input and concentration on post-amputation phantom limb pain. *Journal of Neurology, Neurosurgery and Psychiatry, 27,* 58-65.

Morgenstern, F. S. (1970). Chronic pain: A study of some general features which play a role in maintaining a state of chronic pain after amputation. In O. W. Hill (Ed.), *Modern trends in psychosomatic medicine* (Vol. 2, pp. 225-245). London: Butterworth.

Muraoka, M., Komiyama, H., Hosoi, M., Mine, K., & Kubo, C. (1996). Psychosomatic treatment of phantom limb pain with post-traumatic stress disorder: A case report. *Pain, 66,* 385-388.

Nikolajsen, L., Ilkjaer, S., Krøner, K., Christensen, J. H., & Jensen, T. S. (1997). Randomised trial of epidural bupivacaine and morphine in prevention of stump and phantom pain in lower-limb amputation. *Lancet, 350,* 1353-1357.

Parkes, C. M. (1973). Factors determining the persistence of phantom pain in the amputee. *Journal of Psychosomatic Research, 17,* 97-108.

Parkes, C. M., & Napier, M. M. (1975). Psychiatric sequelae of amputation [Special publication]. *British Journal of Psychiatry, 9,* 440-446.

Pilowsky, I., & Kaufman, A. (1965). An experimental study of atypical phantom pain. *British Journal of Psychiatry, 111,* 1185-1187.

Poeck, K. (1964). Phantoms following amputation in early childhood and in congenital absence of limbs. *Cortex, 1,* 269-275.

Ramachandran, V. S. (1994). Phantom limbs, neglect syndromes, repressed memories, and Freudian psychology. *International Review of Neurobiology, 37,* 291-333.

Ramachandran, V. S., & Rogers-Ramachandran, D. (1996). Synaesthesia in phantom limbs induced with mirrors. *Proceedings of the Royal Society of London B, 263,* 377-386.

Riddoch, G. (1941). Phantom limbs and body shape. *Brain, 64,* 197-222.

Riese, W., & Bruck, G. (1950). Le membre fantôme chez l'enfant. *Revue Neurologique, 83,* 221-222.

Roger, A. G. (1989). Use of amitriptyline (Elavil) for phantom limb pain in younger children. *Journal of Pain and Symptom Management, 4,* 96.

Rosen, V. H. (1950). The role of denial in acute postoperative affective reactions following removal of body parts. *Psychosomatic Medicine, 12,* 356-361.

Schilder, P. (1950). *The image and appearance of the human body: Studies in the constructive energies of the psyche.* New York: International Universities Press.

Seigel, E. F. (1979). Control of phantom limb pain by hypnosis. *American Journal of Clinical Hypnosis, 21,* 285-286.

Sherman, R. A. (1976). Case reports of treatment of phantom limb pain with a combination of electromyographic biofeedback and verbal relaxation techniques. *Biofeedback and Self Regulation, 1,* 353.

Sherman, R. A. (1989). Stump and phantom limb pain. *Neurologic Clinics, 7,* 249-264.

Sherman, R. A., Gall, N., & Gormly, J. (1979). Treatment of phantom limb pain with muscular relaxation training to disrupt the pain-anxiety-tension cycle. *Pain, 6,* 47-55.

Sherman, R. A., Sherman, C. J., & Bruno, G. M. (1987). Psychological factors influencing chronic phantom limb pain: An analysis of the literature. *Pain, 28,* 285-295.

Sherman, R. A., Sherman, C. J., & Parker, L. (1984). Chronic phantom and stump pain among American veterans: Results of a study. *Pain, 18,* 83-95.

Shukla, G. D., Sahu, S. C., Tripathi, R. P., & Gupta, D. K. (1982). A psychiatric study of amputees. *British Journal of Psychiatry, 141,* 50-53.

Simmel, M. L. (1956a). On phantom limbs. *Archives of Neurology and Psychiatry, 75,* 637-647.

Simmel, M. L. (1956b). Phantoms in patients with leprosy and in elderly digital amputees. *American Journal of Psychology, 69,* 529-545.

Simmel, M. L. (1959). Phantoms, phantom pain and 'denial.' *American Journal of Psychotherapy, 13,* 603-613.

Simmel, M. L. (1961). The absence of phantoms for congenitally missing limbs. *American Journal of Psychology, 74,* 467-470.

Simmel, M. L. (1962). Phantom experiences following amputation in childhood. *Journal of Neurology, Neurosurgery and Psychiatry, 25,* 69-78.

Skoyles, J. R. (1990). Is there a genetic component to body schema? *Trends in Neuroscience, 13,* 409.

Smith, O. A., & DeVito, J. L. (1984). Central neural integration for the control of autonomic responses associated with emotion. *Annual Review of Neuroscience, 7,* 43-65.

Sohn, D. L. (1914). The psychic complex in congenital deformity. *New York Medical Journal, 100,* 959-961.

Solomon, G. F., & Schmidt, K. M. (1978). A burning issue: Phantom limb pain and psychological preparation of the patient for amputation. *Archives of Surgery, 113,* 185-186.

Spanos, N. P., Carmanico, S. J., & Ellis, J. A. (1994). Hypnotic analgesia. In R. Melzack & P. D. Wall (Eds.), *The textbook of pain* (pp. 1349-1366). Edinburgh: Churchill Livingstone.

Steigerwald, F., Brass, J., & Krainick, J. U. (1981). The analysis of personality factors in the prediction of phantom limb pain. In J. Siegfried & M. Zimmermann (Eds.), *Phantom and stump pain* (pp. 84-88). New York: Springer-Verlag.

Stengel, E. (1965). Pain and the psychiatrist. *British Journal of Psychiatry, 111,* 795-802.

Szasz, T. S. (1975). *Pain and pleasure* (2nd ed.). New York: Basic Books.

Tasker, R. R., Organ, L. W., & Hawrylyshyn, P. A. (1982). *The thalamus and midbrain of man.* Springfield, IL: Thomas.

Tebbi, C. K., & Mallon, J. C. (1987). Long-term psychosocial outcome among cancer amputees in adolescence and early adulthood. *Journal of Psychosocial Oncology, 5,* 69-82.

Tebbi, C. K., Petrilli, A. S., & Richards, M. E. (1989). Adjustment to amputation among adolescent oncology patients. *American Journal of Pediatric Hematology/Oncology, 11,* 276-280.

Tennen, H., Rohrbaugh, M., Press, S., & White, L. (1981). Reactance theory and therapeutic paradox: A compliance-defiance model. *Psychotherapy: Theory, Research and Practice, 18,* 14-22.

Turgay, A., & Sonuvar, B. (1983). Emotional aspects of

arm or leg amputation in children. *Canadian Journal of Psychiatry, 28*, 294–297.

Turner, J. A., & Clancy, S. (1986). Strategies for coping with chronic low back pain: Relationship to pain and disability. *Pain, 24*, 355–364.

Varni, J. W., Rubenfeld, L. A., Talbot, D., & Setoguchi, Y. (1989a). Determinants of self-esteem in children with congenital/acquired limb deficiencies. *Developmental and Behavioral Pediatrics, 10*, 13–16.

Varni, J. W., Rubenfeld, L. A., Talbot, D., & Setoguchi, Y. (1989b). Family functioning, temperament, and psychologic adaptation in children with congenital or acquired limb deficiencies. *Pediatrics, 84*, 323–330.

Varni, J. W., Rubenfeld, L. A., Talbot, D., & Setoguchi, Y. (1989c). Stress, social support, and depressive symptomatology in children with congenital/acquired limb deficiencies. *Journal of Pediatric Psychology, 14*, 515–530.

Varni, J. W., & Setoguchi, Y. (1991). Psychosocial factors in the management of children with limb deficiencies. *Physical Medicine and Rehabilitation Clinics of North America, 2*, 395–404.

Varni, J. W., Setoguchi, Y., Talbot, D., & Rubenfeld Rappaport, L. (1991). Effects of stress, social support, and self-esteem on depression in children with limb deficiencies. *Archive of Physical Medicine and Rehabilitation, 72*, 1053–1058.

Vetter, R. J., & Weinstein, S. (1967). The history of the phantom in congenitally absent limbs. *Neuropsychologia, 5*, 335–338.

Wall, P. D. (1981). On the origin of pain associated with amputation. In J. Siegfried & M. Zimmermann (Eds.), *Phantom and stump pain* (pp. 2–14). New York: Springer-Verlag.

Wall, P. D., & Gutnick, M. (1974). Properties of afferent nerve impulses originating from a neuroma. *Nature, 248*, 740–743.

Weeks, G. R., & L'Abate, L. (1982). *Paradoxical psychotherapy: Theory and practice with individuals, couples, and families.* New York: Brunner/Mazel.

Weinstein, S. (1962). *Phantoms in paraplegia.* Paper presented at the Eleventh Annual Conference on Clinical Spinal Cord Injury.

Weinstein, S., & Sersen, E. A. (1961). Phantoms in cases of congenital absence of limbs. *Neurology, 11*, 906–911.

Weinstein, S., Sersen, E. A., & Vetter, R. J. (1964). Phantoms and somatic sensation in cases of congenital aplasia. *Cortex, 1*, 276–290.

Weiss, S. A. (1958). The body image as related to phantom sensations: A hypothetical conceptualization of seemingly isolated findings. *Annals of the New York Academy of Science, 74*, 25–29.

Wesley, E. L. (1953). Perseverative behavior in a concept-formation task as a function of manifest anxiety and rigidity. *Journal of Abnormal and Social Psychology, 48*, 129–134.

Wilkins, K., McGrath, P. J., Finley, G. A., & Katz, J. (1998). Phantom limb sensations and phantom limb pain in child and adolescent amputees. *Pain, 78*, 7–12.

Chapter 19

Cancer Pain

KAREN L. SYRJALA
JANET ABRAMS

Cancer patients require psychosocial approaches to understanding and managing their pain because standard medical approaches do not adequately resolve many of their pain problems. While the disease itself causes significant pain in up to 80% of advanced disease cancer patients and in 30–60% of patients in active treatment, everyone with cancer will experience pain as a result of some combination of procedures, treatment, and the disease (Cherny, 1998; Cleeland et al., 1994).

Although clinicians and researchers estimate that 90–95% of cancer pain can be effectively managed with medical treatment, as many as half of all patients do not receive adequate relief (Cleeland et al., 1994; Zhukovsky, Gorowski, Hausdorff, Napolitano, & Lesser, 1995). Explanations for this gap between our ability to relieve pain and actual rates of pain relief are almost entirely nonmedical: (1) reluctance of patients to take prescribed medications, (2) reluctance of patients to discuss their pain, (3) inadequate assessment, (4) inadequate patient knowledge about what to tell their doctors and what it is possible to treat, and (5) myths that disrupt communication between patients, their family members, and health care providers (Von Roenn, Cleeland, Gonin, Hatfield, & Pandya, 1993; Ward et al., 1993).

Even with optimal management, some pain problems are not well addressed by any available medical treatments. To give two examples, very brief procedure-related pain or unpredictable neuropathic pain can be quite disturbing to patients, but both health care providers and patients are reluctant to use medications that have duration of action far past the pain duration. Medications also may either provide inadequate relief or take effect after the pain has begun to resolve on its own. In these circumstances, psychological and cognitive strategies can be used to directly relieve pain. In other circumstances, cognitive strategies and an understanding of psychosocial factors as they interact with pain can be used to relieve the overall suffering of the patient or to improve medical management.

Although we readily affirm that psychosocial approaches are needed in the treatment of cancer pain, it is more challenging to define the role that psychosocial factors play in elucidating cancer pain problems. Pain clearly leads to greater psychological dysfunction, but effects in the opposite direction are less stable and more modest. Of all psychosocial factors, emotional distress is most consistently associated with pain report. Ahles, Blanchard, and Ruchdeschel (1983) compared cancer patients with pain to cancer patients without pain and found that those with pain reported higher levels of depression, anxiety, and hostility; but relationships were not stable across all measures of anxiety. These investigators further determined that medication use and activity level in cancer patients with pain were related to the affective dimension of the McGill Pain Questionnaire but not to more global measures of anxiety or depression such as the

Beck Depression Inventory or the Symptom Checklist 90. With similar results, Schacham, Reinhardt, Raubertas, and Cleeland (1983) found weak associations between pain and general mood and overall low levels of distress in the cancer patients they assessed. Correlations of pain with anxiety were inconsistent, anger was not related to pain, and depression was most strongly correlated with pain. Spiegel and Bloom (1983b) report significant relationships between pain level, mood, and beliefs about pain, but these variables explained only a small percentage of the variance in pain. Dalton and Feuerstein (1988) note that, though intensity of pain reports cannot be fully explained by the extent of pathology, biobehavioral factors are themselves only modest predictors of cancer pain report.

Our own research concurs with these earlier studies. We evaluated psychosocial status in 358 patients prior to their receiving cancer treatment that would result in significant pain. Results indicated a very modest predictive relationship between psychosocial factors and later pain report (Syrjala & Chapko, 1995). Distress specific to treatment was most strongly associated with pain report, predicting about 5% of the variance in pain. Lower levels of self-efficacy specific to pain also predicted higher pain report in men, and less use of support-seeking coping predicted more pain in women. Depression and general anxiety prior to treatment were not associated with later pain report. However, patients who reported more anger were slightly more likely to report more pain later. Similarly, very small associations existed between the social factors of lower income and education levels, predicting more pain in bivariate analyses. In regression analyses, only 5% of the variance in pain report could be predicted from psychosocial variables, most of this from treatment-specific distress. In contrast, 22% of the variance in pain could be explained by observable tissue damage.

Looking at the relationship of pain and depression from the standpoint of depression as a predictor of pain, Cleeland (1984) reported no difference in pain intensity or functional status in depressed and nondepressed cancer patients. Likewise, Stam, Goss, Rosenal, Ewens, and Urton (1985) found that mood did not change before and after radiation therapy, whereas pain scores did change over time.

The relationship between pain and social environment in cancer patients has been explored only peripherally. Stam and colleagues (1985) reported a weak relationship between social network and pain interference with daily activities in can-

cer patients, and Spiegel and Bloom (1983b) found little relationship between pain intensity and social support, social functioning, or coping in breast cancer patients.

These findings suggest some specificity of affective distress in response to pain rather than pain resulting in or resulting from broad symptoms of psychological disturbance. Data from the studies described above indicate that most pain reported by cancer patients cannot be presumed to be elevated consistently by psychosocial factors. However, this does not mean that patients have no psychological responses to unrelieved pain.

Pain is among the most significant contributors to emotional distress for cancer patients (Heim & Oei, 1993; Lancee et al., 1994; Massie & Holland, 1990). Over time, unrelieved pain can engender feelings of helplessness, hopelessness, and irritability. These feelings often lead to depression. Worries and fears that one will not be able to cope can result in anxiety reactions and feelings of loss of control that make patients more susceptible to phobias or panic attacks. Having to cope with numerous symptoms along with pain can also contribute to generalized distress (Portenoy et al., 1994).

The emotional consequences of uncontrolled pain can be extreme. Cancer patients with severe, unrelieved pain are more likely to consider and to commit suicide (Breitbart, 1989; Foley, 1991). Levin, Cleeland, and Dar (1985) found that 69% of cancer patients would consider suicide if their pain were not adequately controlled. Of physicians who have assisted cancer patients in dying, unremitting pain, with inability to perform self-care, was identified as the essential requirement for meeting these requests (Emanuel et al., 1998).

The seriousness of these emotional responses needs to be recognized and treated. These are not simply emotions "to be expected," since the majority of cancer patients are not anxious or depressed (Derogatis et al., 1983). Medical explanations for the physical symptoms do not mean that psychological or psychosocial treatments will not help. For patients with severe pain, pain should be treated immediately, with psychiatric symptoms treated concurrently or treated if they remain after pain is better controlled. In other words, never assume that pain reported as somatic has a psychological etiology and never treat the "emotional pain" and wait to see whether the physical pain then resolves. Conversely, clinical depression should be treated concurrently with pain; there should be no delay to see whether pain relief also relieves the depression. Because of the overlap in somatic symptoms of cancer and depression, an assessment of depression and anxiety should require that affective and cognitive symptoms are present in addition to somatic symptoms. Even when medications or disease are causing or contributing to the symptoms, depression can be very successfully treated pharmacologically and psychotherapeutically.

FACTORS TO CONSIDER IN TREATING CANCER PAIN

In working with cancer patients, there are medical factors that influence psychological responses and psychosocial factors that influence pain treatment. Recognizing these will improve the care of the patient.

Stage or Progression of the Disease

Psychological reactions and social needs of a patient vary depending on the stage of disease and the pace at which the disease is expected to progress. These reactions influence receptiveness to pain treatments. The majority of cancer patients do not have psychiatric disorders and cope well with their illness (Derogatis et al., 1983). Still, the most distressing time for patients is when the disease recurs (Silberfarb, Maurer, & Crouthamel, 1980), usually indicating progression to an advanced stage and further reducing survival prognosis by at least 50%. With recurrence, patients sometimes feel a sense of personal failure, loss of confidence in themselves and their providers, and uncertainty about treatment choices, since previous efforts did not work. Earlier in disease course, patients tend to have more optimism and more motivation to participate in their care. Newly diagnosed patients may be most open to cognitive methods. They also may be more reluctant to take analgesics because of fear and may be more confident of their own ability to influence their pain with nonpharmacological methods. Alternatively, these patients may be in shock or trauma from the barrage of treatments and changes in life plans, making them more vulnerable to emotional and cognitive responses to sensation. As the disease advances toward end stage, patients become continuously fatigued, cognition tends to become less sharp, focus turns from the world to a smaller nucleus of people and concerns, and interest in comfort predominates. These patients may be less able to engage in self-control methods of pain management and more willing to use analgesic options. Patients themselves may have less concern about addiction or tolerance, but families may remain concerned enough to withhold analgesics. Patients have far greater need for the physical and emotional support of family and therefore are less able to manage conflicts over medication if they occur.

Concurrent Illness and Symptoms

A critical factor to consider in working with cancer patients with pain is that these people usually experience multiple somatic symptoms along with the pain; they are also likely to be depleted in energy and often in concentration. Particularly with advanced disease, patients commonly report 4 to 11 symptoms at one time (Portenoy et al., 1994). Clearly, fatigue, nausea, and difficulty attending to new learning can interfere with taking medications, understanding medical care, and using cognitive intervention methods. These symptoms disrupt attention and motivation. For patients with severe fatigue, multiple other symptoms, or severe pain, we adapt nonpharmacological methods to be very brief and include the family or we return at a time when symptoms are under better control and cognitive status is improved.

Differing Nature and Implications of Pain Problems

Few persistent pain problems are so closely associated with death in patients', families', and providers' thoughts than cancer disease-related pain. The uncertainty about severity or duration of pain and the unpredictability of outcomes add to the emotional impact. In contrast, pain related to procedures or treatment can be quite predictable both in quality and duration. Procedure and treatment-related pain may be less associated with death, but these discomforts can cause distress because of the belief that patients have a choice in deciding to proceed with a treatment. From this standpoint, patients sometimes have a "gut level" feeling of discord. On the one hand, they feel a sense of control in having made a choice to proceed with treatment, but at the same time, experiences are so entirely unfamiliar that severe dissonance can occur because patients initially feel much worse as a result of the treatments they choose. This incongruity can result in distress that magnifies the experience of suffering. Patients may initially have difficulty labeling or expressing these internal conflicts. Great relief for the affective component of pain can be offered by helping the patient to express these contradictions and then using the strategies described in the subsequent section, "Treatment Approaches." These cognitive strategies enhance perceived control, support belief in one's success in managing difficulties, and support the appropriateness of decisions, given the knowledge available at the time.

In disease progression-related pain, such reassurance is not so easy. Instead we must empathize with, and allow expression of, the difficulties in not knowing how the pain, or life, will progress. Furthermore, pain is associated with invasion of the body by disease and is often accompanied by fear of death. We provide as much assurance about what is predictable as is possible, whether it is about the pain or about other aspects of care. A primary reassurance given in these situations is that the patient will not be alone, that the care providers will be prepared to respond to whatever does occur, and that the focus will always be on the patient's safety and comfort. With the patient, we then recognize the areas over which he or she has control, and we attempt to enhance this control by increasing the awareness the patient has about the pain and options for treatment. It is most important to understand, when responding to a patient's specific pain issue, that uncertainty about the future and loss of control over one's body or one's life are the most emotionally difficult aspects of living with cancer (Syrjala & Chapko, 1995). Not knowing what the future will bring surpasses pain or fear of pain in patient reports of what is most difficult to tolerate. Addressing this uncertainty by informing the patient of possible outcomes and acknowledging how difficult it is not to know can help the patient and family cope with both this uncertainty and pain.

Psychological Health and Coping Style of Patients

The large majority of cancer patients have led functional lives with reasonably successful coping. Although many may have pain that is expected to be chronic in duration, the vast majority, while having entrenched beliefs about pain, do not have the entrenched modes of coping with pain that result in dysfunctional patterns. Thoughts, feelings, and behaviors are the targets of psychosocial interventions for managing cancer pain. In cancer, expectations, fear, anxiety, guilt, and hopelessness are particularly intertwined with pain in patients' thoughts. For example, a cancer patient may worriedly complain of leg pain during a follow-up visit with his oncologist. When questioned, the patient reports that the last time he experienced a similar pain, it presaged his relapse. As worry about a recurrence escalates, his focus on pain increases accordingly. When the physician asks the patient what activity he did in the past 2 days, the patient remembers that he walked a much greater distance than usual. This brief conversation suggests another explanation for the leg pain, the meaning of the pain changes, and, as the threat from the pain decreases, so does the patient's experience of the pain. If the patient is given a basic instruction to contact the provider with new pain problems, the provider can intervene early to prevent maladaptive patterns of explaining or coping with the pain.

Mitigating factors in the patient's experience of pain are often not so benign as in the above example, yet it does help to clarify the frequent association between how a cancer patient may think and what he or she experiences. If patients change how they think about their pain, if they can take charge of how they feel and act in relation to the pain, even if the action is to take medication appropriately, then they can significantly improve their comfort. For example, we move people's thoughts from: "This pain is so bad. What if it just keeps getting worse and worse until I'll finally be glad to die?" to "I'm hurting. What can I do? I'll take another pill before the pain gets too bad. Then I'll try some soothing breathing and imagery while I'm waiting for the pill to work."

A major challenge that must be met by nearly all patients is a sense of being alone with the disease. Some aspects of this aloneness cannot be eradicated. However, knowing that they are not alone with their pain can help patients to cope.

Although we and others have found that most cancer patients do not have the maladaptive cognitions and behaviors often found in depression (Derogatis et al., 1983; Syrjala, Donaldson, Davis, Kippes, & Carr, 1995), some of the standard cognitive-behavioral methods can still be of benefit to a majority of patients. Thus we have simplified a number of strategies for use with generally psychologically healthy people. As patients understand what is happening to them, their symptoms begin to seem more manageable, and their sense of control over their situation increases. They become active participants in their care. For some patients, the introduction of more specialized interventions can offer treatments that patients can learn to do themselves, thus facilitating even more active participation in their own symptom management.

For patients who do have maladaptive cognitions or behavior patterns, the full use of standard cognitive-behavioral and psychosocial methods, as used in chronic nonmalignant pain, can be equally effective with cancer patients if adapted to incorporate the issues described previously. One such difficult situation is the patient with a personality disorder who may require greater amounts of time and treatment strategies beyond the direct management of pain. For adaptations that can improve success in working with these patients, the reader is referred to Weisberg and Keefe (Chapter 4, this volume). Adaptations are also needed with patients who have major depression or anxiety. Another difficult adaptation of treatment is required with patients who have histories of substance abuse, most commonly alcohol; sometimes this history is many years old, other times substances are being used at present.

Chemically Dependent Patients

Addiction as a result of cancer pain treatment is extremely rare, on the order of 1:2000–4000 (Porter & Jick, 1980). Rapidly escalating opioid use in the vast majority of cases indicates progressive disease rather than either tolerance or addiction (Foley, 1993). Those patients who develop patterns of pain medication use that have addictive characteristics most frequently have histories of substance abuse. However, patients with histories of heavy substance use will also have different needs for pain management, even when using medications appropriately. Distinguishing the factors that contribute to high-dose medication use can be taxing in these patients.

Whether a patient has an active substance abuse pattern or a past history, some recognition of this factor is needed if patients are to receive adequate treatment. With non-cancer populations, abuse history might make pharmacological treatment less likely. With cancer patients, treatment approaches are selected largely unrelated to this issue, but then treatment planning, monitoring, and expectations must be adapted to the individual's chemical dependency history. These patients require thorough assessment of their pattern of use. Even with this assessment, patients may deny use or problems related to substances.

Surprises occur, such as in the case of the patient recently referred for evaluation who indicated minimal alcohol use and no other substance use in her initial evaluation. In this case, the standard preprocedure dosing of light sedation had no effect, and the patient required many times the standard dose to achieve the anesthetic levels needed to proceed. During the procedure, she was treated with the same intent, light sedation; nonetheless, the time and care spent in monitoring, the concern of the treating physician, and all future treatment planning with this patient required consideration of her high cross-tolerance with sedatives and opioids. Further examination of her substance use was undertaken; it was necessary to confront her with the evidence from the procedure and to express about the need to provide her with adequate pain relief and safe treatment. Although she denied abuse, she acknowledged high-volume daily alcohol and anxiolytic use, a family history of substance abuse, and behavior patterns that indicated a tendency to use escape, avoidance, or denial strategies in coping. This history indicated that treatment planning had to incorporate strategies that did not rely on patient self-report, that treatment monitoring would require greater care and more time than usual, and that drug requirements for pain relief would likely be far higher than the normal range. In this case, monitoring plans were made with interdisciplinary collaboration between oncology, nursing, anesthesiology, psychology, and psychiatry. Criteria were set for self-care behaviors that she needed to maintain if she were to receive medication when she reported pain. Around the clock, long-acting anxiolytics were started to replace intermittent anxiolytics she took for anxiety and insomnia. Other than informing her of the possible hazards of drinking during treatment and recommending that she therefore taper her alcohol use, there was little pressure about her drinking. Chemotherapy and disease progression tend to make alcohol less well tolerated and less enjoyable. She was monitored for withdrawal symptoms. The patient and all staff working with her were informed of the criteria and plan for monitoring behaviors and responding to medication requests. The severity of the patient's disease-related pain, treatment-related pain, and necessary procedures made medications essential, and the issues of addiction had to be dealt with concurrently using a strict behavioral plan rather than denying the patient access to analgesics, anxiolytics, or sedatives. Any treatment of the addiction itself had to wait until cancer was no longer the primary problem.

With the prevalence of alcoholism, a common problem is a history of heavy alcohol use with interim years of sobriety or an ongoing pattern of heavy drinking that is not identified as a problem. In either of these cases, patients are often even more concerned than the usual patient about the addiction potential of opioid analgesics. Yet cross-tolerance with alcohol is likely to mean that these patients require higher than usual doses of opioids to get equivalent relief. In these cases, the concerns of the patient, family, and providers require particular attention to the education strategies described subsequently, as well as closer monitoring to evaluate adequacy of treatment and of the educational materials that have been adapted to focus on the specific needs and circumstances of the patient.

Caregiver/Family Role in the Patient's Disease Course

In today's changing health care system, more demands than ever are placed on family members. A patient's cancer diagnosis puts the entire family into crisis (Abrams, Roth-Roemer, Cowan, & Syrjala, 1997; Doherty, Colangelo, & Hovander, 1991; Lewis, 1986, 1990; Wellisch, 1985). Families greatly affect patient care by providing emotional support, bringing patients to appointments, attending medical appointments with the patient, and preparing meals and medications for the patient. A caregiver's beliefs about pain medications can enhance or sabotage the intended treatment. Family members interpret and remember what was communicated at the medical appointment. They direct patients toward or away from treatment. They deny prescribed medications when they believe that taking the medication is not in the patient's best interest. The absence of caregivers often impedes care for the isolated patient. The role of the family caregivers must be considered when working with a cancer patient in pain.

TREATMENT CHOICES AND ADHERENCE

Lack of adherence to prescribed treatment is an underrecognized problem in cancer pain. Because the majority of patients are motivated to increase their chance to live, health care providers expect that patients take medications as prescribed. Although patients may be extremely compliant with cancer therapies, we find a very different story with regard to symptom-related medications. In this arena, patients act on their own beliefs or their families' beliefs; they are much more likely to reduce doses, to skip doses, and to simply stop taking a medication because they do not like a side effect or are afraid of dependence or tolerance. Whereas drug-seeking behaviors or addiction occur rarely (Porter & Jick, 1980), frequent problems occur when patients do not take medications. Cancer patients generally take from 4 to 40 pills a day, and they may refuse medication for the sole reason that they will not add another pill to their regimen.

Another source of reluctance to take medications that relieve pain stems from side effects that are regrettably common on initial dosing (Bruera, Macmillan, Hanson, & MacDonald, 1989; Sjøgren, 1997). Patients do not like being too sleepy to drive; they worry, appropriately, about constipation and mental clouding. Nausea and vomiting are the most aversive of symptoms, and it is very hard to convince patients to take medicines that have caused these effects previously. To complicate matters further, if patients choose not to take a medication because of side effects, they are unlikely to continue to complain about the original pain problem, since they believe they have to choose between the pain and the side effect.

The literature on compliance makes it clear just how difficult it is to assess this area, much less to intervene. At the same time, the literature unequivocally shows that patients in general are quite different in their medication usage from what their health care providers have intended (DiMatteo et al., 1993). Because cancer patients feel that their lives depend on their oncologists, they wish to be "good patients" (Ward et al., 1993); therefore, they often do not inform their health care providers when they depart from prescribed treatments or even when they have questions about treatment. Patients want to know everything equally on all topics; they have difficulty sorting out the relative importance of information (Beisecker & Beisecker, 1990). As a result, they may not ask questions or may not provide information that a health care provider considers important or obvious.

As with all of us, when we think we know an answer, we do not ask the question. Thus patients have said: "I know they save morphine until you're dying" or "I know morphine is addicting." The physician or nurse will never hear a question from these patients, will not know these thoughts are on these patients' minds, but these patients may do anything possible not to take morphine.

The topic of pain is emotionally laden for cancer patients, who frequently believe pain is inevitable (Ward et al., 1993). If pain is inevitable, untreatable, and frightening, what is the use in talking or even thinking about it? These beliefs often originate from a prior experience with a friend or family member years earlier when treatment options were less diverse or available. The importance of personal beliefs in influencing pain treatment behavior, the difficulty patients have in knowing what to ask their physicians or nurses, and the resistance patients have to taking more pills all attest to the importance of using psychosocial methods to assure that patients do not suffer unnecessarily.

These many aspects of patient participation in their own treatment demonstrate the complexities of care and the many opportunities for treatment to go awry. Communication strategies involving assessment, information, and education methods are invaluable for assuring that patients and health care providers work together to maximize patient comfort.

TREATMENT APPROACHES

Nonpharmacological methods used to assist cancer patients in managing pain are not unique to this population. Nonetheless, psychosocial and cognitive strategies all benefit from an understanding of the context in which these methods are used. For instance, assessment is a standard medical technique, but the application we describe requires the health care provider to consider not just the data collected from the patient but also the impact of the questions on the patient and the metacommunication that occurs in the process of the assessment. In this assessment process, the effort is not greater, but the result can surpass what occurs in a standard medical pain evaluation.

All of the following methods are intended to be integrated with medical care rather than used as alternatives to medical care. By and large these are verbal approaches that require patients' interest, willingness to be involved, and ability to maintain adequate attention and to provide some feedback. Consequently, all of these methods work best when they are used earlier in treatment as a part of a comprehensive treatment plan, when patients are motivated, not excessively fatigued, and not distracted by severe pain. These requirements are not so different from what is needed of any patient

with pain who must be involved in his or her care. Even to take pills as prescribed, a patient must understand the prescription, must ask questions when information is unclear, and must be willing to follow the treatment recommended. When employed in an integrated fashion, psychosocial approaches optimize the comfort of the patient by facilitating all aspects of care.

Most of these strategies are targeted for use with any patient who is experiencing discomfort. Because we know that psychological factors are influential but not causal in the maintenance of cancer pain symptoms (Elliott, Elliott, Murray, Braun, & Johnson, 1996; Syrjala & Chapko, 1995), we know that any patient can benefit from these strategies, not just those patients in psychological distress or those who have psychiatric diagnoses (Spiegel & Bloom, 1983a; Syrjala et al., 1995; Syrjala et al., 1996). Of course, those patients who are in continuous, severe pain will benefit from aggressive medical treatment prior to use of nonmedical methods. Patients with delirium or severe psychiatric disruption will need additional care beyond the methods we detail (see Weisberg & Keefe, Chapter 4, this volume). Patients who are depressed or highly anxious will benefit from the methods described combined with treatment directed to the affective symptoms. Further details of these methods are available elsewhere (Syrjala & Abrams, 1996; Syrjala & Roth-Roemer, 1998).

Communication Methods

Communication is the most basic intervention used in cancer care. At a time when illness-related concerns become the focus of patient and family thinking, communication with the medical staff is given enormous significance. Words and behaviors are repeated, overinterpreted, and scrutinized for underlying messages. Most often, the family uses the medical team as a basis for their spoken and unspoken rules, beliefs, and behaviors (Rait & Lederberg, 1989). Health care providers routinely convey information, they listen, they reassure patients and family members, and they actively educate patients about both the pain and potential treatments. Each of these interactions can enhance patients' beliefs in their ability to cope with the symptoms they have, can foster adherence to the medical plan, or conversely can escalate patient fear or helpless feelings, often without signaling to the health care provider that this is happening.

Assessment

Pain assessment is the cornerstone of all pain treatment. It begins the process of communication that determines medical treatment and also begins to teach patients how to think about their pain. By asking the same questions at each assessment and giving the patient some options for answers, the physician and patient begin to develop a common language for communication. Instead of "what does your pain feel like?" the following question makes the patient's job easier and targets the information a care provider needs to know: "Does your pain feel burning, shooting, electric, or like pins and needles, or is it an aching, gnawing, pressing, or throbbing kind of pain? What words best describe how it feels?" The patient begins recognizing different qualities in pain, and the provider begins to determine whether intervention should be oriented to neuropathic and/or somatic or visceral treatments. Inadequate assessment is the first step to inadequate treatment (Cleeland et al., 1994; Cleeland & Syrjala, 1992; Von Roenn et al., 1993). Adequate assessment may well be the first step toward facilitating patient adherence and participation in treatment.

In our recent study of an educational intervention for cancer-related pain (Syrjala et al., 1996), a patient called to thank us profusely for "teaching me so much about pain—it changed my life and gave me a mission for the time I have left." We thanked her, but we were quite confused when we realized that she was in the control group that did not receive the pain education. With further discussion, she told us how much she learned from the assessment of her pain in the study. It gave her a new language for talking to her doctor, which led to much improved pain relief.

Education

Whereas information provides facts, education requires an interactive process in which patients must learn and then use knowledge to direct their own behavior. Education does more than label an experience; it allows patients to take the information presented to them, adapt it to their situation, and then adjust their coping accordingly. Education involves both the telling of facts and a discussion of patients' questions and concerns. For example, the patient who is underusing prescribed opioids for fear of becoming addicted may be more likely to use the appropriate amount of drug after he or she has had a chance to discuss worries, has learned

that addiction is not a concern, and has asked questions about this information.

Patients who are given information but then seem not to hear it often frustrate clinicians. Anxiety, unfamiliarity, and the medications we use in cancer treatment may affect our patients' ability to retain educational information. Benzodiazapines used for sleep or anxiety or as antiemetics impair memory (Curran, Gardiner, Java, & Allen, 1993; Danion et al., 1992; Hanks, O'Neill, Simpson, & Wesnes, 1995; Patat et al., 1995). Data also indicate that opioids, although they have minimal effects on most areas of function, do restrict learning and retention of new information (Cleeland et al., 1996; Kerr et al., 1991). So although patients may appear to comprehend information immediately during their office visit, they may not be able to retain this information for later recall at home. In addition to these medical aspects of learning interference, the anxiety and helplessness brought about by a cancer diagnosis, compounded by the experience of unremitting pain, can also make information retention a difficult task. Recognizing these limitations can help us to consider ways to overcome them.

Concerns about negative effects of educating patients sometimes arise from fears that discussing possible side effects will oversensitize patients to symptoms. Available research indicates that informing cancer patients about possible side effects of therapy does not increase the occurrence of side effects or have other adverse effects (Howland, Baker, & Poe, 1984; Wilson, 1981).

Education can be particularly helpful in addressing patient fears. Mounting evidence supports the observation that patients and their families not only fear cancer pain but also believe that pain cannot be effectively controlled without unacceptable consequences. A survey in Wisconsin (Doyle, Cleeland, & Joranson, 1991) found that 72% of the respondents believed that cancer pain can get so bad that a person might consider suicide; 39% thought that strong pain killers are an indication that a patient is close to death. In relation to effects of opioids, 70% expressed concerns about tolerance, and 70% expressed concerns about mental confusion. These concerns can interfere with adequate pain treatment. When patients who return home to treat themselves believe that opioids are dangerous, they will not adhere to their physicians' prescriptions no matter how effective the treatment might be.

In view of the many time demands on physicians' practices, it is important to note that written materials, videos, and communication with nurses can be acceptable substitutes for education directly from the physician, as long as the information is reinforced by the physicians' communications. Numerous booklets, books, and videotapes are available to use as educational tools with patients and should be incorporated into routine oncology practice (Agency for Health Care Policy and Research, 1994; Ferrell & Rhiner, 1993; Levy, Rimer, Keintz, MacElwee, & Kedziera, 1991; Syrjala, Abrams, DuPen, Niles, & Rupert, 1997). Written materials are particularly valuable because they reduce the burden of having to retain information solely in memory. Education should be addressed when pain is just reaching the point at which opioids are needed.

Everyday Reframing

Reframing means, quite simply, thinking about a threatening situation in a different way that reduces its threat. If health care providers remember that their exact words will be retained and repeated over and over by patients and families and if they use this fact to actively choose words to influence patient and family perception, this will be one of the simplest and most helpful strategies they can use. Although most patients and families look for statements that offer hope, they will also hang on to negative information. It can be extremely valuable, when providing feedback about the patient's condition, to include statements about what is going well without being misleading. Specific positive accomplishments are always possible to find.

Reframing provides an opportunity to look at the situation from a more neutral or positive perspective. The essence of reframing is to (1) acknowledge and validate the problems; (2) widen the perspective to include things that are not problems and to include specific accomplishments of the patient; and (3) give the patient credit for the accomplishment so that the patient feels recognized and proud of what he or she is doing. For example: "You've been able to walk a little bit each day; that's wonderful, it will help you keep your strength." For a very ill patient for whom getting out of bed is a huge effort, the acknowledgment may be quite different: "You've been able to get a sponge bath, that must have taken a lot of energy and effort." Although the accomplishment may seem quite small, the patient knows how much energy the activity took and will appreciate having this recognized. In this way the clinician can acknowledge

the problems that are of concern to the patient and his or her family while recognizing that, no matter how difficult the situation, there are things that are not problems and that they are doing a good job. This simple, positive perspective can do much to contribute to feelings of control, self-efficacy, and overall good feelings for patients and their families.

Expressing Thoughts and Feelings

Presence of distress, especially distress specific to the pain or cancer situation, will contribute to the patient's perception of pain (Syrjala & Chapko, 1995). Patients who are preoccupied will not hear information and will not learn what they need to about their treatment. Consequently, they will be less likely to adhere to treatment. These will be the patients who require more attention and time in the future and who will have poorer pain relief. As we discuss in the later section on structured support, talking and expressing concerns has been nearly as effective as more advanced techniques in relieving cancer pain (Spiegel & Bloom, 1983a; Syrjala et al., 1995).

Advanced Cognitive-Behavioral Interventions

There are times when routine, brief strategies are not enough to manage chronic or recurring pain. At such times, it can be helpful to consult with a psychologist or other behavioral medicine specialist who can help the patient learn more specialized cognitive-behavioral pain management techniques.

Active Coping

Active coping strategies essentially teach patients to notice when they have a recurring problem or worry and to focus on finding something to do about the problem, even if they cannot entirely make it go away. Fawzy and colleagues (1993) trained malignant melanoma patients in active coping and communication skills and found that those who received the training lived longer. The first step in active coping is to identify the problem and to take one problem at a time. Then several steps are followed to resolve the problem. The patient should:

- *Collect information.* Talk to doctors, nurses, social workers, other patients, and his or her family. Ask them to explain the situation. Ask them what can be done. Ask them what else can be done if the first steps don't work. Keep asking until useful options are found. Ask for or look for information to read, experts to talk to, or other sources of information.

- *List what can be done to resolve the problem.* Use the information from others as well as his or her own ideas.
- *Check off these options when they are done.*
- Once available actions have been taken, *talk to people who can offer emotional support.* Being alone with pain, fear, or another problem can be the most difficult aspect of a problem.

When a patient has accomplished these steps, it is time to use methods to eliminate the problem from his or her mind. At this point, we encourage the use of distraction, imagery, and reframing to change thoughts, to ease emotions, and to introduce emotionally positive actions that add to quality of life.

Distraction

Distraction skills are taught with an emphasis on focusing attention away from discomfort. We work with patients to identify which distractions work best for them and help them to plan when, where, and how they will use specific strategies. Examples of commonly used distraction techniques include spending time with and talking to family and friends, listening to music, getting a massage, walking, or taking a bath. Regardless of the distraction, these positive activities provide a sense of achievement that reminds patients of their control over their own experience.

Distraction is not the same as denial, which implies an inability to recognize reality. Nor is it the same as avoidance, which implies an unwillingness or inability to cope with reality. Denial can be beneficial in situations in which nothing can be done to change the circumstances and in which focusing on fears just increases anxiety (Lazarus & Folkman, 1984). Avoidance, on the other hand, seems unhelpful as a coping strategy and is related to greater levels of distress (Vitaliano et al., 1990). Distraction as an active coping strategy involves a willingness to accept reality while engaging in a positive portion of it.

Imagery/Hypnosis

Imagery is one of the most easily accepted, most useful noninvasive methods for managing pain. Nearly everyone enjoys and responds to pleasant

place images, which provide patients with an opportunity to turn their focus away from their pain and discomfort for a time. In turn, their enjoyment of the experience enhances the likelihood they will continue to use imagery. We incorporate suggestions for increased comfort and well-being or for analgesia in the painful area (for details, see Syrjala & Abrams, 1996). Analgesic suggestions transform the pain by introducing numbness or watching the pain as it changes color and shape, moves to a distant location, or decreases in intensity (Dahlgren, Kurtz, Strube, & Malone, 1995; Kiernan, Dane, Phillips, & Price, 1995; Syrjala et al., 1995; Syrjala & Abrams, 1996).

To assist patients in applying these skills on their own, we teach them the steps for using imagery and provide suggestions about how easy and automatic relaxation and imagery can be (Syrjala, Danis, Abrams, & Keenan, 1992). It is the intentional use of suggestion that is the primary distinction between imagery and hypnosis (Barber, 1990; Hilgard & Hilgard, 1975; Syrjala & Abrams, 1996). For the purposes of pain management, research does not yet allow us to clearly distinguish effects of hypnosis from those of relaxation and imagery. Because of the negative connotations of hypnosis for some patients, we usually use the term "relaxation with imagery" (Hendler & Redd, 1986).

Although all of the interventions described in this chapter show evidence of effectiveness in relieving cancer pain, the strongest controlled clinical trial data validate the efficacy of support combined with imagery or hypnosis (Spiegel & Bloom, 1983a; Syrjala, Cummings, & Donaldson, 1992; Syrjala et al., 1995). In a meta-analysis of cognitive-behavioral interventions for pain that was not limited to cancer pain, Fernandez and Turk (1989) found that all strategies were effective but that imagery consistently showed the largest effect size.

Patient-Directed Reframing

Just as the messages we give to patients are powerful, so are the messages patients give to themselves. Using this awareness, we help patients prepare self-statements to use in the face of major stressors. We prepare these statements by first exploring the messages a person naturally gives him- or herself. Many patients initially deny having any helpless or self-defeating thoughts. With an accepting approach, exploration, and some provision of examples from other patients, most people acknowledge specific fears or concerns that sometimes enter their minds about what might go wrong. After teaching them to identify negative self-talk, times when they expect the worst, or situations that really bother them, we teach four forms of reframing that patients can do for themselves:

1. Focus on what they have accomplished, rather than on what remains to be done.
2. Find something positive that they will gain from the situation and focus on that: "This is hard, but I've learned I'm stronger than I ever imagined."
3. Focus on what they would do to help someone else in the same situation: If this were happening to your close friend, what would you do to help him or her?
4. Focus on the temporary nature of what is difficult: "This is difficult, but I know this will not last forever. In a week it will be hard to remember how this felt."

Patients develop their own alternative phrases to remind themselves both that there are areas in which they have control and that they are cared for. Many patients use their religious beliefs to enhance their self-statements with soothing thoughts that reduce the aloneness nearly all cancer patients feel. Finally, we work out statements to reinforce that they are doing as well as possible in this exceptional experience. It is important to emphasize that this approach is most effective when it is individualized. Specific self-statements and reframes must be adapted by, and developed with, each patient.

In discussing any cognitive modifications such as this with patients and families, it is essential to assure them that these messages alone will neither cure them nor kill them. They need not struggle to maintain only the "right" or only positive thoughts. Fears and helpless thoughts are normal and should be understood and tolerated as normal. At the same time, we encourage patients to use these thoughts to help them identify when they need more information or when they need reassurance from someone else whose knowledge or support they value.

Structured Support

Cancer patients and their families report using support more often than any other coping strategy (Dunkel-Shetter, Feinstein, Taylor, & Falke, 1992). The value of support is being increasingly recognized in numerous studies examining the relationship of social support to physical and emotional well-being. Recent research demonstrates that cancer patients who receive active psychological support, with or without skills training, from groups or individuals report less pain and live longer (Fawzy et al., 1993; Spiegel, 1989; Spiegel & Bloom, 1983a; Syrjala et al., 1995). Spiegel and Bloom (1983a) randomly assigned breast cancer patients to one of three groups: support groups alone, support groups plus brief hypnosis training, and no psychological treatment. Patients participated in the support groups for 1 year. Both support groups reported significantly less pain and suffering than the no-treatment group. We have found similar results in our research: Patients receiving imagery or coping skills training reported significantly less pain than standard treatment patients but not significantly less pain than patients who received structured support with skills training (Syrjala et al., 1995). Researchers are exploring whether these support interventions have effects on survival and function through adherence to treatment, through education, or through improved health-related behaviors or whether they have neuroendocrine or immunological effects that enhance survival (Fawzy et al., 1993; Fawzy, Fawzy, Arndt, & Pasnau, 1995; Redd et al., 1991; Spiegel, 1989).

CONCLUSIONS

Research indicates that psychosocial interventions, when integrated with standard medical care, do reduce cancer pain. In a meta-analysis of 116 psychoeducational intervention studies conducted within the past 2 decades, Devine and Westlake (1995) concluded that psychoeducational interventions were effective not only in increasing knowledge but also in significantly reducing cancer symptom severity, including pain, anxiety, depression, mood, nausea, and vomiting. Similarly, a recent review article (Fawzy et al., 1995) on a mix of randomized and nonrandomized psychosocial interventions for cancer patients supports the integrated use of psychological interventions. The authors conclude that a variety of structured interventions, including education, relaxation/imagery/hypnosis, active coping training, and psychosocial support, is effective in cancer symptom management when integrated into the overall medical care of the cancer patient; however, no specific methods were singled out as more effective than others. Our research and that of Fawzy and colleagues clearly indicate that long-term treatment is not necessary, that brief, focused interventions can be effective (Fawzy et al., 1995, Syrjala, Cummings, & Donaldson, 1992; Syrjala & Chapko, 1995).

Studies such as these indicate that attention to psychosocial factors helps cancer patients to manage disease-related pain and treatment-related pain. Specific content may be less important than providing patients with skills for self-management of symptoms, conveying that they have the ability to cope with the pain and the disease and that they will not be left to cope alone, even if the process is difficult or the outcome is death.

ACKNOWLEDGMENT

This work was supported by grants from the National Cancer Institute (Nos. CA63030, CA78990, and CA68139).

REFERENCES

Abrams, J. R., Roth-Roemer, S., Cowan, J. E., & Syrjala, K. L. (1997). Impact of bone marrow transplant on family caregivers. *Annals of Behavioral Medicine, 19,* S172.

Agency for Health Care Policy and Research. (1994). *Clinical practice guideline on management of cancer pain: No. 9. Patient guide* (AHCPR Publication No. 94–0595). Rockville, MD: U.S. Department of Health and Human Services.

Ahles, T. A., Blanchard, E. B., & Ruchdeschel, J. C. (1983). The multidimensional nature of cancer-related pain. *Pain, 17,* 277–288.

Barber, J. (1990). Hypnosis. In J. J. Bonica, C. R. Chapman, W. E. Fordyce, & J. Loeser (Eds.), *The management of pain* (2nd ed., pp. 1733–1741). Philadelphia: Lea & Febiger.

Beisecker, A. E., & Beisecker T. D. (1990). Patient information-seeking behaviors when communicating with doctors. *Medical Care, 28,* 19–28.

Breitbart, W. (1989). Suicide. In J. C. Holland & J. H. Rowland (Eds.), *Handbook of psychooncology* (pp. 291–299). New York: Oxford University Press.

Bruera, E., Macmillan, K., Hanson, J., & MacDonald, R. N. (1989). The cognitive effects of the administration of narcotic analgesics in patients with cancer pain. *Pain, 39,* 13–16.

Cherny, N. I. (1998). Cancer pain: Principles of assessment and syndromes. In A. Berger, R. K. Portenoy, & D. E. Weissman (Eds.), *Principles and practice of supportive oncology* (pp. 3–42). Philadelphia: Lippincott.

Cleeland, C. S. (1984). The impact of pain on the patient with cancer. *Cancer, 54,* 2635–2641.

Cleeland, C. S., Gonin, R., Hatfield, A. K., Edmonson, J. H., Blum, R. H., Stewart, J. A., & Pandya, K. J. (1994). Pain and its treatment in outpatients with metastatic cancer. *New England Journal of Medicine, 330,* 592–596.

Cleeland, C. S., Nakamura, Y., Howland, E. W., Morgan, N. R., Edwards, K. R., & Backonja, M. (1996). Effects of oral morphine on cold pressor tolerance time and neuropsychological performance. *Neuropsychopharmacology, 15*(3), 252–262.

Cleeland, C. S., & Syrjala, K. L. (1992). How to assess cancer pain. In D. C. Turk & R. Melzack (Eds.), *Handbook of pain assessment* (pp. 362–387). New York: Guilford Press.

Curran, H. V., Gardiner, J. M., Java, R. I., & Allen, D. (1993). Effects of lorazepam upon recollective experience in recognition memory. *Psychopharmacology, 110,* 374–378.

Dahlgren, L. A., Kurtz, R. M., Strube, M. J., & Malone, M. D. (1995). Differential effects of hypnotic suggestion on multiple dimensions of pain. *Journal of Pain and Symptom Management, 10,* 464–470.

Dalton, J. A., & Feuerstein, M. (1988). Biobehavioral factors in cancer pain. *Pain, 33,* 137–147.

Danion, J. M., Peretti, S., Grange, D., Bilik, M., Imbs, J. L., & Singer, L. (1992). Effects of chlorpromazine and lorazepam on explicit memory, repetition priming, and cognitive skill learning in healthy volunteers. *Psychopharmacology, 108,* 345–351.

Derogatis, L. R., Morrow, G. R., Fetting, J., Penman, D., Piasetsky, S., Schmale, A. M., Henrichs, M., & Carnicke, C. L. (1983). The prevalence of psychiatric disorders among cancer patients. *Journal of the American Medical Association, 249,* 751–757.

Devine, E. C., & Westlake, S. K. (1995). The effects of psychoeducational care provided to adults with cancer: Meta-analysis of 116 studies. *Oncology Nursing Forum, 22,* 1369–1377.

DiMatteo, M. R., Sherbourne, C. D., Hays, R. D., Ordway, L., Kravitz, R. L., McGlynn, E. A., Kaplan, S., & Rogers, W. H. (1993). Physicians' characteristics influence patients' adherence to medical treatment: Results from the Medical Outcomes Study. *Health Psychology, 12*(2), 93–102.

Doherty, W. J., Colangelo, N., & Hovander, D. (1991). Priority setting in family change and clinical practice: The family FIRO model. *Family Process, 30,* 227–240.

Doyle, D. M., Cleeland, C. S., & Joranson, D. E. (1991, October). *Wisconsin public attitudes toward cancer pain: Changes over a seven-year period.* Paper presented at the Tenth Annual Meeting of the American Pain Society, New Orleans, LA.

Dunkel-Shetter, C., Feinstein, L. G., Taylor, S. E., & Falke, R. L. (1992). Patterns of coping with cancer. *Health Psychology, 11,* 79–87.

Elliott, B. A., Elliott, T. E., Murray, D. M., Braun, B. L., & Johnson, K. M. (1996). Patients and family members: The role of knowledge and attitudes in cancer pain. *Journal of Pain and Symptom Management, 12,* 209–220.

Emanuel, E. J., Daniels, E. R., Fairclough, D. L., & Clarridge, B. R. (1998). The practice of euthanasia and physician-assisted suicide in the United States: Adherence to proposed safeguards and effects on physicians. *Journal of the American Medical Association, 280*(6), 507–513.

Fawzy, F. I., Fawzy, N. W., Arndt, L. A., & Pasnau, R. O. (1995). Critical review of psychosocial interventions in cancer care. *Archives of General Psychiatry, 52,* 100–113.

Fawzy, F. I., Fawzy, N. W., Hyun, C. S., Elashoff, R., Guthrie, D., Fahey, J. L., & Morton, D. L. (1993). Malignant melanoma: Effects of an early structured psychiatric intervention, coping, and affective state on recurrence and survival 6 years later. *Archives of General Psychiatry, 50*(9), 681–689.

Fernandez, E., & Turk, D. C. (1989). The utility of cognitive coping strategies for altering pain perception: A meta-analysis. *Pain, 38,* 123–135.

Ferrell, B., & Rhiner, M. (1993). *Managing cancer pain at home.* Duarte, CA: City of Hope National Medical Center.

Foley, K. M. (1991). The relationship of pain and symptom management to patient requests for physician-assisted suicide. *Journal of Pain and Symptom Management, 6,* 289–297.

Foley, K. M. (1993). Changing concepts of tolerance to opioids: What the cancer patient has taught us. In C. R. Chapman & K. M. Foley (Eds.), *Current and emerging issues in cancer pain: Research and practice* (pp. 331–350). New York: Raven Press.

Hanks, G. W., O'Neill, W. M., Simpson, P., & Wesnes, K. (1995). The cognitive and psychomotor effects of opioid analgesics: II. A randomized controlled trial of single doses of morphine, lorazepam and placebo in healthy subjects. *European Journal of Clinical Pharmacology, 48,* 455–460.

Heim, H. M., & Oei, T. P. (1993). Comparison of prostate cancer patients with and without pain. *Pain, 53*(2), 159–162.

Hendler, C. S., & Redd, W. H. (1986). Fear of hypnosis: The role of labeling in patients' acceptance of behavioral interventions. *Behavior Therapy, 17,* 2–13.

Hilgard, E. R., & Hilgard, J. R. (1975). *Hypnosis in the relief of pain.* Los Altos, CA: Kaufmann.

Howland, J. S., Baker, M. G., & Poe, T. (1984). Does patient education cause side effects?: A controlled trial. *Journal of Family Practice, 31,* 62–64.

Kerr, B., Hill, H., Coda, B., Calogero, M., Chapman, C. R., Hunt, E., Buffington, V., & Mackie, A. (1991). Concentration-related effects of morphine on cognition and motor control in human subjects. *Neuropsychopharmacology, 5,* 157–166.

Kiernan, B. D., Dane, J. R., Phillips, L. H., & Price, D. D. (1995). Hypnotic analgesia reduces R-III nociceptive reflex: Further evidence concerning the multifactorial nature of hypnotic analgesia. *Pain, 60,* 39–47.

Lancee, W. J., Vachon, M. L., Ghadirian, P., Adair, W., Conway, B., & Dryer, D. (1994). The impact of pain and impaired role performance on distress in persons with cancer. *Canadian Journal of Psychiatry, 39,* 617–622.

Lazarus, R. S., & Folkman, S. (1984). *Stress, appraisal, and coping.* New York: Springer.

Levin, D. N., Cleeland, C. S., & Dar, R. (1985). Public attitudes towards cancer pain. *Cancer, 56,* 2337–2339.

Levy, M. H., Rimer, B., Keintz, M. K., MacElwee, N., & Kedziera, P. (1991). *No more pain.* Philadelphia: Fox Chase Cancer Center.

Lewis, F. M. (1986). The impact of cancer on the family: A critical analysis of the research literature. *Patient Education Counsel, 8,* 269–289.

Lewis, F. M. (1990). Strengthening family supports: Cancer and the family. *Cancer, 65,* 752–759.

Massie, M. J., & Holland, J. C. (1990). Depression and the cancer patient. *Journal of Clinical Psychiatry, 51,* 12–17.

Patat, A., Perault, M. C., Vandel, B., Ulliac, N., Zieleniuk, I., & Rosenzweig, P. (1995). Lack of interaction between a new antihistamine, mizolastine, and lorazepam on psychomotor performance and memory in healthy volunteers. *British Journal of Clinical Pharmacology, 39,* 31–38.

Portenoy, R., Thaler, H. T., Kornblith, A. B., Lepore, J. M., Friedlander-Klar, H., Kiyasu, E., Sobel, K., Coyle, N., Kemeny, N., Norton, L., & Scher, H. (1994). The Memorial Symptom Assessment Scale: An instrument for the evaluation of symptom prevalence, characteristics and distress. *European Journal of Cancer, 30,* 1326–1336.

Porter, J., & Jick, H. (1980). Addiction rare in patients treated with narcotics. *New England Journal of Medicine, 302,* 123–128.

Rait, D., & Lederberg, M. (1989). The family of the cancer patient. In J. C. Holland & J. H. Rowland (Eds.), *Handbook of psychooncology* (pp. 585–597). New York: Oxford University Press.

Redd, W. H., Silberfarb, P. M., Andersen, B. L., Andrykowski, M. A., Bovbjerg, D. H., Burish, T. G., Carpenter, P. J., Cleeland, C., Doglin, M., Levy, S. M., Mitnick, L., Morrow, G. R., Schover, L. R., Spiegel, D., & Stevens, J. (1991). Physiologic and psychobehavioral research in oncology. *Cancer, 67,* 813–822.

Schacham, S., Reinhardt, L. C., Raubertas, R. F., & Cleeland, C. S. (1983). Emotional states and pain: Intraindividual and interindividual measures of association. *Journal of Behavioral Medicine, 6,* 405–419.

Silberfarb, P. M., Maurer, L. H., & Crouthamel C. S. (1980). Psychosocial aspects of neoplastic disease: I. Functional status of breast cancer patients during different treatment regimens. *American Journal of Psychiatry, 137,* 450–455.

Sjøgren, P. (1997). Psychomotor and cognitive functioning in cancer patients. *Acta Anasthesiologica Scandinavica, 41,* 159–161.

Spiegel, D. (1989). Effect of psychosocial treatment on survival of patients with metastatic breast cancer. *Lancet, 14,* 888–891.

Spiegel, D., & Bloom, J. R. (1983a). Group therapy and hypnosis reduce metastatic breast carcinoma pain. *Psychosomatic Medicine, 45,* 333–339.

Spiegel, D., & Bloom, J. R. (1983b). Pain in metastatic breast cancer. *Cancer, 52,* 341–345.

Stam, H., Goss, C., Rosenal, L., Ewens, S., & Urton, B. (1985). Aspects of psychological distress and pain in cancer patients undergoing radiation therapy. In H. L. Fields (Ed.), *Advances in pain research and therapy* (Vol. 9, pp. 569–573). New York: Raven Press.

Syrjala, K. L., & Abrams, J. R. (1996). Hypnosis and imagery in the treatment of pain. In R. J. Gatchel & D. C. Turk (Eds.), *Psychological approaches to pain management: A practitioner's handbook* (pp. 231–258). New York: Guilford Press.

Syrjala, K. L., Abrams, J. R., Cowan, J., Hansberry, J., Robison, J., Cross, J., Roth-Roemer, S., DuPen, A., DuPen, S., Stillman, M., Cleeland, C. S., & Fredrickson, M. (1996). Is educating patients and families the route to relieving cancer pain? In *8th World Congress on Pain Abstracts* (p. 167). Seattle: IASP Press.

Syrjala, K. L., Abrams, J. R., DuPen, A., Niles, R., & Rupert, J. (1997). *Relieving cancer pain* (2nd ed.). Seattle, WA: Academy Press.

Syrjala, K. L., & Chapko, M. K. (1995). Evidence for a

biopsychosocial model of cancer treatment-related pain. *Pain, 61,* 69–79.

Syrjala, K. L., Cummings, C., & Donaldson, G. W. (1992). Hypnosis or cognitive behavioral training for the reduction of pain and nausea during cancer treatment: A controlled clinical trial. *Pain, 48,* 137–146.

Syrjala, K. L., Danis, B., Abrams, J. R., & Keenan, R. (1992). *Coping skills for bone marrow transplantation.* Seattle, WA: Printex Press.

Syrjala, K. L., Donaldson, G. W., Davis, M. W., Kippes, M. E., & Carr, J. E. (1995). Relaxation and imagery and cognitive-behavioral training reduce pain during cancer treatment: A controlled clinical trial. *Pain, 63,* 189–198.

Syrjala, K. L., & Roth-Roemer, S. L. (1998). Nonpharmacologic approaches to pain. In A. Berger, R. K. Portenoy, & D. E. Weissman (Eds.), *Principles and practice of supportive oncology* (pp. 77–91). Philadelphia: Lippincott.

Vitaliano, P. P., Maiuro, R. D., Russo, J., Katon, W., DeWolfe, D., & Hall, G. (1990). Coping profiles associated with psychiatric, physical health, work, and family problems. *Health Psychology, 9,* 348–376.

Von Roenn, J. H., Cleeland, C. S., Gonin, R., Hatfield, A. K., & Pandya, K. J. (1993). Physician attitudes and practice in cancer pain management: A survey from the Eastern Cooperative Oncology Group. *Annals of Internal Medicine, 119,* 121–126.

Ward, S. E., Goldberg, N., Miller-McCauley, V., Mueller, C., Nolan, A., Pawlik-Plank, D., Robbins, A., Stormoen, D., & Weissman, D. E. (1993). Patient-related barriers to management of cancer pain. *Pain, 52,* 319–324.

Wellisch, D. K. (1985). Family therapy and cancer: Keeping house on a foundation of quicksand. In M. R. Lansky (Ed.), *Family approaches to major psychiatric disorders* (pp. 122–147). Washington, DC: American Psychiatric Press.

Wilson, J. F. (1981). Behavioral preparation for surgery: Benefit or harm? *Journal of Behavioral Medicine, 4,* 79–102.

Zhukovsky, D. S., Gorowski, E., Hausdorff, J., Napolitano, B., & Lesser, M. (1995). Unmet analgesic needs in cancer patients. *Journal of Pain and Symptom Management, 10,* 113–119.

Chapter 20

HIV, AIDS, and Pain

WILLIAM BREITBART

With the introduction of highly active antiretroviral therapies (i.e., combination therapies including protease inhibitors), the face of the AIDS epidemic, particularly for those who can avail themselves of and/or tolerate these new therapies, is indeed changing. Death rates from AIDS in the United States have dropped dramatically in the last 2 years, and rates of serious opportunistic infections and cancers are declining. Despite these hopeful developments, the future is still unclear, and millions of patients with HIV disease worldwide will continue to die of AIDS and to suffer from the enormous burden of physical and psychological symptoms. Even with the advances in AIDS therapies, pain continues to be an issue in the care of patients with HIV disease. As the epidemiology of AIDS changes in the United States, the challenge of managing pain in AIDS patients with a history of substance abuse is becoming an ever-growing challenge. Studies conducted between 1990 and 1995 have documented that pain in individuals with HIV infection or AIDS is highly prevalent, diverse, and varied in syndromal presentation; associated with significant psychological and functional morbidity; and alarmingly undertreated (Breitbart, 1996, 1997; Breitbart, Rosenfeld, et al., 1996; Breitbart, McDonald, et al., 1996; Hewitt et al., 1997; Larue, Fontaine, & Colleau, 1997; Lebovits et al., 1989; McCormack, Li, Zarowny, & Singer, 1993; O'Neill & Sherrard, 1993; Rosenfeld et al., 1996; Singer et al., 1993). Pain management needs to be more integrated into the total

care of patients with HIV. This chapter describes the prevalence and types of pain syndromes encountered in patients with HIV disease, and reviews the psychological and functional impact of pain, as well as the barriers to adequate pain treatment in this population. Finally, principles of pain management, with particular emphasis on the management of pain in HIV-infected patients with a history of substance abuse, are outlined. As will be discussed, an interdisciplinary pain management program for chronic pain (covered in greater detail by Gatchel & Turk, Chapter 27, this volume) is important to use with these patients. Moreover, other significant psychological variables involved in the management of pain with these patients will be reviewed.

PREVALENCE OF PAIN IN AIDS

Estimates of the prevalence of pain in HIV-infected individuals have been reported to range from 30% to over 90%, with the prevalence of pain increasing as disease progresses (Breitbart et al., 1991; Breitbart, Rosenfeld, et al., 1996; Breitbart, McDonald, et al., 1996; Kimball & McCormick, 1996; Larue et al., 1997; Lebovits et al., 1989; Schofferman & Brody, 1990; Singer et al., 1993), particularly in the latest stages of illness.

Studies suggest that approximately 30% of ambulatory HIV-infected patients in early stages of HIV disease (pre-AIDS; Category A or B dis-

315

ease) experience clinically significant pain and that as many as 56% have had episodic painful symptoms of less clear clinical significance (Breitbart, McDonald, et al., 1996; Larue et al., 1997; Singer et al., 1993). In a prospective cross-sectional survey of 438 ambulatory AIDS patients in New York City, 63% reported "frequent or persistent pain of at least two weeks' duration" at the time of assessment (Breitbart, McDonald, et al., 1996). The prevalence of pain in this large sample increased significantly as HIV disease progressed, with 45% of AIDS patients with Category A3 disease, 55% of those with Category B3 disease, and 67% of those with Category C1, 2, or 3 disease reporting pain. Patients in this sample of ambulatory AIDS patients also were more likely to report pain if they had other concurrent HIV-related symptoms (e.g. fatigue, wasting) or had received treatment for an AIDS-related opportunistic infection or if they had not been receiving antiretroviral medications (e.g., AZT, ddI, ddC, d4t).

In a study of pain in hospitalized patients with AIDS in a public hospital in New York City, over 50% of patients required treatment for pain, with pain being the presenting complaint in 30% of patients and the second most common presenting problem after fever (Lebovits et al., 1989). In a French multicenter study, 62% of hospitalized patients with HIV had clinically significant pain (Larue, et al., 1997). Schofferman and Brody (1990) reported that 53% of patients with far-advanced AIDS cared for in a hospice setting had pain, while Kimball and McCormick (1996) reported that up to 93% of AIDS patients in their hospice experienced at least one 48–hour period of pain during the last 2 weeks of life.

Larue and colleagues (1994) demonstrated that patients with AIDS being cared for by hospice at home had prevalence rates and intensity ratings for pain that were comparable to, and even exceeded, those of cancer patients. Breitbart, Rosenfeld, and colleagues (1996) reported that ambulatory AIDS patients in their New York City sample reported a mean pain intensity "on average" of 5.4 (on the 0–10 numerical rating scale of the Brief Pain Inventory) and a mean pain "at its worst" of 7.4. In addition, as with pain prevalence, the intensity of pain experienced by patients with HIV increases significantly as disease progresses. AIDS patients with pain, like their counterparts with cancer pain, typically describe an average of 2.5 to 3 concurrent pains at a time (Breitbart, Rosenfeld, et al., 1996; Hewitt et al., 1997).

PAIN SYNDROMES IN HIV/AIDS: OVERVIEW

Pain syndromes encountered in AIDS are diverse in nature and etiology. The most common pain syndromes reported in studies to date include painful sensory peripheral neuropathy, pain due to extensive Kaposi's sarcoma, headache, oral and pharyngeal pain, abdominal pain, chest pain, arthralgias and myalgias, and painful dermatological conditions (Breitbart et al., 1991; Breitbart, McDonald, et al., 1996; Hewitt et al., 1997; Larue et al., 1994; Lebovits et al., 1989; Schofferman & Brody, 1990; Singer et al., 1993; O'Neill & Sherrard, 1993; Penfold & Clark, 1992). In a sample of 151 ambulatory AIDS patients who underwent a research assessment that included a clinical interview, neurological examination, and review of medical records (Hewitt et al., 1997), the most common pain diagnoses included headaches (46% of patients, 17% of all pains), joint pains (arthritis, arthralgias, etc.; 31% of patients, 12% of pains), painful polyneuropathy (distal symmetrical polyneuropathy; 28% of patients, 10% of pains), and muscle pains (myalgia, myositis; 27% of patients, 12% of pains). Other common pain diagnoses included skin pain (Kaposi's sarcoma, infections; 25% of patients—30% of homosexual males in the sample had pain from extensive KS lesions), bone pain (20% of patients), abdominal pain (17% of patients), chest pain (13%), and painful radiculopathy (12%). Patients in this sample had a total of 405 pains (averaging 3 concurrent pains), with 46% of patients diagnosed with neuropathic-type pain, 71% with somatic pain, 29% with visceral pain, and 46% with headache (classified separately because of controversy as to pathophysiology). When pain type was classified by pains (as opposed to patients), 25% were neuropathic pains, 44% were nociceptive-somatic, 14% were nociceptive-visceral, and 17% were idiopathic-type pains. Patients in this study who had lower CD4+ cell counts were significantly more likely to be diagnosed with polyneuropathy and headache. Hewitt and colleagues (1997) demonstrated that although pains of a neuropathic nature (e.g., polyneuropathies, radiculopathies) certainly make up a large proportion of pain syndromes encountered in AIDS patients, pains of a somatic and/or visceral nature are also extremely common clinical problems.

Pain syndromes seen in HIV disease can be categorized into three types (see Table 20.1): (1) those directly related to HIV infection or to consequences of immunosuppression; (2) those due to

AIDS therapies; and (3) those unrelated to AIDS or AIDS therapies (Breitbart, 1997; Hewitt et al., 1997). In studies to date, approximately 45% of pain syndromes encountered are directly related to HIV infection or to consequences of immunosuppression; 15–30% are due to therapies for HIV- or AIDS-related conditions, as well as diagnostic procedures; and the remaining 25–40% are unrelated to HIV or its therapies (Hewitt et al., 1997).

We have reported on the experience of pain in women with AIDS (Breitbart et al., 1995; Hewitt et al., 1997). Although preliminary in nature, our studies suggest that women with HIV disease experience pain more frequently than men with HIV disease and report somewhat higher levels of pain intensity. This may in part be a reflection of the fact that women with AIDS-related pain are twice as likely to be undertreated for their pain compared to men (Breitbart, Rosenfeld, et al., 1996). Women with HIV disease have unique pain syndromes of a gynecological nature specifically related to opportunistic infectious processes and cancers of the pelvis and genito-urinary tract (Marte & Allen, 1991). Women with AIDS were significantly more likely to be diagnosed with radiculopathy and headache in one survey (Hewitt et al., 1997).

Children with HIV infection also experience pain (Strafford et al., 1991). HIV-related conditions in children that are observed to cause pain include: meningitis and sinusitis (headaches); otitis media; shingles; cellulitis and abscesses; severe candida dermatitis; dental caries; intestinal infections, such

TABLE 20.1. Pain Syndromes in AIDS Patients

Pain related to HIV/AIDS
  HIV neuropathy
  HIV myelopathy
  Kaposi's sarcoma
  Secondary infections (intestines, skin)
  Organomegaly
  Arthritis/vasculitis
  Myopathy/myositis

Pain related to HIV/AIDS therapy
  Antiretrovirals, antivirals
  Antimyocobacterials, PCP prophylaxis
  Chemotherapy (vincristine)
  Radiation
  Surgery
  Procedures (bronchoscopy, biopsies)

Pain unrelated to AIDS
  Disk disease
  Diabetic neuropathy

as mycobacterium avium intracellular (MAI) and cryptosporidium; hepatosplenomegaly; oral and esophageal candidiasis; and spasticity associated with encephalopathy that causes painful muscle spasms.

SPECIFIC PAIN SYNDROMES ENCOUNTERED IN PATIENTS WITH HIV DISEASE

The following section reviews, in detail, the various painful manifestations of HIV disease. The important review by O'Neill and Sherrard (1993) forms the basis of this section on specific pain syndromes in HIV disease.

Gastrointestinal Pain Syndromes

Many of the opportunistic infections and HIV-associated neoplasms may present as pain referable to the gastrointestinal tract. Generally the pain will be alleviated by specific treatment of the causative diseases. Adequate analgesia should be provided during diagnostic assessment (O'Neill & Sherrard, 1993).

Oropharyngeal Pain

Oral cavity and throat pain is very common, accounting for approximately 20% of the pain syndromes encountered in one study (Lebovits et al., 1989). The sources of oral cavity pain have been well described (Cook, 1990; O'Neill & Sherrard, 1993; Rabeneck et al., 1990). Oropharyngeal candidiasis occurs in up to 75% of HIV-positive individuals and, although frequently asymptomatic, it is the most common cause of oral cavity pain. Bacterial infections are mainly seen as necrotizing gingivitis and can arise in HIV-positive patients even though they maintain a good standard of oral hygiene (O'Neill & Sherrard, 1993). Dental abscesses occur more commonly in HIV-infected individuals than in the general population. Oral ulcerations are extremely common and can be the result of herpes simplex virus (HSV), cytomegalovirus (CMV), Epstein–Barr virus (EBV), atypical and typical mycobacterial infection, cryptococcal infection, or histoplasmosis. Frequently, no infectious agent can be identified, and these painful aphthous ulcers are a clinically challenging problem (O'Neill & Sherrard, 1993). Up to 75% of patients with cutaneous Kaposi's sarcoma also have intraoral lesions, most commonly on the palate, although these seldom cause pain (O'Neill & Sherrard, 1993).

Esophageal Pain

About one-third of patients with HIV disease experience esophageal symptoms such as dysphagia or pain on swallowing (odynophagia), often due to esophageal candidiasis. Esophageal candidiasis occurs in between 25% and 75% of patients with HIV disease (Connolly et al., 1989; Eisner & Smith, 1990; Bonacini, Young, & Lane, 1991) and may present as dysphagia or odynophagia. Ulcerative esophagitis, which can be quite painful, is usually a result of CMV infection but can be idiopathic. Infectious causes of esophagitis include herpes simplex, Epstein–Barr virus, mycobacteria, cryptosporidium, and *Pneumocystis carinii* (Connolly et al., 1989; Bonacini et al., 1989; de Silva, Stoopack, & Raufman, 1990; Goodman, Pinero, Rance, Mansell, & Uribe-Botero, 1989; Kazlow, Shah, Benkov, Dische, & LeLeiko, 1986; Kitchen et al., 1990). Kaposi's sarcoma and lymphoma both have been reported to invade the esophagus resulting in dysphagia, pain, and ulceration (O'Neill & Sherrard, 1993). Zidovudine has also been reported to be a cause of esophageal ulceration (Edwards, Turner, Gold, & Cooper, 1990).

Abdominal Pain

Abdominal pain is the primary site of pain in 12–25% of patients with HIV disease (Barone, Gunold, Nealson, & Arvanitis, 1986; Lebovits et al., 1989; Hewitt et al., 1997). Infectious causes of abdominal pain predominate, and include cryptosporidiosis, shigella, salmonella and campylobacter enteritis, CMV ileitis, and mycobacterial (MAI) infection. Perforation of the small and large intestine secondary to CMV infection has been described (Barone et al., 1986). Repeated intussusception of the small intestine has been seen in association with campylobacter infection (Balthazar, Reich, & Pachter, 1986). Lymphoma in the gastrointestinal (GI) tract can present with abdominal pain and intestinal obstruction (Davidson et al., 1991). Kaposi's sarcoma spreads to the GI tract of 40–50% of AIDS patients with cutaneous lesions (Friedman, Wright, & Altman, 1985). Rarely, intestinal Kaposi's sarcoma may cause obstruction, bleeding, perforation, and diarrhea (Potter et al.,

1984). Other causes of abdominal pain in HIV-positive patients (O'Neill & Sherrard, 1993) include ileus, organomegaly, spontaneous aseptic peritonitis, toxic shock, herpes zoster, and Fitzhugh–Curtis syndrome (perihepatitis in association with tubal gonococcal or chlamydia infection).

Biliary Tract and Pancreatic Pain

Cholecystitis may occur in HIV-infected patients as a result of opportunistic infection, CMV and cryptosporidiosis being the most common infectious agents. Extrahepatic biliary tract obstruction secondary to Kaposi's sarcoma or MAI infection has been reported (O'Neill & Sherrard, 1993). Sclerosing cholangitis (CMV, cryptosporidiosis), also known as AIDS cholangiopathy, is another cause of right upper quadrant or epigastric pain (Cello, 1989). Opportunistic liver infections (CMV, MAI, fungal infections), as well as drug-induced hepatic toxicities (ddI, pentamidine), are sources of hepatitis and abdominal or right upper quadrant pain (Bonacini, 1992).

Pancreatitis is often related to adverse effects of HIV-related therapies, in particular the antiretroviral agents didanosine (ddI) and dideoxycytidine (ddC). Between 7% and 10% of patients on ddI develop pancreatitis, and lower rates are reported with other antiretrovirals. Intravenous pentamidine is also associated with pancreatitis. Infectious causes of pancreatitis include CMV infection, MAI infection, cryptococcal infection (Wilcox, Forsmark, Grendell, & Darragh, & Cello, 1990). Rarely, lymphoma or Kaposi's sarcoma may involve the pancreas, resulting in pancreatitis.

Anorectal Pain

Painful anorectal diseases are common, occurring in about one-third of homosexual men with HIV disease (Wexner, Smithy, Milson, & Dailey, 1986). Infectious causes of anorectal pain include perirectal abscesses, CMV proctitis, fissure-in-ano, and HSV infection. A small increase has been noted in anal/anorectal carcinoma in HIV-positive homosexual men (Rabkin & Blattner, 1991).

Chest Pain Syndromes

Chest pain is a common complaint in patients with HIV disease, comprising approximately 13% of the pain syndromes encountered in a sample of ambulatory AIDS patients (Hewitt et al., 1997). Sources of chest pain in patients with HIV disease are similar to those encountered in the general population, that is, cardiac, esophageal, lung and pleura, and chest wall; the etiologies may be somewhat unique, such as opportunistic infections or cancers. In immunosuppressed patients, infectious causes of chest pain should be considered, particularly in the presence of fever and some localizing sign such as dysphagia, dyspnea, or cough. Infectious causes of chest pain include pneumocystis pneumonia (with or without a pneumothorax), esophagitis (CMV, candidiasis, herpes simplex), pleuritis/pericarditis (viral, bacterial, tuberculous), and postherpetic neuralgia. Opportunistic cancers (Kaposi's sarcoma, lymphoma) invading the esophagus, pericardium, chest wall, lung, and pleura may be sources of chest pain. Rarely, pulmonary embolus or bacterial endocarditis may be the cause of chest pain.

Neurological Pain Syndromes in AIDS

Pain syndromes originating in the nervous system include headache, painful peripheral neuropathies, radiculopathies, and myelopathies. HIV is highly neurotropic, invading central and peripheral nervous system structures early in the course of HIV disease. As many as 40–75% of patients with late-stage AIDS have a neurological complication (Dalakas & Pezeshkpour, 1988; Cornblath & McArthur, 1988; Levy, Bredesen, & Rosenblum, 1988; Snider et al., 1983) either directly due to HIV itself (e.g., AIDS dementia, HIV peripheral neuropathy, HIV myelopathy) or secondary to opportunistic infection (e.g., CNS toxoplasmosis, CMV neuropathy) cancer (e.g., CNS lymphoma), or medication side effects (toxic neuropathies due to ddI [didanosine], ddC [zalcitabine], D_4T [stavudine], or AZT [zidovudine]-induced headache). Headache is a frequent symptom in HIV-infected patients and may be an important indication of disease of the central nervous system, including opportunistic infections and cancers. Rarely, cerebrovascular events (e.g., thalamic stroke) occurring in hypercoagulable states can result in central pain syndromes.

Headache

Headache is extremely common, reported by approximately 40–50% of patients with HIV disease, particularly in later stages of illness (Hewitt et al., 1997; Goldstein, 1990). Headache poses a diagnostic

dilemma for physicians in that the underlying cause may range from benign stress and tension to life-threatening central nervous system infection (O'Neill & Sherrard, 1993). The differential diagnosis of headache in patients with HIV disease includes HIV encephalitis and atypical aseptic meningitis, opportunistic infections of the nervous system, AIDS-related central nervous system neoplasms, sinusitis, tension, migraine, and AZT-induced headache (Richman et al., 1987). Toxoplasmosis and cryptococcal meningitis are the two most commonly encountered opportunistic infections of the central nervous system in patients with HIV disease (Levy et al., 1988). Cerebral toxoplasmosis usually presents with persistent headache, sometimes associated with focal signs, change in mental status, or seizures. Diagnosis is based on radiological imaging (magnetic resonance imaging is more sensitive than computed tomography), with a characteristic appearance of multiple deep ring-enhancing lesions and a clinical response to a trial of empiric treatment for toxoplasmosis. A brain biopsy is sometimes necessary to establish a definitive diagnosis and to differentiate cerebral toxoplasmosis from cerebral lymphoma. Cryptococcal meningitis usually presents with symptoms of headache, neck stiffness, and recurring fever, although focal neurological signs may occur. Other opportunistic infections of the central nervous system that can present as headache in the AIDS patient include CMV, HSV and herpes zoster, progressive multifocal leukoencephalopathy (papovavirus), candida albicans, mycobacterium tuberculosis, MAI, and neurosyphilis. Headache related to sinus infection is common in immunocompetent patients with HIV disease who present with headache but have no focal neurologic signs. Opportunistic cancers of the central nervous system include central nervous system lymphoma, metastatic systemic lymphoma, and metastatic intracranial Kaposi's sarcoma. These can present, particularly in the immunocompromised patient with HIV disease, with signs of increased intracranial pressure with or without focal neurological signs, as well as fever and meningismus. More benign causes of headache in the patient with HIV disease include zidovudine (AZT)-induced headache, occurring in 15–30% of patients; tension headache; migraine with or without aura; and unclassifiable or idiopathic headache (Lipton et al., 1991).

Neuropathies Encountered in HIV-Infected Patients

Pain syndromes of a neuropathic nature occur in approximately 40% of AIDS patients with pain

(Hewitt et al., 1997). Although several types of peripheral neuropathy have been described in patients with HIV/AIDS (Table 20.2), the most common painful neuropathy encountered is the predominantly sensory neuropathy (PSN) of AIDS, affecting up to 30% of people with HIV infection (Cornblath & McArthur, 1988; Parry, 1988; Levy, Bredesen, & Rosenblum, 1985; Snider et al., 1983). Other potentially painful neuropathies encountered in HIV/AIDS patients, however, can be caused by viral and nonviral infectious processes (mononeuritis multiplex, including polyneuritis cranialis, polyradiculopathy of the lower limbs, cauda equina syndrome, and plexopathies caused by CMV, HZV, MAI), immune-mediated inflammatory demyelination (acute and chronic Guillain–Barré syndrome), a variety of medical conditions (diabetic neuropathy, postherpetic neuralgia, entrapment neuropathies), nutritional deficiencies (B6, B12), toxins (alcohol) and HIV-related therapies (e.g., ddI [didanosine], ddC [zalcitabine]). Several antiretroviral drugs, such as ddI, ddC, and D$_4$T (stavudine), chemotherapy agents used to treat Kaposi's sarcoma (vincristine), as well as a number of medications used in the treatment of PCP, mycobacterial infection, and other HIV-associated infections, can cause painful toxic neuropathy (O'Neill & Sherrard,

1993; Lefkowitz & Breitbart, 1992; Griffin, Wesselingh, Griffin, Glass, & McArthur, 1994).

Predominantly Sensory Neuropathy (PSN) of AIDS. The most frequently encountered neuropathy is a symmetrical predominantly sensory painful peripheral neuropathy. This is a late manifestation, occurring most often in patients with an AIDS-defining illness, but it has been reported earlier in the course of the disease (Cornblath & McArthur, 1988). Prevalence in hospice populations ranges from 19% to 26% (Schofferman & Brody, 1990; Moss, 1990; Singh, Fermie, & Peters, 1992). It is the only peripheral sensory neuropathy that has been postulated to be a direct result of HIV infection of the peripheral nervous system (Cornblath & McArthur, 1988). The predominant symptom in about 60% of patients is pain in the soles of the feet. Paresthesia is frequent and usually involves the dorsum of the feet in addition to the soles. Most patients have signs of peripheral neuropathy (most commonly, absent or reduced ankle jerks and elevated thresholds to pain and vibration sense); and while the signs progress, the symptoms often remain confined to the feet (Simpson & Wolfe, 1991; Cornblath & McArthur, 1988; Lange, Britton, Younger, & Hays, 1988). Although the patients' complaints are predominantly sensory, electrophysiological studies demonstrate both sensory and motor involvement.

Immune-Mediated Neuropathies. Acute Guillain–Barré syndrome has been described in association with seroconversion (group-I infection) but may occur at any time. Both acute and chronic inflammatory demyelinating polyneuropathies are predominantly motor, and sensory abnormalities are rare (Parry, 1988). Mononeuritis multiplex presents with sensory or motor deficits in the distribution of multiple spinal, cranial, or peripheral nerves (Dalakas & Pezeshkpour, 1988) and may progress into a chronic inflammatory demyelinating polyneuropathy (Parry, 1988).

Infectious Neuropathies. Polyradiculopathies (associated with CMV infection) often present with radicular pain and follow a distinct course (Fuller, Jacobs, & Guiloff, 1989). The onset is usually subacute and the deficit initially confined to sacral and lumbar nerve roots. Both sensory and motor functions are involved, and there is usually early involvement of sphincters. Progression is relentless (Parry, 1988).

TABLE 20.2. Neuropathies Encountered in HIV/AIDS-Infected Patients

Predominantly sensory neuropathy (PSN) of AIDS

Immune-mediated
   Inflammatory demyelinating polyneuropathies (IDPs)
      Acute (Guillain–Barré syndrome)
      Chronic inflammatory demyelinating polyneuropathy (CIDP)

Infectious
   Cytomegalovirus polyradiculopathy
   Cytomegalovirus multiple mononeuropathy
   Herpes zoster
   Mycobacterial (MAI)

Toxic/nutritional
   Alcohol, vitamin deficiencies (B6, B12)
   Antiretrovirals: ddI (didanosine), ddC (zalcitabine), D$_4$T (stavudine)
   Antivirals: foscarnet
   PCP prophylaxis: dapsone
   Antibacterial: metronidazole
   Antimycobacterials: INH (isoniazid), rifampin, ethionamide
   Antineoplastics: vincristine, vinblastine

Other medical conditions
   Diabetic neuropathy
   Postherpetic neuralgia

Toxic/Nutritional Neuropathies. Toxic and nutritional neuropathies in patients with HIV disease have been reported with the following: alcohol; vitamin deficiencies (B6, B12); antiretroviral drugs—ddI (didanosine), ddC (zalcitabine), and D4T (stavudine); antivirals—foscarnet; PCP prophylaxis—dapsone; antibacterial drugs—metronidazole; antimycobacterial drugs—isoniazid, rifampin, and ethionamide; and antineoplastics—vincristine and vinblastine (Simpson & Wolfe, 1991; Griffin et al., 1994).

Painful Neuropathies According to Stage of HIV Infection. The type of neuropathy varies with the stage of infection. The acute or seroconversion phase of HIV disease is associated with mononeuritides, brachial plexopathy, and acute demyelinating polyneuropathy. The latent or asymptomatic phase (CD4+ T lymphocytes > 500/mm^3) is characterized by acute and chronic demyelinating polyneuropathies. The transition phase (200–500 CD4+ cells) is characterized by herpes zoster (shingles) and mononeuritis multiplex. The late phase of HIV disease (< 200 CD4+ cells) is characterized by HIV predominantly sensory polyneuropathy, CMV polyneuropathy, mononeuritis multiplex, autonomic neuropathy, mononeuropathies secondary to meningeal disease, and antiretroviral induced toxic neuropathies (Griffin et al., 1994).

Rheumatological Pain Syndromes

In studies conducted by the Memorial Sloan-Kettering group (Hewitt, et al., 1997), over 50% of pain syndromes were classified as rheumatological in nature, including various form of arthritis, arthropathy, arthralgia, myopathy, myositis, and myalgias. In another study, 72% of patients with different stages of HIV infection had painful symptoms involving the musculoskeletal system (Berman, Espinoza, Diaz, Aguilar, & Rolando, 1988).

Arthritis and Arthropathies

HIV disease has been associated with several types of painful arthritis and arthropathies, including nonspecific arthralgias, reactive arthritis, psoriatic arthritis, HIV-associated arthritis, and, rarely, aseptic arthritis (Espinoza, Aguilar, Berman, Gutierrez, & Vasey, 1989; Kaye, 1989). The most frequently reported arthritis is a reactive arthritis, or Reiter's syndrome (Winchester, Bernstein, Fischer, Enlow, & Solomon, 1987; Foster et al., 1988; Kaye, 1989),

often unresponsive to nonsteroidal anti-inflammatory drug therapies (NSAIDs). Reiter's syndrome can present with persistent oligoarthritis primarily affecting the large joints of the lower limbs, sacroiliitis, urethritis, conjunctivitis, keratoderma blenorrhagica, circinate balanitis, and oral ulceration. Many patients are positive for HLA-B27 antigen. Diarrhea is a common precipitating event. Nonspecific arthralgias are common (Berman et al., 1989; Kaye, 1989; Espinoza et al., 1989). Acute HIV infection may present with a polyarthralgia in association with a mononucleosis-like illness. There is also a syndrome of acute severe and intermittent articular pain, often referred to as HIV-associated painful articular syndrome, which commonly affects the large joints of the lower limbs and shoulders. Psoriasis and psoriatic arthritis have been reported in patients with HIV infection (Johnson, Duvic, Rapini, & Rios, 1986; Espinoza et al., 1988). The arthritis is typically seen in conjunction with the skin changes of psoriasis, and authors suggest it may follow a disease course that proves refractory to conventional therapy (O'Neill & Sherrard, 1993). An HIV-associated arthritis has also been described (Rynes et al., 1988), which typically presents as an oligoarthritis affecting the joints of the lower limbs. Synovial fluid is noninflammatory, and biopsy shows a mild chronic synovitis. There is no associated infection to suggest a reactive arthritis, and the patients reported have been HLA-B27 negative. It appears that this arthritis is caused by the HIV virus itself (Espinoza et al., 1989). Septic arthritis has been reported in patients with HIV disease, including arthritis due to bacterial infections, and infections with Cryptococcus neoformans and Sporothrix schenckii (Espinoza et al., 1989; Kaye, 1989).

Myopathy and Myositis

Muscle pain is very common in patients with HIV disease. Several types of myopathy and myositis have been described in HIV-infected patients, including HIV-associated myopathy or polymyositis, necrotizing noninflammatory myopathy both in association with zidovudine and without zidovudine, pyomyositis, and microsporidiosis myositis (Dalakas, Pezeshkpour, Gravell, & Sever, 1986; Gorand, Henry, & Guiloff, 1988; Panegyres, Ran, Kakulas, Armstrong, & Hollingsworth, 1988; Watts, Hoffbrand, Paton, & Davie, 1987; Nelson, Daniels, Dean, Barton, & Gazzard, 1992; Ledford et al., 1985; Rienhart et al., 1990). Polymyositis may occur at any stage of HIV infection; it is thought to be the result of direct viral infection of muscle cells (Kaye, 1989) and may present with a subacute onset of proximal muscle weakness and myalgia (Dalakas et al., 1986). Electromyographic evidence of myopathy, a raised serum creatinine kinase, and biopsy evidence of polymyositis are common in symptomatic patients. Drugs used in the treatment of HIV disease may also be associated with the development of myalgia (Richman et al., 1987) and myositis (Bessen, Greene, Louie, Sietzman, & Weinberg, 1988; Gorand et al., 1988). Zidovudine has been particularly implicated. In these patients, symptoms frequently improve following discontinuation of zidovudine therapy (O'Neill & Sherrard, 1993).

PAIN'S IMPACT ON QUALITY OF LIFE

Pain, in patients with HIV disease, has a profound negative impact on physical and psychological functioning, as well as overall quality of life (Rosenfeld et al., 1996; Larue et al., 1997). In a study of the impact of pain on psychological functioning and quality of life in ambulatory AIDS patients (Rosenfeld et al., 1996), depression was significantly correlated with the presence of pain. In addition to being significantly more distressed, depressed, and hopeless, those with pain were twice as likely to have suicidal ideation (40%) as those without pain (20%). HIV-infected patients with pain were more functionally impaired (Rosenfeld et al., 1996). Such functional interference was highly correlated to levels of pain intensity and depression. Patients with pain were more likely to be unemployed or disabled and reported less social support. Larue and colleagues (1997) reported that HIV-infected patients with pain intensities greater than 5 (on a 0–10 numerical rating scale) reported significantly poorer quality of life during the week preceding their survey than patients without pain. Pain intensity had an independent negative impact on HIV patients' quality of life, even after adjustment for treatment setting, stage of disease, fatigue, sadness, and depression. Singer and colleagues (1993) also reported an association between the frequency of multiple pains, increased disability, and higher levels of depression. Psychological variables, such as the amount of control people believe they have over pain, emotional associations and memories of pain, fears of death, depression, anxiety, and hopelessness, contribute to the experience of pain in people with AIDS and can increase suffering

(Breitbart, 1993; Rosenfeld et al., 1996). Our group also reported (Payne et al., 1994) that negative thoughts related to pain were associated with greater pain intensity, psychological distress, and disability in ambulatory patients with AIDS. Those AIDS patients who felt that pain represented a progression of their HIV disease reported more intense pain than those who did not see pain as a threat.

MANAGEMENT OF PAIN IN AIDS

Assessment Issues

The initial step in pain management is a comprehensive assessment of pain symptoms. The health professional working in the AIDS setting must have a working knowledge of the etiology and treatment of pain in AIDS. This would include an understanding of the different types of AIDS pain syndromes discussed previously, as well as a familiarity with the parameters of appropriate pharmacological treatment. A close collaboration of the entire health care team is optimal when attempting to adequately manage pain in the AIDS patient. A careful history and physical examination may disclose an identifiable syndrome (e.g., herpes zoster, bacterial infection, or neuropathy) that can be treated in a standard fashion (Watson, Chipman, Reed, Evans, & Birkett, 1992; Kishore-Kumar et al., 1990). A thorough staffing by an interdisciplinary pain management team is essential in order to evaluate all of the significant physical and psychosocial issues involved in the pain process. A comprehensive pain management program can then be prescribed (again, a review of such an interdisciplinary pain management program approach is presented by Gatchel & Turk, Chapter 27, this volume. For example, a standard pain history (Portenoy & Foley, 1989; Foley, 1985) may provide valuable clues to the nature of the underlying process and, indeed, may disclose other treatable disorders. A description of the qualitative features of the pain, its time course, and any maneuvers that increase or decrease pain intensity should be obtained. Pain intensity (current, average, at best, at worst) should be assessed to determine the need for weak versus potent analgesics and as a means to serially evaluate the effectiveness of ongoing treatment. Pain descriptors (e.g., burning, shooting, dull, or sharp) will help determine the mechanism of pain (somatic, nociceptive, visceral nociceptive, or neuropathic) and may suggest the likelihood of response to various classes of traditional and adjuvant analgesics (nonsteroidal anti-inflammatory drugs, opioids, antidepressants, anticonvulsants, oral local anesthetics, corticosteroids, etc.; Jacox et al., 1994; World Health Organization, 1986; Portenoy, 1990). Additionally, detailed medical, neurological, and psychosocial assessments (including a history of substance use or abuse) must be conducted. When possible, family members or partners should be interviewed. During the assessment phase, pain should be aggressively treated while pain complaints and psychosocial issues are subject to an ongoing process of reevaluation (Portenoy & Foley, 1989).

Multimodal Approach

Federal guidelines developed by the Agency for Health Care Policy and Research (AHCPR) for the management of cancer pain (Jacox et al., 1994) also address the issue of management of pain in AIDS and state: "The principles of pain assessment and treatment in the patient with HIV positive/AIDS are not fundamentally different from those in the patient with cancer and should be followed for patients with HIV-positive/AIDS." In contrast to pain in cancer, pain in HIV disease may more commonly have an underlying treatable cause (O'Neill & Sherrard, 1993).

Optimal management of pain in AIDS is multimodal and requires phamacological, psychotherapeutic, cognitive-behavioral, anesthetic, neurosurgical, and rehabilitative approaches. A multidimensional model of AIDS pain that recognizes the interaction of cognitive, emotional, socioenvironmental, and nociceptive aspects of pain suggests a model for multimodal intervention.

Pharmacotherapies for Pain in AIDS

The World Health Organization (WHO; 1986) has devised guidelines for analgesic management of cancer pain that the AHCPR has endorsed for the management of pain related to cancer or AIDS (Jacox et al., 1994). These guidelines, also known widely as the "WHO analgesic ladder," have been well validated (Ventafridda, Caraceni, & Gamba, 1990). This approach advocates selection of analgesics based on the severity, as well as the type, of pain (i.e., neuropathic vs. nonneuropathic pain). For pain of mild to moderate severity, nonopioid analgesics such as NSAIDs (nonsteroidal antiinflammatory drugs) and acetaminophen are recommended. For pain that is persistent and moderate to severe in intensity, opioid analgesics of increasing potency (such as morphine) should be utilized. Adjuvant agents, such as laxatives and psychostimulants, are useful in preventing, as well as treating, opioid side effects such as constipation or sedation, respectively. Adjuvant analgesic drugs, such as the antidepressant analgesics, are suggested for considered use, along with opioids and NSAIDs, in all stages of the analgesic ladder (mild, moderate, or severe pain), but they have their most important clinical application in the management of neuropathic pain.

This WHO approach, although not yet validated for AIDS, has been recommended by the AHCPR and clinical authorities in the field of pain management and AIDS (Jacox et al., 1993; O'Neill & Sherrard, 1993; Singer et al., 1993; Lefkowitz & Breitbart, 1992; American Pain Society, 1992; Lebovits et al., 1989; Schofferman & Brody, 1990). Clinical reports describing the successful application of the principles of the WHO analgesic ladder to the management of pain in AIDS, with particular emphasis on the use of opioids, have also recently appeared in the literature (Newshan & Wainapel, 1993; Schofferman & Brody, 1990; McCormack et al., 1993; Anand, Carmosino, & Glatt, 1994; Patt & Reddy, 1993; Kimball & McCormick, 1996; Lefkowitz & Newshan, 1997; Kaplan, 1996).

Nonopioid Analgesics

The nonopioid analgesics (Table 20.3) are prescribed principally for mild to moderate pain or to augment the analgesic effects of opioid analgesics in the treatment of severe pain. The use of NSAIDs in patients with AIDS must be accompanied by heightened awareness of toxicity and adverse effects. NSAIDs are highly protein-bound, and the free fraction of available drug is increased in AIDS patients who are cachectic, wasted, and hypoalbuminic, often resulting in toxicities and adverse effects. Patients with AIDS are frequently hypovolemic, on concurrent nephrotoxic drugs, and experiencing HIV nephropathy, and so are at increased risk for renal toxicity related to NSAIDs. The antipyretic effects of the NSAIDs may also interfere with early detection of infection in patients with AIDS.

The major adverse effects associated with NSAIDs include gastric ulceration, renal failure, hepatic dysfunction, and bleeding. The nonacetylated salicylates, such as salsalate, sodium salicylate, and choline magnesium salicylate theoretically have fewer gastrointestinal (GI) side effects and

TABLE 20.3. Oral Analgesics for Mild to Moderate Pain in AIDS

Analgesic (by class)	Starting dose (mg)	Duration (hr)	Plasma half-life (hr)	Comments
Nonsteroidal				
Aspirin	650	4–6	4–6	The standard for comparison among nonopioid analgesics
Ibuprofen	400–600	–	–	Like aspirin, can inhibit platelet function
Choline magnesium trisalicylate	700–1,500	–	–	Essentially no hematological or gastrointestinal side effects
Weaker opioids				
Codeine	32–65	3–4	–	Metabolized to morphine, often used to suppress cough in patients at risk of pulmonary bleed
Oxycodone	5–10	3–4	–	Available as a single agent and in combination with aspirin or acetaminophen
Propoxyphene	65–130	4–6	–	Toxic metabolite norpropoxy accumulates with repeated dosing

might be considered in cases in which GI distress is an issue. Prophylaxis for NSAID-associated GI symptoms include H2 antagonist drugs (cimetidine, 300 mg three to four times daily, or ranitidine, 150 mg twice daily); misoprostol, 200 mg four times daily; omeprazole, 20 mg daily; or an antacid. Patients should be informed of these symptoms, issued guaiac cards with reagent, and taught to check their stool weekly. NSAIDs affect kidney function and should be used with caution. NSAIDs can cause a decrease in glomerular filtration, acute and chronic renal failure, interstitial nephritis, papillary necrosis, and hyperkalemia (Murray & Brater, 1990). In patients with renal impairment, NSAIDs should be used with caution, because many (i.e., ketoprofen, feroprofen, naproxen, and carpofen) are highly dependent on renal function for clearance. The risk of renal dysfunction is greatest in patients with advanced age, preexisting renal impairment, hypovolemia, concomitant therapy with nephrotoxic drugs, and heart failure. Prostaglandins modulate vascular tone, and their inhibition by the NSAIDs can cause hypertension as well as interference with the pharmacological control of hypertension (Radeck & Deck, 1987). Caution should be used in patients receiving B-adrenergic antagonists, diuretics, or angiotensin-converting enzyme inhibitors. Several studies have suggested that there is substantial biliary excretion of several NSAIDs, including indomethacin and sulindac. In patients with hepatic dysfunction, these drugs should be used with caution. NSAIDs, with the exception of the nonacetylated salicylates (e.g., sodium salicylate, choline magnesium trisalicylate), produce inhibition of platelet aggregation (usually reversible, but irreversible with aspirin). NSAIDs should be used with extreme caution or avoided in patients who are thrombocytopenic or who have clotting impairment.

Opioid Analgesics

Opioid analgesics are the mainstay of pharmacotherapy for pain of moderate to severe intensity in the patient with HIV disease (Table 20.4). Several reports describing the safe and effective use of opioid drugs in the management of moderate to severe pain in populations of patients with HIV disease (including patients with a history of injection drug use as their HIV transmission factor) have begun to appear in the literature (Newshan & Wainapel, 1993; Patt & Ready, 1993; Anand et al., 1994; Kimball & McCormick, 1996; Kaplan et al., 1996; Lefkowitz & Newshan, 1997). Kaplan and colleagues (1996) conducted a multicenter study in which 44 patients with moderate to severe AIDS-related pain were treated with sustained-release oral morphine in an open-label prospective study of patients treated for up to 18 days. For patients who completed treatment, pain intensity decreased by 65%. The quality of life was reported good for 80% of these patients, and acceptability of therapy was 96%. In addition, 92% of side effects were resolved. The total morphine dose re-

TABLE 20.4. Opioid Analgesics for Moderate to Severe Pain in AIDS

Analgesic	Equianalgesic route	Dose (mg)	Analgesic onset (hr)	Duration (hr)	Plasma half-life (hr)	Comments
Morphine	PO	30–60[a]	1–1½	4–6	2–3	Standard of comparison for the narcotic analgesics.
	IM, IV, SC	10	½–1	3–6		
	PO	90–120	1–1½	8–12	–	Long-acting sustained-release form.
Oxycodone	PO	20–30	1	3–6	2–3	In combination with aspirin or acetaminophen, it is considered a weaker opioid; as a single agent, it is comparable to the strong opioids, such as morphine.
	PO	20–40	1	8–12	2–3	Available in immediate-release and sustained-release preparation.
Hydromorphone	PO	7.5	½–1	3–4	2–3	Short half-life; ideal for elderly patients. Comes in suppository and injectable forms.
	IM, IV	1.5	¼–½	3–4	2–3	
Methadone	PO	20	½–1	4–8	15–30	Long half-life; tends to accumulate with initial dosing, requires careful titration. Good oral potency.
	IM, IV	10	½–1	–	15–30	
Levorphanol	PO	4	½–1½	3–6	12–16	Long half-life; requires careful dose titration in first week. Note that analgesic duration is only 4 hours.
	IM	2	½–1		12–16	
Meperidine	PO	300	½–1½	3–6	3–4	Active toxic metabolite, ormeperidine, tends to accumulate (plasma half-life is 12–16 hours), especially with renal impairment and in elderly patients, causing delirium, myoclonus, and seizures.
	IM	75	½–1	3–4	3–4	
Fentanyl transdermal system	TD	0.1	12–18	48–72	20–22	Transdermal patch is convenient, bypassing GI analgesia until depot is formed. Not suitable for rapid titration.
	IV	.01		–	–	

[a]30 mg for repeat around-the-clock dosing; 60 mg for single dose or intermittent dosing.

Note. PO, oral; IM, intramuscular; IV, intravenous; SC, subcutaneous; TD, transdermal.

mained stable through the course of the study. In a pilot study, Lefkowitz and Newshan (1997) reported similar findings on the effectiveness and safety of the transdermal fentanyl patch in a small sample of patients with AIDS-related pain.

Principles that are useful in guiding the appropriate use of opioid analgesics for pain (Portenoy, 1990; Foley & Inturrisi, 1987; American Pain Society, 1992) include the following: (1) choose an appropriate drug; (2) start with lowest dose possible; (3) titrate dose; (4) use "as needed" doses selectively; (5) use an appropriate route of administration; (6) be aware of equivalent analgesic doses; (7) use a combination of opioid, nonopioid, and adjuvant drugs; (8) be aware of tolerance; and (9) understand physical and psychological dependence. In choosing the appropriate opioid analgesic for cancer pain, Portenoy (1990) highlights the following important considerations: (1) opioid class; (2) "weak" versus "strong" opioids; (3) pharmacokinetic characteristics; (4) duration of analgesic effect; (5) favorable prior response; and (6) opioid side effects.

Opioid analgesics are divided into two classes, the agonists and the agonist–antagonists, based on their affinity to opioid receptors. Pentazocine, butorphanol, and nalbuphine are examples of opioid analgesics with mixed agonist–antagonist properties. These drugs can reverse opioid effects and precipitate an opioid withdrawal syndrome in patients who are opioid-tolerant or dependent. They are of limited use in the management of chronic pain in AIDS. Oxycodone (in combination with either aspirin or acetaminophen), hydrocodone, and codeine are the so-called "weaker" opioid analgesics and are indicated for use in step 2 of the WHO ladder for pain of mild to moderate intensity. More severe pain is best managed with morphine or another of the stronger opioid analgesics, such as hydromorphone, methadone, levorphanol, or fentanyl. Oxycodone, as a single agent without aspirin or acetaminophen, is available in immediate and sustained-release forms and is considered a "stronger" opioid in these forms.

The oral route has often been described as the preferred route of administration of opioid analgesics from the perspectives of convenience and cost. However, the transdermal route of administration has gained rapid acceptance among clinicians and patients. Patients with HIV infection are burdened with the task of taking anywhere from 20–40 tablets of medication per day and often need to follow complicated regimens in which medication has to be taken on an empty stomach and so

forth. In a study on patient-related barriers to pain management in AIDS patients (Breitbart et al., 1998), the vast majority of AIDS patients endorsed a preference to utilize a pain intervention that required a minimal number of additional pills (e.g., sustained-release preparations of oral opioids) or interventions that did not require taking pills at all (i.e., transdermal opioid system). Immediate release oral morphine or hydromorphone preparations require that the drug be taken every 3 to 4 hours. Longer acting, sustained-release oral morphine preparations and oxycodone preparations are available that provide up to 8 hours or more of analgesia, minimizing the number of daily doses required for the control of persistent pain. Rescue doses of immediate-release, short-acting opioid are often necessary to supplement the use of sustained-release morphine or oxycodone, particularly during periods of titration or pain escalation. The transdermal fentanyl patch system (Duragesic) also has applications in the management of severe pain in AIDS (Patt & Reddy, 1993; Lefkowitz & Newshan, 1997). Each transdermal fentanyl patch contains a 48–72 hour supply of fentanyl, which is absorbed from a depot in the skin. Levels in the plasma rise slowly over 12–18 hours after patch placement; so with the initial placement of a patch, alternative opioid analgesia (either oral, rectal, or parenteral) must be provided until adequate levels of fentanyl are attained. The elimination half-life of this dosage form of fentanyl is long (21 hours), and so it must be noted that significant levels of fentanyl will remain in the plasma for about 24 hours after the removal of a transdermal patch. The transdermal system is not optimal for rapid dose titration of acutely exacerbated pain; however, a variety of dosage forms is available. As with sustained-release morphine preparations, all patients should be provided with oral or parenteral rapidly acting short duration opioids to manage breakthrough pain. The transdermal system is convenient and can minimize the reminders of pain associated with repeated oral dosing of analgesics. In AIDS patients, it should be noted that the absorption of transdermal fentanyl can be increased with fever, resulting in increased plasma levels and shorter duration of analgesia from the patch.

It is important to note that opioids can be administered through a variety of routes: oral, rectal, transdermal, intravenous, subcutaneous, intraspinal, and even intraventrularly (Patt & Reddy, 1993). There are advantages and disadvantages, as well as indications for use of these various routes. Further discussion of such alternative delivery routes as the intraspinal route are beyond the scope of this chapter; however, interested readers are directed to the Agency for Health Care Policy and Research *Clinical Practice Guideline: Management of Cancer Pain* (Jacox et al., 1994), available free of charge through 1-800-4cancer.

The opioids are extremely effective analgesics, and their side effects are common and can be minimized if anticipated in advance. Sedation is a common CNS side effect, especially during the initiation of treatment. Sedation usually resolves after the patient has been maintained on a steady dosage. Persistent sedation can be alleviated with a psychostimulant, such as dextroamphetamine, pemoline, or methylphenidate. All are prescribed in divided doses in early morning and at noon. Additionally, psychostimulants can improve depressed mood and enhance analgesia (Bruera, Chadwick, Brennels, Hanson, & MacDonald, 1987; Breitbart, 1992). Delirium, of either an agitated or a somnolent variety, can also occur while on opioid analgesics and is usually accompanied by attentional deficits, disorientation, and perceptual disturbances (visual hallucinations and, more commonly, illusions). Myoclonus and asterixis are often early signs of neurotoxicity that accompany the course of opioid-induced delirium. Meperidine (Demerol), when administered chronically in patients with renal impairment, can lead to a delirium due to accumulation of the neuroexcitatory metabolite normeperidine (Kaiko et al., 1983). Opioid-induced delirium can be alleviated through the implementation of three possible strategies: (1) lowering the dose of the opioid drug presently in use, (2) changing to a different opioid, or (3) treating the delirium with low doses of high-potency neuroleptics, such as haloperidol. The third strategy is especially useful for agitation and clears the sensorium (Breitbart, 1989). For agitated states, intravenous haloperidol in doses starting at between 1 mg. and 2 mg. is useful, with rapid escalation of dose if no effect is noted. Gastrointestinal side effects of opioid analgesics are common. The most prevalent are nausea, vomiting, and constipation (Portenoy, 1990). Concomitant therapy with prochlorperazine for nausea is sometimes effective. Because all opioid analgesics are not tolerated in the same manner, switching to anoter narcotic can be helpful if an antiemetic regimen fails to control nausea. Constipation caused by narcotic effects on gut receptors is a problem frequently encountered, and it tends to be responsive to the regular use of senna derivatives. A careful review of medications is imperative because anticholinergic drugs such as the tricyclic antidepressants can worsen opioid-induced constipation and can cause bowel obstruction. Respiratory depression is a worrisome but rare side effect of the opioid analgesics. Respiratory difficulties can almost always be avoided if two general principles are adhered to: (1) start opioid analgesics in low doses in opioid–naive patients, and (2) be cognizant of relative potencies when switching opioid analgesics, routes of administration, or both.

Adjuvant Analgesics

Adjuvant analgesics are the third class of medications frequently prescribed for the treatment of chronic pain and have important applications in the management of pain in AIDS (Table 20.5). Adjuvant analgesic drugs are used to enhance the analgesic efficacy of opioids, treat concurrent symptoms that exacerbate pain, and provide independent analgesia. They may be used in all stages of the analgesic ladder. Commonly used adjuvant drugs include antidepressants, neuroleptics, psychostimulants, anticonvulsants, corticosteroids, and oral anesthetics (Jacox et al., 1994; Breitbart, 1992; Portenoy, 1998).

Antidepressants

The current literature supports the use of antidepressants as adjuvant analgesic agents in the management of a wide variety of chronic pain syndromes, including cancer pain, postherpetic neuralgia, diabetic neuropathy, fibromyalgia, headache, and low back pain (Butler, 1986; France, 1987; Ventafridda et al., 1987; Getto, Sorkness, & Howell, 1987; Magni, Arsie, & Deleo, 1987; Walsh, 1986). The antidepressants are analgesic through a number of mechanisms that include antidepressant activity (France, 1987), potentiation or enhancement of opioid analgesia (Botney & Fields, 1983; Malseed & Goldstein, 1979; Ventafridda, Branchi, et al., 1990), and direct analgesic effects (Spiegel, Kalb, & Pasternak, 1983). The leading hypothesis suggests that both serotonergic and noradrenergic properties of the antidepressants are probably important and that variations among individuals in pain (as to the status of their own neurotransmitter systems) is an important variable (Watson et al., 1992). Other possible mechanisms of antidepressant analgesic activity that have been proposed include adrenergic and serotonin receptor effects (Gram, 1983), adenosinergic effects (Merskey & Hamilton, 1989), antihistaminic effects (Gram,

TABLE 20.5. Psychotropic Adjuvant Analgesic Drugs for AIDS Pain

Generic name	Approximate daily dosage range (mg)	Route
Tricyclic antidepressants		
Amitriptyline	10–150	PO,IM
Nortriptyline	10–150	PO
Imipramine	15.5–150	PO,IM
Desipramine	10–150	PO
Clomipramine	10–150	PO
Doxepin	12–150	PO,IM
Heterocyclic and noncyclic antidepressants		
Trazodone	125–300	PO
Maprotiline	50–300	PO
Serotonin reuptake inhibitors		
Fluoxetine	20–80	PO
Paroxetine	10–60	PO
Sertraline	50–200	PO
Newer agents		
Nefazodone	100–500	PO
Venlafaxine	75–300	PO
Psychostimulants		
Methylphenidate	2.5–20 bid	PO
Dextroamphetamine	2.5–20 bid	PO
Pemoline	13.75–75 bid	PO
Phenothiazines		
Fluphenazine	1–3	PO,IM
Methotrimeprazine	10–20 q6h	IM,IV
Butyrophenones		
Haloperidol	1–3 PO	PO,IV
Pimozide	2–6 bid	PO
Antihistamines		
Hydroxyzine	50 q4h–q6h	PO
Anticonvulsants		
Carbamazepine	200 tid–400 tid	PO
Phenytoin	300–400	PO
Valproate	500 tid–1,000 tid	PO
Gabapentin	300 tid–1,000 tid	PO
Oral local anesthetics		
Mexiletine	600–900	PO
Corticosteroids		
Dexamethasone	4–16	PO,IV
Benzodiazepines		
Alprazolam	0.25–2.0 tid	PO
Clonazepam	0.5–4 bid	PO

Note. PO, oral; IM, intramuscular; IV, intravenous; q4h, every 4 hours; q6h, every 6 hours; bid, twice a day; tid, three times a day.

1983), and direct neuronal effects, such as inhibition of paroxysmal neuronal discharge and decreasing sensitivity of adrenergic receptors on injured nerve sprouts (Devor, 1983).

There is substantial evidence that the tricyclic antidepressants in particular are analgesic and useful in the management of chronic neuropathic and nonneuropathic pain syndromes. Amitriptyline is the tricyclic antidepressant most studied and has been proved effective as an analgesic in a large number of clinical trials addressing a wide variety of chronic pain syndromes, including neuropathy, cancer pain, fibromyalgia, and others (Pilowsky, Hallet, Bassett, Thomas, & Penhall, 1982; Watson et al., 1992; Max et al., 1987; Sharav, Singer, Dione, & Dubner, 1987; Ventafridda et al., 1987; France, 1987). Other tricyclics that have been shown to have efficacy as analgesics include imipramine (Young & Clarke, 1985; Sindrup, Gram, Brosen, Eshoj, & Mogenson, 1990), desipramine (Kishore-Kumar et al., 1990; Max et al., 1992), nortriptyline (Gomez-Perez et al., 1985), clomipramine (Langohr, Stohr, & Petruch, 1982; Tiegno et al., 1987), and doxepin (Hammeroff et al., 1982).

The heterocyclic and noncyclic antidepressant drugs—such as trazodone, mianserin, maprotiline, and the newer specific serotonin reuptake inhibitors (SSRIs), fluoxetine and paroxetine—may also be useful as adjuvant analgesics for chronic pain syndromes (Davidoff, Guarracini, Roth, Silva, & Yarkong, 1987; Breitbart, 1992; Spiegel et al., 1983; Costa, Mogos, & Toma, 1985; Eberhard et al., 1988; Watson et al., 1992; Feighner, 1985; Hynes et al., 1985; Max, 1992; Ventafridda et al., 1987; Sindrup et al., 1990). Fluoxetine, a potent antidepressant with specific serotonin reuptake inhibition activity (Feighner, 1985), has been shown to have analgesic properties in experimental animal pain models (Hynes et al., 1985) but failed to show analgesic effects in a clinical trial for neuropathy (Max, 1992). Several case reports suggest fluoxetine may be a useful adjuvant analgesic in the management of headache (Diamond & Frietag, 1989) and fibrositis (Geller, 1989). Paroxetine, a newer SSRI, is the first antidepressant of this class shown to be a highly effective analgesic in a controlled trial for the treatment of diabetic neuropathy (Sindrup et al., 1990). Newer antidepressants such as sertraline, venlafaxine, and nefazodone may also eventually prove to be clinically useful as adjuvant analgesics. Nefazodone, for instance, has been demonstrated to potentiate opioid analgesics in an animal model (Pick, Paul, Eison, & Pasternak, 1992).

Given the diversity of clinical syndromes in which the antidepressants have been demonstrated to be analgesic, trials of these drugs can be justified in the treatment of virtually every type of chronic pain (Portenoy, 1998). The established benefit of several of the antidepressants in patients with neuropathic pains (Max et al., 1997; Max, Sindrup et al., 1990), however, suggests that these drugs may be particularly useful in populations, such as cancer and AIDS patients, in which an underlying neuropathic component to the pain(s) often exists (Portenoy, 1998). Although studies of the analgesic efficacy of these drugs in HIV-related painful neuropathies have not yet been conducted, the drugs are widely applied clinically, using the model of diabetic and postherpetic neuropathies.

Although antidepressant drugs are analgesic in both neuropathic and nonneuropathic pain models, their clinical use is most commonly in combination with opioid drugs, particularly for moderate to severe pain. Antidepressant adjuvant analgesics have their most broad application as "coanalgesics," potentiating the analgesic effects of opioid drugs (Jacox et al., 1994). The "opioid sparing" effects of antidepressant analgesics has been demonstrated in a number of trials, especially in cancer populations with neuropathic, as well as nonneuropathic, pain syndromes (Walsh, 1986; Ventafridda et al., 1987).

The dose and time course of onset of analgesia for antidepressants when used as analgesics appears to be similar to their use as antidepressants. There is compelling evidence that the therapeutic analgesic effects of amitriptyline are correlated with serum levels, as are the antidepressant effects, and that analgesic treatment failure is due to low serum levels (Max et al., 1987). A high-dose regimen of up to 150 mg of amitriptyline or higher is suggested (Max et al., 1987). The proper analgesic dose for paroxetine is likely in the 40–60 mg range, with the major analgesic trial utilizing a fixed dose of 40 mg (Sindrup et al., 1990). There is anecdotal evidence to suggest that the debilitated medically ill (cancer, AIDS patients) often respond (re: depression or pain) to lower doses of antidepressant than are usually required in the physically healthy, probably because of impaired metabolism of these drugs (Breitbart, 1992). As to the time course of onset of analgesia, a biphasic process appears to occur. There are immediate or early analgesic effects that occur within hours or days, and these are probably mediated through inhibition of synaptic reuptake of catecholamines. In addition, there are later, longer analgesic effects that peak over a

2- to 4-week period that are probably due to receptor effects of the antidepressants (Pilowsky et al., 1982; Max et al., 1987).

Neuroleptics and Benzodiazepines

Neuroleptic drugs, such as methotrimeprazine, fluphenazine, haloperidol, and pimozide, may play a role as adjuvant analgesics (Beaver et al., 1966; Gomez-Perez et al., 1985; Maltbie et al., 1979; Lechin et al., 1989) in AIDS patients with pain; however, their use must be weighed against what appears to be an increased sensitivity to the extrapyramidal side effects of these drugs in AIDS patients with neurological complications (Breitbart, Marotta, & Call, 1988). Anxiolytics, such as alprazolam and clonazepam, may also be useful as adjuvant analgesics, particularly in the management of neuropathic pains (Fernandez & Levy, 1990; Swerdlow & Cundhill, 1981; Caccia, 1975).

Psychostimulants

Psychostimulants, such as dextroamphetamine, methylphenidate, and pemoline, may be useful antidepressants in patients with HIV infection or AIDS who are cognitively impaired (Fernandez & Levy, 1990; Bruera et al., 1987). Psychostimulants also enhance the analgesic effects of the opioid drugs (Bruera et al., 1989). Psychostimulants are also useful in diminishing sedation secondary to narcotic analgesics, and they are potent adjuvant analgesics. Bruera et al. (1987) demonstrated that a regimen of 10 mg methylphenidate with breakfast and 5 mg with lunch significantly decreased sedation and potentiated the effect of narcotics in patients with cancer pain. Methylphenidate has also been demonstrated to improve functioning on a number of neuropsychological tests, including tests of memory, speed, and concentration, in patients receiving continuous infusions of opioids for cancer pain (Bruera et al., 1987). Dextroamphetamine has also been reported to have additive analgesic effects when used with morphine in postoperative pain (Forrest, 1977). In relatively low doses, psychostimulants stimulate appetite, promote a sense of well-being, and improve feelings of weakness and fatigue in cancer patients.

Pemoline is a unique alternative psychostimulant that is chemically unrelated to amphetamine but may have similar usefulness as an antidepressant and adjuvant analgesic in AIDS patients (Breitbart & Mermelstein, 1992). Advantages of pemoline as a psychostimulant in AIDS pain patients include the lack of abuse potential, the lack of federal regulation through special triplicate prescriptions, the mild sympathomimetic effects, and the fact that it comes in a chewable tablet form that can be absorbed through the buccal mucosa and thus can be used by AIDS patients who have difficulty swallowing or who have intestinal obstruction. Clinically, pemoline is as effective as methylphenidate or dextroamphetamine in the treatment of depressive symptoms and in countering the sedating effects of opioid analgesics. There are no studies of pemoline's capacity to potentiate the analgesic properties of opioids. Pemoline should be used with caution in patients with liver impairment, and liver function tests should be monitored periodically with longer term treatment.

Anticonvulsants

Selected anticonvulsant drugs appear to be analgesic for the lancinating dysesthesias that characterize diverse types of neuropathic pain (Portenoy, 1998). Clinical experience also supports the use of these agents in patients with paroxysmal neuropathic pains that may not be lancinating and, to a far lesser extent, in those with neuropathic pains characterized solely by continuous dysesthesias. Although most practitioners prefer to begin with carbamazepine because of the extraordinarily good response rate observed in trigeminal neuralgia, this drug must be used cautiously in AIDS patients with thrombocytopenia, those at risk for marrow failure, and those whose blood counts must be monitored to determine disease status. If carbamazepine is used, a complete blood count should be obtained prior to the start of therapy, after 2 and 4 weeks, and then every 3-4 months thereafter. A leukocyte count below 4,000 is usually considered to be a contraindication to treatment, and a decline to less than 3,000, or an absolute neutrophil count of less than 1,500 during therapy, should prompt discontinuation of the drug. Other anticonvulsant drugs may be useful for managing neuropathic pain in AIDS patients, including phenytoin, clonazepam, valproate, and gabapentin (Portenoy, 1998).

Several newer anticonvulsants have been used in the treatment of neuropathic pain, particularly in patients with reflex sympathetic dystrophy. These drugs include gabapentin, lamotrigine, and felbamate. Of these newer anticonvulsants, anecdotal experience has been most favorable with gabapentin, which is now being widely used by pain specialists to treat neuropathic pain of various types. Gabapentin has a relatively high degree of safety, with no known drug–drug interactions and a lack of hepatic metabolism (Portenoy, 1998). Treatment with gabapentin is usually initiated at a dose of 300 mg/day and then gradually increased to a dose range of 900–3,200 mg/day in three divided doses.

Corticosteroids

Corticosteroid drugs have analgesic potential in a variety of chronic pain syndromes, including neuropathic pains and pain syndromes resulting from inflammatory processes (Portenoy, 1998). Like other adjuvant analgesics, corticosteroids are usually added to an opioid regimen. In patients with advanced disease, these drugs may also improve appetite, nausea, malaise, and overall quality of life. Adverse effects include neuropsychiatric syndromes, gastrointestinal disturbances, and immunosuppression.

Baclofen

Baclofen is a GABA-agonist that has proven efficacy in the treatment of trigeminal neuralgia (Fromm, 1989). On this basis, a trial of this drug is commonly employed in the management of paroxysmal neuropathic pains of any type. Dosing is generally undertaken in a manner similar to the use of the drug for its primary indication, spasticity. A starting dose of 5 mg two to three times per day is gradually escalated to 30–90 mg/day and sometimes higher if side effects do not occur. The most common adverse effects are sedation and confusion.

Oral Local Anesthetics

Local anesthetic drugs may be useful in the management of neuropathic pains characterized by either continuous or lancinating dysesthesias. Controlled trials have demonstrated the efficacy of tocainide (Lindstrom & Lindblom, 1987) and mexiletine (Chabal, Jacobson, Madano, Chaney, & Ballell, 1992), and there is clinical evidence that suggests similar effects from flecainide (Dunlop, Davies, Hockley, & Turner, 1989) and subcutaneous lidocaine (Brose & Cousins, 1991). It is reasonable to undertake a trial with oral local anesthetic in patients with continuous dysesthesias who fail to respond adequately to, or who cannot tolerate, the tricyclic antidepressants and with patients with lancinating pains

refractory to trials of anticonvulsant drugs and baclofen. Mexiletine is preferred in the United States (Portenoy, 1998).

Psychological Interventions

A variety of physical and psychological therapies may also prove useful in the management of HIV-related pain. Physical interventions range from bed rest and simple exercise programs to the application of cold packs or heat to affected sites. Other nonpharmacologic interventions include whirlpool baths, massage, the application of ultrasound, and transcutaneous electrical nerve stimulation (TENS). Increasing numbers of AIDS patients have resorted to acupuncture to relieve their pain, with anecdotal reports of efficacy.

Several psychological interventions have demonstrated potential efficacy in alleviating HIV-related pain, including hypnosis, relaxation, distraction techniques such as biofeedback and imagery, and cognitive-behavioral techniques. They are often utilized in an interdisciplinary pain-management program. Because anxiety/stress and pain perception are closely related, these psychological interventions may have a significant impact on the pain process indirectly through reducing anxiety/stress rather than through any pathophysiology per se. Of course, future research is needed to delineate such anxiety/stress–pain cycle issues more carefully. Where nonpharmacological and standard pharmacological treatments fail, anesthetic and even neurosurgical procedures (such as nerve block, cordotomy, and epidural delivery of analgesics) are additional options available to the patient who appreciates the risks and limitations of these procedures.

It should also be noted that, as part of interdisciplinary pain management, programs for education and counseling, as well as support groups focusing on the management of grief, depression, anger, feelings of helplessness, and other related issues, are often administered to patients. Many such programs have been developed (e.g., Morokoff, Holmes-Johnson, & Weiss, 1987). Such programs again act to defuse some of the anxiety and stress that can significantly affect the threshold or experience of pain.

Finally, psychological impairment and emotional complications of AIDS patients are often exacerbated by the experience of chronic pain. These issues, as well as the common problems of substance abuse (discussed in a subsequent section of this chapter), need to be addressed within the context of an interdisciplinary program.

UNDERTREATMENT OF PAIN IN AIDS

Reports of dramatic undertreatment of pain in AIDS patients have appeared in the literature (Lebovits et al., 1989; McCormack et al., 1993; Breitbart, Rosenfeld, et al. 1996; Larue et al., 1997). These studies suggest that all classes of analgesics, particularly opioid analgesics, are underutilized in the treatment of pain in AIDS. Our group has reported (Breitbart, McDonald, et al., 1996) that less than 8% of individuals in our cohort of ambulatory AIDS patients reporting pain in the severe range (8–10 on a numerical rating scale of pain intensity) received a strong opioid, such as morphine, as recommended by published guidelines (i.e., the WHO analgesic ladder). In addition, 18% of patients with "severe" pain were prescribed no analgesics whatsoever, 40% were prescribed a nonopioid analgesic (e.g., NSAID), and only 22% were prescribed a "weak" opioid (e.g., acetaminophen in combination with oxycodone). Utilizing the Pain Management Index (PMI; Zelman, Cleeland, & Howland, 1987), a measure of adequacy of analgesic therapy derived from the Brief Pain Inventory's record of pain intensity and strength of analgesia prescribed, we further examined adequacy of pain treatment. Only 15% of our sample received adequate analgesic therapy based on the PMI. This degree of undermedication of pain in AIDS (85%) far exceeds published reports of undermedication of pain (using the PMI) in cancer populations of 40% (Cleeland et al., 1994). Larue and colleagues (1997) report that in France, 57% of patients with HIV disease reporting moderate to severe pain did not receive any analgesic treatment at all, and only 22% received a "weak" opioid.

Although opioid analgesics are underutilized, it is clear that adjuvant analgesic agents, such as the antidepressants, are also dramatically underused (Breitbart, Rosenfeld, et al., 1996; Larue et al., 1997; McCormack et al., 1993; Lebovits et al., 1989). Breitbart, Rosenfeld, and colleagues (1996) report that less than 10% of AIDS patients reporting pain received an adjuvant analgesic drug (e.g., antidepressants, anticonvulsants) despite the fact that approximately 40% of the sample had neuropathic-type pain. This class of analgesic agents is a critical component of the WHO analgesic lad-

der, particularly in managing neuropathic pain, and is vastly underutilized in the management of HIV-related pain.

BARRIERS TO PAIN MANAGEMENT IN AIDS

A number of different factors have been proposed as potential influences on the widespread undertreatment of pain in AIDS, including patient-, clinician-, and health care system-related barriers (Breitbart, Rosenfeld, et al., 1996; Passik et al., 1994; Breitbart et al., 1998; Breitbart, Rosenfeld, & Kaim, in press). Sociodemographic factors that have been reported to be associated with undertreatment of pain in AIDS include gender, education, and substance abuse history (Breitbart, McDonald, et al., 1996). Women, less educated patients, and patients who reported injection drug use as their HIV risk transmission factor are significantly more likely to receive inadequate analgesic therapy for HIV-related pain.

Breitbart et al. (1998) surveyed 200 ambulatory AIDS patients utilizing a modified version of the Barriers Questionnaire (BQ; Ward et al., 1993), which assesses a variety of patient-related barriers to pain management (resulting in patient reluctance to report pain or take opioid analgesics). Results of this study demonstrated that patient-related barriers (as measured by BQ scores) were significantly correlated with undertreatment of pain (as measured by the PMI) in AIDS patients with pain. Additionally, BQ scores were significantly correlated with higher levels of psychological distress and depression, indicating that patient-related barriers contributed to undertreatment for pain and poorer quality of life. The most frequently endorsed BQ items were those concerning the addiction potential of opioids, side effects and discomfort related to opioid administration, and misconceptions about tolerance. Although there were no age, gender, or HIV risk transmission factor associations with BQ scores, nonwhite and less educated patients scored higher on the BQ. Several additional "AIDS specific" patient-related barriers examined (Passik et al, 1994; Breitbart et al., 1998) reveal that 66% of patients are trying to limit their overall intake of medications (i.e., pills) or utilize nonpharmacologic interventions for pain, 50% of patients cannot afford to fill a prescription for analgesics or have no access to pain specialists, and about 50% are reluctant to take opioids for pain out of a concern that family, friends, or physicians will assume they are misusing or abusing these drugs.

In a survey of approximately 500 AIDS care providers (Breitbart et al., in press), clinicians (primarily physicians and nurses) rated the barriers to AIDS pain management they perceived to be the most important in the care of AIDS patients. The most frequently endorsed barriers were those regarding lack of knowledge about pain management or access to pain specialists and concerns regarding the use and addiction potential of opioid drugs in the AIDS population. The top five barriers endorsed by AIDS clinicians included lack of knowledge regarding pain management (51.8%); reluctance to prescribe opioids (51.5%); lack of access to pain specialists (50.9%); concern regarding drug addiction and/or abuse (50.5%); and lack of psychological support or drug treatment services (43%). Patient reluctance to report pain and to take opioids were less commonly endorsed barriers, with about 24% of respondents endorsing those barriers. In contrast, past surveys of oncologists (Von Roenn, Cleeland, Gonin, Hatfield, & Pandya, 1993) rated patient reluctance to report pain or take opioids as two of the top four barriers. Like AIDS care providers, oncologists also highly endorsed a reluctance to prescribe opioids, even to a population of cancer patients with a significantly lower prevalence of past or present substance abuse disorders. Both oncologists and AIDS care providers report that they have inadequate knowledge of pain management and pain assessment skills.

Pain Management and Substance Abuse in AIDS

Individuals who inject drugs are among the AIDS exposure categories with the highest rate of increase over the past 5 years, especially in large urban centers. Pain management in the substance-abusing AIDS patient is perhaps the most challenging of clinical goals. Fears of addiction and concerns regarding drug abuse affect patient compliance, physician management of pain, and use of narcotic analgesics, often leading to the undermedication of HIV-infected patients with pain. Of course, this is an important issue in the treatment of chronic pain patients in general; it is not specific only to AIDS patients. Interdisciplinary pain-management programs have been developed to take into account such substance abuse problems and their psychosocial sequelae. Detoxification efforts and the "weaning" of psychological dependence always

need to be considered whenever treating a chronic pain patient.

Studies of patterns of chronic narcotic analgesic use in patients with cancer, burns, and postoperative pain, however, have demonstrated that, although tolerance and physical dependence commonly occur, addiction, that is, psychological dependence and drug abuse, are rare and almost never occur in individuals who do not have histories of drug abuse (Kanner & Foley, 1981; Porter & Jick, 1980; Perry & Heidrich, 1982). More relevant to the clinical problem of pain management in AIDS patients, however, is the issue of managing pain in the growing segment of HIV-infected patients who have a history of substance abuse or who are actively abusing drugs. The use of opioids specifically for pain control in patients with HIV infection and a history of substance abuse raises several difficult pain treatment questions, including how to treat pain in people who have a high tolerance to narcotic analgesics; how to mitigate this population's drug-seeking and potentially manipulative behavior; how to deal with patients who may offer unreliable medical histories or who may not comply with treatment recommendations; and how to counter the risk of patients spreading HIV while high and disinhibited.

Perhaps of greatest concern to clinicians is the possibility that they are being lied to by a substance-abusing AIDS patient complaining of pain. Clinicians must rely on a patient's subjective report, which is often the best or only indication of the presence and intensity of pain, as well as the degree of pain relief achieved by an intervention. Physicians who believe they are being manipulated by drug-seeking patients often hesitate to use appropriately high doses of narcotic analgesics to control pain. The fear is that the clinician is being "duped" into prescribing narcotic analgesics, which will then be abused or sold. Clinicians do not want to contribute to or help sustain addiction. This leads to an immediate defensiveness on the part of the clinician and an impulse to avoid prescribing opioids and even to avoid full assessment of a pain complaint. Because concerns are often raised regarding the credibility of AIDS patients' reports of pain, particularly where there is a history of injection drug use, Breitbart and colleagues (1997) conducted a study of 516 ambulatory AIDS patients, in which they compared the report of pain experience and the adequacy of pain management among patients with and without a history of substance abuse. This study found that there were no significant differences in the report of pain experience (i.e., pain prevalence, pain intensity, and pain-related functional interference) among patients who reported injection drug use (IDU) as their HIV transmission risk factor and those who reported other transmission factors (non-IDU). Furthermore, there were no differences in the report of pain experience among patients who acknowledged current substance abuse, those in methadone maintenance, and those who were in drug-free recovery. The description of HIV-related pain was comparable among IDU and non-IDU groups. What was different was the treatment received by these two groups. Patients in the IDU group were significantly more undermedicated for pain compared to the non-IDU grou.

Unfortunately, the existence or severity of pain cannot be objectively proven. The clinician must accept and respect the report of pain in spite of the possibility of being duped and proceed in the evaluation, assessment, and management of pain. Experience from the cancer pain literature suggests that it is possible to adequately manage pain in substance abusers with life-threatening illness and to do so safely and responsibly, utilizing opioid analgesics and several sound principles of pain management outlined here (Table 20.6; Macaluso, Weinberg, & Foley, 1988; McCaffery & Vourakis,

---

TABLE 20.6. An Approach to Pain Management in Substance Abusers with HIV Disease

1. Substance abusers with HIV disease deserve pain control; we have an obligation to treat pain and suffering in all of our patients.

2. Accept and respect the report of pain.

3. Be careful about the label "substance abuse"; distinguish between tolerance, physical dependence, and "addiction" (psychological dependence or drug abuse).

4. Not all "substance abusers" are the same; distinguish between active users, individuals in methadone maintenance, and those in recovery.

5. Individualize pain treatment.

6. Utilize the principles of pain management outlined for all patients with HIV disease and pain (WHO ladder).

7. Set clear goals and conditions for opioid therapy: set limits, recognize drug abuse behaviors, make consequences clear, use written contracts, establish a single prescriber.

8. Use a multidimensional approach: pharmacological and nonpharmacological interventions, attention to psychosocial issues, team approach.

1992; Portenoy & Payne, 1992; American Pain Society, 1992). Most clinicians experienced in working with this population of patients recommend that practitioners set clear and direct limits. Although this is an important aspect of the care of IV-drug-using people with HIV disease, it is by no means the whole answer. As much as possible, clinicians should attempt to eliminate the issue of drug abuse as an obstacle to pain management by dealing directly with the problems of opiate withdrawal and drug treatment. Clinicians should err on the side of believing patients when they complain of pain and should utilize knowledge of specific HIV-related pain syndromes to corroborate the report of a patient perceived as being unreliable.

The clinician must be familiar with and understand the current terminology relevant to substance abuse and addiction. It is important to distinguish between the terms "tolerance," "physical dependence," and "addiction" or "abuse" (psychological dependence). Tolerance is a pharmacological property of opioid drugs defined by the need for increasing doses to maintain an (analgesic) effect. Physical dependence is characterized by the onset of signs and symptoms of withdrawal if narcotic analgesics are abruptly stopped or a narcotic antagonist is administered. Tolerance usually occurs in association with physical dependence. Addiction or abuse (also often termed psychological dependence) is a psychological and behavioral syndrome in which there is drug craving, compulsive use (despite physical, psychological, or social harm to user), other aberrant drug-related behaviors, and relapse after abstinence (American Pain Society, 1992). The term "pseudoaddiction" has been coined to describe the patient who exhibits behavior that clinicians associate with addiction, such as requests for higher doses of opioid, but that is in fact due to uncontrolled pain and inadequate pain management (Weissman & Haddox, 1989).

The clinician must also distinguish between the "former" addict who has been drug-free for years, the addict in a methadone maintenance program, and the addict who is actively abusing illicit and/or prescription drugs. Addicts who are actively using and those on methadone maintenance who have pain must be assumed to have some tolerance to opioids, they may require higher starting and maintenance doses of opioids. Preventing withdrawal is an essential first step in managing pain in this population. In addition, "active" addicts with AIDS will understandably require more in the way of psychosocial support and services to adequately deal with the distress of their pain and illness. Former addicts may pose the challenge of refusing opioids for pain because of fears of relapse. Such patients can be assured that opioids, when prescribed and monitored responsibly, may be an essential part of pain management and that the use of the drug for pain is quite different from the abuse of similar drugs. Some authorities emphasize the importance of conducting a comprehensive pain assessment in order to define the pain syndrome. Specific pain syndromes often respond best to specific interventions (i.e., neuropathic pains respond well to antidepressants or anticonvulsants). Adequate assessment of the cause of pain is essential in all AIDS patients, particularly in the substance abuser. It is critical that adequate analgesia be provided while diagnostic studies are underway. Often treatments directed at the underlying disorder causing pain are very effective as well. For example, headache from CNS toxoplasmosis responds well to primary treatments and steroids.

When deciding on an appropriate pharmacological intervention in the substance abuser, it is advisable to follow the WHO analgesic ladder. This approach advocates selection of analgesics based on severity of pain; however, clinicians also often take into account the nature of the pain syndrome in selecting analgesics. For mild to moderate pain, NSAIDs are indicated. The NSAIDs are continued with adjuvant analgesics (antidepressants, anticonvulsants, neuroleptics, steroids) if a specific indication exists. Patients with moderate to severe pain or those who do not achieve relief from NSAIDs are treated with a "weak" opioid, often in combination with NSAIDs and adjuvant drugs, if indicated.

It has been pointed out that it is critical to apply appropriate pharmacological principles to opioid use. One should avoid using agonist–antagonist opioid drugs. The use of PRN dosing often leads to excessive drug-centered interactions with staff that are not productive. Although patients should not necessarily be given the specific drug or route they want, every effort should be made to give patients more of a sense of control and a sense of collaboration with the clinician. Often a patient's report of beneficial or adverse effects of a specific agent are useful to the clinician.

The management of pain in substance-abusing AIDS patients requires a team approach. Again, an interdisciplinary pain-management approach is needed. Early involvement of pain specialists, psychologists, and substance abuse specialists is critical. Nonpharmacological pain interventions should be appropriately applied, not as a substitute for opioids but as an important adjunct. Realistic goals for treatment must be set, and problems related to inappropriate behavior relating to the handling of prescription and interactions with staff should be anticipated. Hospital staff must be educated and made aware that such difficult patients evoke feelings that if acted on could interfere with providing good care. Clear limit setting is helpful for both the patient and treating staff. Sometimes written rules about what behaviors are expected and what behaviors are not tolerated, along with the consequences of those behaviors, should be provided. The use of urine toxicology monitoring, restricting visitors, and placing strict limits on amount of drug per prescription can all be very useful. It is important also to remember that rehabilitation or detoxification from opioids is not appropriate during an acute medical crisis and should not be attempted at that time. Once more stable medical conditions exist, referral to a drug rehabilitation program may be very useful. Constant assessment and reevaluation of the effects of pain interventions must also take place in order to optimize care. Special attention should be given to points in treatment at which routes of administration are changed or at which opioids are being tapered. It must be made clear to patients what drugs and/or regimen would be introduced to control pain when opioids are tapered or withdrawn and what options are available if that nonopioid regimen is ineffective.

Finally, it is important to recognize that substance abusers with AIDS are quite likely to have comorbid psychiatric symptoms, as well as multiple other physical symptoms that can all contribute to increased pain and suffering. Adequate attention must be paid to these physical and psychological symptoms for pain management to be optimized.

SUMMARY

Pain in AIDS, even in this era of protease inhibitors and decreased AIDS death rates, is a clinically significant problem contributing greatly to psychological and functional morbidity. Pain can be adequately treated, and so it must be a focus of care in the AIDS patient. Indeed, a major contribution of psychology has been the development of effective interdisciplinary pain-management programs for these patients experiencing chronic pain. A major future goal is to make AIDS patients more aware of the existence and the potential efficacy of pain reduction of such interdisciplinary pain-management programs. Substance abusers and women are particularly undertreated segments of the AIDS pain population and need special attention. Managing pain in AIDS patients with a history of substance abuse is a particularly challenging problem that AIDS care providers will be facing with increasing frequency. Again, interdisciplinary pain-management programs have a strong psychological component that can deal with such significant psychiatric and psychosocial issues.

ACKNOWLEDGMENTS

This work is supported by National Institute of Mental Health Grant No. MH49034, National Cancer Institute Grant No. CA57790, the Faculty Scholars Program, Open Society Institute, Project on Death in America, and the Emily Davie and Joseph S. Kornfeld Foundation.

REFERENCES

Anand, A., Carmosino, L., & Glatt, A. E. (1994). Evaluation of recalcitrant pain in HIV-infected hospitalized patients. *Journal of Acquired Immune Deficiency Syndromes, 7,* 52–56.

American Pain Society. (1992). *Principles of analgesic use in the treatment of acute pain and cancer pain* (3rd ed.). Skokie, IL: American Pain Society.

Balthazar, B. J., Reich, C. B., & Pachter, H. L. (1986). The significance of small bowel intussusception in acquired immune deficiency syndrome. *American Journal of Gastroenterology,* (Suppl. 1), 1073–1075.

Barone, S. E., Gunold, B. S., Nealson, T. F., & Arvanitis, M. L. (1986). Abdominal pain in patients with acquired immune deficiency syndrome. *Annals of Surgery, 204,* 619–623.

Beaver, W. T., Wallerstein, S. L., Houde, R. W., et al. (1966). A comparison of the analgesic effect of methotrimeprazine and morphine in patients with cancer. *Clinical Pharmacological Therapy, 7,* 436–466.

Berman, A., Espinoza, L. R., Diaz, J. D., Aguilar, J. L., & Rolando, T. (1988). Rheumatic manifestations of human immunodeficiency virus infection. *American Journal of Medicine, 89,* 59–64.

Bessen, I. J., Greene, J. B., Louie, E., Sietzman, P., & Weinberg, H. (1988). Severe polymyositis-like syndrome associated with zidovudine therapy of AIDS and ARC. *New England Journal of Medicine, 318,* 708.

Bonacini, M. (1992). Hepatobiliary complications in patients with human immunodeficiency virus infection. *American Journal of Medicine, 92,* 404–411.

Bonacini, M., Young, T., & Laine, L. (1991). The causes of esophageal symptoms in human immunodeficiency virus infection. *Archives of Internal Medicine, 151,* 1567–1572.

Botney, M., & Fields, H. C. (1983). Amitriptyline potentiates morphine analgesia by direct action on the central nervous system. *Annals of Neurology, 13,* 160–164.

Breitbart, W. (1989). Psychiatric management of cancer pain. *Cancer, 63,* 2336–2342.

Breitbart, W. (1990). Psychiatric aspects of pain and HIV disease. *Focus: A Guide to AIDS Research and Counseling, 5*(9), 1–3.

Breitbart, W. (1992). Psychotropic adjuvant analgesics for cancer pain. *Psychooncology, 7,* 133–145.

Breitbart, W. (1993). Suicide risk and pain in cancer and AIDS patients. In R. Chapman & K. M. Foley (Eds.), *Current emerging issues in cancer pain: Research and practice* (pp. 49–65). New York: Raven Press.

Breitbart, W. (1996). Pharmacotherapy of pain in AIDS. In G. Wormser (Ed.), *A clinical guide to AIDS and HIV* (pp. 359–378). Philadelphia: Lippincott-Raven.

Breitbart, W. (1997). Pain in AIDS. In J. Jensen, J. Turner, & Z. Wiesenfeld-Hallin (Eds.), *Proceedings of the Eighth World Congress on Pain: Vol. 8. Progress in pain research and management* (pp. 63–100). Seattle, WA: IASP Press.

Breitbart, W., Marotta, R. F., & Call, P. (1988). AIDS and neuroleptic malignant syndrome. *Lancet, 2,* 1488.

Breitbart, W., McDonald, M., Rosenfeld, B., Passik, S., Calle, J., Thaler, H., & Portenoy, H. (1995). Pain in women with AIDS [Abstract No. 95739]. *Proceedings of the 14th Annual Meeting of the American Pain Society,* Los Angeles, CA.

Breitbart, W., McDonald, M. V., Rosenfeld, B., Passik, S. D., Hewitt, D., Thaler, H., Portenoy, R. K. (1996). Pain in ambulatory AIDS patients: I. Pain characteristics and medical correlates. *Pain, 68,* 315–321.

Breitbart, W., & Mermelstein H. (1992). Pemoline: An alternative psychostimulant in the management of depressive disorder in cancer patients. *Psychosomatics, 33,* 352–356.

Breitbart, W., Passik, S., Bronaugh, T., et al. (1991, October). Pain in the ambulatory AIDS patient: Prevalence and psychosocial correlates. Abstract presented at the annual meeting of the Academy of Psychosomatic Medicine, Atlanta, Georgia.

Breitbart, W., Passik, S., McDonald, M., Rosenfeld, B., Smith, M., Kaim, M., & Funesti-Esch, J. (1998). Patient-related barriers to pain management in ambulatory AIDS patients. *Pain, 76,* 9–16.

Breitbart, W., Rosenfeld, B., & Kaim, M. (in press). Clinician-related barriers to pain management in AIDS. *Journal of Pain and Symptom Management.*

Breitbart, W., Rosenfeld, B., Passik, S., Kaim, M., Funesti-Esch, J., & Stein, K. (1997). A comparison of pain report and adequacy of analgesic therapy in ambulatory AIDS patients with and without a history of substance abuse. *Pain, 72,* 235–243.

Breitbart, W., Rosenfeld, B., Passik, S., McDonald, M., Thaler, H., & Portenoy, R. (1996). The undertreatment of pain in ambulatory AIDS patients. *Pain, 65,* 239–245.

Brose, W. G., & Cousins, M. J. (1991). Subcutaneous lidocaine for treatment of neuropathic cancer pain. *Pain, 45*(2), 145–148.

Bruera, E., Breuneis, C., Patterson, A. H., & MacDonald, R. N. (1989). Use of methylphenidate as an adjuvant to narcotic analgesics in patients with advanced cancer. *Journal of Pain and Symptom Management, 4,* 3–6.

Bruera, E., Chadwick, S., Brennels, C., Hanson, J., & MacDonald, R. N. (1987). Methylphenidate associated with narcotics for the treatment of cancer pain. *Cancer Treatment Reports, 71,* 67–70.

Butler, S. (1986). Present status of tricyclic antidepressants in chronic pain therapy. In C. Benedetti C. R. Chapman, & G. Moricco (Eds.), *Advances in pain research and therapy* (Vol. 7, pp. 173–196). New York: Raven Press.

Caccia, M. R. (1975). Clonazepam in facial neuralgia and cluster headache: Clinical and electrophysiological study. *European Journal of Neurology, 13,* 560–563.

Cello, J. P. (1989). Acquired immune deficiency cholangiopathy: Spectrum of disease. *American Journal of Medicine, 86,* 539–546.

Chabal, C., Jacobson, L., Madano, A., Chaney, E., & Ballell, A. V. (1992). The use of oral mexiletine for the treatment of pain after peripheral nerve injury. *Anesthesiology, 76*(4), 513–517.

Cleeland, C. S., Gonin, R., Hatfield, A. L., et al. (1994). Pain and its treatment in outpatients with metastic cancer: The Eastern Cooperative Group's outpatient study. *New England Journal of Medicine, 330,* 592–596.

Connolly, G. M., Hawkins, D., Harcourt-Webster, J. N., Parsons, P. A., Husain, O. A. N., & Gazzard, B. G. (1989). Oesophageal symptoms, their causes, treatment and prognosis in patients with the acquired immunodeficiency syndrome. *Gut, 30,* 1033–1039.

Cook, G. C. (1990). The mouth in human immunodeficiency virus (HIV) Infection. *Quarterly Journal of Medicine, 76,* 655–657.

Cornblath, D. R., & McArthur, I. C. (1988). Predominantly sensory neuropathy in patients with AIDS and AIDS-related complex. *Neurology, 38,* 794–796.

Costa, D., Mogos, I., & Toma, T. (1985). Efficacy and safety of mianserin in the treatment of depression of woman with cancer. *Acta Psychiatrica Scandinavia, 72,* 85–92.

Dalakas, M. C., & Pezeshkpour, G. A. (1988). Neuromuscular diseases associated with human immunodeficiency virus infection. *Annals of Neurology, 23*(Suppl.), S38–48.

Dalakas, M. C., Pezeshkpour, G. H., Gravell, M., & Sever, J. L. (1986). Polymyositis associated with AIDS retrovirus. *Journal of the American Medical Association, 256,* 2381–2383.

Davidoff, G., Guarracini, M., Roth, E., Sliwa, J., & Yarkony, G. (1987). Trazodone hydrochloride in the treatment of dysesthetic pain in traumatic myelopathy: A randomized, double-blind placebo-controlled study. *Pain, 29,* 151–161.

Davidson, T., Allen-Mersh, T. G., Miles, A. J. G., Gazzard, B., Wastell, C., et al. (1991). Emergency laparotomy in patients with AIDS. *British Journal of Surgery, 789,* 924–926.

de Silva, R., Stoopack, P. M., & Raufman, J. P. (1990). Esophageal fistulas associated with mycobacterial infection in patients at risk for AIDS. *Radiology, 175,* 449–453.

Devor, M. (1983). Nerve pathophysiology and mechanisms of pain in causalgia. *Journal of the Autonomic Nervous System, 7,* 371–384.

Diamond, S., & Frietag, F. G. (1989). The use of fluoxetine in the treatment of headache. *Clinical Journal of Pain, 5,* 200–201.

Dunlop, R., Davies, R. J., Hockley, J., & Turner, P. (1989). [Letter to the editor]. *Lancet, 1,* 420–421.

Eberhard, G., von Khorring, L., Nilsson, H. L., et al. (1988). A double-blind randomized study of clomimpramine versus maprotiline in patients with idiopathic pain syndromes. *Neuropsychobiology, 19,* 25–32.

Edwards, P., Turner, J., Gold, J., Cooper, D. A. (1990). Esophageal ulceration induced by zidovudine. *Annals of Internal Medicine, 112,* 65–66.

Eisner, M. S., & Smith, P. D. (1990). Etiology of odynophagia and dysphagia in patients with the acquired immunodeficiency syndrome. *Arthritis and Rheumatism, 33,* A446.

Espinoza, L. R., Berman, A., Vasey, F. B., Cahalin, C., Nelson, R., et al. (1988). Psoriatic arthritis and acquired immunodeficiency syndrome. *Arthritis and Rheumatism, 31,* 1034–1040.

Espinoza, L. R., Aguilar, J. L., Berman, A., Gutierrez, F., & Vasey, F. B. (1989). Rheumatic manifestations associated with human immunodeficiency virus infection. *Arthritis and Rheumatism, 32*(12), 1615–1622.

Feighner, J. P. (1985). A comparative trial of fluoxetine and amitriptyline in patients with major depressive disorder. *Journal of Clinical Psychiatry, 46,* 369–372.

Fernandez, F., & Levy, J. K. (1990). Psychiatric diagnosis and pharmacotherapy of patients with HIV infection. In A. Tasman, S. M. Goldfinger, & G. A. Kaufman (Eds.), *Review of psychiatry* (Vol. 9). Washington, DC: American Psychiatric Press.

Foley, K. M. (1985). The treatment of cancer pain. *New England Journal of Medicine, 313,* 84–95.

Foley, K. M., & Inturrisi, C. E. (1987). Analgesic drug therapy in cancer pain: Principles and practice. In R. Payne & K. M. Foley (Eds.), *Cancer pain medical clinics of North America* (pp. 207–232). Philadelphia: Saunders.

Forrest, H. (1977). Dextroamphetamine with morphine for the treatment of post-operative pain. *New England Journal of Medicine, 296,* 712–715.

Forster, S. M., Seifert, M. H., Keat, A. C., Rowe, I. F., Thomas, B. J., et al. (1988). Inflammatory joint disease and human immunodeficiency virus infection. *British Medical Journal, 296,* 1625–1627.

France R. D. (1987). The future for antidepressants: Treatment of pain. *Psychopathology, 20,* 99–113.

Friedman, S. I., Wright, T. L., & Altman, D. F. (1985). Gastrointestinal Kaposi's sarcoma in patients with acquired immunodeficiency syndrome. Endoscopic and autopsy findings. *Gastroenterology, 89,* 102–108.

Fromm, G. H. (1989). Trigeminal neuralgia and related disorders. In R. H. Portenoy (Ed.), *Pain: Mechanisms and syndromes: Vol. 7. Neurologic clinics* (pp. 305–319). Philadelphia: Saunders.

Fuller, G. N., Jacobs, J. M., & Guiloff, R. J. (1989). Association of painful peripheral neuropathy in AIDS with cytomegalovirus infection. *Lancet, 334,* 937–941.

Geller, S. A. (1989). Treatment of fibrositis with fluoxetine hydrochloride (Prozac). *American Journal of Medicine, 87,* 594–595.

Getto, C. J., Sorkness, C. A., & Howell, T. (1987). Antidepressant and chronic malignant pain: A review. *Journal of Pain Symptom Control, 2,* 9–18.

Goldstein, J. (1990). Headache and acquired immunodeficiency syndrome. *Neurology Clinics, 8,* 947–961.

Gomez-Perez, F. J., Riell, J. A., Dies, H., Rodriguez-Rivera, I. G., Gonzales-Barranco, J., & Lozano-Casteneda, O. (1985). Nortriptyline and fluphenazine in the symptomatic treatment of diabetic neuropathy: A double-blind cross-over study. *Pain, 23,* 395–400.

Goodman, P., Pinero, S. S., Rance, R. M., Mansell,

P. W. A., & Uribe-Botero, G. (1989). Mycobacterial oesophagitis in AIDS. *Gastrointestinal Radiology*, 14, 103–105.

Gorand, D. A., Henry, K., & Guiloff, R. J. (1988). Necrotising myopathy and zidovudine. *Lancet*, 331, 1050.

Gram, L. F. (1983). Receptors, pharmacokinetics and clinical effects. In G. D. Burrows, et al. (Eds.), *Antidepressants* (pp. 81–95). Amsterdam: Elsevier.

Griffin, J. W., Wesselingh, S. L., Griffin, D. E., Glass, J. D., & McArthur, J. C. (1994). Peripheral nerve disorders in HIV infection: Similarities and contrasts with CNS disorders. In R. W. Price & S. W. Perry (Eds.), *HIV, AIDS and the brain* (pp. 159–182). New York: Raven Press.

Hammeroff, S. R., Cork, R. C., Scherer, K., et al. (1982). Doxepin effects on chronic pain, depression and plasma opioids. *Journal of Clinical Psychiatry*, 2, 22–26.

Hewitt, D., McDonald, M., Portenoy, R., Rosenfeld, B., Passik, S., & Breitbart W. (1997). Pain syndromes and etiologies in ambulatory AIDS patients. *Pain*, 70, 117–123.

Hynes, M. D., Lochner, M. A., Bemis, K., et al. (1985). Fluoxetine, a selective inhibitor of serotonin uptake, potentiates morphine analgesia without altering its discriminative stimulus properties or affinity for opioid receptors. *Life Sciences*, 36, 2317–2323.

Jacox, A., Carr, D., Payne, R., Berde, C. B., Breitbart, W., Cain, J. M., Chapman, C. R., Cleeland, C. S., Ferrell, B. R., Finley, R. S., Hester, N. O., Stratton Hill, J. R. C., Leath, W. D., Lipman, A. G., Logan, C. L., McGarvey, C. L., Miastrowsky, C. A., Mulder, D. S., Paice, J. A., Shapiro, B. S., Silberstein, E. B., Smith, R. S., Stover, J., Tsou, C. V., Vecchiarelli, L., & Weissman, D. E. (1994). *Clinical Practice Guideline Number 9: Management of cancer pain* (AHCPR Publication No. 94–0592). Washington, DC: U. S. Department of Health and Human Services, Agency for Health Care Policy and Research.

Johnson, T. M., Duvic, M., Rapini, R. P., & Rios, A. (1986). AIDS exacerbates psoriasis. *New England Journal of Medicine*, 313, 1415.

Kaiko, R., Foley, K., Grabinski, P., Wallenstein, S. L., Rogers, A. C., & Houde, R. W. (1983). Central nervous system excitation effects of meperidine in cancer patients. *Annals of Neurology*, 13, 180–183.

Kanner, R. M., & Foley, K. M. (1981). Patterns of narcotic use in a cancer pain clinic. *Annals of the New York Academy of Science*, 362, 161–172.

Kaplan, R., Conant, M., Cundiff, D., Maciewicz, R., Ries, K., Slagle, S., Slywka, J., & Buckley, B. (1996). Sustained-release morphine sulfate in the management of pain associated with acquired immune deficiency syndrome. *Journal of Pain and Symptom Management*, 12, 150–160.

Kaye, B. R. (1989). Rheumatologic manifestations of infection with human immunodeficiency virus. *Annals of Internal Medicine*, 111, 158–167.

Kazlow, P. G., Shah, K., Benkov, K. J., Dische, R., & LeLeiko, N. S. (1986). Esophageal cryptosporidiosis in a child with acquired immune deficiency. *Gastroenterology*, 91, 1301–1303.

Kimball, L. R., & McCormick, W. C. (1996). The pharmacologic management of pain and discomfort in persons with AIDS near the end of life: Use of opioid analgesia in the hospice setting. *Journal of Pain and Symptom Management*, 11, 88–94.

Kishore-Kumar, R., Max, M. B., Scafer, S. C., et al. (1990). Desipramine relieves post-herpetic neuralgia. *Clinical Pharmacological Therapy*, 47, 305–312.

Kitchen, V. S., Helbert, M., Francis, N. D., et al. (1990). Epstein-Barr virus associated oesphageal ulcers in AIDS. *Gut*, 31, 1223–1225.

Lange, D. J., Britton, C. B., Younger, D. S., & Hays, A. P. (1988). The neuromuscular manifestations of human immunodeficiency virus infections. *Archives of Neurology*, 45, 1084–1088.

Langohr, H. D., Stohr, M., & Petruch, F. (1982). An open and double-blind crossover study on the efficacy of clonipramine (anafranil) in patients with painful mono- and polyneuropathies. *European Journal of Neurology*, 21, 309–315.

Larue, F., Brasseur, L., Musseault, P., Demeulemeester, R., Bonifassi, L., & Bez, G. (1994). Pain and HIV infection: A French national survey [Abstract]. *Journal of Palliative Care*, 10, 95.

Larue, F., Fontaine, A., & Colleau, S. (1997). Underestimation and undertreatment of pain in HIV disease: Multicentre study. *British Medical Journal*, 314, 23–28.

Lebovits, A. K., Lefkowitz, M., & McCarthy, D., et al. (1989). The prevalence and management of pain in patients with AIDS. A review of 134 cases. *Clinical Journal of Pain*, 5, 245–248.

Lechin, F., Vander Dijs, B., Lechin, M. E., et al. (1989). Pimozide therapy for trigeminal neuralgia. *Archives of Neurology*, 9, 960–964.

Ledford, D. K., Overman, M. D., Gonzalvo, A., Cali, A., Mester, S. W., et al. (1985). Microsporidiosis myositis in a patient with the acquired immunodeficiency syndrome. *Annals of Internal Medicine*, 102, 628–630.

Lefkowitz, M., & Breitbart, W. (1992). Chronic pain and AIDS. In R. H. Wiener (Ed.), *Innovations in pain medicine* (pp. 36-1–36-18). Orlando, FL: Paul Deutsch Press.

Lefkowitz, M., & Newshan, G. (1997, October). *An evaluation of the use of duragesic for chronic pain in patients with AIDS*. Abstract presented at the annual meeting of the American Pain Society, New Orleans, Louisiana.

Levy, R. M., Bredesen, D. E., & Rosenblum, M. L. (1985). Neurological manifestations of the AIDS experience at UCSF and review of the literature. *Journal of Neurosurgery*, 62, 475–495.

Levy, R. M., Bredesen, D. E., & Rosenblum, M. L. (1988). Opportunistic central nervous system pathology in patients with AIDS. *Annals of Neurology*, 23, S7–S12.

Lindstrom, P., & Lindblom, T. (1987). The analgesic tocainide for trigeminal neuralgia. *Pain*, 28, 45–50.

Lipton, R. B., Feraru, E. R., Weiss, G., et al. (1991). Headache in HIV-I-related disorders. *Headache*, 31, 518–522.

Macaluso, C., Weinberg, D., Foley, K. M. (1988). Opioid abuse and misuse in a cancer pain population. *Journal of Pain and Symptom Management*, 3, 54.

Magni, G., Arsie, D., & Deleo, D. (1987). Antidepressants in the treatment of cancer pain. A survey in Italy. *Pain*, 29, 347–353.

Malseed, R. T., & Goldstein, F. J. (1979). Enhancement of morphine analgesics by tricyclic antidepressants. *Neuropharmacology*, 18, 827–829.

Maltbie, A. A., Cavenar, S. O., Sullivan, J. L., et al. (1979). Analgesia and haloperidol: A hypothesis. *Journal of Canadian Psychiatry*, 40, 323–326.

Marte, C., & Allen, M. (1991). HIV-related gynecologic conditions: Overlooked complications. *Focus: A Guide to AIDS Research and Counseling, 7*, 1–3.

Max, M. B. (1992). Effects of desipramine, amitryptyline, and fluoxetine on pain and diabetic neuropathy. *New England Journal of Medicine, 326*, 1250–1256.

Max, M. B., Culnane, M., Schafer, S. C., Gracely, R. H., et al. (1987). Amitryptyline relieves diabetic neuropathy pain in patients with normal and depressed mood. *Neurology, 37*, 589–596.

McCaffery, M., & Vourakis, C. (1992). Assessment and relief of pain in chemically dependent patients. *Orthopedic Nursing, 11*, 13–27.

McCormack, J. P., Li, R., Zarowny, D., & Singer, J. (1993). Inadequate treatment of pain in ambulatory HIV patients. *Clinical Journal of Pain, 9*, 247–283.

Mersky, H., & Hamilton, J. T. (1989). An open trial of possible analgosis effects of dipyridamole. *Journal of Pain and Symptom Management, 4*, 34–37.

Morokoff, P. J., Holmes-Johnson, E., & Weiss, C. S. (1987). A psychological program for HIV-seropositive persons. *Patient Education and Counseling, 10*, 287–300.

Moss, V. (1990). Palliative care in advanced HIV disease: Presentation, problems and palliation. *AIDS, 4*, S235–S242.

Murray, M. D., & Brater, D. C. (1990). Adverse effects of nonsteroidal anti-inflammatory drugs on renal function. *Annals of Internal Medicine, 112*, 559–560.

Nelson, M. R., Daniels, D., Dean, R., Barton, S., & Gazzard, B. G. (1992). Staphylococcus aureus psoas abscess in a patient with AIDS. *International Journal of Sexually Transmitted Diseases and AIDS, 3*, 294.

Newshan, G., & Wainapel, S. (1993). Pain characteristics and their management in persons with AIDS. *Journal of the Association of Nurses in AIDS Care, 6*(1), 53–59.

O'Neill, W. M., & Sherrard, J. S. (1993). Pain in human immunodeficiency virus disease: A review. *Pain, 54*, 3–14.

Panegyres, P. K., Ran, N., Kakulas, B. A., Armstrong, J. A., & Hollingsworth, P. (1988). Necrotising myopathy and zidovudine. *Lancet, 331*, 1050–1051.

Parry, G. J. (1988). Peripheral neuropathies associated with human immunodeficiency virus infection. *Annals of Neurology, 23*(Suppl.), 349–553.

Passik, S., Breitbart, W., Rosenfeld, B., McDonald, M., Thaler, H., & Portenoy, R. (1994, November). AIDS specific patient-related barriers to pain management. Abstract presented at the annual meeting of the American Pain Society, Miami, Florida.

Patt, R. B., & Reddy, S. R. (1993, November). Pain and the opioid analgesics: Alternate routes of administration. *News Journal of the Physicians' Association for AIDS Care*, pp. 453–458.

Payne, D., Jacobsen, P., Breitbart, W., Passik, S., Rosenfeld, B., & McDonald, M. (1994, November). *Negative thoughts related to pain are associated with greater pain, distress and disability in AIDS pain.* Abstract presented at the annual meeting of the American Pain Society, Miami, Florida.

Penfold, R., & Clark, A. J. M. (1992). Pain syndromes in HIV infection. *Canadian Journal of Anaesthesiology, 39*, 724–730.

Perry, S., & Heidrich, G. (1982). Management of pain during debridement: A survey of US burn units. *Pain, 13*, 267–78.

Pick, C. G., Paul, D., Eison, M. S., & Patsernak, G. (1992).

Potentiation of opioid analgesia by the antidepressant nefazodone. *European Journal of Pharmacology, 2*, 375–381.

Pilowsky, I., Hallet, E. C., Bassett, E. L., Thomas, P. G., & Penhall, R. K. (1982). A controlled study of amitryptyline in the treatment of chronic pain. *Pain, 14*, 169–179.

Portenoy, R. K. (1990). Pharmacologic approaches to the control of cancer pain. *Journal of Psychosocial Oncology, 8*, 75–107.

Portenoy, R. K. (1998). Adjuvant analgesics in pain management. In D. Doyle, G. W. C. Hanks, & N. MacDonald (Eds.), *Oxford textbook of palliative medicine* (2nd ed., pp. 361–390). New York: Oxford University Press.

Portenoy, R., & Foley, K. M. (1989). Management of cancer pain. In J. C. Holland & J. H. Rowland (Eds.), *Handbook of psychooncology* (pp. 369–382). New York: Oxford University Press.

Portenoy, R. K., & Payne, R. (1992). Acute and chronic pain. In J. H. Lowinson, P. Ruiz, & R. B. Millman (Eds.), *Comprehensive textbook of substance abuse* (pp. 691–721). Baltimore: Williams & Wilkins.

Porter, J., & Jick, H. (1980). Addiction rare in patients treated with narcotics. *New England Journal of Medicine, 302*, 123.

Potter, D. A., Danforth, D. N., Macher, A. M., Longo, D. L., Stewart, L., et al. (1984). Evaluation of abdominal pain in the AIDS patient. *Annals of Surgery, 199*, 332–339.

Rabeneck, L., Popovic, M., Gartner, S., et al. (1990). Acute HIV infection presenting with painful swallowing and esophageal ulcers. *Journal of the American Medical Association, 263*, 2318–2322.

Rabkin, C. S., & Blattner, W. A. (1991). HIV infection and cancers other than non-Hodgkin lymphoma and Kaposi's sarcoma. *Cancer Surveys, 10*, 151–160.

Radeck, K., & Deck, C. (1987). Do nonsteroidal anti-inflammatory drugs interfere with blood pressure control in hypertensive patients? *Journal of General Internal Medicine, 2*, 108–112.

Richman, D. D., Fischl, M. A., Grieco, M. H., et al. (1987). The toxicity of azidothymidine (AZT) in the treatment of patients with AIDS and AIDS-related complex. *New England Journal of Medicine, 317*, 192–197.

Rienhart, W. F., Sprenger, H. G., Mooyaart, E. L., Tamsma, J. T., Kengen, R. A., & Weits, J. (1990). Nontropical pyomyositis as a cause of subacute, multifocal myalgia in the Acquired Immunodeficiency Syndrome. *Arthritis and Rheumatism, 33*(11), 1728–1732.

Rosenfeld, B., Breitbart, W., McDonald, M. V., Passik, S. D., Thaler, H., & Portenoy, R. K. (1996). Pain in ambulatory AIDS patients: II. Impact of pain on psychological functioning and quality of life. *Pain, 68*, 323–328.

Rynes, R. I., Goldenberg, D. L., DiGiacomo, R., Olson, R., Hussain, M., et al. (1988). Acquired immunodeficiency syndrome-associated arthritis. *American Journal of Medicine, 84*, 810–816.

Schofferman, J., & Brody, R. (1990). Pain in far advanced AIDS. In K. M. Foley et al. (Eds.), *Advances in pain research and therapy* (Vol. 16, pp. 379–386). New York: Raven Press.

Sharav, Y., Singer, E., Dione, R. A., & Dubner, R. (1987). The analgesic effect of amitriptyline on chronic facial pain. *Pain, 31*, 199–209.

Simpson, D. M., & Wolfe, D. E. (1991). Neuromuscular complications of HIV infection and its treatment. *AIDS, 5,* 917–926.

Sindrup, S. H., Gram, L. F., Brosen, K., Eshoj, O., & Mogenson, E. F. (1990). The selective serotonin reuptake inhibitor paroxetine is effective in the treatment of diabetic neuropathy symptoms. *Pain, 42,* 135–144.

Singer, E. J., Zorilla, C., Fahy-Chandon, B., et al. (1993). Painful symptoms reported for ambulatory HIV-infected men in a longitudinal study. *Pain, 54,* 15–19.

Singh, S., Fermie, P., & Peters, W. (1992, July). *Symptom control for individuals with advanced HIV infection in a subacute residential unit: Which symptoms need palliating?* (Poster Abstract No. POD 5248). Poster session presented at the International Conference on AIDS/III STD World Congress, Amsterdam, The Netherlands.

Snider, W. D., Simpson, D. M., Nielsen, S., et al. (1983). Neurological complications of AIDS: Analysis of 50 patients. *Annals of Neurology, 14,* 403–418.

Spiegel, K., Kalb, R., & Pasternak, G. W. (1983). Analgesic activity of tricyclic antidepressants. *Annals of Neurology, 13,* 462–465.

Strafford, M., Cahill, C., Schwartz, T., et al. (1991). Recognition and treatment of pain in pediatric patients with AIDS [Abstract]. *Journal of Pain and Symptom Management, 6,* 146.

Swerdlow, M., Cundhill, J. G. (1981). Anticonvulsant drugs used in the treatment of lacerating pains: A comparison. *Anesthesia, 36,* 1129–1134.

Tiegno, M., Pagnoni, B., Calmi, A., et al. (1987). Chlorimipramine compared to pentazocine as a unique treatment in post-operative pain. *Journal of Clinical Pharmacology Research, 7,* 141–143.

Ventafridda, V., Bonezzi, C., Caraceni, A., et al. (1987). Antidepressants for cancer pain and other painful syndromes with deafferentation component: Comparison of amitriptyline and trazodone. *Italian Journal of Neurological Sciences, 8,* 579–587.

Ventafridda, V., Branchi, M., Ripamonti, C., et al. (1990). Studies on the effects of antidepressant drugs on the antinociceptive action of morphine and on plasma morphine in rat and man. *Pain, 43,* 155–162.

Ventrafridda, V., Caraceni, A., Gamba, A. (1990). Field testing of the WHO Guidelines for Cancer Pain Relief: Summary report of demonstration projects. In K. M. Foley, J. J. Bonica, & V. Ventrafridda (Eds.), *Proceedings of the Second International Congress on Pain: Vol 16. Advances in pain research and therapy* (pp. 155–165). New York: Raven Press.

Von Roenn, J. H., Cleeland, C. S., Gonin, R., Hatfield, A. L., Pandya, K. J. (1993). Physician attitudes and practice in cancer pain management: A survey from the Eastern Cooperative Oncology Group. *Annals of Internal Medicine, 119,* 121–126.

Walsh, T. D. (1986). Controlled study of imipramine and morphine in chronic pain due to advanced cancer. In K. M. Foley, et al. (Eds.), *Advances in pain research and therapy* (Vol. 16, pp. 155–165). New York: Raven Press.

Ward, S. E., Goldberg, N., Miller-McCauley, C., Mueller, C., Nolan, A., Pawlik-Plank, D., Robbins, A., Stormoen, D., & Weissman, D. E. (1993). Patient-related barriers to management of cancer pain. *Pain, 52,* 319–324.

Watson, C. P., Chipman, M., Reed, K., Evans, R. J., & Birkett, N. (1992). Amitriptyline versus maprotiline in post herpetic neuralgia: A randomized double-blind, cross-over trial. *Pain, 48,* 29–36.

Watts, R. A., Hoffbrand, B. I., Paton, D. F., Davie, J. C. (1987). Pyomyositis associated with human immunodeficiency virus infection. *British Medical Journal, 194,* 1524–1525.

Weissman, D. E., & Haddox, J. D. (1989). Opioid pseudo-addiction and iatrogenic syndrome. *Pain, 36,* 363–366.

Wexner, S. D., Smithy, W. B., Milsom, J. W., & Dailey, T. H. (1986). The surgical management of anorectal diseases in AIDS and pre-AIDS patients. *Diseases of the Colon and Rectum, 29,* 719–723.

Wilcox, C. M., Forsmark, C. E., Grendell, J. H., Darragh, T. M., Cello, J. P. (1990). Cytomegalovirus-associated acute pancreatic disease in patients with acquired immunodeficiency syndrome. *Gastroenterology, 99,* 263–267.

Winchester, R., Bernstein, D. H., Fischer, H. D., Enlow, R., Solomon, G. (1987). The co-occurrence of Reiter's syndrome and acquired immunodeficiency. *Annals of Internal Medicine, 106,* 19–26.

World Health Organization. (1986). *Cancer pain relief.* Geneva: Author,

Young, R. J., & Clarke, B. F. (1985). Pain relief in diabetic neuropathy: The effectiveness of imipramine and related drugs. *Diabetic Medicine, 2,* 363–366.

Zelman, D., Cleeland, C., & Howland, E. (1987). Factors in appropriate pharmacolgical management of cancer pain: A cross-institutional investigation. *Pain* (Suppl.), S136.

Part III

ISSUES IN PREVENTION AND MANAGEMENT

Chapter 21

Coping with Pain

JENNIFER L. BOOTHBY
BEVERLY E. THORN
MICHAEL W. STROUD
MARK P. JENSEN

More than 30 years ago, the gate control theory of pain taught us that how much we are hurt or damaged does not bear a one-to-one relationship with how much pain we experience; nociception and pain are not the same (Melzack & Wall, 1965). Nociception is the activation of peripheral sensory fibers when tissue is damaged or is about to be damaged. Pain is a sensory or emotional experience associated with or described in terms of tissue damage (Merskey & Bogdale, 1994). Melzack and Wall (1965) identified several variables that might moderate the relationship between nociception and pain, and a growing body of research has shown that these variables influence pain experience over and above any effects of physical damage. These include cognitive factors such as attention and perception of control over pain (Turk, Meichenbaum, & Genest, 1983; Weisenberg, 1977), as well as factors involving the immediate environment, such as specific people or context (see review in Jensen, 1997). How others respond to a person when he or she communicates pain has also been shown to predict pain behaviors and disability over and above pain severity or intensity (Flor, Turk, & Rudy, 1989; Flor, Kerns, & Turk, 1987; Romano et al., 1995). Gate control theory and the research that supports it confirm what many pain clinicians see every day—the disability and pain

experiences of people with chronic pain have relatively little to do with nociception or tissue damage and much to do with how patients and the people around them respond to the pain.

Many of the variables that influence pain and disability fall under the construct of coping, and many models of pain and illness give coping responses an important, if not central, role in understanding and predicting adjustment to pain and illness (cf. Arathuzik, 1991; Tunks & Bellissimo, 1988; Turk et al., 1983; Unruh, 1996; Weir, Browne, Roberts, Tunks, & Gafni, 1994). Testing these models and identifying the associations between specific coping responses and adjustment have been important areas of research in chronic pain. Although the findings from this research have important theoretical implications, they also have immediate applications for the practicing pain clinician and the individuals he or she serves. Identification of those pain-coping strategies that have the greatest influence on adjustment provides the clinician with an empirical rationale for deciding which coping strategies (if any) to teach and encourage and which to discourage.

Much of the research on pain and coping performed prior to 1991 was reviewed by Jensen, Turner, Romano, and Karoly (1991). The conclusions of that article were (1) that the use of coping strategies categorized as "active" (e.g., exercise, activity, ignoring pain) may be associated with better psychological and physical functioning, whereas the use of passive coping strategies (withdrawal, resting, medication use) predicts poorer functioning; (2) that the coping strategy of wishful thinking (e.g., passively hoping that things will get better) is associated with lower levels of positive affect and physical functioning; and (3) that although other coping strategies may play an important role in adjustment to chronic pain, the limited number of studies and the paucity of true experimental designs made it difficult to draw specific conclusions regarding their relative importance. The goal of this chapter is to provide an update of that 1991 review and determine what has been learned since that time regarding the importance of coping in adjustment to chronic pain.

The chapter begins with a brief review of Lazarus and Folkman's transactional model of stress and coping (Lazarus & Folkman, 1984), which provides a useful framework for conceptualizing the most important issues involved in the coping process. Research examining the relationships between composite measures of coping (basically, categories of coping) and adjustment to chronic pain are then reviewed. This is followed by a discussion of research examining the relationships between individual measures of coping and adjustment. Finally, we discuss the clinical implications.

A TRANSACTIONAL MODEL
OF STRESS AND COPING

Perhaps the most common framework used to conceptualize coping is Lazarus and Folkman's (1984) transactional model of stress. The transactional model outlines several important factors and processes involved in coping with stress. First, dispositional variables such as personality, stable social roles, and/or biological parameters can affect a person's interaction with a stressor. These dispositional variables certainly influence how that person will cope and how the coping responses ultimately influence adjustment. In addition to the dispositional variables that influence reactions to stress, people also engage in a series of ever-changing appraisal processes that influence their emotional responses to the stressor, including whether, and which, coping responses will be attempted. One category of appraisals, labeled primary appraisals by Lazarus and Folkman, are those relating to judgments about whether a potential stressor is irrelevant, benign-positive, or stressful. Lazarus and Folkman identify three types of stressful appraisals: those that suggest the event poses a threat, those that suggest the event poses a challenge, or those that suggest the event will result in possible harm or loss. Appraisals regarding potential harm produce negative emotions such as fear and anxiety, whereas those focusing on the challenging aspects of the event(s) might produce feelings of eagerness or excitement, particularly when the person believes that effective coping responses are possible. Beliefs about coping options and their possible effectiveness are called secondary appraisals in Lazarus and Folkman's model. Finally, coping responses, which Lazarus and Folkman define as "constantly changing cognitive and behavioral efforts to manage specific external and/or internal demands that are appraised as taxing or exceeding the resources of the person" (1984, p. 141), ultimately influence important adaptational outcomes, such as social functioning, morale, and somatic health. This chapter focuses on the hyothesized link between coping responses and adaptational outcomes as they relate to chronic pain.

STRESS AND COPING
AND CHRONIC PAIN

In Lazarus and Folkman's (1984) model, stress is neither an event nor the response of a person to events. Rather, stress is defined as the relationship between life events and a person's responses to those events. They write, "Psychological stress is a particular relationship between the person and the environment that is appraised by the person as taxing or exceeding his or her resources and endangering his or her well-being" (p. 19). In this conceptualization, an event that is not appraised as stressful is not considered a stressor. Using this model of stress, nociceptive stimulation or even pain experience would not be considered stressors, nor would any of a person's physiological responses (e.g., decreased immune function, increased blood pressure) to pain. Pain would only be considered a stressor when, and if, a person believes that this pain taxes or exceeds his or her ability to manage it.

In addition, a person with chronic pain must deal with more than just daily pain. He or she must deal with many changes, such as feelings of dependency, marital strain or divorce, and/or losing a job and income. Many, if not all, of these pain-related losses may be appraised as taxing or exceeding the person's resources. Thus each of these losses may contribute to the "stress" of a person with chronic pain. In the broadest sense, coping with chronic pain means coping with these multiple stressors.

COMPOSITE MEASURES OF COPING: THEIR RELATIONSHIP TO ADJUSTMENT

The concept of coping has been variously categorized as emotion-focused versus problem-focused (Lazarus & Folkman, 1984), passive versus active (Brown & Nicassio, 1987), and illness-focused versus wellness-focused (Jensen, Turner, Romano, & Strom, 1995). In addition to these rationally derived categories, some researchers have attempted to identify coping categories, or composites, using factor analyses of the instruments used to assess coping. Both approaches have tended to result in the classification of coping dimensions or composites into two basic types: those coping responses that have generally been assumed to be maladaptive (passive, emotion-focused, illness-focused) and those efforts that are thought to be adaptive (active, problem-focused, and wellness-focused) in managing pain and its impact. These composites appear to reflect how clinicians think about the coping options available to persons with chronic pain. In general, clinicians treating chronic pain tend to discourage the use of "maladaptive" strategies and to teach and encourage the use of "adaptive" strategies (Jensen et al., 1995).

We begin the review of the empirical literature with an examination of how these composite measures of coping relate to adjustment among individuals with chronic pain. However, some cautionary statements regarding the interpretation of this research are in order. There may not be consistent overarching dimensions of coping made up of individual coping responses that are strongly related. Three sets of findings support that conclusion. First, the relationships among most measures of coping are generally weak to moderate (e.g., Blalock, DeVellis, & Giorgino, 1995; Lennon, Dohrenwend, Zautra, & Marbach, 1990; Robinson et al., 1997). Second, empirically derived coping composites, even when using the same measures in very similar populations, rarely replicate exactly (see Jensen et al., 1991). Third, when researchers do find significant associations between composite measures of coping and some measure of functioning, it is rare for all of the individual coping

strategies that make up the coping composite to contribute to the significant association (e.g., Geisser, Robinson, & Henson, 1994). More often, significant associations between coping composites and functioning are due to the significant association between one or two members of the coping composite rather than to the composite as a whole.

In addition, research that uses coping composites may have limited utility. Such research cannot tell us how specific coping strategies are related to functioning. Even if a specific category or dimension of coping predicted important outcomes in every study, it is more difficult to teach groups of individual coping strategies than to teach specific strategies. Moreover, it may not be practical to teach or encourage a whole group of coping responses that fall under a category of coping when only one or two of the coping responses that make up the composite actually contribute to the prediction of adjustment. It is more practical to teach and encourage specific coping strategies (for example, relaxation, cognitive restructuring, and task persistence) than categories of coping. Similarly, discouraging specific strategies (rest, catastrophizing) is easier than telling the patient to avoid all passive strategies.

There are two reasons to use coping composites in research (Jensen et al., 1991). First, in those research studies with limited numbers of subjects, multiple analyses of individual coping measures increase the risk of concluding that significant associations exist when they might have occurred in the sample by chance alone (Type I errors). Using composites is therefore a way to limit this type of error. Second, by decreasing the number of predictors in an analysis, the use of composites can increase the power of statistical tests. Thus composite measures may provide a more sensitive test for theoretical models of coping and adjustment to chronic pain. The associations between the individual coping responses and adjustment may then be presented for descriptive and practical purposes, not for hypothesis testing (see Jensen, Turner, & Romano, 1994, for an example of this approach). With these issues in mind, we can now review the research that has examined how coping composites predict adjustment.

The research using composite measures of coping that has been conducted since 1991 largely replicates the findings of that conducted prior to 1991—coping composites predict both concurrent and subsequent psychological and physical functioning among individuals with chronic pain. A review of this research follows, organized by type of study: correlational, longitudinal, treatment-outcome, and experimental. In general, and replicating the research performed prior to 1991, coping composites labeled as "maladaptive" tend to be associated positively with measures of dysfunction, and those thought to be "adaptive" tend to be associated negatively with measures of dysfunction. These findings support the potential role that coping responses play in adjustment to chronic pain.

Correlational Studies

In a correlational study comparing the validity of a two-factor "active" versus "passive" solution for the Coping Strategy Questionnaire (CSQ; Rosenstiel & Keefe, 1983) and the Vanderbilt Pain Management Inventory (VPMI; Brown & Nicassio, 1987), passive coping was found to be predictive of distress and depression, whereas active coping was predictive of activity level (Snow-Turek, Norris, & Tan, 1996). Another correlational study using two samples of rheumatoid arthritis patients found that those who used "adaptive coping" strategies (as defined by the use of CSQ Coping Self-Statements in one sample and by the use of active coping as measured by the VPMI in a second sample) reported less negative and more positive affect (Zautra et al., 1995). Those who reported using "maladaptive" strategies (as defined by high scores on the CSQ Catastrophizing subscale in one sample and the use of passive coping strategies measured by the VPMI in the second) reported more negative and less positive affect. Patients with higher levels of pain were more likely to use maladaptive strategies, and those with more pain-related limitations were more likely to use maladaptive and less likely to use adaptive strategies for coping (Zautra et al., 1995). However, another study using the adaptive coping composite of the CSQ did not find adaptive coping to be predictive of response to lumbar sympathetic nerve blocks or response to interdisciplinary pain rehabilitation (Connally & Sanders, 1991).

Factor analysis of the CSQ in five studies found a superordinate factor that was labeled Coping Attempts by the investigators. Although the specific scales that loaded on it differed from one study to the next, this factor tended to contain the following subscales: Calming or Coping Self-Statements, Reinterpreting Pain Sensations, Ignoring Pain Sensations, Increasing Activity Level, and Diverting Attention. Predictive validity of the Coping Attempts factor using various pain outcome measures

has generally shown weak but occasionally statistically significant associations to positive adaptation. One study found that children with sickle cell disease who scored high on this factor showed less activity reduction during painful episodes and more uptime overall than children with low scores (Gil et al., 1993). Another study of children with sickle cell disease found that higher scores on Coping Attempts were related to fewer emergency room visits and lower rates of reduction in household activity over the course of 9 months (Gil, Williams, Thompson, & Kinney, 1991). Martin et al. (1996) reported that adult fibromyalgia patients scoring high on this factor reported greater physical and total disability but lower levels of psychosocial disability as measured by the Symptom Impact Profile. Still other authors reported that the Coping Attempts factor in fibromyalgia patients was not predictive of any pain outcome measures (Nicassio, Schoenfeld-Smith, Radojevic, & Schuman, 1995). Beckham, Keefe, Caldwell, and Roodman (1991) also found that the Coping Attempts factor was not related to outcome measures of adjustment in a sample of rheumatoid arthritis patients.

A factor labeled Pain Control and Rational Thinking has also been obtained from the CSQ. Controlling for demographic variables and medical status, Beckham et al. (1991) found that rheumatoid arthritis patients who scored higher on this factor were more likely to report lower levels of pain, depression, and physical and psychological disability. Similar findings were reported with a sample of children having juvenile chronic arthritis. Children with higher scores on Pain Control and Rational Thinking had lower ratings of pain intensity after controlling for age, disease duration, and disease activity. Higher scores on this factor were also associated with the report of fewer pain locations (Schanberg, Lefebvre, Keefe, Kredich, & Gil, 1997). Keefe and colleagues (1991) found that rheumatoid arthritis patients recovering from knee replacement surgery who scored higher on Pain Control and Rational Thinking reported lower levels of pain and less psychological disability. Lenhart and Ashby (1996) found that two CSQ-derived composites labeled Helplessness and Avoidance were associated with higher levels of disability after controlling for age and compensation status.

A composite labeled the Composite Coping Index (CCI) is derived from the Cognitive Coping Strategies Inventory (CCSI; Butler, Damarin, Beaulieu, Schwebel, & Thorn, 1989). The CCI is created by summing six scales that reflect cognitive strategies thought to be adaptive (internal and external attention diversion, imaginative inattention, imaginative transformation/context; imaginative transformation/sensation; somatization) and subtracting a seventh scale that measures catastrophizing. In the original cross-validation study, the composite measure of coping was negatively related to self-ratings of pain intensity and nurses' ratings of patients' ability to tolerate postsurgical pain. The Catastrophizing subscale was positively correlated with self-ratings of postsurgical pain (Butler et al., 1989). In a later study, however, the CCI was not significantly related to analgesic use among women undergoing breast surgery, although the Catastrophizing subscale was (Jacobsen & Butler, 1996).

Kleinke (1992) described the development of a measure of four pain coping composites that he labeled Self-Management (active strategies such as coping self-statements, distracting activities, and exercise), Helplessness (catastrophizing thoughts and withdrawal), Social Support (seeking emotional support from others), and Medical Remedies (using various coping strategies associated with acute pain conditions, such as guarding, application of heat or cold, and taking medications). In a group of chronic pain patients, Self-Management and Social Support were negatively associated with measures of psychological distress and positively associated with a measure of activity level, whereas Helplessness showed the opposite pattern. Medical Remedies was negatively associated with activity level.

Coping strategy composites usually considered maladaptive have been associated with negative outcome. For example, a correlational study reported that higher rates of Negative Thinking were related to higher rates of psychological distress and reduction in household activity and that higher scores on Passive Adherence were associated with more frequent emergency room visits and reduction in household, social, and school activities (Gil et al., 1991). Another correlational study using sickle cell patients found that patients reporting poorer adjustment used Negative Thinking, Passive Adherence, and palliative coping responses more often than patients considered to have adjusted well to disease-related pain (Thompson, Gil, Abrams, & Phillips, 1992). Geisser, Robinson, and Henson (1994) found that Pain Avoidance predicted concurrent interference of pain with activities, affective distress, and pain severity. Analyses of individual strategies loading on this factor demonstrated that this relationship was due to the use of Praying/Hoping rather than the use of Diverting Attention (the other strategy loading on this factor).

Longitudinal Studies

In a study of patients with newly developed musculoskeletal pain, the use of passive coping (as measured by the VPMI) was found to be related to higher pain intensity at the end of 26 weeks (Potter and Jones, 1992). In a study of rheumatoid arthritis patients, Smith and Wallston (1992) reported that passive coping with pain (as measured by the VPMI) was positively related to psychosocial impairment over a 4-year period and was negatively related to perceived quality of emotional support; active coping strategies were relatively unrelated to any of the variables investigated. Another longitudinal study of temporomandibular joint pain patients found that patients reporting more use of passive coping strategies (as measured by the VPMI) at 3-month follow-up were more likely to report greater pain interference in daily activities at 12 months. Increases in the use of active coping (as measured by the CSQ) were associated with absence of jaw disability after 3 months (Turner, Whitney, Dworkin, Massoth, & Wilson, 1995). A study of patients with low back pain using a similar design found that use of active coping (as measured by the CSQ) was related to increased uptime at 3-month follow-up. However, active coping was unrelated to pain outcomes at 6 months (Spinhoven & Linssen, 1991).

Longitudinal studies with sickle cell patients have found that the CSQ composite factors labeled Negative Thinking and Passive Adherence were related to poor outcome. Gil, Abrams, Phillips, and Williams (1992) found that sickle cell patients who reported more Negative Thinking and Passive Adherence at baseline also reported less uptime, higher rates of activity reduction, and more frequent and longer hospitalizations over a 9-month period than patients with lower scores on these measures. Another study found that patients who increased their use of Negative Thinking over a 9-month period increased their number of health care contacts, whereas those who decreased their use of Negative Thinking had fewer health contacts during the same period (Gil et al., 1993). A longitudinal study of chronic pain patients reported that patients scoring higher on the CSQ factor labeled Pain Control and Rational Thinking were less likely to report distress and more likely to return to work (Dozois, Dobson, Wong, Hughes, & Long, 1996).

Following multidisciplinary treatment in an inpatient setting, chronic pain patients relying on the use of Pain Control and Rational Thinking reported lower overall pain levels than patients who used other coping strategies. Improvements in Negative Thinking and coping strategies at posttreatment were related to better outcomes in pain report, emotional distress, and activity discomfort (Tota-Faucette, Gil, Williams, Keefe, & Goli, 1993).

Treatment Outcome Studies

Most treatment outcome studies measure coping strategy use at pre- and posttreatment; however, treatment is not targeted specifically at changing coping strategies as such. Rather, treatment is generally less specific, involving a multidisciplinary effort or a general cognitive/behavioral approach. In one study, the effectiveness of stress management training, disease education, and standard medical care was compared in a group of rheumatoid arthritis patients. Patients trained in stress management techniques reported less helplessness, more frequent coping attempts, higher self-efficacy, and higher confidence in their pain-coping abilities following treatment. These gains were maintained at 3-month and 15-month follow-up (Parker et al., 1995). In another study, fibromyalgia patients were assigned to either group treatment with a cognitive/educational focus, group treatment with a focus on education and discussion, or a wait-list control group. Aggregate measures of pain coping were created by content analysis and correlational analysis of various pain questionnaires. Both treatment groups reported greater "pain coping" and "pain control" compared to the control group. These authors did not find changes in catastrophizing, pain intensity, relaxation, activity level, or pain behavior over the course of treatment (Vlaeyen et al., 1996). Turner and Jensen (1993) compared three treatment strategies and a wait-list control group in a group of patients with low back pain. Patients receiving relaxation training, cognitive therapy, or a combination of the two did not differ from the control group with respect to maladaptive thinking or depression. Both treatment groups showed improvement on all other noncoping pain-related outcome measures. A group of headache patients received cognitive-behavioral therapy (CBT), a component of which was specifically aimed at reducing catastrophizing self-statements. Two treatment approaches and a wait-

list control group were compared. The treatment groups either were given time-specific goals for the use of coping strategies or were instructed to use coping strategies for as long as possible. Both treatment groups reported more frequent use of adaptive coping strategies and less frequent catastrophizing (as measured by the CCSI) compared to their pretreatment levels. Patients who received specific time goals for coping also showed lower intake of non-narcotic analgesics and lower pain levels from pre- to posttreatment (James, Thorn, & Williams, 1993). Another study with rheumatoid arthritis patients found that those receiving CBT increased pain coping as measured by the Pain Coping Inventory, whereas patients receiving occupational therapy and those on a waiting list for treatment showed no changes (Kraaimaat, Brons, Geenen, & Bijlsma, 1995). A group of sickle cell patients receiving cognitive coping skills training reported higher levels of Coping Attempts and lower levels of Negative Thinking, as measured by the CSQ, following treatment. Patients receiving only disease education did not show significant changes in their use of coping strategies (Gil et al., 1996). Chronic pain patients participating in a 7-week multidisciplinary pain treatment program improved coping skills (as measured by the McGill Pain Questionnaire [MPQ]) and decreased analgesic consumption (Skinner et al., 1990).

As a group, the treatment outcome studies provide strong evidence that a variety of chronic pain treatment programs have an effect on coping responses. This raises the possibility, consistent with cognitive-behavioral models, that treatment programs may be effective, at least in part, because of changes they produce in how individuals respond to their pain problem and pain experience.

Experimental Studies

Few true experiments have examined the effect of coping strategies on pain intensity or pain tolerance. As noted earlier, it is difficult to encourage or discourage the use of "categories" of coping; therefore, the few experimental studies that manipulate coping do so by comparing individual strategies (see the next section). In a study manipulating goals for the use of coping strategies taught in session, Thorn and Hansell (1993) found that subjects given specific time goals for coping with cold pressor pain tolerated the pain longer than those told to "last as long as you can."

Summary of the Composite Research

Research using composites is consistent with the hypothesis that general categories of coping play a role in adaptation to chronic pain. Existing research indicates that measures of "adaptive" coping strategies, which often include categories of coping labeled Active Coping, Coping Attempts, and Pain Control and Rational Thinking, predict concurrent and future functioning, whereas "maladaptive" strategy composites, which include categories of coping labeled Passive Coping, Negative Thinking, and Pain Avoidance, predict concurrent and future dysfunction.

INDIVIDUAL COPING STRATEGIES AND ADJUSTMENT TO CHRONIC PAIN

Research examining the association between individual coping responses and adjustment can indicate the relative importance of specific coping strategies. As a result, this research may be of more use to the practicing clinician than research involving composite measures. Even if passive strategies are generally maladaptive, some are probably more maladaptive than others and should therefore be targeted for change first. Similarly, active strategies appear to be generally adaptive. However, analysis of specific coping strategies (reported in this section) clearly indicates that some active strategies may play a minor role at best in adjustment to chronic pain. Given the difficulties associated with lasting behavior change, it would appear far more practical to alter behaviors and beliefs that demonstrate consistent and strong associations with adjustment than those that have a minimal association with functioning.

Research prior to 1991 provided some indication of the relationship between specific coping strategies and adjustment (Jensen et al., 1991). Coping strategies identified as potentially maladaptive for chronic pain patients included the use of wish-fulfilling fantasy and pain-contingent rest and paying greater attention to pain. Social comparison, or viewing oneself as better off than others, was the single strategy identified as possibly adaptive. Catastrophizing was consistently shown to predict both psychological and physical dysfunction across samples and studies. Since 1991, a great deal of additional research has examined the associations between specific coping strategies and adjustment. We review this work in the subsections

that follow, organized by the specific coping strategies studied.

Catastrophizing

Catastrophizing is commonly defined as use of excessive and exaggerated negative self-statements when in pain. Examples of such statements on the CSQ and CCSI, respectively, are "It's awful and I feel that it overwhelms me" and "I find myself expecting the worst." There is some discussion in the literature regarding whether catastrophizing might be better considered an appraisal (a primary appraisal reflecting the threat of pain to one's well-being) than a coping response per se (Jensen et al., 1991). Because of its inclusion in the most frequently used measure of pain coping (the CSQ) and because of its strong and consistent link to important adaptation outcomes (see the following discussion), we choose to include it in this review. Ultimately, whether catastrophizing is labeled as a coping strategy or an appraisal is not as important as the question of whether or not it leads to dysfunction. If it proves to be maladaptive it should be discouraged, and research examining the impact of catastrophizing on adjustment is therefore important to the practicing clinician.

A great deal of research performed since 1991 confirms a consistent relationship between catastrophizing responses and adjustment to chronic pain. Studies employing concurrent correlation and regression analyses have found catastrophizing to be associated with higher levels of psychological distress (Geisser, Robinson, & Henson, 1994; Geisser, Robinson, Keefe, & Weiner, 1994; Harkapaa, 1991; Hill, 1993; Jensen, Turner, & Romano, 1992; Robinson et al., 1997; Ulmer, 1997), higher rates of analgesic use and postoperative pain (Jacobsen & Butler, 1996), poorer physical functioning and disability (Hill, Niven, & Knussen, 1995; Martin et al., 1996; Robinson et al., 1997), higher ratings of pain intensity (Geisser, Robinson, & Henson, 1994; Geisser, Robinson, Keefe, & Weiner, 1994; Harkapaa, 1991; Hill, 1993; Hill et al., 1995; Lefebvre, Lester, & Keefe, 1995; Lester, Lefebvre, & Keefe, 1996; Robinson et al., 1997; Sullivan, Bishop, & Pivik, 1995; Ulmer, 1997; Wilkie & Keefe, 1991), more reports of pain interference in daily activities (Geisser, Robinson, & Henson, 1994; Lin & Ward, 1996; Robinson et al., 1997), lower levels of general activity (Robinson et al., 1997), higher rates of psychosocial dysfunction (Hill et al., 1995; Jensen et al., 1992), and reduced ability to work (Lester et al., 1996). Among a group of chronic pain patients who participated in multidisciplinary treatment, decreases in catastrophizing from pretreatment to 6-month follow-up predicted decreases in depression and pain-related physician visits over the same period. Changes in catastrophizing did not predict changes in disability, however (Jensen et al., 1994).

Jensen et al. (1992) reported that, in a sample of chronic pain patients, catastrophizing was related to psychosocial dysfunction only for those patients with short and medium pain duration. Similarly, patients with acute pain and patients with chronic pain that is considered to be inconsistent with known physiological and anatomical principles, that has vague symptoms, or that is poorly localized were found to report higher levels of catastrophizing and other maladaptive pain-coping strategies than patients with chronic pain that is more congruent with known medical principles (Hadjistavropoulos & Craig, 1994). In a 9-month longitudinal study, chronic pain patients who scored higher on a measure of catastrophizing were less likely to be employed than patients scoring lower on this measure (Dozois et al., 1996). With respect to experimental pain studies, catastrophizers have also been found to report higher levels of pain and more emotional distress (Sullivan et al., 1995).

Although catastrophizing has been shown to predict outcome in nearly all studies examined, it does not always do so. Jensen et al. (1992) found that catastrophizing did not contribute to the prediction of disability in a group of chronic pain patients when pain-related variables (pain intensity, site, duration), and many other pain-coping strategies (the other ratings and scales of the CSQ) were controlled.

Results from treatment-outcome studies are promising with respect to catastrophizing. A treatment-outcome study found that either cognitive or relaxation treatment combined with treatment designed to increase health behavior and activity levels was more effective in decreasing the use of catastrophizing than treatment aimed at health behavior and activity levels alone (Vlaeyen, Haazen, Schuerman, Kole-Snijders, & van Eek, 1995). Another study examining the effectiveness of group multimodal treatment for fibromyalgia patients found that patients improved on various outcome measures, with the greatest change emerging on the Catastrophizing subscale of the CSQ. These treatment gains were maintained at 2-year follow-up (Bennett et al., 1996). Headache patients were less likely to catastrophize following cognitive-behavioral

treatment (James et al., 1993; ter Kuile, Spinhoven, Linssen, & van Houwelingen, 1995), and those patients who engaged in more catastrophizing following treatment reported higher levels of psychological distress. In summary, it appears that a variety of nonspecific short-term treatments are effective in reducing the use of catastrophizing by pain patients.

Praying/Hoping

Several studies have found praying and hoping to be associated with poorer adjustment to chronic pain. An example of a praying-and-hoping coping response on the CSQ is "I have faith in doctors that someday there will be a cure for my pain." In a study of patients with chronic low back pain who were undergoing a work-hardening program, more frequent use of praying/hoping at pretreatment was related to greater subjective disability and lower functional capacity (maximum lift) at posttreatment (Dozois et al., 1996). Praying and hoping was also found to be correlated with higher levels of overall disability (Ashby & Lenhart, 1994; Hill et al., 1995; Jensen et al., 1992), more pain interference in daily life (Geisser, Robinson, & Henson, 1994; Lester et al., 1996; Lin & Ward, 1996; Robinson et al., 1997), pain severity (Geisser, Robinson, & Henson, 1994; Harkapaa, 1991; Hill, 1993; Hill et al., 1995; Robinson et al., 1997), and affective distress (Geisser, Robinson, & Henson, 1994; Hill, 1993) among individuals with a variety of pain conditions. In a group of chronic pain patients who received multidisciplinary treatment, decreases in the use of praying and hoping from pretreatment to 6-month follow-up predicted decreases in depression and pain-related physician visits over the same period. Changes in praying/hoping did not predict changes in disability (Jensen et al., 1994). However, other studies have found praying/hoping to be unrelated to pain severity (Lester et al., 1996), disability (Swimmer, Robinson, & Geisser, 1992), psychological functioning (Dozois et al., 1996; Harkapaa, 1991; Jensen et al., 1992; Robinson et al., 1997), psychosocial dysfunction (Hill et al., 1995; Jensen et al., 1992), general activity level (Robinson et al., 1997), and return to work following a work-hardening program (Dozois et al., 1996). Following participation in a work-hardening program, male patients with low back pain improved in the use of all coping strategies measured by the CSQ with the exception of prayer and diverting attention. The use of prayer as a means of coping with chronic pain was unaffected by the treatment program (Dozois, Dobson, Wong, Hughes, & Long, 1995).

As a group, these studies suggest that praying or hoping is associated with important adjustment measures at some times but not at others. When a significant association emerged, however, praying and hoping was positively associated with dysfunction and negatively associated with measures of adaptation. Because of the correlational nature of this research, it is not possible to determine whether people pray and hope more when they are having a more difficult time (compared to when they are functioning well) or whether praying and hoping actually contribute to greater dysfunction. Certainly this research indicates the need to study the coping response of praying and hoping in more detail.

Reinterpreting Pain

Responses on the CSQ and CCSI that are typical of individuals who use reinterpreting pain as a coping strategy include "I don't think of it as pain but rather as a dull or warm feeling" and "If my pain feels shooting I try and pretend that it is only tingling," respectively. Buckelew et al. (1992) found that Reinterpreting Pain Sensations was the only coping strategy on the CSQ to be associated with lower pain reports in patients undergoing EMG or nerve conduction studies. Other authors found that headache patients who increased their use of reinterpreting pain following training in either cognitive self-hypnosis or autogenic techniques reported lower pain levels (ter Kuile, Spinhoven, & Linssen, 1995). However, in a study examining the work-return rates among chronic pain patients following treatment, individuals who scored higher on Reinterpreting Pain Sensations were significantly less likely than those using other strategies to be employed at 9-month follow-up (Dozois et al., 1996). Still other authors have noted that chronic pain patients who use reinterpreting pain as a coping strategy have higher rates of psychosocial dysfunction (Hill et al., 1995; Jensen et al., 1992).

Overall, reinterpreting pain sensations tends to show weak and nonsignificant associations with most functional variables, such as interference of pain with activities or ability to work (Geisser, Robinson, & Henson, 1994; Lester et al., 1996), affective distress (Dozois et al., 1996; Geisser, Robinson, & Henson, 1994; Hill, 1993), physi-

cal disability (Dozois et al., 1996; Hill et al., 1995; Jensen et al., 1992), functional capacity (Dozois et al., 1996), psychosocial dysfunction (Jensen et al., 1992), and pain severity (Geisser, Robinson, & Henson, 1994; Hill, 1993; Hill et al., 1995; Lester et al., 1996). Robinson et al. (1997) who created new scale scores from the original CSQ items, constructed a scale labeled Distancing From Pain that included four items from the original CSQ Reinterpreting Pain Sensations scale. This new scale failed to show significant associations with general activity level, interference of pain with activities, pain severity, or affective distress in a large group of chronic pain patients (Robinson et al., 1997). As a group, these studies suggest that reinterpreting pain sensations plays at most a minor role in adjustment to chronic pain. However, it may be a useful strategy for coping with acute pain.

Ignoring Pain

Ignoring pain occasionally displays significant associations with functioning. An example of this coping strategy on the CSQ is "I tell myself it doesn't hurt." Ignoring pain was found to be associated with greater pain interference in daily life among a group of patients with low back pain (Lin & Ward, 1996) but was associated with lower pain interference in a group of chronic pain patients (Robinson et al., 1997). Higher use of the strategy of ignoring pain at pretreatment was found to predict return to work at 9 months following a work-hardening program (Dozois et al., 1996). More frequent use of this strategy has been shown to be associated with lower ratings of pain (Geisser, Robinson, & Henson, 1994; Hill, 1993) and with higher levels of general activity (Robinson et al., 1997).

However, the majority of studies indicate that ignoring pain does not predict pain interference with activities or ability to work (Geisser, Robinson, & Henson, 1994; Lester et al., 1996), physical disability (Dozois et al., 1996; Hill et al., 1995; Jensen et al., 1992), psychosocial dysfunction (Hill et al., 1995; Jensen et al., 1992), psychological functioning (Dozois et al., 1996; Geisser, Robinson, & Henson, 1994; Hill, 1993; Jensen et al., 1992; Robinson et al., 1997), or pain severity (Hill et al., 1995; Lester et al., 1996; Robinson et al., 1997). Moreover, changes in the strategy of ignoring pain from pretreatment to 6-month follow-up were unrelated to changes in disability, depression, or number of physician visits over the same time period (Jensen et al., 1994). Thus ignoring pain probably has little influence on adjustment for the majority of individuals with chronic pain.

Distraction/Diverting Attention

Distraction is another coping strategy that bears an inconsistent relationship to functioning in chronic pain patients. An item from the CCSI illustrating this coping strategy is "If possible, I would try and read a book or magazine to take my mind off the pain." More frequent use of distraction has been linked to less perceived disability (Schmitz, Saile, & Nilges, 1996) and greater overall feelings of well-being (Van Lankveld, Van't Pad Bosch, Van De Putte, Naring, & Van Der Staak, 1994). Among children with musculoskeletal pain, a factor called Cognitive Refocusing was associated with lower pain reports and fewer depressive symptoms (Varni et al., 1996). Greater use of distraction and emotional-support seeking were found to be related to more positive mood among rheumatoid arthritis patients only for those patients experiencing lower levels of pain. For patients reporting more intense pain, these strategies were associated with less positive mood (Affleck, Urrows, Tennen, & Higgins, 1992). McCracken (1997) reported that attention to pain as measured by the Pain Vigilance and Awareness Questionnaire significantly predicted distress, disability, and health care utilization in a group of chronic pain patients when pain intensity was controlled. Hill (1993) found more frequent use of diverting attention from pain to be associated with greater pain severity and higher levels of psychological distress in a group of individuals with phantom limb pain. Distraction also predicted higher levels of pain severity and interference with daily activities in a group of chronic pain patients (Robinson et al., 1997).

In contrast, Dozois et al. (1996) failed to find a relationship between pretreatment use of distraction and posttreatment disability, functional capacity, distress, or employment status at 9 months following a work-hardening program. Moreover, other researchers have failed to identify significant associations between the use of distraction and pain interference with activities or ability to work (Geisser, Robinson, & Henson, 1994; Lester et al., 1996), general activity level (Robinson et al., 1997), disability (Hill et al., 1995; Jensen et al., 1992, Swimmer et al., 1992), affective distress/depression (Geisser, Robinson, & Henson, 1994; Harkapaa, 1991; Jensen et al., 1992; Robinson

et al., 1997), psychosocial dysfunction (Hill et al., 1995; Jensen et al., 1992), or pain severity (Geisser, Robinson, & Henson, 1994; Harkapaa, 1991; Hill et al., 1995; Lester et al., 1996). Diverting attention was one of only two coping strategies to be unaffected by participation in a work-hardening program (Dozois et al., 1995). Changes in the use of the diverting-attention strategy from pretreatment to 6-month follow-up were also found to be unrelated to changes in disability, depression, or number of physician visits over the same time period for a group of chronic pain patients (Jensen et al., 1994).

In an experiment specifically manipulating distraction, participants undergoing pressure pain were either instructed to use cognitive distraction or sensation monitoring or were given no instructions. Those receiving instruction in cognitive distraction showed greater pain tolerance (Stevens, 1992). In a similar study, instruction in either distraction or sensation monitoring was superior to no instruction in modifying pain tolerance and intensity (Stevens & Terner, 1993). Distraction may therefore be a similar strategy to ignoring pain—not particularly helpful for chronic pain but perhaps useful for managing acute pain episodes. On the other hand, preliminary research raises the possibility that paying attention to pain, at least among individuals with chronic pain, may prove maladaptive (McCracken, 1997).

Positive Coping Self-Statements

Certain studies have found positive self-statements to be associated with adaptive functioning. Examples of positive coping self-statements on the CSQ and CCSI, respectively, are "I see it as a challenge and don't let it bother me" and "I concentrate on convincing myself that I will deal with the pain and that it will get better in the near future." More frequent use of coping self-statements has been shown to be associated with lower levels of pain severity (Hill, 1993), less depressed mood (Van Lankveld et al., 1994), less psychological distress (Hill, 1993), and higher levels of general activity (Robinson et al., 1997). This is not a consistent finding, however. The use of positive coping self-statements did not predict posttreatment disability, functional status, distress, or return to work 9 months following participation in a work-hardening program (Dozois et al., 1996). Several studies have not found the use of coping self-statements to be associated with interference of pain with activities or ability to work (Geisser, Robinson, &

Henson, 1994; Lester et al., 1996; Robinson et al., 1997), with disability (Hill et al., 1995; Jensen et al., 1992; Swimmer et al., 1992), with affective distress/depression (Geisser, Robinson, & Henson, 1994; Harkapaa, 1991; Jensen et al., 1992; Robinson et al., 1997), with psychosocial dysfunction (Hill et al., 1995; Jensen et al., 1992), or with pain severity (Geisser, Robinson, & Henson, 1994; Harkapaa, 1991; Hill et al., 1995; Lester et al., 1996; Robinson et al., 1997). In a multidisciplinary program, changes in coping self-statements from pretreatment to 6-month follow-up were unrelated to changes in disability, depression, or number of physician visits over the same time period (Jensen et al., 1994). As a group, these findings suggest that the use of positive coping self-statements tends not to have a significant relation to functioning. When associations do emerge, their use is more likely to be adaptive than maladaptive.

Engaging in Distracting Activities

Increasing Activities, a scale from the CSQ that represents a tendency to engage in distracting activities when in pain, rarely predicts functioning. It is important to note that this scale does not reflect engaging in regular exercise, a behavior critical in preventing deconditioning of chronic pain patients. Research has shown scores on this scale to be unrelated to interference of pain with activities or ability to work (Geisser, Robinson, & Henson, 1994; Lester et al., 1996), to disability (Dozois et al., 1996; Hill et al., 1995; Jensen et al., 1992; Swimmer et al., 1992), to affective distress/depression (Dozois et al., 1996; Geisser, Robinson, & Henson, 1994; Jensen et al., 1992), to psychosocial dysfunction (Jensen et al., 1992), to functional capacity (Dozois et al., 1996), or to pain severity (Geisser, Robinson, & Henson, 1994; Hill et al., 1995; Lester et al., 1996). However, Hill (1993) found distracting activities to predict higher levels of pain severity and psychological distress among individuals with phantom limb pain, and Hill et al. (1995) replicated these findings with regard to pain severity. Overall, increasing distracting activities likely has little influence on adjustment to chronic pain.

Other Strategies

Of five coping strategies assessed by the Ways of Coping Scale (WOCS; Folkman, Lazarus, Dunkel-

Schetter, DeLonges, & Gruen, 1985, a precursor to the Ways of Coping Checklist, Vitaliano, Russo, Carr, Maiuro, & Becker, 1985), only one, escape avoidance, predicted poor physical and psychosocial health in a group of women with osteoarthritis (Burke & Flaherty, 1993). Examples of items in the Escape Avoidance scale are "Wished that the situation would go away, or somehow be over," and "Hoped a miracle would happen." Scores on both the Avoidance and Wishful Thinking scales of the Ways of Coping Checklist–Revised (Vitaliano et al., 1985) distinguished depressed from nondepressed low back pain patients, and in each case the depressed patients used these passive strategies more frequently (Weickgenant et al., 1993). The use of self-blame, social support-seeking, and problem-focused coping were the same across the two groups. The Wishful Thinking scale was also shown to predict lower levels of positive affect and physical functioning in research prior to 1991 (Jensen et al., 1991).

Blalock et al. (1995) examined the association between 11 specific coping strategies (assessed by the 72-item Coping Strategies Inventory [CSI], Tobin, Holroyd, Reynolds, & Wigal, 1989; plus 10 items from the Coping Orientation to Problems Experienced Scale [COPE]; Carver, Scheier, & Weintraub, 1989) in predicting subsequent psychological functioning over a 6-month period among a group of adults with osteoarthritis. The authors controlled for pain level, initial psychological functioning, and physical functioning, in addition to relevant sociodemographic variables. They examined three dimensions of psychological functioning: positive affect, negative affect, and depression. More frequent use of problem solving at the initial assessment predicted an increase in positive affect 6 months later. More frequent use of social support, self-criticism, and social withdrawal and less frequent use of problem avoidance and turning to religion predicted higher levels of negative affect 6 months later. Finally, more frequent use of social support and social withdrawal and less frequent use of problem avoidance at the initial assessment predicted higher levels of depression 6 months later. In these analyses, use of cognitive restructuring, emotional expression, wishful thinking, and information seeking at the initial assessment were not significantly related to changes in psychological functioning.

Jaspers, Heuvel, Stegenga, and de Bont (1993) examined the association between eight scales from the Coping with Specific Symptoms Questionnaire (CSSQ; Asma & Jaspers, 1990), a Dutch coping measure, and a number of functioning measures in a group of individuals with temporomandibular joint osteoarthrosis or synovitis. Use of all the coping strategies, problem-focused coping, expression of emotions, avoidance, comforting thinking, wishful thinking, and palliative coping were positively associated with psychological distress. Three of the scales, Expression of Emotions, Comforting Thinking, and Palliative Coping, were positively associated with interference with activities and negative mood. Comforting Thinking was positively associated with pain severity, and Wishful Thinking was similarly associated with pain severity, as well as general activity level.

Van Lankveld et al. (1994) assessed a number of general coping strategies in a group of rheumatoid arthritis patients, including several strategies that have not been investigated specifically by other researchers: optimism, pacing (adapting one's level of activity), and creative solution seeking. General optimism was associated positively with general well-being and cheerful mood and negatively with depressed mood. Pacing also predicted depressed mood (positive relationship) and cheerful mood (negative relationship). Creative solution seeking was unrelated to mood or well-being in these patients.

Jensen et al. (1995) correlated the frequency of coping strategies, as rated by patients and spouses, with patient disability and activity level, as rated by spouses. Frequency of use of three coping strategies thought to be maladaptive (guarding, or not moving specific painful body parts; asking for assistance; and sedative–hypnotic medication use) bore moderate to strong positive relations with patient disability. Guarding and sedative medication use were negatively associated with patient activity level. The associations between strategies thought to be adaptive (relaxation, task persistence, exercise/stretch, coping self-statements, and seeking social support) and spouse-reported patient disability and activity level were not as strong as those between maladaptive strategies and disability. Of 14 coefficients examined, only one was of moderate strength and significant: that between spouse ratings of patient use of task persistence and spouse-rated patient disability ($r = -.38$).

In a study relating examination of pretreatment-to-follow-up changes in some of these coping strategies to changes in disability, depression, and number of physician visits, only changes in the use of muscle-strengthening exercise predicted changes in depression (Jensen et al., 1994). Changes in opioid medication use, aerobic exercise, stretching exercise, and keeping busy were unrelated to changes in functioning. However, these investigators acknowledged that the measures of these coping strategies were single ratings, which may attenuate their reliability and validity.

It was noted in Jensen et al. (1991) that social comparison (viewing oneself as better off than others) was a strategy identified as possibly adaptive. In an experiment designed specifically to manipulate social comparison, participants undergoing cold pressor pain were asked to rate their pain intensity at quit point while being given bogus information about other participants' quit-point pain ratings. Those participants given relatively intense comparative values (i.e., they were manipulated to view themselves as better off than others) gave relatively lower pain intensity ratings than participants not given this feedback, confirming that this type of social comparison may be adaptive in terms of pain behavior (Wilson, Chaplin, & Thorn, 1995).

Summary of Research Examining Individual Measures of Coping

Since 1991, many more studies have examined the ability of measures of individual coping responses to predict functioning among individuals with chronic pain than were published prior to 1991. The findings show that the strength of the relationships between specific coping responses and functioning can vary widely, with some coping responses rarely able to predict functioning, some demonstrating occasional (but consistent when significant) relationships to adjustment, and one demonstrating a consistent and strong relationship to functioning.

In nearly every study, more frequent catastrophizing responses predict higher levels of distress and disability among chronic pain patients. Frequently, the relationships found are in the moderate to strong range. Ignoring pain, reinterpreting pain, and distraction or diverting attention, on the other hand, rarely predict important measures of functioning among chronic pain patients, although these strategies may be useful in coping with acute pain episodes. Although praying/hoping, positive self-statements, rest, and wishful thinking do not show as strong and consistent a relationship to functioning as catastrophizing, several investigators have found that these coping responses do predict functioning in some situations. When significant, the directions of the relationships found are consistent. Praying/hoping, pain-contingent rest, and wishful thinking are associated with greater dysfunction, whereas the use of positive coping self-statements tends to be associated with lower dysfunction.

Preliminary research has examined a large number of other coping strategies, including the use of guarding, task persistence, asking for assistance, relaxation, regular exercise, medication use, seeking social support, and pacing, among others. In some cases these have been shown to predict patient functioning, making further explorations into their possible role in adjustment to chronic pain worth pursuing.

An important limitation of much of the extant research is its correlational nature. Although the absence of strong associations between a coping response and a measure of adjustment may be used as evidence against one influencing the other, the presence of a significant association cannot be used as evidence that the coping response influences the adjustment measure or that the adjustment measure predicts the coping response. As an analogy, imagine a gold miner who needs to choose where to dig and that he or she has a device that indicates where gold definitely is not and also where it might be. Although the use of such a device cannot guarantee that the miner will strike gold every time he or she digs, it is helpful nevertheless because it can save the miner time by telling him or her where to avoid digging. Correlational studies can be seen as such a device; they tell us that reinterpreting pain, ignoring pain, and distracting activities may not be very helpful for chronic pain patients—at least not in influencing psychological functioning and disability. There is little gold here. On the other hand, correlational studies do tell us that further explorations to determine the role that catastrophizing, praying/hoping, positive coping self-statements, pain-contingent rest, and wishful thinking might play in adjustment to chronic pain may yield large dividends. Discovery of the gold (causal relationships) will require longitudinal studies, process analyses of outcome studies, and true experiments.

Treatment-outcome studies aimed specifically at changing individual coping strategies would be particularly useful. The vast majority of treatment-outcome studies reviewed did not target specific coping strategies but rather offered a form of more "generic" treatment. The results from these outcome studies tend to suggest that broad-based, generic treatment can effect changes in coping. Studies that compare treatments that focus specifically on changing coping with nonspecific treatments would help elucidate the mechanism that promotes changes in coping strategy use and, ostensibly, adaptive outcome. Likewise, more true experiments that manipulate specific coping strategies would help identify those strategies that are truly useful in terms of adaptive coping with pain.

Another important gap in the research is that most if not all of the studies conducted to this point have used patients with chronic pain who are seeking treatment for intractable pain. It would be useful to study individuals who do not seek treatment for their chronic pain. Analysis of the spontaneous coping strategies used by these "adaptive copers" might shed further light on which specific methods for coping offer promise for further study.

CLINICAL IMPLICATIONS

Final conclusions regarding whether the specific coping strategies examined in the coping research are ultimately adaptive or maladaptive (that is, influence functioning one way or another) or are merely reflective of functioning (that is, covary with functioning but have no causal impact on functioning) must wait until true experiments can be performed. Nevertheless, the research that has been accomplished to date does have direct practical clinical implications. First, the research suggests that there are coping strategies that are not related to functioning, such as reinterpretation of pain sensations, ignoring pain, and distraction. Time spent teaching or encouraging the use of these strategies among chronic pain patients is possibly time that is wasted and that could be more profitably spent on other coping strategies.

Second, despite the lack of experimental research, the strong and consistent associations found between catastrophizing and important adjustment measures among chronic pain patients provides evidence that catastrophizing may be harmful. This conclusion is entirely consistent with a large body of treatment-outcome research that demonstrates the effectiveness of cognitive restructuring (a treatment that teaches the identification and elimination of maladaptive cognitions such as catastrophizing and encourages a more realistic appraisal of events) for decreasing depression specifically but also for increasing functioning among chronic pain patients. In short, cognitive restructuring should be considered an important (if not essential) component of chronic pain treatment, especially for those individuals who evidence higher than average levels of catastrophizing.

Based on the preliminary evidence of a negative association between wishful thinking and praying/hoping and positive adaptation, chronic pain treatment should probably also encourage patients to take a very active role in their recovery. Merely wishing, waiting, or hoping that things will get better has the potential to interfere with improvement. Also based on preliminary findings, it may be a good idea to discourage the use of pain-contingent rest, guarding, and use of sedative-hypnotic medication as strategies for dealing with pain. Although such strategies are certainly appealing and may produce short-term reductions in discomfort, both pain-contingent rest and guarding have the potential for reducing physical functioning and leading to more pain and discomfort in the long run by weakening muscles and tendons (Fordyce, 1976). Similarly, use of sedative–hypnotics may allow short-term relief by minimizing or decreasing the affective dimension of pain. However, such a strategy probably has little benefit for long-term adaptation, especially if it provides just enough relief to decrease motivation for learning and practicing other strategies that provide long-term benefit.

SUMMARY

The research performed since 1991 on coping with chronic pain has provided continued evidence for the potential importance of coping responses to important adaptation outcomes among chronic pain patients. Moreover, a substantial number of studies have provided greater insight into the specific coping strategies and how they relate to adjustment. Research has continued to demonstrate consistent negative relationships between the response of catastrophizing and concurrent functioning, and preliminary evidence indicates that praying/hoping, pain-contingent rest, guarding, and use of sedative–hypnotic medication may be maladaptive. Although research is preliminary, possible adaptive strategies include coping self-statements, positive social comparisons, regular exercise, seeking social support, and task persistence. Certainly, the research indicates that ignoring pain, reinterpreting pain sensations, and engaging in distracting activities when in pain play a minor role if any in adjustment to chronic pain.

Further research is needed to examine the influence of changes in specific coping strategies on subsequent functioning. This is particularly needed for those coping strategies/responses that show the greatest likelihood of influencing adjust-

ment (i.e., that have shown the strongest and most consistent relationships to functioning). In particular, research attempting to manipulate the use of catastrophizing will help finalize our understanding of the contribution of this maladaptive coping strategy to patients' functioning. Likewise, additional research aimed at further understanding the importance of coping self-statements as they relate to adaptation to pain would be useful.

REFERENCES

Affleck, G., Urrows, S., Tennen, H., & Higgins, P. (1992). Daily coping with pain from rheumatoid arthritis: Patterns and correlates. *Pain, 51,* 221–229.

Arathuzik, D. (1991). The appraisal of pain and coping in cancer patients. *Western Journal of Nursing Research, 13,* 714–731.

Ashby, J. S., & Lenhart, R. S. (1994). Prayer as a coping strategy for chronic pain patients. *Rehabilitation Psychology, 39,* 205–209.

Asma, M. J. O. van, & Jaspers, J. P. C. (1990). Coping en psychopathologie: de constructie van een vragenlijst. *Gedradg en Gezongheid, 18,* 140–144.

Beckham, J. C., Keefe, F. J., Caldwell, D. S., & Roodman, A. A. (1991). Pain coping strategies in rheumatoid arthritis: Relationships to pain, disability, depression, and daily hassles. *Behavior Therapy, 22,* 113–124.

Bennett, R. M., Burckhardt, C. S., Clark, S. R., O'Reilly, C. A., Wiens, A. N., & Campbell, S. M. (1996). Group treatment of fibromyalgia: A 6 month outpatient program. *Journal of Rheumatology, 23,* 521–528.

Blalock, S. J., DeVellis, B. M., & Giorgino, K. B. (1995). The relationship between coping and psychological well-being among people with osteoarthritis: A problem-specific approach. *Annals of Behavioral Medicine, 17,* 107–115.

Brown, G. K., & Nicassio, P. M. (1987). Development of a questionnaire for the assessment of active and passive coping strategies in chronic pain patients. *Pain, 31,* 53–63.

Buckelew, S. P., Conway, R. C., Shutty, M. S., Lawrence, J. A., Grafing, M. R., Anderson, S. K., Hewett, J. E., & Keefe, F. J. (1992). Spontaneous coping strategies to manage acute pain and anxiety during electrodiagnostic studies. *Archives of Physical Medicine and Rehabilitation, 73,* 594–598.

Burke, M., & Flaherty, M. J. (1993). Coping strategies and health status of elderly arthritic women. *Journal of Advanced Nursing, 18,* 7–13.

Butler, R. W., Damarin, F. L., Beaulieu, C. L., Schwebel, A. I., & Thorn, B. E. (1989). Assessing cognitive coping strategies for acute pain. *Psychological Assessment: A Journal of Consulting and Clinical Psychology, 1,* 41–45.

Carver, C. S., Scheier, M. F., & Weintraub, J. K. (1989). Assessing coping strategies: A theoretically based approach. *Journal of Personality and Social Psychology, 56,* 267–283.

Connally, G. H., & Sanders, S. H. (1991). Predicting low back pain patients' response to lumbar sympathetic nerve blocks and interdisciplinary rehabilitation: The role of pretreatment overt pain behavior and cognitive coping strategies. *Pain, 44,* 139–146.

Dozois, D. J. A., Dobson, K. S., Wong, M., Hughes, D., & Long, A. (1995). Factors associated with rehabilitation outcome in patients with low back pain (LBP): Prediction of employment outcome at 9-month follow-up. *Rehabilitation Psychology, 40,* 243–259.

Dozois, D. J. A., Dobson, K. S., Wong, M., Hughes, D., & Long, A. (1996). Predictive utility of the CSQ in low back pain: Individual vs. composite measures. *Pain, 66,* 171–180.

Flor, H., Kerns, R. D., & Turk, D. C. (1987). The role of spouse reinforcement, perceived pain, and activity levels of chronic pain patients. *Journal of Psychosomatic Research, 31,* 251–259.

Flor, H., Turk, D. C., & Rudy, T. E. (1989). Relationship of pain impact and significant other reinforcement of pain behaviors: The mediating role of gender, marital status, and marital satisfaction. *Pain, 38,* 45–50.

Folkman, S., Lazarus, R., Dunkel-Schetter, I., DeLonges, A., & Gruen, R. (1985). *Ways of Coping Scales, Set Number One (Community Sample).* Berkeley: University of California, Department of Psychology.

Fordyce, W. E. (1976). *Behavioral methods for chronic pain and illness.* St. Louis, MO: Mosby.

Geisser, M. E., Robinson, M. E., & Henson, C. D. (1994). The Coping Strategies Questionnaire and chronic pain adjustment: A conceptual and empirical reanalysis. *The Clinical Journal of Pain, 10,* 98–106.

Geisser, M. E., Robinson, M. E., Keefe, F. J., & Weiner, M. L. (1994). Catastrophizing, depression and the sensory, affective and evaluative aspects of chronic pain. *Pain, 59,* 79–83.

Gil, K. M., Abrams, M. R., Phillips, G., & Williams, D. A. (1992). Sickle cell disease pain: 2. Predicting health care use and activity level at 9-month follow-up. *Journal of Consulting and Clinical Psychology, 60,* 267–273.

Gil, K. M., Thompson, R. J., Jr., Keith, B. R., Tota-Faucette, M., Noll, S., & Kinney, T. R. (1993). Sickle cell disease pain in children and adolescents: Change in pain frequency and coping strategies over time. *Journal of Pediatric Psychology, 18,* 621–637.

Gil, K. M., Williams, D. A., Thompson, R. J., Jr., & Kinney, T. R. (1991). Sickle cell disease in children and adolescents: The relation of child and parent pain coping strategies to adjustment. *Journal of Pediatric Psychology, 16,* 643–663.

Gil, K. M., Wilson, J. J., Edens, J. L., Webster, D. A., Abrams, M. A., Orringer, E., Grant, M., Crawford, W. C., & Janal, M. N. (1996). The effects of cognitive coping skills training on coping strategies and experimental pain sensitivity in African American adults with sickle cell disease. *Health Psychology, 15,* 3–10.

Hadjistavropoulos, H. D., & Craig, K. D. (1994). Acute and chronic low back pain: Cognitive, affective, and behavioral dimensions. *Journal of Consulting and Clinical Psychology, 62,* 341–349.

Harkapaa, K. (1991). Relationships of psychological distress and health locus of control beliefs with the use of cognitive and behavioral coping strategies in low back pain patients. *Clinical Journal of Pain, 7,* 275–282.

Hill, A. (1993). The use of pain coping strategies by patients with phantom limb pain. *Pain, 55,* 347–353.

Hill, A., Niven, C. A., & Knussen, C. (1995). The role of coping in adjustment to phantom limb pain. *Pain, 62,* 79–86.

Jacobsen, P. B., & Butler, R. W. (1996). Relation of cognitive coping and catastrophizing to acute pain and analgesic use following breast cancer surgery. *Journal of Behavioral Medicine, 19,* 17–29.

James, L. D., Thorn, B. E., & Williams, D. A. (1993). Goal specification in cognitive behavioral therapy for chronic headache pain. *Behavior Therapy, 24,* 305–320.

Jaspers, J. P. C., Heuvel, F., Stegenga, B., & de Bont, L. G. M. (1993). Strategies for coping with pain and psychological distress associated with temporomandibular joint osteoarthrosis and internal derangement. *Clinical Journal of Pain, 9,* 94–103.

Jensen, M. P. (1997). Validity of self-report and observation measures. In T. S. Jensen, J. A. Turner, & Z. Weisenfeld-Hallin (Eds.), *Proceedings of the Eighth World Congress on Pain: Vol. 8. Progress in pain research and management* (pp. 637–661). Seattle, WA: IASP Press.

Jensen, M. P., Turner, J. A., & Romano, J. M. (1992). Chronic pain coping measures: Individual vs. composite scores. *Pain, 51,* 273–280.

Jensen, M. P., Turner, J. A., & Romano, J. M. (1994). Correlates of improvement in multidisciplinary treatment of chronic pain. *Journal of Consulting and Clinical Psychology, 62,* 172–179.

Jensen, M. P., Turner, J. A., Romano, J. M., & Karoly, P. (1991). Coping with chronic pain: A critical review of the literature. *Pain, 47,* 249–283.

Jensen, M. P., Turner, J. A., Romano, J. M., & Strom, S. E. (1995). The Chronic Pain Coping Inventory: Development and preliminary validation. *Pain, 60,* 203–216.

Keefe, F. J., Caldwell, D. S., Martinez, S., Nunley, J., Beckham, J., & Williams, D. A. (1991). Analyzing pain in rheumatoid arthritis patients: Pain coping strategies in patients who have had knee replacement surgery. *Pain, 46,* 153–160.

Kleinke, C. L. (1992). How chronic pain patients cope with pain: Relation to treatment outcome in a multidisciplinary pain clinic. *Cognitive Therapy and Research, 16,* 669–685.

Kraaimaat, F. W., Brons, M. R., Geenen, R., & Bijlsma, J. W. J. (1995). The effect of cognitive behavior therapy in patients with rheumatoid arthritis. *Behaviour Research and Therapy, 33,* 487–495.

Lazarus, R. S., & Folkman, S. (1984). *Stress, appraisal, and coping.* New York: Springer.

Lefebvre, J. C., Lester, N., & Keefe, F. J. (1995). Pain in young adults: II. The use and perceived effectiveness of pain-coping strategies. *Clinical Journal of Pain, 11,* 36–44.

Lenhart, R. S., & Ashby, J. S. (1996). Cognitive coping strategies and coping modes in relation to chronic pain disability. *Journal of Applied Rehabilitation Counseling, 27,* 15–18.

Lennon, M. C., Dohrenwend, B. P., Zautra, A. J., & Marbach, J. J. (1990). Coping and adaptation to facial pain in contrast to other stressful life events. *Journal of Personality and Social Psychology, 59,* 1040–1050.

Lester, N., Lefebvre, J. C., & Keefe, F. J. (1996). Pain in

young adults: III. Relationships of three pain-coping measures to pain and activity interference. *Clinical Journal of Pain, 12,* 291–300.

Lin, C., & Ward, S. E. (1996). Perceived self-efficacy and outcome expectancies in coping with chronic low back pain. *Research in Nursing and Health, 19,* 299–310.

Martin, M. Y., Bradley, L. A., Alexander, R. W., Alarcon, G. S., Triana-Alexander, M., Aaron, L. A., & Alberts, K. R. (1996). Coping strategies predict disability in patients with primary fibromyalgia. *Pain, 68,* 45–53.

McCracken, L. M. (1997). Attention to pain in persons with chronic pain: A behavioral approach. *Behavior Therapy, 28,* 271–284.

Melzack, R., & Wall, P. D. (1965). Pain mechanisms: A new theory. *Science, 150,* 971–979.

Merskey, H., & Bogdale, N. (Eds.). (1994). *Classification of chronic pain: Descriptions of chronic pain syndromes and definitions of pain terms.* Seattle, WA: IASP Press.

Nicassio, P. M., Schoenfeld-Smith, K., Radojevic, V., & Schuman, C. (1995). Pain coping mechanisms in fibromyalgia: Relationship to pain and functional outcomes. *Journal of Rheumatology, 22,* 1552–1558.

Parker, J. C., Smarr, K. L., Buckelew, S. P., Stucky-Ropp, R. C., Hewett, J. E., Johnson, J. C., Wright, G. E., Irvin, W. S., & Walker, S. E. (1995). Effects of stress management on clinical outcomes in rheumatoid arthritis. *Arthritis and Rheumatism, 38,* 1807–1818.

Potter, R. G., & Jones, J. M. (1992). The evolution of chronic pain among patients with musculoskeletal problems: A pilot study in primary care. *British Journal of General Practice, 42,* 462–464.

Robinson, M. E., Riley, J. L., Myers, C. D., Sadler, I. J., Kvaal, S. A., Geisser, M. E., & Keefe, F. J. (1997). The Coping Strategies Questionnaire: A large sample, item level factor analysis. *Clinical Journal of Pain, 13,* 43–49.

Romano, J. M., Turner, J. A., Jensen, M. P., Friedman, L. S., Bulcroft, R. A., Hops, H., & Wright, S. F. (1995). Chronic pain patient–spouse behavioral interactions predict patient disability. *Pain, 63,* 353–360.

Rosenstiel, A. K., & Keefe, F. J. (1983). The use of coping strategies in low back pain patients: Relationship to patient characteristics and current adjustment. *Pain, 17,* 33–40.

Schanberg, L. E., Lefebvre, J. C., Keefe, F. J., Kredich, D. W., & Gil, K. M. (1997). Pain coping and the pain experience in children with juvenile chronic arthritis. *Pain, 73,* 181–189.

Schmitz, U., Saile, H., & Nilges, P. (1996). Coping with chronic pain: Flexible goal adjustment as an interactive buffer against pain-related distress. *Pain, 67,* 41–51.

Skinner, J. B., Erskine, A., Pearce, S., Rubenstein, I., Taylor, M., & Foster, C. (1990). The evaluation of a cognitive behavioural treatment programme in outpatients with chronic pain. *Journal of Psychosomatic Research, 34,* 13–19.

Smith, C. A., & Wallston, K. A. (1992). Adaptation in patients with chronic rheumatoid arthritis: Application of a general model. *Health Psychology, 11,* 151–162.

Snow-Turek, A. L., Norris, M. P., & Tan, G. (1996). Active and passive coping strategies in chronic pain patients. *Pain, 64,* 455–462.

Spinhoven, P., & Linssen, A. C. G. (1991). Behavioral

treatment of chronic low back pain: I. Relation of coping strategy use to outcome. *Pain, 45,* 29–34.

Stevens, M. J. (1992). Interaction of coping style and cognitive strategies in the management of acute pain. *Imagination, Cognition, and Personality, 11,* 225–232.

Stevens, M. J., & Terner, J. L. (1993). Moderators of cognitive coping derived from attentional and parallel processing models of pain. *Imagination, Cognition, and Personality, 12,* 341–353.

Sullivan, M. J. L., Bishop, S. R., & Pivik, J. (1995). The Pain Catastrophizing Scale: Development and validation. *Psychological Assessment, 7,* 524–532.

Swimmer, G. I., Robinson, M. E., & Geisser, M. E. (1992). Relationship of MMPI cluster type, pain coping strategy, and treatment outcome. *Clinical Journal of Pain, 8,* 131–137.

ter Kuile, M. M., Spinhoven, P., & Linssen, A. C. G. (1995). Responders and nonresponders to autogenic training and cognitive self-hypnosis: Prediction of short- and long-term success in tension-type headache patients. *Headache, 35,* 630–636.

ter Kuile, M. M., Spinhoven, P., Linssen, A. C. G., & van Houwelingen, H. C. (1995). Cognitive coping and appraisal processes in the treatment of chronic headaches. *Pain, 64,* 257–264.

Thompson, R. J., Jr., Gil, K. M., Abrams, M. R., & Phillips, G. (1992). Stress, coping, and psychological adjustment of adults with sickle cell disease. *Journal of Consulting and Clinical Psychology, 60,* 433–440.

Thorn, B. E., & Hansell, P. L. (1993). Goals for coping with pain mitigate time distortion. *American Journal of Psychology, 106,* 211–225.

Tobin, D. L., Holroyd, K. A., Reynolds, R. V., & Wigal, J. K. (1989). The hierarchical factor structure of the Coping Strategies Inventory. *Cognitive Therapy and Research, 13,* 343–361.

Tota-Faucette, M. E., Gil, K. M., Williams, D. A., Keefe, F. J., & Goli, V. (1993). Predictors of response to pain management treatment. *Clinical Journal of Pain, 9,* 115–123.

Tunks, E., & Bellissimo, A. (1988). Coping with the coping concept: A brief comment. *Pain, 34,* 171–174.

Turk, D. C., Meichenbaum, D., & Genest, M. (1983). *Pain and behavioral medicine: A cognitive-behavioral perspective.* New York: Guilford Press.

Turner, J. A., & Jensen, M. P. (1993). Efficacy of cognitive therapy for chronic low back pain. *Pain, 52,* 169–177.

Turner, J. A., Whitney, C., Dworkin, S. F., Massoth, D., & Wilson, L. (1995). Do changes in patient beliefs and coping strategies predict temporomandibular disorder treatment outcomes? *Clinical Journal of Pain, 11,* 177–188.

Ulmer, J. F. (1997). An exploratory study of pain, coping, and depressed mood following burn injury. *Journal of Pain and Symptom Management, 13,* 148–157.

Unruh, A. (1996). Gender variations in clinical pain experience. *Pain, 65,* 123–167.

Van Lankveld, W., Van't Pad Bosch, P., Van De Putte, L., Naring, G., & Van Der Staak, C. (1994). Disease-specific stressors in rheumatoid arthritis: Coping and well-being. *British Journal of Rheumatology, 33,* 1067–1073.

Varni, J. W., Waldron, S. A., Gragg, R. A., Rappoff, M. A., Bernstein, B. H., Lindsley, C. B., & Newcomb,

M. D. (1996). Development of the Waldron/Varni Pediatric Pain Coping Inventory. *Pain, 67,* 141–150.

Vitaliano, P. P., Russo, J., Carr, J. E., Maiuro, R. D., & Becker, J. (1985). The Ways of Coping Checklist: Revision and psychometric properties. *Multivariate Behavioral Research, 20*(1), 3–26.

Vlaeyen, J. W. S., Haazen, I. W. C. J., Schuerman, J. A., Kole-Snijders, A. M. J., & van Eek, H. (1995). Behavioural rehabilitation of chronic low back pain: Comparison of an operant treatment, an operant-cognitive treatment and an operant-respondent treatment. *British Journal of Clinical Psychology, 34,* 95–118.

Vlaeyen, J. W. S., Teeken-Gruben, N. J. G., Goossens, M. E. J. B., Rutten-van Molken, M. P. M. H., Pelt, R. A. G. B., van Eek, H., & Heuts, P. H. T. G. (1996). Cognitive-educational treatment of fibromyalgia: A randomized clinical trial: I. Clinical effects. *Journal of Rheumatology, 23,* 1237–1245.

Weickgenant, A. L., Slater, M. A., Patterson, T. L., Atkinson, J. H., Grant, I., & Garfin, S. R. (1993). Coping activi-ties in chronic low back pain: Relationship with depression. *Pain, 53,* 95–103.

Weir, R., Browne, G., Roberts, J., Tunks, E., & Gafni, A. (1994). The meaning of illness questionnaire: Further evidence for its reliability and validity. *Pain, 58,* 377–386.

Weisenberg, M. (1977). Pain and pain control. *Psychological Bulletin, 84,* 1008–1044.

Wilkie, D. J., & Keefe, F. J. (1991). Coping strategies of patients with lung cancer-related pain. *Clinical Journal of Pain, 7,* 292–299.

Wilson, J. J., Chaplin, W. F., & Thorn, B. E. (1995). The influence of different standards on the evaluation of pain: Implications for assessment and treatment. *Behavior Therapy, 26,* 217–239.

Zautra, A. J., Burleson, M. H., Smith, C. A., Blalock, S. J., Wallston, K. A., DeVellis, R. F., DeVellis, B. M., & Smith, T. W. (1995). Arthritis and perceptions of quality of life: An examination of positive and negative affect in rheumatoid arthritis patients. *Health Psychology, 14,* 399–408.

Chapter 22

Pain Management in Primary Care: An Individualized Stepped-Care Approach

MICHAEL VON KORFF

Primary medical care is "the point of entry into the health care system and the locus of responsibility for organizing care for patients and for populations over time" (Starfield, 1992). Primary care is where most patients seeking medical care for common pain conditions are seen. For example, back pain, headache, abdominal pain, chest pain, and neck pain are each among the 20 most common reasons for visiting primary care physicians in the United States (American Academy of Family Physicians, 1987).

PRIMARY CARE: A CRITICAL CONTEXT

Cost-effective organization of health care services depends on a well-organized and effective primary care service. Primary care is population-based—it aspires to serve the entire population and their most common health care needs. It is the setting of first contact, an accessible setting in which early intervention is possible. It tries to provide continuity of care and comprehensive services. The physician knows the patient, assumes ongoing responsibility, and attends to psychological and social factors in illness, as well as diagnosing and treating disease. Primary care physicians often care for other family members as well and may have a broader understanding of the social circumstances of the patient. They act as gatekeepers to specialty care,

referring patients who may require specialized services while controlling access to costly or potentially harmful specialty services that are not warranted by medical need. Primary care aspires to be cost-effective—to provide essential services to the large numbers of persons seeking care at a cost that the patient and society can afford (Starfield, 1992; Von Korff, 1994).

This chapter focuses on back pain because it is the most common chronic pain condition seen by primary care physicians, and it is often considered a vexing problem in clinical practice. In primary care settings, the management of chronic pain in general and back pain in particular is fraught with unresolved difficulties (Von Korff, 1994). Chronic back pain patients are often stereotyped by primary care physicians as difficult, dependent, and poorly motivated (Klein, Najman, Kohrman, & Munro, 1982; Cherkin, MacCornack, & Berg, 1988). Primary care physicians have been criticized for suboptimal use of pain medications (both over- and underprescribing) and for failure to use behavioral methods of pain management (Portenoy, 1989; Melzack, 1990; Turk, Holzman, & Kerns, 1986). There is also concern that primary care physicians may sanction disability, provide a gateway to misuse of pain medications, and discourage self-care by implicitly promising a medical solution to chronic pain (Fordyce, 1976; Osterweis, Kleinman, & Mechanic, 1987).

Whereas patients expect doctors to explain the cause of the back pain, control pain, and assist their return to normal activities, primary care physicians tend to view their role as providing diagnostic screening and palliative care until back pain resolves on its own (Cherkin et al., 1988). Given these discordant expectations, it is not surprising that the care of back pain is regarded by both patients and physicians as fraught with difficulties, frustrations, and misunderstandings (Cherkin & MacCornack, 1989; Deyo & Diehl, 1986).

THE COSTS OF BACK PAIN CARE

Cypress (1983) estimated in 1977–1978 that there were approximately 16 million physician visits for back pain per year in the United States. Given the large volume of patients seen for back pain, modest differences in the costs of an episode of back pain care can have large economic implications. The type of provider has been shown to have a significant effect on the costs of care. Carey et al. (1995) found that time to functional recovery was similar for acute back pain patients seen by orthopedic surgeons, chiropractors, and primary care physicians in North Carolina. However, after adjusting for case-mix differences, the mean costs of an episode of back pain care were about $500 for urban primary care physicians, whereas they were about $750 for orthopedic surgeons and $800 for urban chiropractors.

Among primary care physicians, there is evidence that differences in practice style are also associated with significant differences in costs. Von Korff, Barlow, Cherkin, and Deyo (1994) found that primary care physicians whose back-pain-practice style was characterized by infrequently prescribing bed rest and prescription pain relievers had significantly lower costs for back pain care over the following year (mean cost of care was $428) compared to physicians whose practice style was characterized by frequently prescribing pain medications and bed rest (mean cost $768). Again, costs differed, but long-term functional outcomes did not. In this cohort of patients, 21% of back pain patients accounted for 66% of the costs of back pain care, pointing to the importance of cost-effective management of the high-cost patient in determining the total costs of care (Engel, Von Korff, & Katon, 1996). These data suggest that a well-organized primary care service for back pain may be essential for controlling the costs of back pain care on a population basis.

A RESEARCH AGENDA FOR PRIMARY CARE

In 1995, an International Forum for Primary Care Research on Low Back Pain, held in Seattle, Washington, convened leading researchers studying the management of back pain in primary care settings. Through a group consensus process (Borkan & Cherkin, 1996), priorities for future research were identified. Among the top priorities were:

> Defining meaningful subgroups of back pain patients and criteria for classification.
> Developing strategies for containing and reversing back pain disability and costs.
> Developing and testing effective psychosocial interventions for back pain.
> Developing and testing new ways for primary care physicians to manage back pain.
> Developing self-care approaches that enhance self-reliance among persons with recurrent or chronic back pain.
> Determining how patient and provider beliefs and expectations influence the outcomes of care.

This chapter addresses these priorities by developing an individualized stepped-care model for management of back pain in the primary care setting. Underlying these research priorities was the sense that back pain management in primary care needed to move toward a more effective and satisfying balance between medical management and self-care. The objective of this chapter is to provide a framework for seeking a more effective balance between medical management and self-care of back pain in the primary care setting.

BACK PAIN: A RECURRENT-CHRONIC CONDITION

Management of back pain in primary care settings has often been based on the assumption that back pain is either acute or chronic and that the large majority of patients present with acute pain. When patients present with an acute exacerbation of back pain, many primary care physicians assume that the prognosis is quite favorable. Management has emphasized palliative interventions while the "tincture of time" allows the underlying injury to resolve.

In contrast, management of chronic back pain is an area of uncertainty for many primary care physicians. There is increased awareness of the importance of avoiding prolonged bed rest and encouraging patients to engage in physical exercise (Deyo, Diehl, & Rosenthal, 1986; Bigos et al., 1994). But in medical encounters, the benefits of physical exercise may be mentioned only briefly, without collaborative planning of how and when the patient should exercise (Turner, LeResche, Von Korff, & Ehrlich, 1998). Although there is growing awareness that patients with chronic back pain may be emotionally distressed (Von Korff & Simon, 1996) and experiencing problems in work and family life, interventions that enhance patients' abilities to cope with chronic back pain are not routinely available in primary care (Von Korff, 1994).

Chronic back pain is typically defined as an episode lasting 3 months or more, whereas episodes of shorter duration are considered acute (Nachemson & Bigos, 1984). Long-term outcome studies of primary care patients have found that a recurrent course is far more typical than either an acute or a chronic course and that primary care back pain patients experience chronic phases of back pain more often than previously believed (Von Korff, Deyo, Cherkin, & Barlow, 1993; Von Korff & Saunders, 1996). For example, Bergquist-Ullman and Larsson (1977) found that at 1-year follow-up of persons with acute or subacute back pain, 62% experienced at least one recurrence. In this study, 12% of study patients had back pain on more than half the days in the 1-year follow-up period (after excluding patients with chronic back pain at baseline). Von Korff and Saunders (1996) reported that among unselected primary care back pain patients assessed 1 year after a primary care visit, over 80% reported back pain in the prior 6 months and 60% reported back pain in the prior week. In this study, 32% characterized their back pain problem as "persistent" at 1-year follow-up, and 29% reported back pain on more than half the days in the prior 6 months. Hence recurrent back pain is typical and chronic back pain is common among primary care patients.

Recurrent back pain shares features of both acute pain (episodes are time-limited) and chronic pain (the condition persists over long periods of time and the significance of the underlying injury or disease is uncertain). There is evidence that intermittent back pain episodes can result in significant interference with activities (Von Korff et al., 1993). Given the episodic nature of back pain, it is questionable whether a primary descriptor of patient status (acute/chronic pain) should be based only on the duration of a single episode

(Von Korff & Saunders, 1996). Classification of cases on the basis of episode duration does not consider critical features of pain, such as its intensity and the degree of interference with activities. It may be more useful to differentiate cases based on their usual level of pain intensity, the degree of interference with activities, and the persistence of pain over an extended period of time (Von Korff, Ormel, Keefe, & Dworkin, 1992).

Prognostic information that adequately prepares patients for relapses and for times when back pain is chronic may be important in preparing patients to adequately adapt to a recurrent or chronic condition. For example, a patient who has been told to expect to be better within a week may become worried when back pain is still present 2 or 3 months later, which is often the case. However, since it is difficult to predict with a high degree of reliability which patients will experience continuing activity limitations and which patients will have a favorable short-term outcome, effective management may need to match the level of care to the patient's outcome. For example, most patients may not want or need any service beyond the initial primary care visit for back pain, but patients found to have continuing activity limitations a month or two after the visit may need an appropriate intervention that addresses their ongoing difficulties.

Given that back pain is typically recurrent and often chronic, assessment and management in primary care should be appropriate for patients with a prior history of back pain episodes and high likelihood of experiencing back pain episodes in the future. Thus care may need to prepare patients for managing future flare-ups of back pain and to provide adequate support for effective management of a chronic or recurrent pain condition.

SELF-MANAGEMENT IS ESSENTIAL FOR RECURRENT AND CHRONIC PAIN

In management of a recurrent or chronic illness, collaboration between patients and health care providers is important for effective and cost-effective management (Von Korff, Gruman, Schaefer, Curry, & Wagner, 1997). For back pain care, it is also what patients and providers often prefer. In a primary care study carried out at Group Health Cooperative of Puget Sound (Turner et al., 1998), primary care back pain patients and their physicians were asked, "Who should direct patient care for back pain?" The large majority of both patients and physicians said that it should be either a shared responsibility or that the patient should direct care mostly (see Table 22.1). Only 5% of physicians and 12% of patients said that the clinician should mostly or totally direct back pain care. Collaborative management of chronic illness has been defined as "care that strengthens and supports self-care in chronic illness while assuring that effective medical, preventive and health maintenance interventions take place" (Von Korff et al., 1997).

For the large majority of back pain patients in primary care, outcomes are more dependent on effective self-care (e.g., exercise, sustaining work activities, appropriate use of pain medications) than on the quality of the diagnostic or therapeutic interventions of physicians. Clark, Becker, Janz, Lorig, Rawkowski, and Anderson (1991), Lorig (1993) and others (Von Korff et al., 1997) have identified the core tasks of self-care of chronic illness that are directly applicable to self-care of chronic pain. Effective self-care of a chronic illness involves engaging in health promoting activities (e.g., exercise); minimizing the impacts of illness on daily activities; monitoring illness and adapting to changes (e.g., flare-ups); collaborating with health care providers in developing a management plan; and carrying out or adhering to a management plan and to specific treatments.

In the following sections, an individualized "stepped-care" model is developed that provides a framework for strengthening and supporting self-care of back pain in primary care settings.

ENHANCING PATIENT READINESS FOR SELF-CARE

Important self-care tasks in managing back pain include restoring and sustaining activities in work and family life, engaging in regular physical exercise, managing the effects of back pain on emotions

and interactions with others, pacing physical activities, using effective body mechanics to reduce risks of a flare-up, and making appropriate use of health care services and pharmacological treatments for back pain. Given the primary importance of these self-care tasks in determining the outcomes of back pain, a key question is how health care providers can strengthen and support patient self-care skills and their readiness to integrate these self-care behaviors into their daily routine.

Kerns, Rosenberg, Jamison, Caudill and Haythornthwaite (1997) have recently applied the "stages of change" model to assessing readiness for self-care of chronic pain. This model (Prochaska & DiClemente, 1983) holds that behavior change occurs in the following stages:

> *Precontemplation*—the person is not yet considering changing a target behavior.
> *Contemplation*—the person is considering changing the behavior.
> *Preparation*—the person is making plans to change the behavior.
> *Action*—the person has begun to change the behavior.
> *Maintenance*—the behavior has become part of the person's routine.

A key implication of the stages of change framework is that behavior change interventions are more likely to be effective if they are individualized to the person's level of readiness. Although the stage of change model is a useful heuristic for guiding behavior change interventions, this model has important limitations in its application to readiness for management of chronic pain. Most significantly, self-care of chronic pain involves an interrelated set of behaviors and attitudes (Turk, Meichenbaum, & Genest, 1983), and patient readiness to adopt different self-care behaviors in that set may differ. For example, a patient may be quite self-reliant in managing the impacts of back pain on work performance but not ready to engage in regular exercise. Readiness for self-care may be behavior-specific, rather than reflecting a global readiness for self-care.

In efforts to support self-care of chronic illness, patient-centered approaches may be more successful than directive advice (Anderson, 1995). In an audiotape study of 76 back pain visits (described in greater detail in a subsequent section and in Turner et al., 1998), it was common for physicians to recommend exercise in a directive fashion. However, it was uncommon for physicians

TABLE 22.1. Who Should Direct Back Pain Care?: Responses of Primary Care Back Pain Patients and Their Clinicians (n = 76)

Response	% of clinicians	% of patients
Patient entirely	4	7
Patient mostly	28	26
Shared	52	51
Clinician mostly/totally	5	12
Someone else	11	4

to ask patients if they were interested in increasing their level of exercise, what kinds of exercise they were already doing or had done in the past, what kinds of exercise they preferred, or what kind of exercise they were most likely to be able to sustain. When patients spontaneously mentioned exercises they were already doing, the physicians did not consistently offer praise and encouragement that might increase the likelihood of maintaining the behavior. Because patients differ in their preferences for particular self-care behaviors, providing options and choices is important, along with tailoring advice to the patient's level of readiness.

AN INDIVIDUALIZED STEPPED-CARE MODEL FOR MANAGING BACK PAIN

Pain management in the primary care setting faces three significant challenges:

1. The time available for assessment and management of patients in any one contact is relatively brief.
2. Primary care physicians see patients varying widely in severity and chronicity of their pain condition (Von Korff et al., 1992).
3. It cannot be reliably determined at the time of the initial primary care visit whether a particular patient is likely to have a favorable outcome requiring only acute palliative care or a less favorable long-term outcome that might benefit from subsequent interventions to support effective self-care.

These three challenges can be addressed by an individualized stepped-care approach.

Stepped care has been used for management of a wide range of medical and behavioral conditions, including hypertension (SHEP Cooperative Research Group, 1991), alcohol dependence (Donovan & Marlatt, 1993), nicotine dependence (Hurt, 1993), cholesterol reduction (Oster et al., 1995), and bulimia (Treasure, Schmidt, Tiller, Todd, & Turnbill, 1996). The essence of a stepped-care approach is that care is modified based on the patient's outcome. For example, a patient whose hypertension is not adequately controlled on a first-line medication may be stepped up to a second-line medication (SHEP Cooperative Research Group, 1991). Or patients who do not experience

a good outcome after receiving minimal self-care intervention may be stepped up to more intensive services (Treasure et al., 1996; Donovan & Marlatt, 1993).

The stepped-care approach described in this chapter addresses specific patient worries, difficulties, and activity limitations associated with back pain (see Table 22.2). A form of stepped-care is proposed in which care is personalized to each patient's specific concerns, activity limitations, preferences, and level of readiness, and the level of care is guided by the severity and duration of activity limitations of the patient observed at outcome. Tiemens (1999) has called this combination of stepped-care and matching *individualized stepped care.* Abrams et al. (1996) initially proposed the integration of stepped care and treatment matching strategies for treatment of tobacco dependence. In individualized stepped care, the level and intensity of care is guided by the observed outcome, but treatment matching may also occur based on specific patient concerns and activity limitations, on patient preferences and readiness, or when a patient's initial status merits aggressive intervention.

TABLE 22.2. An Individualized Stepped-Care Model of Managing Back Pain in Primary Care

Step 1. For all back pain patients

Identify and address specific patient worries.
Identify and support the patient's motivation for self-care.

Step 2. For moderately impaired back pain patients

Support management of common activity limitations.
    Identify difficulties and goals.
    Support planning to overcome difficulties and to achieve goals.
    Support the patient's motivation for exercise.

Referral to a low-cost self-care program is a desirable option for Step 2.

Step 3. For severely impaired back pain patients

Address work performance difficulties.
    Identify work difficulties.
    Prescribe early return to work (with light duty if necessary).
    Consider graded exercise and strengthening.
    Refer for active intervention if return to work is at risk.

Identify and treat clinical depression.

Step 1: Identify and Address Patient Worries, Support Self-Care

At Step 1, the clinician focuses on identifying and addressing specific patient worries and supporting the patient's motivation for self-care. Step 1 is applied to all patients seeking primary care for back pain. For many primary care patients, worries, concerns, and attitudes toward self-care may be readily influenced by brief counseling in the primary care visit or by minimal educational interventions offered in the primary care setting.

Common worries of back pain patients concern health status and physical activity. Table 22.3 provides data on the percent of primary care back pain patients who agree with statements concerning specific worries about health status and about physical activity. These patients had volunteered to participate in a randomized controlled trial of an educational intervention to improve self-care. They had all had at least one back pain visit before their most recent visit. They were interviewed about 2 months after their most recent back pain visit.

It was common for these patients to be worried about long-term disability and to fear that back pain might mean there was something seriously wrong with their backs. A smaller proportion of patients were worried that their back pain might be due to a serious disease. It was common for patients to be worried that a wrong movement could cause a serious problem and to believe that avoiding unnecessary movement was a safe way to prevent pain from worsening. A minority of patients thought that they might injure themselves if they exercised or that it was unsafe to be physically active.

There are a number of approaches to reducing these common worries of primary care patients that could become a routine part of the primary care visit. To reduce worries about serious disease, the primary care physician should explain the "red flags" for serious disease and how the history and diagnostic examination exclude serious conditions (infection, cancer, etc.). Patients can then be asked to identify any residual worries so that they can be discussed specifically. Providing clear and personalized information relevant to a patient's specific worries can be helpful. Ensuring that patients understand that it is safe and beneficial to resume normal activities as the flare-up subsides and explaining why this is helpful is also important. In general, recommending actions that counter a patient's worries is likely to be beneficial. Providing advice on sensible ways of resuming physical activities may be helpful in reducing worries about physical activity while preparing patients for the likelihood of additional flare-ups and residual pain in the future.

Step 1 should also identify and support the patient's motivation for self-care. Although physicians sometimes assume that back pain patients seek care to obtain a diagnosis, specific treatments, and/or prescription pain medications, patients are often motivated to seek care for reasons that are generally consistent with self-care. Primary care back pain patients were asked to rate the importance of different objectives for their visit (Turner et al., 1998). Visit objectives most often rated extremely or very important were receiving information on managing the back pain problem, on reducing pain without prescription medications, on resuming normal activities as quickly as possible, and on preventing recurrences (see Table 22.4). A major-

TABLE 22.3. Percentage of Primary Care Back Pain Patients Agreeing with Statements Concerning Worries about Back Pain 2 Months after Their Primary Care Visit

Health worries (n = 250)	
I might become disabled for a long time by back pain.	60%
I wouldn't have this much pain if there weren't something dangerously wrong.	45%
Back pain might be due to a serious disease.	19%
Worries about physical activity (n = 226)	
The wrong movement could lead to a serious problem.	64%
Avoiding unnecessary movements is the safest way to prevent pain from worsening.	51%
I might injure myself if I exercise.	31%
It's not safe to be physically active.	13%

Note. Back pain patients volunteered to participate in a self-care intervention study with previous back pain visits.

TABLE 22.4. Percentage of Primary Care Back Pain Patients Rating Visit
Objectives as Extremely or Very Important (n = 76)

Objective for the visit	Percent
To receive information on . . .	
How to manage back pain	85
How to reduce back pain without prescription drugs	83
What you can do to get back to your usual activities as quickly as possible	81
How to prevent a recurrence of back pain	76
The likely course of back pain	76
The cause of back pain	64
Receive . . .	
A medical diagnosis	68
Reassurance that you don't have a serious disease	52
A medical treatment that permanently cures your back pain	51
A prescription medicine to relieve your current back pain	35
An X-ray or other diagnostic test	34
A referral to a physical therapist	30
A referral to a medical specialist	27
A note to excuse absence from work	12

ity of patients also rated receiving a medical diagnosis, receiving information on the cause of back pain, and reassurance that back pain was not due to a serious disease as extremely or very important. While these objectives call on the medical competence of the clinician, addressing them is likely to increase the readiness of most patients for self-care. A common patient objective that seems less consistent with self-care is receiving a medical treatment that permanently cures the back pain problem, which was rated as extremely or very important by 51% of the study patients. For the large majority of primary care back pain patients, this is an unrealistic expectation that deserves discussion and clear feedback on the limits of medical diagnosis and treatment of back pain problems. In general, the most commonly rated goals of primary care back pain patients in this study were consistent with fostering back pain self-care.

The patient's readiness for self-care can be enhanced in many ways during the initial primary care visit. Patients can be given more realistic information about the likelihood of recurrences and told that chronic back pain is a common problem that does not need to be disabling. Such prognostic information needs to be combined with unambiguous information that chronic or recurrent back pain is bothersome but that it is rarely indicative of serious disease or pathology. Reviewing the "red flags" that indicate when medical care is necessary for back pain (Bigos et al., 1994) can help patients

understand that medical care for back pain is usually optional and that medical treatment offers nothing more than sensible self-care for the large majority of patients. Readiness for self-care may be enhanced by asking patients how they are managing back pain, followed by offering strong support for effective self-care strategies that the patient is already trying. Enumerating things that the patient can do to manage activity limitations can help patients identify alternatives to a "medical cure." Finally, developing a plan for managing flare-ups may help patients prepare for their next severe episode of back pain.

Step 2: Support Management of Common Activity Limitations

For patients who continue to experience moderate to severe activity limitations several weeks after the initial primary care visit, interventions that support active management of difficulties may be warranted. Active management means identifying the patient's difficulties, helping the patient identify goals for overcoming those difficulties, developing action plans for achieving those goals, and providing ongoing support and follow-up for patients carrying out an action plan (Von Korff et al., 1997). Although some of these tasks can be done in the primary care visit, supporting active management is likely to require supportive interventions outside the primary care visit itself. Our research team is currently testing such interventions with primary care back pain patients with positive results in two large randomized controlled trials (Von Korff et al., in press).

Step 3: Address Work Performance Difficulties, Identify and Treat Clinical Depression

The majority of primary care back pain patients do not experience significant interference with work activities, nor are they clinically depressed. However, in a long-term follow-up study of primary care back pain patients from Group Health Cooperative of Puget Sound, we found that 2–3% reported being unable to work at follow-up 1 to 5 years after the primary care visit and that a similar percent reported receiving worker's compensation for back pain (see Table 22.5). About 8% reported having been unable to obtain or keep full-time work due to back pain in the prior year at long-term follow-up. At long-term follow-up, almost 15% reported 14 or more days in the prior 6 months when they were unable to carry out their usual activities (work, school, or housework) due to back pain. And about 19–25% reported that they accomplished less at work in the prior 2 weeks due to back pain. At baseline, 22% had SCL-90 depres-

sion scores that placing them in the top 10% of depression symptom severity, whereas about 15–17% had elevated depression levels at 1 and 2 years. By 5 years, the percent clinically depressed was similar to population norms (11.2 %). These data indicate that a significant minority of primary care back pain patients experience continuing difficulties with work performance, ranging from reduced performance and missed days to a much smaller set of patients who are work-disabled. And a significant minority are clinically depressed. Step 3 of the stepped-care model addresses the needs of these more severely impaired patients.

Because Step 3 focuses attention on a much smaller number of more severely impaired patients, more active and aggressive intervention is called for. Step 3 requires the primary care physician to ask a limited number of screening questions to identify patients who have significant work performance difficulties or who are clinically depressed. For those patients meriting active intervention to restore work performance, actions of the primary care physician may include prescribing early return to work, with light duty if necessary; considering a graded exercise and strengthening, or work-hardening, program; or, when return to work is questionable, referring the patient for active intervention to maximize the likelihood of return to work. For patients who are clinically depressed, active pharmacological or psychotherapeutic treat-

TABLE 22.5. Indicators of Interference with Work Activities and Clinical Depression among Unselected Primary Care Back Pain Patients, 1 Month, 1 Year, 2 Years, and 5 Years after the Index Visit

	Baseline (n = 1,213)	1 year (n = 1,128)	2 years (n = 1,024)	5 years (n = 819)
Unable to work	3.8%	2.0%	2.9%	2.8%
Receiving worker's compensation for back pain				
Currently	3.5%	1.5%	2.0%	2.6%
Ever in lifetime	13.8%			
Unable to obtain or keep full-time work due to back pain				
In the past year	8.5%	11.0%	7.5%	7.5%
Ever in lifetime	15.9%			
Days kept from usual activities (work, school, housework) in the prior 6 months due to back pain				
1 or more	65.0%	41.3%	40.9%	42.0%
7 or more	45.9%	20.8%	18.9%	21.7%
14 or more	35.1%	13.8%	13.3%	14.7%
30 or more	20.8%	9.6%	9.0%	10.4%
90 or more	6.9%	4.8%	4.8%	5.4%
Accomplished less at work in the prior 2 weeks due to back pain (among employed)	32.4%	18.9%	20.5%	25.3%
High SCL-90 Depression score (score of 1.5 or greater)	22.1%	17.3%	15.5%	11.2%

ment is merited for those meeting criteria for major depression (American Psychiatric Association, 1987). For all Step 3 patients with either significant work disability or clinically significant depression, active follow-up by the primary care physician's staff is warranted to monitor restoration of work performance or therapeutic response to depression treatments.

THE ANATOMY OF A BACK PAIN VISIT IN PRIMARY CARE

In the preceding section, an individualized stepped-care model for managing primary care back pain patients was outlined. This section reviews the anatomy of the primary care back pain visit and its process and content. The observed management of back pain in the primary care visit is compared to the proposed stepped-care model. The data presented in this section were derived from a study in which primary care visits were audiotaped and coded for 76 back pain patients (Turner et al., 1998). Information was also collected from patients by interview immediately before the visit and 1 month later.

Structure of the Primary Care Visit

A consistent structure of the back pain visit was observed. The five parts of the prototypical primary care visit were (1) social introduction or greeting, (2) brief history of the problem, (3) physical examination, (4) treatment recommendations, and (5) closing. The visit typically opened with a social interchange or greeting. The clinician then took a brief history of the problem and conducted a physical examination. The history would begin with a general statement such as, "What can I help you with today?" or a back-pain-specific question or statement such as, "Tell me about your back pain." Following the physical examination, the doctor and patient discussed treatment options, after which the visit was closed. This structure allowed the clinician to efficiently take a history, conduct a physical examination, prescribe acute treatments for short-term control of pain, and give advice about self-care within the 10 to 15 minutes typically available. However, as we shall see, the visits did not in general systematically identify or address patient worries, identify functional difficulties, identify goals for overcoming difficulties, develop plans for achieving goals, or systematically identify and ad-

dress significant difficulties in performance of work activities.

Assessing and Addressing Patient Worries

In conducting the physical examinations that were routinely performed for almost every primary care patient participating in the audiotape study, the physicians often did not take the opportunity to explain what they were looking for, nor did they explain what serious conditions had been excluded. In no visit did the clinician systematically explain the "red flags" that indicate that medical attention is necessary, although questions about the presence of some of the red flag signs and symptoms were assessed in most visits. Eleven patients raised disease worries (including such things as arthritis, spinal or nerve problems, kidney problems, osteoporosis, and multiple sclerosis). The coders rating the audiotapes assessed these worries as being fully addressed 50% of the time, partially addressed 28% of the time, and not addressed 22% of the time. According to the rating of the audiotapes, only 22% of the study patients were told to stay active and to avoid bed rest. In general, the primary care physicians were not giving a clear explanation of why engaging in normal activities and physical exercise was safe even when back pain continued, although they often advised that exercise was beneficial. Although patient worries about long-term disability are quite common among back pain patients, this patient concern was rarely discussed by the primary care clinician in a systematic manner. These results suggest that there is considerable room for improvement in eliciting and addressing common patient worries in the primary care visit.

Supporting Self-Care

An intriguing finding of the audiotape study was that 47% of the study patients mentioned three or more things that they were doing to self-manage back pain during the visit. Only 10% of the study patients did not mention anything that they were doing to manage back pain. Among the practices mentioned by the study patients, 85% were considered effective self-care techniques by the study investigators. Although the clinicians rarely discouraged self-care, they often did not actively support the self-care practices mentioned by patients. Thus there appeared to be many missed opportunities to focus the visit on self-care rather than on medical management of back pain. Moreover, when the clinicians gave self-care advice, their recommendations were planned in a collaborative fashion only 17% of the time. The clinician's recommendations were actively accepted by the patient only 25% of the time. The operational definition of collaborative planning was that the clinician explicitly checked to see whether the patient agreed with the recommendation. It was more common for the clinicians to reiterate their recommendations (this occurred for 57% of all recommendations). These results suggest a significant opportunity to change the primary focus of the visit from the clinician's treatment recommendations to supporting and enhancing the patient's self-care practices.

Prognostic Information

The prognostic information given to patients was somewhat ambiguous and not fully in line with the current understanding of the natural history of back pain among primary care patients. Coding of audiotapes determined that 72% of the study patients were told to expect their back pain to improve, but it was generally left ambiguous what "improved" meant. Twenty-three percent were told to expect to be pain-free. In contrast, only 20% were told to expect their back pain to recur, and 11% were told that chronic back pain is not unusual. Thirty-nine percent were given information about how long it takes for back pain to improve. Among these patients, 57% were told to expect their pain to improve within 2 weeks or less. It was unusual for the clinician to make a clear distinction between the worst pain that would be over within a matter of days and residual back pain that would continue for a longer time period.

Examples of overly optimistic prognostic statements included: "Back disorders gradually get better and they usually go away completely, 100%." "The pain itself should get better over several days, at the most a few weeks, but usually its just a few days." "Should just get better in a few days, don't think you have to worry about any long-term problem." Although these favorable prognostic statements are intended to be reassuring, they may have the opposite effect for patients whose pain does not improve as quickly as expected. An example of a more realistic, and perhaps more reassuring, prognostic statement was the following: "Backs can take a while to heal, up to a couple of months. You will probably have a complete resolution, but it may

flare up again. That doesn't mean there is anything seriously wrong." This prognostic statement combines a realistic appraisal of the variable time course of back pain with reassurance that taking a while to get better and experiencing future flare-ups do not indicate that there is something dangerously wrong with the back.

Assessing Patient Goals and Goal Setting

Data on patient goals for the primary care visit reviewed earlier (see Table 22.4) suggest that patients have a multiplicity of goals for the visit and that many of the goals that are highly rated are consistent with patients assuming greater responsibility for self-care. At the same time, many patients endorse goals for the primary care visit that are consistent with medical management of back pain (e.g. receiving a diagnosis, obtaining a permanent medical cure, or being given a prescription pain medication). Given the number of goals that patients have and their heterogeneity, clarification and targeting of goals might be considered an important task for the opening phase of the primary care visit.

In reviewing the audiotapes of primary care back pain visits, it was surprising that the clinicians rarely asked patients to identify or clarify their most important goals for the visit. There was only one case in which the clinician specifically asked a patient to state his or her objectives for the visit. Clarification of patient goals is likely to require an opening question that more specifically elicits these goals and follow-up responses for patients who have difficulty identifying their objectives. A checklist completed by the patient before the visit begins might be an efficient means of helping patients clarify and target their most important goals for the visit.

Assessing Interference with Activities and Work Performance

A stepped-care approach depends on the primary care clinician being able to differentiate patients who are experiencing only limited impairment from those who are moderately to severely impaired at the time of the initial visit and on the capacity of the primary care team to follow up with patients to briefly assess functional recovery 6 to 8 weeks after the primary care visit. Unfortunately, at the time of the initial visit, analysis of the audiotapes revealed uneven assessment of functional status. As shown in Table 22.6, relatively few patients were asked by their clinician about interference with work or family responsibilities. It was more common for patients to mention interference with activities than it was for the clinicians to inquire. But even including times that the problem of interference was raised by the patient, information about whether the patient had taken time off work or housework due to back pain was elicited in only 36% of the visits. It was more common for information about interference with specific activities to be discussed (such as lifting or sitting), but this information was twice as likely to be brought up by the patient as it was to be elicited by the physician. In contrast, a number of kinds of information about pain was discussed in more than 75% of the visits, typically raised by the physician (see Table 22.7). Commonly discussed pain topics included the pattern of the pain, the history of prior episodes, the duration of the current episode, whether pain radiates to the leg, what brought on the current episode, and what makes the pain better and worse. The relative inattention to interference with daily activities and the greater attention to pain may inadvertently foreclose opportunities to focus the visit on self-management strategies that patients can use to improve their performance of daily activities. It is likely that greater attention to pain than to interference with daily activities reflects clinician beliefs in the importance of information about pain for the diagnostic evaluation of the underlying condition.

Among the patients in the audiotape study, 42% rated their interference with work activities in the past week as great (7 or greater on a 0–10 scale), and an additional 23% rated work interference as moderate (4–6). Only 16% indicated that they had no interference with work activities in the prior week. When asked before the visit how important it was to receive information on what could be done to return to normal activities as quickly as possible, 47% rated this as extremely important, an additional 35% rated this as very important, and only 5% rated it as not at all important. These results suggest that there may be an important opportunity to increase the focus of the back pain visit on the performance of work and family activities by the patient and away from the diagnostic significance of the report of pain. By focusing on interference with daily activities, the clinician may create a context in which self-management is brought to the fore and medical management of pain is given less prominence.

Treatment Recommendations and Advice

Table 22.8 summarizes the treatment recommendations made by the clinicians in the latter part of the visit. In general, the treatment recommendations were responsible and in accord with guidelines for conservative management of back pain (Bigos et al., 1994). Typically, patients were managed with some combination of nonsteroidal anti-inflammatory medication, advice about exercise, and referral to physical therapy. Less frequently, muscle relaxant or opioid medications were prescribed. However, the number of distinct treatment recommendations made in these relatively brief visits was quite remarkable. On average, the clinicians made seven different recommendations. As a result of the number of recommendations, the part of the visit in which treatment and self-care advice was offered had a hurried quality. Often, the clinician gave advice without taking time to determine how this fit with the patient's preferences or with the patient's readiness to engage in the recommended self-care behaviors. Given the number of treatment recommendations, one might wonder

TABLE 22.6. Assessment of Activity Limitations in 76 Audiotaped Primary Care Back Pain Visits

	Percent of visits		
Topic	Asked by clinician	Brought up by patient	Total
Has the patient taken time off work or housework due to back pain?	13.2	22.4	35.6
Does back pain interfere with work?	14.5	17.1	31.6
Does back pain interfere with family responsibilities?	2.6	3.9	6.5
Does back pain interfere with social life?	10.5	22.4	32.9
Does back pain interfere with specific activities (e.g., lifting, walking, sitting, driving)?	19.7	40.8	60.5

TABLE 22.7. Assessment of Pain in 76 Audiotaped Primary Care Back Pain Visits

| | Percent of visits | | |
Topic	Asked by clinician	Brought up by patient	Total
Pain pattern	67.1	21.1	88.2
Pain intensity rating	7.9	1.3	9.2
History of prior episodes	67.1	18.4	88.5
Duration of current episodes	53.9	40.8	94.7
Does pain radiate to the leg?	76.3	5.2	81.6
What brought on this episode?	46.1	34.2	80.3
What makes back pain worse?	32.9	43.4	76.3
What helps?	38.2	51.3	89.5

how the patient could recall what advice was given. Although the clinician would often write a prescription and might recommend a book on care of back pain that the patient might purchase, the advice rendered was not typically placed in written form. Patients generally left the visit with no documentation of the recommendations of the physician. If a standardized care plan supported by detailed instructions for the patient were routinely used in the primary care visit, with check-offs for recommended options, the limited time in the visit might be used to discuss patient preferences and readiness in a more collaborative fashion.

CONCLUSION

The current organization of the primary care visit emphasizes a diagnostically focused discussion of pain history and unfocused advice regarding control of symptoms and exercise. The proposed individualized stepped-care model offers an approach

TABLE 22.8. Recommendations Made by the Clinicians in 76 Audiotaped Visits

Recommendations	Percent of patients
Activating recommendations	
Walking, not specifically aerobic	34
Strengthening exercise	30
Stretching	28
Stay active/avoid bed rest	22
Exercise not otherwise specified	20
Flexibility exercise	17
Aerobic exercise	12
Symptom-focused recommendations	
Over-the-counter, nonsteroidal anti-inflammatory drugs	88
Cold	39
Heat	34
"Muscle relaxants"	28
Opioids	14
Massage	11
Other recommendations	
X-ray	18
Chiropractor	7
Physical therapy	54
Mean number of recommendations per patient	7

to focusing the primary care visit on addressing common patient worries, supporting self-care, supporting patient efforts to manage difficulties with daily activities, and, for severely impaired patients, addressing work performance difficulties and treating clinical depression. Full implementation of the proposed stepped-care model is likely to require low-cost self-management interventions in primary care settings and the development of accessible (and reasonably priced) services for managing patients with significant work performance difficulties. The proposed stepped-care model offers a framework that limits the medicalization of back pain care while responding to the worries of the large majority of back pain patients and the functional disabilities of patients significantly impaired by back pain. How primary care services can be organized to implement this stepped-care approach will require rigorous, empirical research testing its effectiveness. However, this approach allows for most patients to be managed within the constraints of the brief primary care visit with changes in the emphasis of the visit. The individualized stepped-care model also permits targeting services that address the functional disabilities of patients whose activity limitations are more severe in cost-effective ways.

ACKNOWLEDGMENTS

This chapter is based on a lecture given at the University of Calgary, December 5, 1997: "Back Pain Management and Outcome in Primary Care: Can We Do Better?" It was supported by grants from the National Institute for Dental Research (No. POI DE08773) and the Agency for Health Care Policy and Research (No. RO1 HS06168).

REFERENCES

Abrams, D. B., Orleans, C. T., Niaura, R. S., Goldstein, M. G., Proschaska, J. O., & Velicer, W. (1996). Integrating individual and public health perspectives for treatment of tobacco dependence under managed health care: A combined stepped-care and matching model. *Annals of Behavioral Medicine, 18*(4), 290–304.

American Academy of Family Physicians. (1987). *Facts about: Family practice*. Kansas City: Author.

American Psychiatric Association. (1987). *Diagnostic and statistical manual of mental disorders* (3rd ed., rev.). Washington, DC: Author.

Anderson, R. M. (1995). Patient empowerment and the traditional medical model: A case of irreconcilable differences? *Diabetes Care, 18*, 412–415.

Bergquist-Ullman, M., & Larsson, U. (1977). Acute low back pain in industry: A controlled prospective study with special reference to therapy and confounding factors. *Acta Orthopaedica Scandinavica, 170*, 1–117.

Bigos, S. J., Bowyer, O. R., Braen, G. R., Brown, K., Deyo, R., Haldeman, S., Hart, J. L., Johnson, E. W., Keller, R., Kido, D., Liang, M. H., Nelson, R. M., Nordin, M., Owen, B. D., Pope, M. H., Schwartz, R. K., Stewart, D. H., Susman, J., Triano, J. J., Tripp, L. C., Turk, D. C., Watts, C., & Weinstein, J. N. (1994). *Acute low back problems in adults. Clinical Practice Guideline No. 14* (AHCPR Publication No. 95-0642). Rockville, MD: U.S. Department of Health and Human Services, Agency for Health Care Policy and Research.

Borkan, J. M., & Cherkin, D. C. (1996). An agenda for primary care research on low back pain. *Spine, 21*, 2880–2884.

Carey, T. S., Garrett, J., Jackman, A., McLaughlin, C., Fryer, J., & Smucker, D. R. (1995). The outcomes and costs of care for acute low back pain among patients seen by primary care practitioners. *New England Journal of Medicine, 333*, 913–917.

Cherkin, D. C., & MacCornack, F. A. (1989). Patient evaluations of low back pain care from family physicians and from chiropractors. *Western Journal of Medicine, 150*, 351–355.

Cherkin, D. C., MacCornack, F. A., & Berg, A. O. (1988). The management of low back pain: A comparison of the beliefs and behaviors of family physicians and chiropractors. *Western Journal of Medicine, 149*, 475–480.

Clark, N. M., Becker, M. H., Janz, N. K., Lorig, K., Rawkowski, W., & Anderson, L. (1991). Self-management of chronic disease by older adults: A review and questions for research. *Journal of Aging and Health, 3*, 3–27.

Cypress, B. K. (1983). Characteristics of physician visits for back symptoms: A national perspective. *American Journal of Public Health, 73*, 389–395.

Deyo, R. A., & Diehl, A. K. (1986). Patient satisfaction with medical care for low-back pain. *Spine, 11*, 28–30.

Deyo, R. A., Diehl, A. K., & Rosenthal, M. (1986). How many days of bed rest for acute low back pain? A randomized clinical trial. *New England Journal of Medicine, 315*, 1064–1070.

Donovan, D. M., & Marlatt, G. A. (1993). Recent developments in alcoholism behavioral treatment. *Recent Developments in Alcoholism, 11*, 397–411.

Engel, C. C., Von Korff, M., & Katon, W. J. (1996). Back pain in primary care: Predictors of high health care costs. *Pain, 65*, 197–204.

Fordyce, W. E. (1976). *Behavioral methods in chronic pain and illness*. St. Louis, MO: Mosby.

Hurt, R. D. (1993). Nicotine dependence—treatment for the 1990s [Editorial]. *Journal of Internal Medicine, 233*, 307–310.

Kerns, R. D., Rosenberg, R., Jamison, R. N., Caudill, M. A., & Haythornthwaite, J. (1997). Readiness to adopt a self-management approach to chronic pain: The Pain Stages of Change Questionnaire. *Pain, 72*, 227–234.

Klein, D., Najman, J., Kohrman, A. F., & Munro, C. (1982). Patient characteristics that elicit negative responses from family physicians. *Journal of Family Practice, 5*, 881–888.

Lorig, K. (1993, Fall). Self-management of chronic illness: A model for the future. *Generations, 11*–14.

Melzack, R. (1990). The tragedy of needless pain. *Scientific American, 262*, 27–33.

Nachemson, A., & Bigos, S. J. (1984) The low back. In J. Cruess & W. R. J. Rennie (Eds.), *Adult orthopedics* (pp. 843–937). New York: Churchill-Livingstone.

Oster, G., Borok, G. M., Menzin, J., Heys, J. F., Epstein, R. S., Quinn, V., Benson, V. V., Dudl, R. J., & Epstein, A. (1995). A randomized trial to assess effectiveness and cost in clinical practice: Rationale and design of the Cholesterol Reduction Intervention Study. *Controlled Clinical Trials, 16*, 3–16.

Osterweis, M., Kleinman, A., & Mechanic, D. (1987). *Pain and disability: Clinical, behavioral and public policy perspectives.* Washington, DC: National Academy Press.

Portenoy, R. K. (1989). Opioid therapy in the management of chronic back pain. In C. D. Tollison (Ed.), *Interdisciplinary rehabilitation of low back pain* (pp. 137–157). Baltimore: Williams & Wilkins.

Prochaska, J. O., & DiClemente, C. C. (1983). Stages and processes of self-change of smoking: Toward an integrative model of change. *Journal of Consulting and Clinical Psychology, 51*, 390–395.

SHEP Cooperative Research Group. (1991). Prevention of stroke in antihypertensive drug treatment in older persons with isolated hypertension: Final results of the Systolic Hypertension in the Elderly Program. *Journal of the American Medical Association, 265*, 3255–3264.

Starfield, B. (1992). *Primary care: Concept, evaluation, policy.* New York: Oxford University Press.

Tiemens, B. (1999). *Management of mental disorders in primary care: The doctor, the patient, and the medical model.* Doctoral dissertation, University of Groningen, The Netherlands.

Treasure, J., Schmidt, U., Tiller, J., Todd, G., & Turnbill, S. (1996). Sequential treatment for bulimia nervosa incorporating a self-care manual. *British Journal of Psychiatry, 168*, 98–98.

Turk, D. C., Holzman, A. D., & Kerns, R. D. (1986). Chronic pain. In K. A. Holroyd & T. L. Creer (Eds.), *Self-management of chronic disease: Handbook of clinical interventions and research* (pp. 441–471). Orlando, FL: Academic Press.

Turk, D. C., Meichenbaum, D., & Genest, M. (1983). *Pain and behavioral medicine: A cognitive-behavioral perspective.* New York: Guilford Press.

Turner, J. A., LeResche, L., Von Korff, M., & Ehrlich, K. (1998). Primary care back pain patient characteristics, visit content and short-term outcomes. *Spine, 23*, 463–469.

Von Korff, M. (1994). Perspectives on management of back pain in primary care. In G. F. Gebhardt & D. L. Hammond (Eds.), *Proceedings of the Seventh World Congress on Pain: Vol. 2. Progress in pain research and management.* Seattle, WA: IASP Press.

Von Korff, M., Barlow, W., Cherkin, D., & Deyo, R. A. (1994). Effects of practice style in managing back pain. *Annals of Internal Medicine, 121*, 187–195.

VonKorff, M., Deyo, R. A., Cherkin, D., & Barlow, W. (1993). Back pain in primary care: Outcomes at one year. *Spine, 18*, 855–862.

Von Korff, M., Gruman, J., Schaefer, J., Curry, S. J., & Wagner, E. H. (1997). Collaborative management of chronic illness. *Annals of Internal Medicine, 127*, 1097–1102.

Von Korff, M., Moore, J. E., Lorig, K., Cherkin, D. C., Saunders, K., Gonzales, V. M., Laurent, D., Rutter, C., & Comite, F. (in press). A randomized trial of a lay-led self-management group intervention for back pain patients in primary care. *Spine.*

Von Korff, M., Ormel, J., Keefe, F., & Dworkin, S. F. (1992). Grading the severity of chronic pain. *Pain, 50*, 133–149.

Von Korff, M., & Simon, G. (1996). The relationship of pain and depression. *British Journal of Psychiatry, 168*(Suppl. 30), 101–108.

Von Korff, M., & Saunders, K. (1996). The course of back pain in primary care. *Spine, 21*, 2833–2837.

Chapter 23

Prevention with Special Reference to Chronic Musculoskeletal Disorders

STEVEN J. LINTON

The prevention of chronic musculoskeletal pain (MSP) is an important challenge for the 21st century. Although chronic neck and back pain are not ordinarily life threatening, they inflict untold suffering and disability. Acute MSP serves an important function as a "warning signal," and it sets boundaries on our behavior. Thus we find that most people at some time during their life will suffer from MSP. However, a surprising number of people develop recurrent or chronic problems that not only cause suffering but also seriously disrupt normal life.

A few facts quickly underscore the pressing need for preventive interventions. Epidemiological studies indicate that as many as 85% of adults will miss work or seek professional care for MSP during their working career (Fordyce, 1995; Nachemson, 1992; Skovron, 1992; Waddell, 1996). For example, we asked a random sample of 35- to 45-year-olds to answer a questionnaire about MSP (Linton, Hellsing, & Halldén, 1998). The 1-year prevalence was, given the age group, an amazing 66%. Naturally, not all of those reporting pain had serious problems, but 25% were deemed to have a significant problem that included intense pain episodes and considerable functional hindrance. Nineteen percent of those with pain had taken sick leave for it during the previous year, and 15% said they had missed work because of the pain but had arranged the absence without being formally on sick leave. With an average number of health-care visits of 3 per person per year, this amounts to several thousand visits, making MSP one of the most common reasons for seeking medical care.

The distribution of the consumption of health care and compensation resources is highly skewed, with a small number of sufferers using the majority of the resources. In our study mentioned previously, just 6% of those reporting pain had more than 50% of the health care visits, a frequent finding in other studies as well (Reid, Haugh, Hazard, & Tripathi, 1997; Von Korff, 1994). There was also a correlation between health care utilization and sick leave, indicating that the same people tend to be high consumers of both entities. Thus less than 10% of the sufferers may consume as much as 70–80% of the resources (Linton, 1994; Reid et al., 1997; Skovron, 1992). Prevention aimed at hindering the development of such problems might then promise better quality of life for patients, as well as savings for health care and compensation systems.

Interestingly, epidemiological studies show that there may be a large number of people with recurrent or chronic pain problems who consume little or no resources. For example, Brattberg, Thorslund, and Wikman (1989) found that about 40% of the adult population reported considerable pain lasting more than 6 months, although many did not seek any health care for it. In a survey of nursing personnel, we found that the majority of nurses reporting moderate to intense pain often or always had not missed a single day of work during the past year for it (Linton & Buer, 1995). Some of these people might benefit from preventive interventions designed to hinder the problem from developing further. These data also demonstrate that many people cope with long-term or recurrent pain with little or no professional help.

It is well known that 85% of people suffering acute back pain return to work within 6 weeks (Reid et al., 1997), but this does not mean that they have recovered fully or permanently. Research shows that over 40% still report considerable pain and dysfunction a year after seeking primary care (Von Korff, 1994). As a result, the natural course appears to be recurrent episodes. For some, this will develop into more frequent and perhaps longer episodes, while a small minority will develop *chronic* pain, that is, of more than 6 months duration. In other words, most people who develop chronic problems requiring extended sick leave and health care apparently have a long history of recurrent problems before the occurrence of a long-term absence.

Because MSP is a common malady that may become recurrent or chronic, there are enormous costs involved. Unfortunately, although most resources pay for various forms of compensation for work loss, only a small fraction finance health care. A recent study in the Netherlands, for example, demonstrated that 93% of all expenditures were related to compensation and that only 7% went for actual care (van Tulder, Koes, & Bouter, 1995). Consider that the cost of back-related compensation alone costs the Netherlands, a country of some 15 million people, $150 million per hour (van Tulder et al., 1995)! The picture is similar in Sweden (Linton, 1998; National Board of Occupational Safety, 1996). Although health care expenditures have increased in absolute value, there is some evidence that the proportion being spent on health care as opposed to compensation has remained largely unchanged (Linton, 1998). And these expenditures may not always provide for early preventive interventions. Health care costs are largely spent on hospital-based diagnostics (e.g., MRIs) and procedures (e.g., surgery). Only a small amount is spent on primary care based interventions (Linton, 1998; van Tulder et al., 1995).

These facts show that MSP is related to considerable suffering and to disruption of normal life. Health care utilization, although costly, makes up a relatively small amount of the total cost and may be too little, too late. Work loss is considerable and accounts for fantastic sums. Although a surprisingly large number of people suffer from recurrent or chronic problems, a relatively small number account for a very significant proportion of the costs. Thus, from a humanitarian as well as a medical and socioeconomic perspective, there is a dire need for prevention.

This need for early and preventive interventions has been recognized by various government authorities around the world in recommendations for early care (Bigos et al., 1994; Fordyce, 1995; Frank, Kerr, et al., 1996; Kendall, Linton, & Main, 1997; National Board of Health and Welfare, 1987; Rosen, 1994; Swedish Council on Technology Assessment in Health Care, 1991). Moreover, in the United States the Department of Health and Human Services has set a goal of increasing to at least 50% the number of worksites offering back-injury-prevention programs (U.S. Department of Health and Human Services, 1991). An important question is, What types of preventive interventions are available and how well do they work?

The aim of this chapter is to provide an overview of various approaches to preventive interventions for MSP in which the focus is on psychological aspects. Back pain is highlighted, since it is a major part of the problem and considerable research is available. MSP is usually not associated with well-defined medical findings, and consequently it is difficult to draw the usual distinction between primary and secondary prevention. Instead, in this review I consider programs that focus on workplace or general populations, as well as those oriented toward patients, for example, in primary care. Because 85% of the population may suffer MSP during their lifetimes, true primary prevention is very difficult. Moreover, because pain serves an important biological function, it would not be wise to "prevent" it from occurring. Thus modern programs focus on "limiting" its occurrence and preventing the development of chronic suffering and dysfunction.

RISK FACTORS AND THE IDENTIFICATION OF THOSE AT RISK

Prevention is based on the early identification of people at risk for developing a given illness. In addition, it is based on altering the causal factors in order to alleviate the risk. Although some "risk" factors may be correlational in nature, that is, they predict the development of the illness but do not in themselves "cause" the problem, risk factors hopefully provide insight into what needs to be "prevented." One feature of researching risk factors is the early identification of people at risk for developing chronic pain and dysfunction. Screening, for example, may be used to help identify patients who may need extra assessment or interventions. Thus screening may help us to concentrate limited resources on those most in need.

Another feature of research on risk factors is isolating important variables that may be altered to hinder the development of chronic problems. As we shall see, a good deal has been done to screen for "at risk" patients, but many interventions to date are based on theory (or belief) rather than on known causal factors. The main reason is that we do not completely understand why MSP problems such as neck and back pain develop. However, advancements are being made and new preventive strategies are being developed.

Risk Factors

A wide variety of risk factors are relevant for MSP, but psychosocial factors appear to be especially important. A number of studies have included, for example, ergonomic, medical, and psychosocial factors and then determined their value for MSP. There is considerable agreement that a host of ergonomic variables is related to various types of MSP. These include heavy work, lifting, bending, twisting, manual handling, and repetitive work (Pope, Andersson, Frymoyer, & Chaffin, 1991; Skovron, 1992). These ergonomic factors have often been interpreted to mean that such movements cause an injury to the spinal system and therefore that physical load should be reduced or avoided. However, physical stress on the spine is not necessarily harmful and may even be beneficial—a fact of the utmost importance for intervention (Burton, Battié, & Main, in press).

Considerable work has also involved medical factors, for example, those recorded in an examination by a general practitioner or specialist. A list of established "red flags" is provided in Table 23.1. However, studies comparing the relative influence of biomechanical, medical, and psychosocial factors are providing mounting evidence that psychosocial factors are of particular importance.

TABLE 23.1. Red Flags for Potentially Serious Medical Conditions

- Features of cauda equina syndrome (urinary retention, bilateral neurological symptoms and signs, saddle anesthesia)—urgent referral required
- Significant trauma
- Weight loss
- History of cancer
- Fever
- Intravenous drug use
- Steroid use
- Patient over 50 years old
- Severe, unremitting nighttime pain
- Pain that gets worse when patient is lying down

Note. Based on ACC and National Health Committee, New Zealand (1997).

Moreover, it appears that psychosocial factors are relevant for the onset of pain and above all for the transition from acute to chronic pain and disability. Let us look briefly at some of the evidence concerning psychosocial factors.

Several reviews have summarized the results of a large number of studies and are of great help in deducing the main results. Table 23.2 presents an overview of some of the important variables as summarized in the New Zealand "Yellow Flags" document (Kendall et al., 1997). Weiser and Cedraschi (1992) found some 16 predictive studies involving healthy, acute, recurrent, or chronic populations. They conclude that distress, preoccupation with symptoms, depression, anxiety, and cognitive factors such as coping and illness beliefs were related to recovery from or development of chronic pain. They also found that job satisfaction and stress were related to outcome.

Which variables are important in the transition from acute to chronic pain? Turk (1997) specifically reviewed this literature and found that a fairly large number of psychological variables play a significant role. Pain severity at onset was found to be a significant predictor of later pain and disability. Anxiety, fear, depression, and psychological distress were found to be related in a number of well-conducted studies. Maladaptive coping, passive cognitions, and stress were also related to chronicity. Last, self-perceived poor health and job satisfaction were found to be important. Turk points out that psychosocial factors are better predictors of chronicity than are clinical or physical factors. However, it is also important to underscore that psychosocial factors may only account for a

TABLE 23.2. An Overview of Psychosocial "Yellow Flags" and Some Pertinent Examples of Each Category

Attitudes and beliefs about the pain

Fear avoidance, that is, belief that activity will cause pain or injury
Belief that pain must be completely abolished before attempting normal activity
Catastrophizing
Belief that pain is uncontrollable
Expectations concerning assessment, treatment, and outcome
Belief that one has poor health or is handicapped

Behaviors

Use of extended rest
Reduced activity or withdrawal from activities of daily life
Avoidance
Report of extremely high-intensity pain
Excessive reliance on aids or appliances
Sleep quality reduced since onset of pain
Substance abuse
Smoking

Compensation

Lack of financial incentive to return to work
Disputes
History of ineffective case management

Diagnosis and treatment

Health professionals sanctioning disability
Conflicting diagnoses
Diagnoses leading to catastrophizing and fear
Dependency, for example, on passive treatments
Health care utilization
Expectation of a "techno-fix"
Lack of satisfaction with previous treatment
Advice to withdraw from daily activities or work

Emotions

Fear of pain or disability
Depression and irritability
Anxiety or heightened awareness of body sensations
Stress
Loss of sense of control

Family

Overprotecting partner
Solicitous behavior from partner
Socially punitive responses
Extent of support in attempts to return to normal activities, including work
History of abuse
History of model for chronic pain behavior

Work

Belief that work is harmful
Unsupportive or unhappy current work environment
Negative experience of management or absence of interest from employer
Specific aspects of psychosocial environment, for example, stress, perceived load, monotony, control, etc.

Note. Based on Kendall et al. (1997).

limited amount of the variability in these studies, demonstrating that it is indeed a complex, multidimensional problem.

Psychosocial variables at the workplace have been frequently researched. Bongers, de Winter, Kompier, and Hildebrandt (1993) have tried to summarize the findings from some 44 cross-sectional and 15 prospective studies that included psychosocial workplace factors. They found that the evidence supports a correlation between job demands, job control, monotonous work, perceived work load, and work under time pressure. Social relations at work were determined to be especially important. They also found that stress symptoms are often associated with MSP. Although their conclusions are drawn in light of some methodological shortcomings, they nevertheless highlight the probable importance of the psychosocial work environment.

An exceptionally salient risk factor is thought to be "fear-avoidance beliefs." This is the fear generated avoidance of certain activities or movements. The fear in turn is related to beliefs that physical activity may exacerbate the pain or cause (re)injury (Lethem, Slade, Troup, & Bentley, 1983; Vlaeyen, Kole-Snijders, Boeren, & van Eek, 1995; Vlaeyen, Kole-Snijders, Rotteveel, Ruesink, & Heuts, 1995). Waddell, Newton, Henderson, Somerville, and Main (1993) developed an instrument to specifically measure this, the Fear Avoidance Beliefs Questionnaire. They found that although there was almost no relationship between pain intensity and disability, there was a strong relationship between fear-avoidance beliefs and disability.

Similarly, McCracken, Gross, Sorg, and Edmands (1993) demonstrated that low back pain patients with high levels of pain-related anxiety had less range of motion than did those with low levels of anxiety. Crombez, Vervaet, Lysens, Eelen, and Baeyens (1996), moreover, found that "avoiders" reported more fear and pain and had lower performance levels on a maximal performance test than did nonavoiders. Vlaeyen, Kole-Snijders, Boeren, and van Eek (1995) have, in addition, found that fear of movement was a better predictor of dysfunction than were biomedical parameters, and they underscored the role of catastrophizing as an instrumental part of a vicious circle involving catastrophizing, fear-avoidance, dysfunction, depression, and pain.

In a recent study, fear-avoidance beliefs and catastrophizing were assessed in pain-free participants from a general population sample (Linton, Buer, Vlaeyen, & Hellsing, in press). In general,

levels of catastrophizing and fear-avoidance were low. However, 1 year later outcome was determined as to whether participants had experienced an episode of neck or back pain. Although catastrophizing was only marginally related to outcome, fear-avoidance beliefs increased the risk of developing a pain episode more than twofold.

Prospective studies may serve to illustrate findings concerning risk factors. Burton, Tillotson, Main, and Hollis (1995) studied 252 consecutive patients with a new episode of low back pain and followed them for 1 year. At consultation patients received a standardized clinical examination, and an interview history was taken. A battery of questionnaires said to measure pain experience, disability, distress, pain beliefs, fear-avoidance, and coping strategies was also completed. Patients were then treated in a standard manner. One year later participants completed a questionnaire measuring pain and disability to determine outcome. Multiple regression analyses were used to deal with the large amount of data and possible intercorrelations, and models were developed for all patients, those with acute as well as those with subacute pain at initial presentation. The psychological variables were by far the most potent predictors in each of these three models. The analysis for acute pain provided the best prediction, as 69% of the variance was accounted for by five variables: the catastrophizing coping strategy, somatic distress, straight leg raise, hoping and praying coping strategy, and leg pain. The authors conclude that the results "show that the psychological status of the patient at presentation has a much stronger influence on outcome than does conventional clinical information" (Burton et al., 1995, p. 726). Catastrophizing, for example, was found to be seven times more important than the best of the clinical or historical variables.

A 10-year follow-up study of employees sheds light on the role of psychological factors in back pain (Leino & Hänninen, 1995). Questionnaires and a clinical examination were administered at the Valmet engineering factories in Jyväskylä, Finland. A total of 411 participants completed both pre- and 10-year follow-up evaluations. At pretest, the psychosocial variables, especially "mental overstrain" and physical workload, were all found to be related to pain as well as to clinical findings made by a physiotherapist. Prospectively, the score on social relations at work produced the most consistent relationship with musculoskeletal morbidity. Poor satisfaction with social relationships at work was an antecedent to pain symptoms and findings. For blue-collar workers, pain was also predicted by work content, work control, and "mental overstrain." Interestingly, physical load was not associated with morbidity. The findings were very similar regardless of anatomical region, which led the authors to suggest a general musculoskeletal reactivity to psychosocial factors. In sum, psychosocial work factors were not only related to pain but also predicted musculoskeletal problems, including neck and back pain 10 years later.

Screening

The data on risk factors suggests that it might be possible to identify people "at risk" of developing chronic pain and disability. Several attempts at developing a screening instrument have been reported. Main, Wood, Hollis, Spanswick, and Waddell (1992) developed a questionnaire based on measures of depression and distress (DRAM) and showed that it accurately identified patients seeking orthopedic care who were at risk of a poor outcome. Patients were classified into one of four categories depending on their scores for depression and distress. These categories were related to outcome, and the DRAM technique was recommended as a screening tool in orthopedic clinics.

Another approach to screening based on questionnaires, the MMPI, and a clinical diagnostic interview has been reported by Gatchel, Polatin, and Kinney (1995). This battery of assessment techniques was employed with patients seeking help for acute back pain in primary care. At a 6-month follow-up outcome was determined as to whether the person was working or not working. They found that scores on a pain and disability measure, personality disorders, and scale 3 (*Hy*) of the MMPI were important factors that correctly classified 87% of the patients, as opposed to a 50% chance level.

The Vermont Screening Questionnaire (Hazard, Haugh, Reid, Preble, & MacDonald, 1996) was developed to help predict long-term compensation cases. The questionnaire consists of 11 items that have been empirically selected from a pool of questions. This questionnaire has been evaluated in a study of 163 people who had recently filed an injury report. A sensitivity of 94% and specificity of 84% were reported (chance = 50%). Thus this instrument may be helpful in determining risk for long-term disability. However, this study only predicted absenteeism in a group filing injury claims, and the study suffered from a large dropout/refusal rate.

As a final example, a screening questionnaire has been developed based on a selection of a variety of psychosocial risk factors (Linton & Halldén, 1997). The instrument contains 24 items covering such areas as background factors, physical function, fear-avoidance beliefs, pain experience, work, psychological factors, and reactions to the pain. The questionnaire has been tested on 137 consecutive primary care patients with acute/subacute neck and/or back pain problems (Linton & Halldén, 1998). A median split of the total score demonstrated a sensitivity of 87% and a specificity of 75% for three classes of sick leave outcome, whereas chance would be 33%. This investigation was conducted with a sample of both acute and subacute patients, and the outcome involved sick leave (three categories) rather than a "working"/"not working" dichotomy. Thus, it is realistic in nature, and the outcome is quite relevant but probably more difficult to predict than mere work status.

The studies on screening all show significantly higher than chance levels of classification. Although the levels are surprisingly high given the nature of the problem, investigations thus far have not tested the instruments on new, independent populations in which we might expect the accuracy to be lower. Nevertheless, these data suggest that screening questionnaires employing psychosocial variables may be a valuable tool in the identification of patients at risk for developing long-term disability.

An alternative approach might be surveillance. This usually involves monitoring symptoms or sick leave. In certain populations, such as at large workplaces, symptoms may be monitored to identify high-risk work areas or individuals with increasing problems. A system of eight simple, self-administered tests to assess physical function, for example, has been found to be sensitive (Hellsing, Linton, & Bryngelsson, 1997). A common method, however, is to monitor sick leave so that all people off work more than a given time (such as 6 weeks) for MSP would be subject to an assessment or treatment. Frank, Brooker, et al. (1996) argue that investigations of risk factors to date are not adequately clear to provide "early predictors of poor long-term outcome that are sufficiently accurate . . . to be clinically useful for targeting high-risk patients" (p. 2919). Instead, they point to critical time periods, based on return-to-work statistics, and assert that those off work after 1 to 2 months' time are at high risk for much longer term disability. In other words, time off work might be monitored and interventions implemented after a given time period. Although a system based on the time aspect may have several advantages, such as being simple to understand, it also has disadvantages. The disadvantages include lack of a system for those not off work and a relatively "late" entry into a preventive intervention, since those off work for 1 or more months usually have a long history of problems (see the previous discussion), as well as the lack of information regarding target variables for intervention.

In fact, screening and surveillance may be combined. Most screening instruments, for example, include items about the history of the problem, such as the length of time off work. The potential advantage of screening is gaining vital information that may increase accuracy at an earlier time point, including factors that may be targeted in an intervention. However, screening probably will never be as accurate as we may wish. Instead, it might best be used as a rough estimate that will help effectively select people in need of further assessment, intervention, or observation.

PREVENTIVE INTERVENTIONS

A wide variety of interventions has been tried in an attempt to prevent the development of chronic pain and disability. Some programs, for example, ergonomic improvements or the enhancement of the psychosocial work environment, have been based on findings from epidemiological studies of risk factors, as well as on theory. However, many of the programs have been based mainly on reasoning rather than on direct evidence concerning risks. This reflects the difficulty of isolating potent risk factors that may be readily altered. I now examine some attempts at prevention.

Interventions Aimed at Workplaces or the General Population

Spitzer (1993) noted that we know very little about primary prevention of MSP, and Frank, Kerr, et al. (1996) conclude that there is little evidence to support the efficacy of primary prevention for back pain. Although a great deal of effort has been put into very early prevention programs, few studies have scientifically evaluated their effects. Moreover, many of the main techniques are not psychological in nature and consequently fall outside the boundaries of this chapter. However, a short overview of programs oriented toward workplaces and the general population is provided as an orientation and because these techniques may be related

to psychological concepts and often involve changing behaviors.

These interventions are generally provided for all members of a given group, such as a certain workplace or age group. Although they may be considered to be primary prevention, the population is in fact "mixed," since many may have experienced symptoms and some have undoubtedly sought care or been off work for their MSP. The goals of the programs are not always clearly stated, but they involve reducing pain levels (e.g., intensity, duration, frequency) and work loss while improving function.

Changing the Work

Ergonomics. This approach is based on an injury model that implies that if occupational loads are reduced, there should also be a reduction in occupational back problems (Burton et al., in press). In this light, exposure to mechanical overload as a single or cumulative factor is said to damage spinal tissue. This in turn results in pain and problems with mobility, and further exposure would be expected to lead to further damage. Although there are epidemiological and laboratory data to support these ideas, the results of interventions based on the model have not been impressive (Burton et al., in press; Skovron, 1992; Westgaard & Winkel, 1997). In fact, Kemmlert, Orelium-Dallner, Kilbom, and Gamberale (1993) have found that a reduction in work load was not related to a reduction in pain problems. Most reports supporting the belief that ergonomical interventions reduce MSP are largely anecdotal (Burton et al., in press; Smedley & Coggon, 1994). Karas and Conrad (1996), for example, searched the literature for scientific evaluations of back injury prevention programs and did not find a single well-designed study concerning ergonomics. However, two uncontrolled studies have shown improvements after initiation of ergonomic improvements (Aaras, 1994; Garg & Owen, 1992).

Clinical experience combined with reports in the literature suggest that when load levels are extreme, such as with very repetitive or heavy work, interventions may be considered. Burton et al. (in press) conclude that despite the lack of proper studies there is some notion that biomechanics-based ergonomic improvements in the workplace have potential. This may be particularly true on the individual level, where workplace adjustments may help a person with pain to cope more effectively and remain on the job despite the problem. Making such improvements may also be important for assisting a worker to return to work despite problems, and it is one way employers show that they value the employee. We also can note, however, that relatively few workplaces in the Western world have jobs that truly entail "heavy work." In fact, programs designed to reduce physical load or otherwise improve the physical work environment may actually make the work more repetitive. Indeed, workload may be reduced to the point where "inactivity" in itself, such as sitting, becomes a risk factor. Moreover, signaling that the work may be harmful and thus in need of modification may inadvertently reinforce fear-avoidance beliefs and behaviors.

Changing the Worker

Interventions designed to change the worker are based on the idea that one can increase resistance to injury. Consequently, offering proper training in work techniques, safety, or increasing muscle strength and enhancing social support at work may serve as protective buffers. Although this sounds sensible, there is surprisingly little research that has actually studied whether these premises are true. However, there is considerable information regarding the utility of some programs in reducing pain and disability.

Education. Education is apparently the most common strategy for prevention, and efforts range from simple pamphlets to multidimensional "back schools." These programs make the assumption that people suffer more than need be because they lack knowledge about a variety of topics as diverse as body mechanics and coping strategies. Back schools usually contain a series of discussions about anatomy, biomechanics, lifting, and postural changes related to work and a program of exercises. They vary from a single session of less than an hour to several sessions (Linton & Kamwendo, 1987; Scheer, Radack, & O'Brien, 1995). In addition, back schools have been incorporated into more elaborate treatment programs, although these are oriented more toward rehabilitation than prevention (Fabio, 1995; Koes, van Tulder, van der Windt, & Bouter, 1994).

Back schools are attractive because they utilize educational principles, may be done with groups, and involve no expensive or complicated technology. In addition, the method appears to have face validity, and patients may enjoy attending the sessions.

However, the utility of back schools has been debated. This is in part because of the fact that back schools as an early intervention make inherent sense, even though they have limited empirical support, and in part because investigations have been conducted in vastly different settings, with everything from healthy to chronic pain participants.

A number of reviews have looked at the effects of educational efforts, including back schools (Cohen, Frank, Bombardier, Peloso, & Guillemin, 1994; Karas & Conrad, 1996; Koes et al., 1994; Lahad, Malter, Berg, & Deyo, 1994; Linton & Kamwendo, 1987; Nordin, Cedraschi, Balagué, & Roux, 1992; Scheer et al., 1995; van der Weide, Verbeek, & van Tulder, 1997). There is some agreement that back schools or other educational techniques may be necessary in some situations but that they do not seem to be sufficient to reduce the problem. Nordin et al. (1992) conclude that education is an important part of working with people but that back schools are a tool that may be used as an adjunct rather than as a sole intervention. Particularly for a population with pain, the evidence suggests the need for a multidisciplinary approach that is much broader and more comprehensive than a simple back school (Fabio, 1995; Koes et al., 1994; Linton & Kamwendo, 1987). There is simply not sufficient evidence to show that back schools on their own are more effective than no treatment (Cohen et al., 1994; Fabio, 1995; King, 1993; Linton & Kamwendo, 1987; Nordin et al., 1992; Scheer et al., 1995)

Despite the large number of years that back schools have been employed, we still do not know whether the basic assumptions hold true. For example, it is not clear whether participants substantially increase their knowledge level. In our own study concerning secretaries at a large hospital, we found that the participants had, on the average, high levels of knowledge before attending a neck school (Kamwendo & Linton, 1991). Perhaps the most central issue is whether participants comply with the advice given, that is, whether they change their behavior. In addition, compliance in performing these behaviors in the long run may be vital for prevention but is difficult to obtain. Finally, few studies have addressed the issue of whether these behavioral changes actually result in a reduction of the problem.

An especially interesting prospective investigation in industry examined the effects of an educational pamphlet (Symonds, Burton, Tillotson, & Main, 1995). The contents were based on psychological conceptions of fear-avoidance. The pamphlet described "confronters" and "avoiders" and contained a very clear message aimed to encourage active coping and the ignoring of normal aches and pain. Examples of positive coping were keeping up daily activities, not relying on medication, being positive, and taking little time off work. One factory received the pamphlet, and two others served as controls. The results showed a reduction in the number of episodes of back pain and the number of days of absence. This study demonstrates that it may, nevertheless, be possible to prevent and reduce back pain disability by employing very specific information that encourages specific behaviors.

Exercise. Exercise is frequently included as a cornerstone in rehabilitation efforts. It is also a common preventive measure for MSP. Although the benefits of training and activity programs are well documented for chronic pain patients, there are still conflicting views as to their value as a strictly preventive measure. A recent review by Gebhardt (1994) searched the literature for studies looking at the effectiveness of exercise for employees. He found six experimental studies that showed a modest result; the overall effect size was .24. Other reviews of the literature have also found limited evidence for the use of exercise in preventing back pain problems (Karas & Conrad, 1996; Lahad et al., 1994; Scheer et al., 1995). It should be kept in mind, however, that there is a paucity of good-quality controlled studies. Furthermore, many studies have been conducted with patients already suffering from considerable pain problems.

As with back schools, there are many fundamental questions that remain to be answered concerning the preventive effects of exercise. These questions range from what type of exercise (for example, to improve physical condition, strength, or mobility) is best, whether patients significantly improve with exercise, whether they continue to exercise after completion of the program, and above all whether this translates into reduced MSP. We studied employees at two large workplaces and randomly assigned volunteers to either a group receiving traditional exercise or one receiving an individualized program designed to enhance compliance (Linton, Hellsing, & Bergström, 1996). We found that compliance was enhanced by our individualized program. However, it took nearly 6 months before the effects were clearly seen. Moreover, although pain was significantly reduced for "compliers," there was no significant difference when compared to noncompliers. Finally, from a psychological point of view, exercise may be a general "health promotion" rather than a specific intervention for MSP. The observed effects may be due to psychological (e.g., decreased anxiety and depression and increased well-being and sense of control), as well as physiological (increased mobility, condition, strength), factors. More work is needed to investigate the best methods for reducing the burden of MSP.

Management and the Psychosocial Work Environment

Given the large number of studies showing that the psychosocial work environment is an important risk for MSP problems, attention has been turned to various ways of improving this aspect of the work environment. This also involves behavior, since such things as social support or management style are dealt with. However, most programs have not been systematically evaluated. Indeed, many programs have not been specific for MSP but have been implemented as a general way to enhance job satisfaction and production. Two areas, however, deserve some specific attention.

First, management style with regard to how a company deals with workplace injuries appears to be quite important. One study indicates that more than 50% of a workplace's costs for injuries depends on how the company manages an injury once it has occurred (Fordyce, 1995). Hunt and Habeck (1993) have examined routines at 220 workplaces in Michigan with more than 100 employees. They found that although ergonomic and wellness programs generally did not have significant effects, management methods that made use of injury data and actively supported participation from management, supervisors, and employees were substantially more successful. These workplaces, for example, maintained an active return-to-work process for employees off work that was flexible to individual needs.

It is not surprising, then, that training programs for supervisors have shown some promise. Wood (1987) taught foremen and personnel managers to contact employees who were absent due to sickness in a supportive way, to document and maintain contact at least every 10 days, and to discuss a return to work. The aim was to enhance recovery and promote return, even though the employee might need special help. Compared to a back school intervention, this program significantly improved return to work. Similar successful programs have been reported as a means of improving return rates after an injury (Håland-Haldorsen, Jensen, Linton, Nygren, & Ursin, 1997; Linton, 1991a; Linton, 1991b).

Programs Aimed at Patients

Some people with MSP will seek care, and the point of first contact with health care providers may be an excellent point for providing early preventive interventions. The fact that many people do not develop a problem requiring care is one reason that this approach is attractive: It may save resources. Another reason is that a shift from traditional medical model-guided "diagnosis and cure" to more active measures might help patients develop more appropriate attitudes toward the problem, as well as help them make important behavioral changes. Finally, as seen in the preceding discussion, it has not been easy to develop potent prevention programs for delivery in broad populations; thus the health care system provides an attractive opportunity to initiate preventive interventions.

The interventions are based on the cognitive-behavioral learning conception of the development of pain, as well as on techniques found to be helpful in rehabilitation. The development of chronic pain has been described in detail elsewhere (Feuerstein & Zastowny, 1996; Fordyce, 1976; Linton, 1994; Linton, Melin, & Götestam, 1984; Philips & Grant, 1991; Turk, 1996), but the main point is that cognitive and behavioral factors appear to be instrumental in its development. Ordinarily, this occurs over a fairly long period of time, which allows ample opportunities for learning of the "sick role." Consequently, the early intervention programs are designed to stop this development by changing cognitions and altering learning patterns.

The time point for intervention has ranged from the first visit at onset to as much as a few months of MSP. The best time for intervention was discussed in the section on risk factors. In a nutshell, the longer one waits, the fewer patients will need care. However, the converse may be that the longer one waits, the more care they may need. Very early programs, consequently, must be inexpensive and relatively easy to administer.

Several attempts at providing preventive interventions for people with subacute MSP have been reported, but not all have been positive. Mitchell and Carmen (1990), for example, provided early activation and education to patients at an average of 41 days postinjury at 12 different centers. Compared to matched controls, these

patients returned to work earlier and accumulated less costs. However, Mitchell and Carmen (1994) discovered in a follow-up that the difference between the groups was no longer significant, although the early activation treatment cost less. In a cohort study of early preventive intervention, Ekberg, Björkqvist, Malm, Bjerre-Kiely, and Axelson (1994) compared a group of patients with subacute neck or shoulder pain receiving an 8-week package of physical training, education, social interaction, and workplace visits with a control group receiving traditional treatment, such as physical therapy, medication, rest, and sick leave. No significant differences were found at the 1- and 2-year follow-ups for measures of sick leave, pain intensity, or the Sickness Impact Profile. These two studies illustrate the potential problems associated with developing early interventions. Because both of the above studies employed personnel not specifically trained in cognitive-behavioral techniques, the disappointing results may be due to the way in which the programs were administered, such as by reinforcing sick behaviors and so forth.

Other early rehabilitation programs have shown positive outcomes. Lindström et al., (1992), for example, provided operant activities training, a back school, and a workplace visit for automobile workers with back pain at 8 weeks off work. They found that these patients required significantly less time to return to work and less sick leave than a control group who received standard medical care. We offered nursing personnel with a history of back pain problems a cognitive-behavioral program that included exercise, ergonomics, and group therapy aimed at improving coping. The program also focused on occupational aspects. The intervention group improved significantly on a variety of variables at the 6-month follow-up as compared to a "treatment as usual" control group. Improvements were maintained at an 18-month follow-up for such variables as pain intensity, fatigue, daily activities, and helplessness.

Indahl, Velund, and Reikeraas (1995) set up a program at a spine clinic for patients who were off work for 12 weeks with low back pain. In all, four contacts were provided in which the patients were examined, radiographs taken, and a great deal of information on self-care and activity given. The intervention was designed to reduce fear, and patients were told that normal activities would enhance healing. Every other patient was assigned to the treatment group (n = 463), and the control group (n = 512) received conventional medical treatment. The intervention resulted in significantly fewer sick leave days. In fact, the intervention group had about half as many days off as the control group and were more than twice as likely to return to work.

Another recent example of an early preventive intervention is the Sherbrooke project in Canada (Loisel et al., 1997). Workplaces with more than 175 workers from the Sherbrooke area were invited to participate. Those with thoracic or lumbar back pain that resulted in sick leave or assignment to light duties for between 1 and 3 months were the focus of the study. The 130 participants were randomly assigned to one of four groups: usual care, clinical intervention only, occupational intervention only, and a full intervention that combined the clinical and occupational interventions. Patients in the usual-care group received ordinary treatment from their doctors. The clinical intervention included a visit to a back pain specialist, a back school, and a multidisciplinary work rehabilitation intervention, ending with a progressive return-to-work program. The occupational intervention, on the other hand, included a visit to an occupational physician that could result in treatment or work recommendations and an ergonomic intervention.

Participants were followed for 1 year with regard to their work absences, pain, and functional status. The full-intervention group returned to work 2.4 times faster and had half as many sick leave days as compared to the usual-care group. Moreover, the effect of the occupational intervention accounted for the greatest part of the improvement. However, pain and function improved in all three intervention groups. The authors conclude that the occupational intervention is of primary importance in preventing the development of chronicity.

A number of programs have been designed for patients with acute pain and are situated in primary care facilities. These have similarities with the above programs for subacute pain but are provided in different settings and for a different patient population. Already in 1986, Fordyce, Brockway, Bergman, and Spengler (1986) reported the results of a program for acute back pain (< 10 days) based on behavioral principles. They found at the 1-year follow-up that those receiving the behaviorally based care were less disabled than the control group receiving usual care.

Haig, Linton, McIntosh, Moneta, and Mead (1990) studied hospital employees with acute MSP (2 days off work) in an occupational health care service. They provided early contact and a program designed to establish good communication with the workplace, as well as to enhance an early modified return to work. They showed a 33% decrease in time off work, as compared to the same time period before the program was started.

In a similar approach in occupational health, Ryan, Krishna, and Swanson (1995) designed a program for mine workers to prevent chronic back pain. This program included an educational part for all employees, special education for supervisors, and a program of early reporting and care. An emphasis was placed on an "on-the-spot" examination and treatment, as well as information to reduce fear and anxiety. In general, workers were advised to return to work and that activity was not harmful. Compared to employees in similar mines, those in program had significantly fewer back pain claims, and, above all, not a single worker developed long-term problems during the 6-year follow-up.

Linton, Hellsing, and Andersson (1993) studied usual care in comparison to an early behaviorally oriented program for first-time sufferers at primary care facilities. The early program reinforced function and other well behaviors and highlighted the importance of maintaining everyday activities and returning to work. There were dramatic differences between the groups with regard to sick leave during the course of the follow-up, and the early care package reduced the risk of developing chronic problems by eightfold.

Finally, Malmivaara et al. (1995) studied 186 patients seeking care for low back pain at an occupational health care clinic in Helsinki, Finland. Patients were randomized to an exercise group or a bed rest group or a group provided with advice to avoid bed rest and continue their daily routines as actively as possible within the limits of their pain. Results were evaluated at 3 and 12 weeks after the intervention. The patients in the group receiving advice had the best results with regard to pain, flexion, disability, and days off work as compared to both the exercise and bed rest groups. Thus it appeared that maintaining daily activity routines was a better preventive strategy than bed rest or back exercises.

Strategies for Prevention

Some strategies for secondary prevention have been previously described, and an overview is presented in Table 23.3 (Linton & Bradley, 1996). Based on the studies described, some additional points may be considered. First, several programs utilized con-

TABLE 23.3. An Overview of Some Strategies Relevant in Health Care Settings for the Secondary Prevention of Chronic Pain

Strategy	Description
1. Early	Time is vital aspect. Intervention should be initiated before disruption of lifestyle, etc., for example, before 12 weeks.
2. Active (health behavior)	Focus on health and behaviors rather than medical, etc., variables. Recommend maintaining daily activity, some training, and return to work.
3. Patient as active partner	As problem cannot be "cured" and as treatment often requires patient to change behaviors, engaging the patient is important.
4. Facilitate communication	Workplace, family, insurance carriers, other medical facilities, etc., are instrumental in enhancing or hindering recovery. Therefore it is important that there is clear communication as well as coordination of services.
5. Follow-up, maintenance	MSP is recurrent and behavioral change is often difficult to maintain. Thus follow-up is of value in evaluating results and adjusting the intervention to maximize results.

Note. Based on Linton and Bradley (1996).

tacts with the workplace as an essential aspect. The Loisel et al. (1997) program dramatically showed that the inclusion of an occupational component was important for obtaining maximal results. Consequently, occupational aspects might be considered as a necessary and central part of prevention rather than as a tagged-on option.

Second, techniques addressing cognitive and emotional aspects, especially anxiety, fear, and beliefs about injury in the acute and subacute phase, appear to be wise strategies. Thorough examinations and considerable information were delivered in several programs in an effort to reduce fear and deal with beliefs about injury. Although none of the studies specifically studied the effects of these, they were an important aspect—indeed the main aspect of some studies (Indahl et al., 1995; Linton et al., 1993).

A third related aspect is recommendations to maintain daily activities. Waddell, Feder, and Lewis (1997) have reviewed the literature and found that advice to stay active and continue ordinary activities despite the pain consistently results in a faster return to work, less disability, and fewer recurrent problems than "treatment as usual."

Together with the strategies in Table 23.3, the preceding observations provide several avenues for attempting to prevent the development of chronic MSP. It should be underscored, however, that these strategies have not been specifically evaluated in scientific investigations but rather derived from the literature. Most have been tested as part of a prevention "package." Nevertheless, they make up a

beginning—as opposed to the final word—of implementing preventive strategies in health care settings. Taken as a whole, the results of early interventions have been encouraging. As pointed out earlier, not all trials have produced significant reductions in suffering or sick leave. Yet several well-designed investigations have demonstrated substantial improvements as compared to treatment as usual. These benefits are mainly seen in the sick leave domain. In part, this is due to the fact that most people with acute or subacute MSP will feel better. However, in the long run, being able to be active, including working, is important for all involved.

Finally, it may be necessary to provide a comprehensive program in order to successfully prevent chronicity. A program may consist, for example, of early identification, perhaps through screening or surveillance; interventions oriented toward various risk factors; acute care routines; and finally, for selected patients, early treatment (rehabilitation). In addition, such a program may need to offer a range of services, from ergonomic advice to skills training, to improve coping.

RECAPITULATION

The literature indicates that psychological variables may be an important key to the effective prevention of chronic MSP. A perusal of the literature demonstrated that several psychosocial variables were related to the onset and, importantly, to the development of chronic problems. At this time, it appears that psychological variables may be equally or more important than information gathered from medical or ergonomical examinations.

In fact, psychological variables have shown promise for identifying patients at risk of developing long-term pain problems. This is valuable, as early identification might allow the allocation of restricted resources to those most in need.

Prevention programs have focused on different settings and populations. Ergonomic changes may be valuable for workers exposed to high levels of loading. However, there is surprisingly little data that demonstrate a clear effect of improving ergonomics at work. Exercise and educational packages aimed at workers or the general population have also been studied. Although these are frequently employed, the results are not usually impressive. They may have value in changing attitudes, as well as in educating people about MSP. Thus programs oriented toward general populations have had difficulty in showing a clear preventive effect. Consequently, these approaches may be necessary, but they do not in themselves appear to be sufficient for preventing MSP problems.

On the other hand, several programs delivered in health care settings have shown some promise in the prevention of chronic MSP. These programs have generally embraced cognitive-behavioral principles and have been oriented toward patients with subacute or acute MSP. Although prevention is not easily obtained and some programs have not been able to show statistically significant improvements as compared to a control condition, several investigations have demonstrated impressive results. Improvements are usually seen in work absences but also in other variables such as function and pain. Since compensation accounts for roughly 90% of the expenditures, this ought to translate into significant financial savings.

Several strategies have been used in attempting to prevent chronic MSP in health care settings. The inclusion of an occupational component appears to be important for long-term results. Moreover, techniques designed to deal with cognitive beliefs and emotional aspects such as fear and anxiety have frequently been employed. Finally, advice to stay active by maintaining everyday routines and returning to work appears to be associated with more rapid recovery and less disability and chronicity than usual treatment.

Given the suffering, size, and cost of the MSP problem, there is every reason to pursue preventive interventions. The evidence to date indicates that it may be possible to successfully prevent chro-

nicity, although we will not succeed with every patient. Moreover, this does not mean that every patient will become pain-free. Yet simple techniques at an early time point appear, on the average, to prevent considerable suffering and disability.

The scientific evaluation of preventive interventions is still in its infancy, and there is a real need for further information. Many of the techniques, for example, have not been specifically studied at all. We still do not know the best time point for intervention nor the best system for early identification. As the cognitive-behavioral strategies outlined have few or no side effects, are relatively cheap, and have shown promise, we may proceed with caution while welcoming new research findings.

REFERENCES

Aaras, A. (1994). The impact of ergonomic intervention on individual health and corporate prosperity in a telecommunications environment. *Ergonomics, 37,* 1679–1696.

Bigos, S. J., Bowyer, O. R., Braen, G. R., Brown, K., Deyo, R., Haldeman, S., Hart, J. L., Johnson, E. W., Keller, R., Kido, D. Liang, M. H., Nelson, R. M., Nordin, M., Owen, B. D., Pope, M. H., Schwartz, R. K., Stewart, D. H., Susman, J., Triano, J. J., Tripp, L. C., Turk, D. C., Watts, C., & Weinstein, J. N. (1994). *Acute low back problems in adults. Clinical Practice Guideline No. 14* (AHCPR Publication No. 95-0642). Rockville, MD: U.S. Department of Health and Human Services, Agency for Health Care Policy and Research.

Bongers, P. M., de Winter, C. R., Kompier, M. A., & Hildebrandt, V. H. (1993). Psychosocial factors at work and musculoskeletal disease. *Scandinavian Journal of Work, Environment, and Health, 19*(5), 297–312.

Brattberg, G., Thorslund, M., & Wikman, A. (1989). The prevalence of pain in a general population: The results of a postal survey in a county of Sweden. *Pain, 37,* 215–222.

Burton, A. K., Battié, M. C., & Main, C. J. (in press). The relative importance of biomechanical and psychosocial factors in low back injuries. In W. Karwowski & W. Marras (Eds.), *Handbook of industrial ergonomics* (pp. 1127–1138). Boca Raton, FL: CRC Press.

Burton, A. K., Tillotson, K. M., Main, C. J., & Hollis, S. (1995). Psychosocial predictors of outcome in acute and subchronic low back trouble. *Spine, 20*(6), 722–728.

Cohen, J. E., Frank, J. W., Bombardier, C., Peloso, P., & Guillemin, F. (1994). Group education interventions for people with low back pain: An overview of the literature. *Spine, 19*(11), 1214–1222.

Crombez, G., Vervaet, L., Lysens, R., Eelen, P., & Baeyens, F. (1996). Do pain expectancies cause pain in chronic low back patients? A clinical investigation. *Behaviour Research and Therapy, 34,* 919–925.

Ekberg, K., Björkqvist, B., Malm, P., Bjerre-Kiely, B., &

Axelson, L. (1994). Controlled two year follow up of rehabilitation for disorders in the neck and shoulders. *Occupational and Environmental Medicine, 51,* 833–838.

Fabio, R. P. D. (1995). Efficacy of comprehensive rehabilitation programs and back school for patients with low back pain: A meta-analysis. *Physical Therapy, 75*(10), 865–878.

Feuerstein, M., & Zastowny, T. R. (1996). Occupational rehabilitation: Multidisciplinary management of work-related musculoskeletal pain and disability. In R. J. Gatchel & D. C. Turk (Eds.), *Psychological approaches to pain management: A practitioner's handbook* (pp. 458–485). New York: Guilford Press.

Fordyce, W. E. (1976). *Behavioral methods for chronic pain and illness.* St. Louis, MO: Mosby.

Fordyce, W. E. (1995). *Back pain in the workplace: Management of disability in nonspecific conditions.* Seattle, WA: IASP Press.

Fordyce, W. E., Brockway, J. A., Bergman, J. A., & Spengler, D. (1986). Acute back pain: A control-group comparison of behavioral vs. traditional management methods. *Journal of Behavioral Medicine, 9,* 127–140.

Frank, J. W., Brooker, A. S., DeMaio, S. E., Kerr, M. S., Maetzel, A., Shannon, H. S., Sullivan, T. J., Norman, R. W., & Wells, R. P. (1996). Disability resulting from occupational low back pain: II. What do we know about secondary prevention? A review of the scientific evidence on prevention after disability begins. *Spine, 21*(24), 2918–2929.

Frank, J. W., Kerr, M. S., Brooker, A. S., DeMaio, S. E., Maetzel, A., Shannon, H. S., Sullivan, T. J., Norman, R. W., & Wells, R. P. (1996). Disability resulting from occupational low back pain: I. What do we know about primary prevention? *Spine, 21*(24), 2908–2917.

Garg, A., & Owen, B. (1992). Reducing back stress to nursing personnel: An ergonomic intervention in a nursing home. *Ergonomics, 35,* 1353–1375.

Gatchel, R. J., Polatin, P. B., & Kinney, R. K. (1995). Predicting outcome of chronic back pain using clinical predictors of psychopathology: A prospective analysis. *Health Psychology, 14*(5), 415–420.

Gebhardt, W. A. (1994). Effectiveness of training to prevent job-related back pain: A meta-analysis. *British Journal of Clinical Psychology, 33,* 571–574.

Haig, A. J., Linton, P., McIntosh, M., Moneta, L., & Mead, P. B. (1990). Aggressive early medical management by a specialist in physical medicine and rehabilitation. *Journal of Occupational Medicine, 32,* 241–244.

Håland-Haldorsen, E. M., Jensen, I. B., Linton, S. J., Nygren, Å., & Ursin, H. (1997). Training work supervisors for reintegration of employees treated for musculoskeletal pain. *Journal of Occupational Rehabilitation, 7*(1), 33–43.

Hazard, R. G., Haugh, L. D., Reid, S., Preble, J. B., & MacDonald, L. (1996). Early prediction of chronic disability after occupational low back injury. *Spine, 21*(8), 945–951.

Hellsing, A. L., Linton, S. J., & Bryngelsson, I. L. (1997). Musculoskeletal health surveillance: Eight simple self-administered tests to add to symptom registration. *Spine, 22*(24), 2977–2982.

Hunt, H. A., & Habeck, R. V. (1993). *The Michigan disability prevention study: Research highlights.* Kalamazoo, MI: Upjohn Institute for Employment Research.

Indahl, A., Velund, L., & Reikeraas, O. (1995). Good prognosis for low back pain when left untampered: A randomized clinical trial. *Spine, 20*(4), 473–477.

Kamwendo, K., & Linton, S. J. (1991). A controlled study of the effect of neck school in medical secretaries. *Scandinavian Journal of Rehabilitation Medicine, 23,* 143–152.

Karas, B. E., & Conrad, K. M. (1996). Back injury prevention interventions in the workplace: An integrative review. *American Association of Occupational Health Nurses Journal, 44*(4), 189–196.

Kemmlert, K., Orelium-Dallner, M., Kilbom, A., & Gamberale, F. (1993). A three-year follow-up of 195 reported occupational over-exertion injuries. *Scandinavian Journal of Rehabilitation Medicine, 25,* 16–24.

Kendall, N. A. S., Linton, S. J., & Main, C. J. (1997). *Guide to assessing psychosocial yellow flags in acute low back pain: Risk factors for long-term disability and work loss.* Wellington, New Zealand: Accident Rehabilitation and Compensation Insurance Corporation of New Zealand and the National Health Committee.

King, P. M. (1993). Back injury prevention programs: A critical review of the literature. *Journal of Occupational Rehabilitation, 3*(3), 145–158.

Koes, B. W., van Tulder, M. W., van der Windt, D., & Bouter, L. M. (1994). The efficacy of back schools: A review of randomised clinical trials. *Journal of Clinical Epidemiology, 47,* 851–862.

Lahad, A., Malter, A. D., Berg, A. O., & Deyo, R. A. (1994). The effectiveness of four interventions for the prevention of low back pain. *Journal of the American Medical Association, 272*(16), 1286–1291.

Leino, P. I., & Hänninen, V. (1995). Psychosocial factors at work in relation to back and limb disorders. *Scandinavian Journal of Work, Environment, and Health, 21*(2), 134–142.

Lethem, J., Slade, P. D., Troup, J. D. G., & Bentley, G. (1983). Outline of a fear-avoidance model of exaggerated pain perceptions. *Behaviour Research and Therapy, 21,* 401–408.

Lindström, I., Öhlund, C., Eek, C., Wallin, L., Peterson, L. E., Fordyce, W. E., & Nachemson, A. L. (1992). The effect of graded activity on patients with subacute low back pain: A randomized prospective clinical study with an operant-conditioning behavioral approach. *Physical Therapy, 72,* 279–293.

Linton, S. J. (1991a). A behavioral workshop for training immediate supervisors: The key to neck and back injuries? *Perceptual and Motor Skills, 73,* 1159–1170.

Linton, S. J. (1991b). The manager's role in employees' successful return to work following back injury. *Work and Stress, 5*(3), 189–195.

Linton, S. J. (1994). The challenge of preventing chronic musculoskeletal pain. In G. F. Gebhart, D. L. Hammond, & T. S. Jensen (Eds.), *Proceedings of the Seventh World Congress on Pain: Vol. 2. Progress in pain and research management* (pp. 149–166). Seattle, WA: IASP Press.

Linton, S. J. (1998). The socioeconomic impact of chronic pain: Is anyone benefitting? *Pain, 75,* 163–168.

Linton, S. J., & Bradley, L. A. (1996). Strategies for the prevention of chronic pain. In R. J. Gatchel & D. C. Turk (Eds.), *Psychological approaches to pain management: A practitioner's handbook* (pp. 438–457). New York: Guilford Press.

Linton, S. J., & Buer, N. (1995). Working despite pain: Factors associated with work attendance versus dysfunction. *International Journal of Behavioral Medicine, 2*(3), 252–262.

Linton, S. J., Buer, N., Vlaeyen, J., & Hellsing, A. L. (in press). Are fear-avoidance beliefs related to a new episode of back pain?: A prospective study. *Psychology and Health.*

Linton, S. J., & Halldén, K. (1997). Risk factors and the natural course of acute and recurrent musculoskeletal pain: Developing a screening instrument. In T. S. Jensen, J. A. Turner, & Z. Wiesenfeld-Hallin (Eds.), *Proceedings of the Eighth World Congress on Pain: Vol. 8. Progress in pain research and management* (pp. 527–536). Seattle, WA: IASP Press.

Linton, S. J., & Halldén, K. (1998). *Can we screen for problematic back pain? A screening questionnaire for predicting outcome in acute and subacute back pain. The Clinical Journal of Pain, 14,* 209–215.

Linton, S. J., Hellsing, A. L., & Andersson, D. (1993). A controlled study of the effects of an early intervention on acute musculoskeletal pain problems. *Pain, 54,* 353–359.

Linton, S. J., Hellsing, A. L., & Bergström, G. (1996). Exercise for workers with musculoskeletal pain: Does enhancing compliance decrease pain? *Journal of Occupational Rehabilitation, 6*(3), 177–190.

Linton, S. J., Hellsing, A. L., & Halldén, K. (1998). A population based study of spinal pain among 35- to 45-year-olds: Prevalence, sick leave, and health-care utilization. *Spine, 23,* 1457–1463.

Linton, S. J., & Kamwendo, K. (1987). Low back schools: A critical review. *Physical Therapy, 67,* 1375–1383.

Linton, S. J., Melin, L., & Götestam, K. G. (1984). Behavioral analysis of chronic pain and its management. *Progress in Behavior Modification, 18,* 1–42.

Loisel, P., Abenhaim, L., Durand, P., Esdaile, J. M., Suissa, S., Gosselin, L., Simard, R., Turcotte, J., & Lemaire, J. (1997). A population based randomized clinical trial on back pain management. *Spine, 22,* 2911–2918.

Main, C. J., Wood, P. L. R., Hollis, S., Spanswick, C. C., & Waddell, G. (1992). The distress and risk assessment method: A simple patient classification to identify distress and evaluate the risk of poor outcome. *Spine, 17,* 42–52.

Malmivaara, A., Häkkinen, U, Aro, T., Heinrichs, M. L., Koskenniemi, L., Kuosma, E., Lappi, S., Paloheimo, R., Servo, C., Vaaranen, V., & Hernberg, S. (1995). The treatment of acute low back pain—bed rest, exercises, or ordinary activity? *New England Journal of Medicine, 332*(6), 351–355.

McCracken, L. M., Gross, R. T., Sorg, P. J., & Edmands, T. A. (1993). Prediction of pain in patients with chronic low back pain: Effects of inaccurate prediction and pain-related anxiety. *Behaviour Research and Therapy, 31,* 647–652.

Mitchell, R. I., & Carmen, G. M. (1990). Results of a multicenter trial using an intensive active exercise program for the treatment of acute soft tissue and back injuries. *Spine, 15,* 514–521.

Mitchell, R. I., & Carmen, G. M. (1994). The functional restoration approach to the treatment of chronic pain in patients with soft tissue and back injuries. *Spine, 19,* 633–642.

Nachemson, A. L. (1992). Newest knowledge of low back pain. *Clinical Orthopaedics, 279,* 8–20.

National Board of Health and Welfare. (1987). *Att förebygga*

sjukdomar i rörelseorganen [*Preventing musculoskeletal pain*]. Stockholm: Socialstyrelsen.

National Board of Occupational Safety. (1996). *Den kostsamma ohälsan* (*The high cost of illness*). Stockholm: Arbetarskyddsstyrelsen.

Nordin, M., Cedraschi, C., Balagué, F., & Roux, E. B. (1992). Back schools in prevention of chronicity. *Baillière's Clinical Rheumatology, 6*(3), 685–703.

Philips, H. C., & Grant, L. (1991). The evolution of chronic back pain problems: A longitudinal study. *Behavior Research and Therapy, 29,* 435–441.

Pope, M. H., Andersson, G. B., Frymoyer, J., & Chaffin, D. G. (1991). *Occupational low back pain: Assessment, treatment, and prevention.* St. Louis: Mosby-Yearbook.

Reid, S., Haugh, L. D., Hazard, R. G., & Tripathi, M. (1997). Occupational low back pain: Recovery curves and factors associated with disability. *Journal of Occupational Rehabilitation, 7*(1), 1–14.

Rosen, M. (1994). *Clinical Standards Advisory Group: Back pain report of a committee on back pain.* London: HMSO.

Ryan, W. E., Krishna, M. K., & Swanson, C. E. (1995). A prospective study evaluating early rehabilitation in preventing back pain chronicity in mine workers. *Spine, 20*(4), 489–491.

Scheer, S. J., Radack, K. L., & O'Brien, D. R. (1995). Randomized controlled trials in industrial low back pain relating to return to work: 1. Acute interventions. *Archives of Physical Medicine and Rehabilitation, 76,* 966–973.

Skovron, M. L. (1992). Epidemiology of low back pain. *Baillière's Clinical Rheumatology, 6*(3), 559–573.

Smedley, J., & Coggon, D. (1994). Will the manual handling regulations reduce the incidence of back disorders? *Occupational Medicine, 44,* 63–65.

Spitzer, W. O. (1993). Low back pain in the workplace: Attainable benefits not attained. *British Journal of Industrial Medicine, 50*(5), 245–250.

Swedish Council on Technology Assessment in Health Care. (1991). *Back pain: causes, diagnostics and treatment.* Stockholm: Author.

Symonds, T. L., Burton, A. K., Tillotson, K. M., & Main, C. J. (1995). Absence resulting from low back trouble can be reduced by psychosocial intervention at the work place. *Spine, 20*(24), 2738–2745.

Turk, D. C. (1996). Biopsychosocial perspective on chronic pain. In R. J. Gatchel & D. C. Turk (Eds.), *Psychological approaches to pain management: A practitioner's handbook* (pp. 3–32). New York: Guilford Press.

Turk, D. C. (1997). The role of demographic and psychosocial factors in transition from acute to chronic pain. In T. S. Jensen, J. A. Turner, & Z. Wiesenfeld-Hallin (Eds.), *Proceedings of the Eighth World Congress on Pain: Vol. 8. Progress in pain research and management* (pp. 185–213). Seattle, WA: IASP Press.

U.S. Department of Health and Human Services. (1991). *Healthy people 2000: National health promotion and disease prevention objectives* (DHHS Publication No. PHS 9-50212). Washington, DC: U.S. Government Printing Office.

van der Weide, W. E., Verbeek, J. H. A. M., & van Tulder, M. W. (1997). Vocational outcome of interventions for low-back pain. *Scandinavian Journal of Work, Environment, and Health, 23,* 165–178.

van Tulder, M. W., Koes, B. W., & Bouter, L. M. (1995). A cost-of-illness study of back pain in the Netherlands. *Pain, 62,* 233–240.

Vlaeyen, J. W. S., Kole-Snijders, A. M. J., Boeren, R. G. B., & van Eek, H. (1995). Fear of movement/(re)injury in chronic low back pain and its relation to behavioral performance. *Pain, 62,* 363-372.

Vlaeyen, J. W. S., Kole-Snijders, A. M. J., Rotteveel, A., Ruesink, R., & Heuts, P. H. T. G. (1995). The role of fear of movement/(re)injury in pain disability. *Journal of Occupational Rehabilitation, 5,* 235-252.

Von Korff, M. (1994). Perspectives on management of back pain in primary care. In G. F. Gebhart, D. L. Hammond, & T. S. Jensen (Eds.), *Proceedings of the Seventh World Congress on Pain: Vol. 2. Progress in pain research and management* (pp. 97-110). Seattle, WA: IASP Press.

Waddell, G. (1996). Low back pain: A twentieth century health care enigma. *Spine, 21*(24), 2820-2825.

Waddell, G., Feder, G., & Lewis, M. (1997). Systematic reviews of bed rest and advice to stay active for acute low back pain. *British Jour*[...] 652.

Waddell, G., Newton, M., Hend[...] & Main, C. J. (1993). A Fe[...] Questionnaire (FABQ) and the ro[...] beliefs in chronic low back pain and[...] *52,* 157-168.

Weiser, S., & Cedraschi, C. (1992). Psychoso[...] in the prevention of chronic low back pain—[...] ture review. *Baillière's Clinical Rheumatology,* [...] 657-684.

Westgaard, R. H., & Winkel, J. (1997). Ergonomic intervention research for improved musculoskeletal health: A critical review. *International Journal of Industrialized Ergonomics, 20,* 463-500.

Wood, E. J. (1987). Design and evaluation of a back injury prevention program within a geriatric hospital. *Spine, 12,* 77-82.

al of General Practice, 47, 647–

389

erson, L., Somerville, D.,
ar-Avoidance Beliefs
e of fear-avoidance
disability. Pain,

cial issues
litera-
6(3),

cal Screening
dromes:

Psychosocial Risk Factors for Poor Surgical Results

ANDREW R. BLOCK

Chronic pain syndromes are a source of tremendous frustration to patients, health care providers, and third-party payers. Chronic pain is almost ubiquitous in incidence, involves tremendous medical, economic, and social costs, and is frequently unresolved despite aggressive, technologically advanced medical intervention. For example, back pain, which occurs each year in approximately 37–51% of individuals in the United States (Von Korff, Dworkin, LeResche, & Kruger, 1988), is this country's leading cause of disability and lost production (Loeser, Bigos, Fordyce, & Violinn, 1990). Furthermore, back pain is associated with $50 billion in direct and indirect costs (Frymoyer, 1993). A number of other chronic pain syndromes also occur with alarming frequency. Chronic pelvic pain has a lifetime occurrence rate of 33% for women in the United States (Walker, Katon, Neraas, Jemelka, & Massoth, 1992). Temporomandibular joint dysfunction occurs in about 12% of the adult population (Dworkin et al., 1990). Headache is the primary cause of over 18 million office visits per year (Stewart & Lipton, 1993).

The search for a cure for chronic pain syndromes can be expensive and frustrating. The patient with unremitting pain may go to many different types of health care providers, often to no avail. As the pain wears on and additional diagnostic efforts are undertaken, many chronic pain patients may be presented with the option of surgery as a means of pain control. If the surgeon can tie the patient's pain to a diagnosable physical lesion, the ideas of removing the offending body part or surgically reducing its effects appear quite plausible. In some cases, patients are so desperate that they want a surgeon to perform "exploratory" surgery, even when no cause for the pain can be identified. A surgical option may seem attractive, as it offers the hope of quick pain control without much additional suffering or effort.

SURGERY FOR RELIEF OF CHRONIC PAIN: POSITIVE AND NEGATIVE RESULTS

Surgery is found as an option in a number of chronic pain syndromes. The syndrome most commonly leading to surgery is low back pain, with approximately 280,000 surgeries performed each year (Taylor, Deyo, Cherkin, & Kreuter, 1994), including laminectomy/discectomy, spinal fusion, and spinal cord stimulation. Another frequent pain-related surgical intervention is implantation of electrical stimulation devices in complex regional pain syndromes (i.e., reflex sympathetic dystrophy; see

Hassenbach, Stanton-Hicks, Schoppa, Walsh, & Covington, 1996). Hysterectomy as a treatment for relief of idiopathic chronic pelvic pain is performed in approximately 70,000–80,000 cases each year (Lee, Dicken, Rubin, & Ory, 1984). Even patients with temporomandibular joint dysfunction may be recommended to undergo surgical procedures such as disk repair or condylectomy.

In this chapter, spine surgery is utilized as a model of pain-related surgical intervention, since procedures on the spine are quite frequent and have been the subject of a large body of research. It is clear that the sometimes Herculean efforts involved in spine surgery may well bring positive results. For example, Malter, Larson, Urban, and Deyo (1996), examining the effectiveness of laminectomy/discectomy, found that those patients receiving surgery had significantly greater quality of life at 5 years postoperation than did patients given conservative care only. Furthermore, the results of this study showed that the cost effectiveness of laminectomy/discectomy exceeded that of medication treatment for hypertension, as well as that of single artery bypass grafting in coronary heart disease.

Unfortunately, the results of surgery for chronic pain syndromes are not uniformly positive. Turner et al. (1992), reviewing all published research on spinal fusion, found that only 65–75% of all patients achieved satisfactory clinical outcomes, poorer outcome being associated with greater numbers of fused levels and the use of instrumentation. Similarly, Hoffman, Wheeler, and Deyo (1993), in a literature review on laminectomy/discectomy, found that the mean success rate of this procedure for relief of spine pain was 67%.

Poor surgical results can have a significant impact on the patient, the physician, the employer, and the insurance company. The patient, of course, continues to remain disabled, with perhaps even greater pain, worsened medication dependence, and more emotional difficulty than prior to the surgery. The pain may be so great or the surgery so unsuccessful that reoperation is required—as is the case for 10% of those who undergo laminectomy/discectomy (Hoffman et al., 1993), and for 23% of those who undergo spinal fusion (Franklin, Haug, Heyer, McKeefrey, & Picciano, 1994). The failed-surgery patient places many demands on the health care system, sometimes requiring increasingly strong medications and expensive multiple treatments. Always there is frustration and discouragement. The patient may feel tremendously let down, the physician angry at the patient for not respond-

ing to treatment, and the employer concerned about the stability of a permanently damaged worker.

In recent years there has been a growing interest in identifying those patients at risk for having a poor response to surgery aimed at relieving their chronic pain. If a means for such identification could be developed, not only would patients be spared the burden of suffering but also significant cost savings could result. If one considers that approximately 235,000 laminectomy/discectomy procedures are performed each year (Taylor et al., 1994) and that approximately 25% of these result in failure, then about 58,750 patients each year continue to experience pain after surgery. The average cost of a laminectomy/discectomy, including hospitalization and postoperative rehabilitation, is about $18,000 (Block, 1996). Therefore, a screening procedure that could correctly predict all laminectomy/discectomy failures would save 58,750 × $18,000 = $1,057,000,000 per year in direct medical costs alone. Additional economic savings would be garnered through avoidance of reoperation, as well as reduction of lost work time and compensation. Avoiding surgical failures also has significant impact on the physician, as it improves overall outcome success and reduces the number of difficult patients in the physician practice.

The body of research on spine surgery outcome has increasingly demonstrated that the strongest predictors of poor results are psychosocial factors. Many elements of the patient's personality, emotional state, and history can combine with current contingencies in the patient's social and vocational environment to militate against good surgical results. This chapter reviews these psychosocial risk factors and concludes with a discussion of the value of including presurgical psychological screening (PPS) within the evaluation of the chronic pain surgery candidate.

PSYCHOLOGICAL RISK FACTORS

Personality and Emotional Factors

Patients with chronic pain arising from spine injuries are frequently the recipients of intensive, technologically sophisticated medical diagnostic tests. Some such tests, including magnetic resonance imaging (MRI), computed tomography (CT scan), X-ray, and myelography, are designed to take a static snapshot of structural abnormalities or problems underlying the patient's pain experience. Other, more invasive, tests attempt diagnosis by linking identifiable pathophysiology to alterations in the pain experience, either through provoking the patient's normal pain (as in discography; see Block, Vanharanta, Ohnmeiss, & Guyer, 1996) or ameliorating the patient's pain (as in selective nerve root blocks and sequential spinal studies; see White & Schofferman, 1995, for thorough discussions of diagnostic procedures). Yet such advanced and expensive procedures of necessity give little attention to the fact that the pain is experienced by individuals who vary widely in their characteristics and coping mechanisms.

Perhaps the most significant influences on spine surgery outcome arise from individual differences in patient personality. Personality traits are defined as "deeply ingrained patterns of behaviors, which include the way one relates to, perceives, and thinks about the environment and oneself that are exhibited in a wide range of social and personal contexts" (American Psychiatric Association, 1994, p. 630). Fortunately, there is an extremely well-researched and widely accepted psychological test for assessment of personality traits in chronic pain patients—the MMPI-2 (Keller & Butcher, 1991). This test has found increasing use in identifying patients whose personalities place them at risk for poor surgical outcome (see Table 24.1).

Studies of the MMPI as a predictor of surgical outcome are of varying quality. Many studies do not report the specific types of surgical procedures being examined. Outcome is assessed at varying intervals, using measures that range from patient self-ratings of pain, medication use, and return to work (e.g., Uomoto, Turner, & Herron, 1988; Doxey, Dzioba, & Mitson, 1988) to surgeon's global ratings of patient outcome (e.g., Long, 1981). However, examination of Table 24.1 reveals that two MMPI scales consistently emerge as predictors of poor surgical outcome: scales *Hs* (Hypochondriasis) and *Hy* (Hysteria). In addition, scales *D* (Depression), *Pt* (Psychasthenia), and *Pd* (Psychopathic Deviate) have been found in some studies to be associated with the failure of spine surgery to relieve pain. A detailed examination of studies examining these scale elevations may be relevant not only to PPS for spine surgery but also to a broad range of pain syndromes.

Pain Sensitivity (MMPI Scales Hs and Hy)

Elevations on these two scales presumably assess a propensity toward excessive focus on, and sensitivity to, physical symptoms and pain (Graham, 1990). Such elevations have been frequently found to be associated with poor outcome in many pain

syndromes, including chronic pelvic pain (Rosenthal, Ling, Rosenthal, & McNeeley, 1984), gastrointestinal disorders (Whitehead, 1993), and conservative treatment of chronic back pain (Kleinke & Spangler, 1988). It is not surprising that such personality traits may negatively affect response to surgery.

One way in which pain sensitivity may complicate the diagnosis and treatment of spine surgery candidates is demonstrated in a study on discography performed in our laboratory (Block et al., 1996). The discogram is a procedure in which radiographic dye is injected into the nucleus of a presumably ruptured disc. The injection achieves two purposes. First, it allows for visualization of the extent of disc rupture through fluoroscopy and the use of use of a postdiscogram CT scan. Second, the injection often provokes the patient's normally occurring pain, perhaps by stimulating nociceptors in the disc itself. Normally, injection of a herniated disc provokes pain, whereas injection of a "normal" disc is not pain-provocative. Frequently, several adjacent discs are examined in the same patient, in order to identify the so-called pain generator. Research has shown, however, that discordant pain (i.e., pain on injection of a normal disc) is frequently experienced (Vanharanta et al., 1987). Our research has found that patients with such discordant pain reports have elevations on scales *Hs* and *Hy* relative to patients with no discordant reports. Such findings are especially significant because an individual patient may show pain reports concordant with an identifiable disc herniation at one level and discordant pain reports at another level. Thus, although discography may identify a "pain generator" in such a patient, the decision to operate is questionable. This study demonstrates that pain sensitivity, as assessed by the MMPI *Hs* and *Hy* scales, can coexist with identifiable pathophysiology and militate against good surgical results.

Depression (MMPI Scale D)

A number of studies reported in Table 24.1 indicate that elevations on the MMPI Depression scale can be significantly associated with poor surgery outcome. Other studies examining depression in surgical candidates with different measures, such as the Beck Depression Inventory, have confirmed that such an emotional state bodes poorly for successful surgery (Junge, Dvorak, & Ahrens, 1995). Such findings are of great significance, since depression and chronic pain share

TABLE 24.1. Studies Examining the Relationship of MMPI to Spine Surgery Outcome

Authors	Subjects	Evaluation interval	MMPI results
Cashion & Lynch (1979)	78 laminectomy patients, no previous surgery	1 year	Significant differences between good and bad outcome, scales Hs, D, K, F, Es
Doxey et al. (1988); Dzioba & Doxey (1984)	116 workers compensation patients, no previous surgery. 74 received surgery, 43 did not	1 year	Hs, Ma, Pt higher in poor outcome patients
Kuperman et al. (1979)	37 discectomy patients, no previous surgery	1 year	Hs, Hy, D, significant R^2 with outcome; R^2 of Hs + Hy + D with outcome = .58
Long (1981)	44 surgery patients, referred because of suspected "nonorganic" factors	6–18 months postsurgery	Hy, Hs, Pd higher in poor outcome group
Pheasant, Gelbert, Goldfarb, & Herron (1979)	90 patients, various procedures	6 months, 1 year	Hs, Hy higher in poor outcome group
Riley et al. (1995)	71 fusion patients, 39% previous surgery, 37% workers compensation	Average 20 months postsurgery	Cluster analysis: poorest outcome in patients with high Hs + Hy, and "depressed–pathological"
Smith & Duerksen (1979)	31 patients, various procedures, 3 previous surgery	Unclear	Hs, Hy, D significant R^2 with outcome
Sorenson & Mors (1988)	57 discectomy patients, no previous surgery	6, 24 months postsurgery	R^2 with poor outcome: Hs = .37, D = .37, Hy = .47; also Sc, Ma
Spengler et al. (1990)	84 discectomy patients, no previous surgery	1 year or more	Hs + Hy significantly associated with poor outcome; also Pd, Sc
Turner, Herron, & Weiner (1986); Uomoto et al. (1988)	106 discectomy patients, 25 previous surgery	1 year	Discrimatory function using MMPI predicted 69.7% of outcome, function including Hs, K, L
Wiltse & Rocchio (1975)	130 chemonucleolysis patients, no previous surgery	1 year	Success predicted by Hs + Hy, not predicted by physical findings

many common symptoms, including sleep disturbance, appetite impairment, decreased concentration and energy, social withdrawal, and lowered self-esteem (Cavanaugh, Clark, & Gibbons, 1983). Furthermore, previous research has shown that up to 85% of chronic pain patients display sufficient symptoms to be given a diagnosis of clinical depression (Lindsay & Wyckoff, 1981). It is well established that depressed individuals more easily perceive negative than positive events (Seligman, 1975) and that depressed pain patients do not perceive the improvements they make (Kremer, Block, & Atkinson, 1983). It appears that, for many surgical candidates, the depression and pain experienced interact, producing a downward physical and emotional spiral from which escape becomes very problematic.

There are, however, two features of depression among chronic pain patients that place qualifications on such pessimistic conclusions. First, clinical depression in some surgical candidates may be a direct reaction to the pain and disability they experience, whereas for other patients, perhaps about 40%, the depression predates their pain (Polatin, Kinney, Gatchel, Lillo, & Mayer, 1993). In general, chronic emotional conditions are more recalcitrant than are reactive types, so that patients whose depression is of more recent onset may be better surgical candidates. Additionally, there are reasons to believe that proper treatment of depression may actually give a boost to surgical results. A large body of research has shown that the use of antidepressant medication in chronic pain patients not only relieves clinical depressive symptomatology (Atkinson, 1989;

McQuay et al., 1996) but may also have anti-nociceptive effects (Onghena & Van Houdenhove, 1992). Furthermore, cognitive-behavioral intervention, when used with depressed chronic pain patients, can lead to increased functional ability and decreased health care utilization (Jensen, Turner, & Romano, 1994), as well as reductions in self-reported pain (Keefe, Salley, & Lefevbre, 1992). To the extent that depression is reactive and is given direct clinical attention, surgical outcome may not be compromised. On the other hand, the patient with chronic depression, especially when this predates the injury and has been resistant to intervention, is at risk for poor surgical results.

Anxiety (MMPI Scale Pt)

Fear, nervousness, worry, obsessive thoughts, and tension are frequent concomitants of chronic pain. Such feelings might be expected to be heightened in patients about to receive spine surgery. Frequently, the surgical candidate has been told by friends or relatives to avoid surgery. There is often trepidation about the ability to return to work or to recover function. Patients often fear the anesthesia, needles, and procedures involved in the surgery itself. For some patients such fears and worries are more chronic in nature. Fishbain, Goldberg, Meagher, Steele, and Rosomoff (1986) found that approximately 25% of chronic pain patients are obsessive–compulsive personality types and that 7% have diagnosable obsessive–compulsive personality disorders. Such protracted problems with anxiety and worry, as well as more reactive anxious emotional states, are tracked by MMPI scale Pt elevations. Examination of Table 24.1 shows that such elevations are associated in a number of studies with reduced spine surgery results. One might expect that more protracted anxious emotional conditions that predate the spine injury would bode more poorly for surgery. Such findings would parallel results seen with depression. Unfortunately, such results are currently lacking, so that high anxiety levels, regardless of their duration, should be considered surgical risk factors.

Anger (MMPI Scale Pd elevations)

Patients with chronic pain frequently experience intense angry feelings (Turk & Fernandez, 1995). These may be directed at any number of subjects. Patients who are injured in motor vehicle accidents are frequently angry at the other driver. Anger may

be directed at physicians or the health care system. Frustrations with insurance coverage may escalate the patient's level of anger. It is also not uncommon for a patient to experience a great deal of self-directed anger. Just as with depression and anxiety, anger may be more chronic in nature. Studies have shown that chronic pain patients frequently have personality disorders in which anger plays a strong component, such as passive–aggressive and antisocial personality disorders (Kuperman, Osmon, Golden, & Blume, 1979).

Anger has been found to have a negative impact on the treatment of chronic pain syndromes. DeGood and Kiernan (1996) found that chronic pain patients who placed blame for the injury on the employer had poorer pain treatment outcomes, as well as higher levels of mood disturbance, than those who did not make such attributions. Turk and Fernandez (1995) have suggested that patients who are angry blame others for their difficulties and that those who are rebellious toward authority figures may respond more poorly to treatment because they fail to form a therapeutic alliance with the health care team. The results in Table 24.1 indicate that anger and rebelliousness, both of which are components of MMPI scale Pd, can be associated with diminished spine surgery outcome. Such emotional and personality characteristics should be considered significant risk factors.

Additional Considerations

Although the four previously listed MMPI scale elevations and their associated emotional conditions are those with the greatest research support, Table 24.1 indicates that negative associations with surgical outcome are also found for other scales (Sorenson & Mors, 1988; Spengler, Ouelette, Battie, & Zeh, 1990). Patients with elevations on these scales should be dealt with carefully.

Intriguing recent research by Riley, Robinson, Geisser, Wittmer, and Smith (1995) has demonstrated the value of examining multiple MMPI scale elevations. In their study, two particular profiles involving multiple scales were found to be associated with diminished surgical results. The first, termed "V-Type," involves elevations on scales Hs and Hy and is consistent with the pain sensitivity concept described previously. The second profile, "Depressed–Pathological," involves extreme elevations on a number of scales, including Sc, Pt, Pa, Hy, D, and Hs. Although this group was small, outcome appeared quite poor. Certainly, patients demonstrating such a significant level of psychopathology would be expected to have difficulties coping with the stress, pain, and psychosocial changes resulting from surgery.

Cognitive Factors

The ways a patient thinks about and copes with the experience of chronic pain can play a large role in determining functional abilities, emotional status, and compliance with treatment recommendations (Jensen et al., 1994). Such "cognitive" aspects of pain, which have been the focus of much chronic pain research in recent years, are divided into two broad areas: coping (specific thoughts and behaviors people use to manage pain and their reaction to pain), and beliefs (thoughts people have regarding the consequences of pain and their ability to cope with pain). Poor coping strategies and negative beliefs have been found to be associated with reduced outcome of treatment for chronic pain in general (Jensen et al., 1994). Such "maladaptive" thoughts include, among others, the following:

> Catastrophizing: Misinterpreting a minor setback as a catastrophe.
> Emotional reasoning: Assuming that one's negative feelings about a situation must be true.
> Personalization: Seeing oneself as the cause of some negative event over which one actually has no influence.

One widely used test of cognitive factors, the Coping Strategies Questionnaire (CSQ), has been applied to patients undergoing spine surgery. Gross (1986) gave the CSQ to 50 laminectomy patients. Results showed that patients scoring high on a positive coping strategy, self-reliance, had decreased postsurgical pain, improved sleep, and better self-rated treatment outcome than less self-reliant individuals. Patients reporting cognitions involving loss of control over pain and catastrophizing had greater postsurgical pain. Although direct research with surgical candidates is limited, the fact that cognitive factors have been shown to significantly affect the outcome of general chronic pain treatment underscores the importance of considering maladaptive cognition as a risk factor for poor surgical outcome.

Behavioral Factors

The experience of chronic back pain involves more than noxious sensation and emotional distress. Pain leads to the emission of a recognizable set of behaviors, including limping, bracing, guarded movement, rubbing the affected area, sighing, and so forth (Keefe & Block, 1982). Such behaviors, perhaps a direct result of painful sensations, often take place within a social context. In this sense, pain behaviors communicate to observers that the patient is experiencing unpleasant sensations. The observer, whether the spouse, the employer, or the physician, often responds to these behaviors. Pain behaviors may provoke such observer responses as taking over the patient's responsibilities, bringing medication, allowing the patient time off from work, and so forth. It is increasingly being recognized that the responses of others, and indeed of the health care system, may be sufficient to maintain pain behaviors "long after the original nociceptive stimulus has been resolved" (Fordyce, 1978, p. 59). In the case of the surgical patient, who obviously has identifiable pathophysiology, such reinforcement of pain behavior may still play a major role in maintaining the patient's pain and physical limitations. These behavioral incentives to remain disabled and disincentives for recovery may be provided to the patient by many sources.

Vocational and Financial Aspects

Job-related injuries may lead to a number of disincentives to improvement or obstacles to recovery. First, patients receiving worker's compensation payments appear to have diminished surgical response. Hudgins (1976) compared clinical outcomes at 1 year postlaminectomy for 76 worker's compensation patients versus an equal number of noncompensation patients. Of the compensation patients, only 10 reported complete pain relief and 14 were unimproved, as compared with the noncompensation group, in which 31 reported complete relief and 4 were unimproved. A number of other authors have found reduced spine surgery results in worker's compensation patients (Davis, 1994; Greenough & Fraser, 1989; Haddad, 1987).

Patients who have been injured on the job may also be less likely to respond well to surgery because they may not enjoy their jobs. Bigos et al. (1991) have found that job dissatisfaction can play a major role in worker's compensation injuries. In a prospective study of 3,000 aircraft manufacturing employees, low levels of job satisfaction were associated with greatly increased risk of job-related injury. Such job dissatisfaction is likely also correlated with poor spine surgery outcome.

An additional vocational factor associated with negative surgical results involves the nature of the patient's job. A number of studies have found that patients who have jobs involving heavy lifting (50 pounds or more frequently) are both more likely to sustain job-related injury and to have poorer results from spine surgery (Davis, 1994; Junge et al., 1995).

Finally, a related financial aspect of many chronic pain-related injuries is associated with reduced outcome. For many patients, the injury may result in a financial settlement. In some cases litigation may be brought against the party who putatively caused the injury. In other cases, the patient may retain a lawyer to help obtain social security disability benefits. For such patients, the financial disincentives to improvement may play a large role in determining outcome. Haddad (1987) found that 77% of worker's compensation patients who were represented by an attorney had poor surgery results versus only 9% of those who did not have an attorney. Poorer surgical outcome is found in patients with a history of lawsuits for medicolegal problems (Finneson & Cooper, 1979; Manniche et al., 1994) and in patients applying for disability pensions (Junge et al., 1995).

Even though vocational and financial issues may exert a strong influence on surgical outcome, this does not mean that patients with job-related injuries are malingering. Surveys of orthopedic and neurosurgeons have found that malingering in back pain patients is rare, occurring in about 5% of patients (Leavitt & Sweet, 1986). Furthermore, malingering is ruled out in the case of most spine surgery candidates. Malingering, according to DSM-IV, involves the intentional production of false or grossly exaggerated physical symptoms (American Psychiatric Association, 1994). Because the spine surgery candidate has a pathophysiological basis for the pain, it would be quite problematic to diagnose malingering. Rather, it seems likely that, due to vocational or incentive-based factors, pain patients may become more pain sensitive and less likely to respond to interventions designed to alleviate pain.

Response of Family Members

Beginning with Fordyce's (1976) pioneering work, the responses of the spouse and other family members have been found to exert a strong influence on the pain patient. Fordyce speculated that the family could reinforce pain and disability by selectively attending to the patient only when pain was reported or displayed, ignoring the patient at other times. Early research in our own laboratory supported this speculation. In the original study (Block, Kremer, & Gaylor, 1980), patients communicated their pain level (on a scale of 0-10) at two times during an interview, once in the presence of the spouse and again in the presence of a "neutral observer," the ward clerk. Patients also responded to questions about the extent to which the spouse reinforced pain behaviors through selective attention. Patients whose spouses were pain "solicitous" reported higher pain levels when the spouse was observing than when the ward clerk was observing. The opposite result was obtained for patients with "nonsolicitous" spouses. Thus this research supported an operant view of chronic pain by demonstrating that the solicitous spouse could act as a "discriminative cue" for the emission of pain behavior by the patient. Subsequent research in a number of laboratories has demonstrated that solicitous spousal response can exert a strong influence on patient pain behavior (Lousberg, Schmidt, & Groenman, 1992). At present the most effective means of examining the extent of spousal reinforcement for pain behavior is the Multidimensional Pain Inventory (MPI; Kerns, Turk, & Rudy, 1985). Surgical candidates whose spouses are shown by the MPI to be solicitous of pain behavior could be expected to have poorer outcome.

Family members may provide emotional disincentives for improvement in another way. Numerous studies have demonstrated that marital distress is high among some chronic pain patients and that the patient's spouse frequently becomes depressed (Romano, Turner, & Clancy, 1989; Schwartz, Slater, Birchler, & Atkinson, 1991). Previous research in our laboratory has shown that such dissatisfied spouses have more negative outcome expectations for the patient and tend to attribute the patient's pain to psychological causes (Block, Boyer, & Silbert, 1985; Block & Boyer, 1984). It is likely that spouses who are dissatisfied would be less supportive of the patient. Social support, particularly from the spouse, has been found to be an important influence on compliance with medical treatment recommendations (O'Brien, 1980) and on recovery from invasive surgery, such as hip replacement (Mutran, Reitzes, Mossey, & Fernandez, 1995). Thus patients who report a high level of marital distress or have unstable or unsupportive marital relationships may have reduced surgical prognosis. It is recommended that marital dissatisfaction be assessed in the surgical candidate, perhaps through the use of the Locke-Wallace Marital Satisfaction Inventory (Locke & Wallace, 1959).

Historical Factors

Every individual who endures spine injury or disease has a lifetime of experiences prior to the onset of pain. The patient's life history, of course, can influence pain perception and response. Patients who do not cope well with adversity may find the stresses involved in dealing with a spine injury to be overwhelming. Furthermore, protracted pain can reactivate many problems the patient experienced earlier in life. For example, patients with a history of very low self-esteem may find that the functional limitations of the spine injury recreate feelings of worthlessness and/or guilt. Research has demonstrated that a number of aspects of the spine surgery candidate's preinjury history, as well as historical problems continuing after the onset of pain, can negatively influence surgical recovery.

Past Psychological Treatment

The existence of diagnosable mental health disorders among chronic pain patients is quite high. Kinney, Gatchel, Polatin, Fogarty, & Mayer (1993), for example, found that among low back pain sufferers, 100% of those with chronic pain, as well as 61% of those with acute pain, had diagnosable psychological conditions. As noted earlier in the discussion of depression, such psychological problems may predate the injury. A number of authors have found or suggested that preexisting psychological problems are associated with reduced spine surgery results (Keel, 1984; Polatin et al., 1993). It would seem likely that more intense preexisting psychological problems (i.e., those leading to inpatient psychiatric treatment) would bode more poorly than would less intense difficulties, although research in this area is lacking.

Physical and Sexual Abuse and Abandonment

Abuse and abandonment are widespread scourges of modern society. Unfortunately, many back pain patients have been victimized by such unconscionable behavior. Haber and Roos (1985) found, for example, that over half of the patients evaluated at

a multidisciplinary pain clinic had a history of such abuse and that for 90% the abuse occurred during adulthood. A recent study by Linton (1997) suggests that experiences of sexual and physical abuse may predispose individuals, especially women, toward chronic pain. This study surveyed nonpatients in Sweden, as well as chronic pain patients, about their history of physical and sexual abuse. Nonpatients were also questioned about any chronic pain symptoms they might have had. For the nonpatient women reporting no pain, frequency of physical abuse was 2% and frequency of sexual abuse was 23%. However, for nonpatient women reporting "pronounced pain," frequency of physical abuse was 8% and frequency of sexual abuse was 46%. Among the female chronic pain patients, 35% had an abuse history. Additional analyses determined that the chances of developing chronic pain were increased fivefold by physical abuse and fourfold by sexual abuse. For men, there appeared to be little association of abuse with pain.

Given these findings, it is perhaps not surprising that sexual and physical abuse have been found to be associated with poor outcome of spine surgery. Schofferman, Anderson, Hinds, Smith, & White (1992) found an 85% failure rate from spine surgery among patients with a strong history of childhood abuse and abandonment, compared to a 5% failure rate among patients lacking such a traumatic history. Therefore, in evaluating the spine surgery candidate, history of physical or sexual abuse should be considered a risk factor.

Substance Abuse

Overuse of narcotic prescription medication, as well as dependence and abuse of alcohol and street drugs, are topics that are underresearched in the area of chronic pain in general and in PPS specifically. It seems likely that patients with protracted pain experience would come to rely on analgesic substances for relief, as well as to improve functional ability. To the extent that such substances are used, the patient's sense of responsibility for symptom control might be diminished, and the belief that pain control depends on external measures might be increased. Thus substance abuse and dependence would seem to exert a potential negative influence on pain treatment outcome. Indeed, Spengler, Freeman, Westbrook, and Miller (1980) examined 30 of their spine surgery failures and found that 25 were "continually abusing medication and alcohol." There is, however, little other direct evidence that substance abuse inhibits surgical recovery. At this point, extensive use of narcotic medication, street drugs, or alcohol should only be considered a risk factor if the patient clearly meets *DSM-IV* criteria for substance abuse.

SUMMARY AND CONCLUSIONS

This chapter has reviewed literature demonstrating that psychosocial factors may influence the outcome of surgeries that are aimed at relief of chronic pain. Table 24.2 summarizes these psychosocial risk factors, which fall into four main categories: personality and emotional factors, cognitive factors, behavioral factors, and historical factors. In general, these risk factors can be assumed to have an additive effect, such that greater numbers of identified risk factors are associated with correspondingly higher risk of poor outcome.

In previous work we have identified a model for quantifying these psychosocial risk factors and combining them with medical risk factors to determine a specific surgical prognosis (see Block, 1996). Although explication of this model is beyond the scope of this chapter, it is clear that psychosocial risk factors militate against good surgical outcome. A study in our laboratory examined outcome in 165 spine surgery candidates (Block, 1997). All participants were given the MMPI, CSQ, and a structured interview prior to surgery. Based

on this evaluation patients were declared to have good, fair, or poor surgical prognosis. Outcome measures, which were given to patients 6 months after surgery, included a pain analogue rating scale, evaluations of continued use of narcotic medication and return to work, and scores on the Oswestry Disability Index. Poor outcome was obtained in 78% of those patients who had been declared to have poor surgical prognosis. These patients were also taking significantly greater levels of narcotics and reporting higher pain levels and had lower levels of self-reported functional ability than did the good prognosis candidates. Such results, combined with the burgeoning research in PPS, suggest that examining psychosocial risk factors in chronic pain patients has the potential to improve overall surgical outcome, avoid iatrogenic problems, and reduce treatment costs.

REFERENCES

American Psychiatric Association. (1987). *Diagnostic and statistical manual of mental disorders* (3rd ed., rev.). Washington, DC: Author.

American Psychiatric Association. (1994). *Diagnostic and statistical manual of mental disorders* (4th ed.). Washington, DC: Author.

Atkinson, J. H. (1989). Psychopharmacologic agents in the treatment of pain syndromes. In C. D. Tollison (Ed.), *Handbook of chronic pain management* (pp. 69–103). Baltimore: Williams & Wilkins.

Bigos, S. J., Battie, M. C., Spengler, D. M., Fisher, L. D., Fordyce, W. E., Hansson, T., Nachemson, A. L., & Worthly, M. D. (1991). A prospective study of work perceptions and psychosocial factors affecting the report of back injury. *Spine, 16,* 1–6.

Block, A. R. (1996). *Presurgical psychological screening in chronic pain syndromes: A guide for the behavioral health practitioner.* Mahwah, NJ: Erlbaum.

Block, A. R. (1997). *Presurgical psychological screening.* Paper presented at the 16th annual meeting of the American Pain Society, New Orleans, LA.

Block, A. R., & Boyer, S. L. (1984). The spouse's adjustment to chronic pain: Cognitive and emotional factors. *Social Science and Medicine, 19,* 1313–1317.

Block, A. R., Boyer, S. L., & Silbert, R. V. (1985). Spouse's perception of the chronic pain patient: Estimates of exercise tolerance. In H. L. Fields, R. Dubner & F. Cervero (Eds.), *Advances in pain research and therapy* (Vol. 9, pp. 897–904). New York: Raven Press.

Block, A. R., Kremer, E., & Gaylor, M. (1980). Behavioral treatment of chronic pain: Variables affecting treatment efficacy. *Pain, 8,* 367–375.

Block, A. R., Vanharanta, H., Ohnmeiss, D., & Guyer, R. D. (1996). Discographic pain report: Influence of psychological factors. *Spine, 21,* 334–338.

Cashion, E. L., & Lynch, W. J. (1979). Personality factors and results of lumbar disc surgery. *Neurosurgery 4,* 141–145.

TABLE 24.2. Psychosocial Risk Factors in Surgery for Chronic Pain

Personality and emotional factors
   Pain sensitivity
   Depression
   Anxiety
   Anger

Cognitive factors
   Catastrophizing and loss of control

Behavioral factors
   Vocational and financial aspects
      Worker's compensation
      Job dissatisfaction
      Heavy lifting
      Financial settlement expected

   Response of family members
      Solicitous spousal responses
      Marital dissatisfaction

Historical factors
   Prior psychological treatment
   Physical and sexual abuse
   Substance abuse

Cavanaugh, S., Clark, D. C., & Gibbons, R. D. (1983). Diagnosing depression in the hospitalized medically ill. *Psychosomatics, 24*, 809–815.

Davis, R. A. (1994). A long-term outcome analysis of 984 surgically treated herniated lumbar discs. *Journal of Neurosurgery, 80*, 514–521.

DeGood, D. E., & Kiernan, B. (1996). Perception of fault in patients with chronic pain. *Pain, 64*, 153–159.

Doxey, N. C., Dzioba, R. B., & Mitson, G. L. (1988). Predictors of outcome in back surgery candidates. *Journal of Clinical Psychology, 44*, 611–622.

Dworkin, S. F., Huggins, K. H., LeResche, L., Von Korff, M., Howard, J., Truelove, E., & Sommers, E. (1990). Epidemiology of signs and symptoms in temporomandibular disorders: Clinical signs in cases and controls. *Journal of the American Dental Association, 120*, 273–281.

Dzioba, R. B., & Doxey, N. C. (1984). A prospective investigation in the orthopedic and psychologic predictors of outcome of first lumbar surgery following industrial injury. *Spine, 9*, 614–623.

Finneson, B. E., & Cooper, V. R. (1979). A lumbar disc surgery predictive score card: A retrospective evaluation. *Spine, 4*, 141–144.

Fishbain, D. A., Goldberg, M., Meagher, B. R., Steele, R., & Rosomoff, H. (1986). Male and female chronic pain patients categorized by DSM-III psychiatric diagnostic criteria. *Pain, 26*, 181–197.

Fordyce, W. E. (1976). *Behavioral methods for chronic pain and illness.* St. Louis: Mosby.

Fordyce, W. E. (1978). Learning process in pain. In R. A. Sternbach (Ed.), *The psychology of pain* (pp. 49–72). New York: Raven Press.

Franklin, G. M., Haug, J., Heyer, N. J., McKeefrey, S. P., & Picciano, J. F. (1994). Outcome of lumbar fusion in Washington State workers' compensation. *Spine, 19*(17), 1897–1904.

Frymoyer, J. W. (1993). Quality: An international challenge to the diagnosis and treatment of disorders of the lumbar spine. *Spine, 18*, 2147–2152.

Graham, J. R. (1990). *The MMPI-2: Assessing personality and psychopathology.* New York: Oxford University Press.

Greenough, C. G., & Fraser, R. D. (1989). The effects of compensation on recovery from low-back injury. *Spine, 14*(9), 947–955.

Gross, A. R. (1986). The effect of coping strategies on the relief of pain following surgical intervention for lower back pain. *Psychosomatic Medicine, 48*, 229–238.

Haber, J., & Roos, C. (1985). Effects of spouse abuse and/or sexual abuse in the development and maintenance of chronic pain in women. *Advances in Pain Research and Therapy, 9*, 889–895.

Haddad, G. H. (1987). Analysis of 2932 workers' compensation back injury cases: The impact of the cost to the system. *Spine, 12*(8), 765–271.

Hassenbach, S. J., Stanton-Hicks, M. Schoppa, D., Walsh, J. G., & Covington, E. C. (1996). Long-term results of peripheral nerve stimulation for reflex sympathetic dystrophy. *Journal of Neurosurgery, 84*, 415–423.

Hoffman, R. M., Wheeler, K. J., & Deyo, R. A. (1993). Surgery for herniated lumbar discs: A literature synthesis. *Journal of General Internal Medicine, 8*, 487–496.

Hudgins, W. R. (1976). Laminectomy for treatment of lumbar disc disease. *Texas Medicine, 72*, 65–69.

Jensen, M. P., Turner, J. A., & Romano, J. M. (1994). Correlates of improvement in multidisciplinary treatment of chronic pain. *Journal of Consulting and Clinical Psychology, 62*(1), 172–179.

Junge, A., Dvorak, J., & Ahrens, S. (1995). Predictors of bad and good outcomes of lumbar disc surgery: A prospective clinical study with recommendations for screening to avoid bad outcomes. *Spine, 20*(4), 460–468.

Keefe, F. J., & Block, A. R. (1982). Development of an observation method for assessing pain behavior in chronic low back pain patients. *Behavior Therapy, 13*, 363–375.

Keefe, F. J., Salley, A. N., & Lefevbre, J. C. (1992). Coping with pain: Conceptual concerns and future directions. *Pain, 51*, 131–134.

Keel, P. J. (1984). Psychosocial criteria for patient selection: Review of studies and concepts for understanding chronic back pain. *Neurosurgery, 15*(6), 935–941.

Keller, L. S., & Butcher, J. N. (1991). *MMPI-2 monographs: Vol. 2. Assessment of chronic pain patients with the MMPI-2.* Minneapolis: University of Minnesota Press.

Kerns, R. D., Turk, D. C., & Rudy, E. E. (1985). The West Haven-Yale Multidimensional Pain Inventory (WHYMPI). *Pain, 23*, 345–356.

Kinney, R. K., Gatchel, R. J., Polatin, P. B., Fogarty, W. T., & Mayer, T. G. (1993). Prevalence of psychopathology in acute and chronic low back pain patients. *Journal of Occupational Rehabilitation, 3*(2), 95–103.

Kleinke, C. L., & Spangler, A. S. (1988). Predicting treatment outcome of chronic back pain patients in a multidisciplinary pain clinic: Methodological issues and treatment implications. *Pain, 33*, 41–48.

Kremer, E. F., Block, A. R., & Atkinson, J. J. (1983). Assessment of pain behavior: Factors that distort self-report. In R. Melzack (Ed.), *Pain management and assessment* (pp. 165–171). New York: Raven Press.

Kuperman, S. K., Osmon, D., Golden, C. J., & Blume, H. G. (1979). Prediction of neurosurgical results by psychological evaluation. *Perceptual and Motor Skills, 48*, 311–315.

Leavitt, F., & Sweet, J. J. (1986). Characteristics and frequency of malingering among patients with low back pain. *Pain, 25*, 357–364.

Lee, N. C., Dicken, R. C., Rubin, G. L., & Ory, H. W. (1984). Confirmation of the preoperative diagnosis for hysterectomy. *American Journal of Obstetrics and Gynecology, 150*, 283–287.

Lindsay, P., & Wyckoff, M. (1981). The depression-pain and its response to antidepressants. *Psychosomatics 22*, 571–577.

Linton, S. J. (1997). A population-based study of the relationship between sexual abuse and back pain: Establishing a link. *Pain, 73*, 47–53.

Locke, J. J., & Wallace, K. M. (1959). Short-term marital adjustment and prediction tests: Their ability and validity. *Journal of Marriage and Family Therapy, 21*, 251–255.

Loeser, J. D., Bigos, S. J., Fordyce, W. E., & Violinn, E. P. (1990). Low back pain. In J. J. Bonica (Ed.), *The management of pain* (Vol. 2, pp. 1448–1482). Philadelphia: Lea & Febiger.

Long, C. (1981). The relationship between surgical outcome and MMPI profiles in chronic pain patients. *Journal of Clinical Psychology, 37*, 744–749.

Lousberg, R., Schmidt, A. J., & Groenman, N. H. (1992). The relationship between spouse solicitousness and pain behavior: Searching for more evidence. *Pain, 51*, 75–79.

Malter, A.D., Larson, E. B., Urban, N., & Deyo, R. A. (1996). Cost-effectiveness of lumbar discectomy for the treatment of herniated intervertebral disc. *Spine, 21,* 1048–1055.

Manniche, C., Asmussen, K. H., Vinterberg, H., Rose-Hansen, E. B. R., Kramhoft, J., & Jordan, A. (1994). Analysis of preoperative prognostic factors in first-time surgery for lumbar disc herniation, including Finneson's and modified Spengler's score systems. *Danish Medical Bulletin, 41,* 110–115.

McQuay, H. J., Tramer, M., Nye, B. A., Carroll, D., Wiffen, P. J., & Moore, R. A. (1996). A systematic review of antidepressants in neuropathic pain. *Pain, 68,* 217–227.

Mutran, E. J., Reitzes, D. C., Mossey, J., & Fernandez, M. E. (1995). Social support, depression and recovery of walking ability following hip fracture surgery. *Journal of Gerontology, 50B,* 5354–5361.

O'Brien, M. E. (1980). Effective social environment and hemodialysis adaptation: A panel analysis. *Journal of Health and Social Behavior, 21,* 360–370.

Onghena, P., & Van Houdenhove, B. (1992) Antidepressant-induced analgesia in chronic non-malignant pain: A meta-analysis of 39 placebo controlled studies. *Pain, 49,* 205–219.

Pheasant, H. C., Gelbert, D., Goldfarb, J., & Herron, L. (1979). The MMPI as predictor of outcome in low-back surgery. *Spine, 4*(1), 78–84.

Polatin, P. B., Kinney, R. K., Gatchel, R. J., Lillo, E., & Mayer, T. G. (1993). Psychiatric illness and chronic low-back pain. The mind and the spine—which goes first? *Spine, 18,* 66–71.

Riley, J. L., Robinson, M. E., Geisser, M. E., Wittmer, V. T., & Smith, A. G. (1995). Relationship between MMPI-2 cluster profiles and surgical outcome in low-back pain patients. *Journal of Spinal Disorders, 8*(3), 213–219.

Romano, J. M., Turner, J. A., & Clancy, S. L. (1989). Sex differences in the relationship of pain patient dysfunction to spouse adjustment. *Pain, 39,* 289–296.

Rosenthal, R. H., Ling, F. W., Rosenthal, T. L., & McNeeley, S. G. (1984). Chronic pelvic pain: Psychological features and laparoscopic findings. *Psychosomatics, 25*(11), 833–841.

Schofferman, J., Anderson, D., Hinds, R., Smith, G., & White, A. (1992). Childhood psychological trauma correlates with unsuccessful lumbar spine surgery. *Spine, 17*(Suppl. 6), S1380–S1384.

Schwartz, L., Slater, M. A., Birchler, G. R., & Atkinson, J. H. (1991). Depression in spouses of chronic pain patients: The role of patient pain and anger, and marital satisfaction. *Pain, 44,* 61–68.

Seligman, M. E. P. (1975). *Helplessness: On depression, development, and death.* San Francisco: Freeman.

Smith, W. L., & Duerksen, D. L. (1979). Personality and the relief of chronic pain: Predicting surgical outcome. *Clinical Neuropsychology, 1,* 35–38.

Sorenson, L. V., & Mors, O. (1988). Presentation of a new MMPI scale to predict outcome after first lumbar diskectomy. *Pain, 34,* 191–194.

Spengler, D. M., Freeman, C., Westbrook, R., & Miller, J. W. (1980). Low-back pain following multiple lumbar spine procedures: Failure of initial selection? *Spine, 5*(4), 356–360.

Spengler, D. M., Ouelette, E. A., Battie, M., & Zeh, J. (1990). Elective discectomy for herniation of a lumbar disc. *Journal of Bone and Joint Surgery [Am], 12,* 230–237.

Stewart, W. F., & Lipton, R. B. (1993). Societal impact of headache. In J. Olesen, P. Tfelt-Hansen, & K. M. A. Welch (Eds.), *The headaches.* New York: Raven Press.

Taylor, V. M., Deyo, R. A., Cherkin, D. C., & Kreuter, W. (1994). Low back pain hospitalization: Recent United States trends and regional variations. *Spine, 19,* 1207–1212.

Turk, D. C., & Fernandez, E. (1995). Personality assessment and the Minnesota Multiphasic Personality Inventory in chronic pain: Underdeveloped and overexposed. *Pain Forum, 4*(2), 104–107.

Turner, J. A., Ersek, M., Herron, L., Haselkorn, J., Kent, D., Ciol, M. A. Marcia, A., & Deyo, R. (1992). Patient outcomes after lumbar spinal fusions. *Journal of the American Medical Association, 268*(7), 907–911.

Turner, J. A., Herron, L., & Weiner, P. (1986). Utility of the MMPI pain assessment index in predicting outcome after lumbar surgery. *Journal of Clinical Psychology, 42,* 764–769.

Uomoto, J. M., Turner, J. A., & Herron, L. D. (1988). Use of the MMPI and MCMI in predicting outcome of lumbar laminectomy. *Journal of Clinical Psychology, 44,* 191–197.

Vanharanta, H., Sachs, B. L., Spivey, M. A., Guyer, R. D., Hochschuler, S. H., Rashbaum, R. F., Johnson, R. G., Ohnmeiss, D., & Mooney, V. (1987). The relationship of pain provocation to lumbar disc deterioration as seen by CT/discography. *Spine, 12,* 295–298.

Von Korff, M., Dworkin, S. F., LeResche, L., & Kruger, A. (1988). An epidemiologic comparison of pain complaints. *Pain, 32,* 173–183.

Walker, E., Katon, W., Neraas, K., Jemelka, R. P., & Massoth, D. (1992). Dissociation in women with chronic pelvic pain. *American Journal of Psychiatry, 149,* 534.

White, A. H., & Schofferman, J. A. (Eds.). (1995). *Spine care.* St. Louis: Mosby.

Whitehead, W. E . (1993). Behavioral medicine approaches to gastrointestinal disorders. *Journal of Consulting and Clinical Psychology, 60*(4), 605–612.

Wiltse, L. L., & Rocchio, P. D. (1975). Preoperative psychological tests as predictors of success of chemonucleolysis in the treatment of low-back syndrome. *Journal of Bone and Joint Surgery [Am], 75,* 478–483.

Chapter 25

The Role of Sex and Gender in Pain Perception and Responses to Treatment

CHRISTINE MIASKOWSKI

Both clinicians and researchers have largely ignored potential or actual differences in how men and women report a variety of symptoms associated with common health problems. In addition, little attention has been paid to how men and women respond to the same therapeutic interventions. In most of the studies that are used to inform clinical practice decisions on a daily basis, researchers have treated the two genders as equals. Most investigators have not asked questions about whether there are between-gender group differences or within-gender group differences in outcomes. In fact, most clinical trials of new pharmacological agents are restricted to male participants because of concerns about exposing women of childbearing years to drugs that might produce teratogenic effects. However, the implementation of the National Institutes of Health funding rules, which mandate the inclusion of women and minorities in clinical trials, will undoubtedly increase the numbers of women who are enrolled in clinical trials (Federal Register, 1994). Hopefully, the inclusion of more women in clinical trials will prompt investigators to evaluate gender differences in their study findings and to report those results that have implications for clinical practice.

The purpose of this chapter is to summarize some of the research studies that have evaluated gender differences in pain perceptions in animals and in humans. In addition, findings from stud-

ies that evaluated gender differences in men's and women's responses to analgesic medications are described. The chapter concludes with a summary of the study findings and a discussion of the implications of these findings for clinical practice and research.

SEX DIFFERENCES IN NOCICEPTIVE RESPONSES IN ANIMALS

Most of the animal studies that evaluated sex differences in behavioral responses to nociceptive stimuli have used electrical stimulation in the form of footshock and thermal stimulation of the tail (i.e., tail-flick test). An evaluation of the research findings on sex differences in nociception in animals suggests that female, compared to male, rats demonstrate greater sensitivity to a range of noxious stimuli (Beatty & Beatty, 1970; Marks & Hobbs, 1972).

Sex Differences in Responses to Electrical Stimulation

Differences in responses to an electrical stimulus (i.e., footshock) can be measured using the spatial preference test (Pare, 1969), the flinch-threshold test, and the jump-threshold test (Beatty & Beatty,

1970; Beatty & Fessler, 1977; Drury & Gold, 1978; Marks, Fargason, & Hobbs, 1972; Marks & Hobbs, 1972). The sensitivity to footshock is mediated primarily through supraspinal mechanisms (Evans, 1961).

The earliest studies that examined for sex differences in responses to footshock demonstrated that the shock thresholds of female rats were significantly lower than those of male rats (Beatty & Beatty, 1970; Marks & Hobbs, 1972; Pare, 1969). The sex differences in response to footshock emerge by 50 days of age and persist throughout life (Beatty & Fessler, 1977).

These early studies using electrical shock failed to evaluate for sex differences based on the hormonal milieu of the animal. Subsequent studies that examined the effects of castration on sex differences in nociceptive thresholds have produced variable results (Beatty & Beatty, 1970; Beatty & Fessler, 1977; Marks et al., 1972; Marks & Hobbs, 1972). Female responses to at least one type of electrical stimulation (i.e., flinch-threshold) appear to depend on the hormonal environment of the female (Drury & Gold, 1978). The effects of castration on the responses of male animals to electrical stimulation requires further investigation.

Sex Differences in Responses to Thermal Stimulation

The tail-flick test is a nociceptive test that measures reactivity to a thermal stimulus and is considered to be mediated primarily at the spinal site (D'Amour & Smith, 1941). Differences in behavioral responses to the tail-flick test between male and female rats, between intact and gonadectomized animals, and among the various stages of the rat's estrous cycle have been evaluated (Kepler, Kest, Kiefel, Cooper, & Bodnar, 1989; Romero, Cooper, Komisaruk, & Bodnar, 1988; Romero, Kepler, Cooper, Komisaruk, & Bodnar, 1987).

A comparison of baseline tail-flick responses between male and female rats demonstrated significantly *higher* tail-flick latencies in females as compared to males (Romero et al., 1988; Romero et al., 1987). These findings are exactly opposite to those observed with electrical stimulation, in which female rats exhibited lower thresholds to footshock. Castration in males failed to produce significant changes in tail-flick latencies, whereas ovariectomy produced significant decreases in tail-flick latencies in female rats (Romero et al., 1988; Romero et al., 1987). At least one study (Kepler et al., 1989) has

demonstrated differences in responses to the tail-flick test during the various phases of the rat's estrous cycle.

In summary, the animal studies that have examined for sex differences in responses to painful stimuli have produced variable results. In some studies (Drury & Gold, 1978; Kepler et al., 1989), female rats' sensitivity to noxious stimuli fluctuated during the phases of the estrous cycle. However, other studies failed to demonstrate any differences in male and female rats' responsiveness to noxious stimuli when the hormonal environment of the rats was evaluated (i.e., an evaluation of the effects of sex steroid hormones during the estrous cycle) or modified (i.e., an evaluation of the effects of castration and sex steroid hormone replacement; Kepler et al., 1989; Romero et al., 1988). Therefore, additional research using animal models is warranted to determine the effect of sex steroid hormones and various neurotransmitters on pain transmission and modulation. The apparent sex differences in animal's responses to noxious stimuli may indicate fundamental sex differences in pain mechanisms and warrant additional investigations. If sex differences in the pain transmission and modulation systems are uncovered through systematic investigations using animal models of acute and chronic pain, these results may shed some light on the apparent gender differences in several clinical pain problems.

GENDER DIFFERENCES IN PAIN PERCEPTION AND RESPONSES TO PAINFUL STIMULI IN HUMANS

Gender differences in pain perception have been the subject of five recent review articles (Berkley, in press; Fillingim & Maixner, 1995; Miaskowski, 1996, 1997; Unruh, 1996). Most of the studies that evaluated gender differences in pain perception were done using experimentally induced pain. The majority of the experimental studies attempted to determine if men and women have different pain thresholds and different levels of pain tolerance. Pain threshold is defined as the minimum amount of stimulation that reliably evokes a report of pain in an individual. Pain tolerance is defined as the time that a continuous stimulus is endured by an individual or the maximally tolerated stimulus intensity that a person can endure.

Results of studies using experimental pain models in humans demonstrate that women exhibit lower pain thresholds than men. In addition, in most of these experimental studies women exhibited less tolerance to noxious stimuli than men did. The most consistent findings demonstrating gender differences in pain thresholds and tolerance are observed when mechanical (Brennum, Kjeldsen, Jensen, & Jensen, 1989; Buchanan & Midgley, 1987; Fisher, 1987; Jensen, Rasmussen, Pedersen, Louis, & Olesen, 1992) and thermal (i.e., cold pressure pain; Hall & Davies, 1991; McCaul & Haugtvedt, 1982) stimuli are used. The findings from the experimental pain studies are often interpreted to mean that women are more sensitive to painful stimuli than men.

At least two plausible explanations can be postulated to explain the gender differences in responses to experimentally induced pain. The hormonal status of the individual may explain some of the gender differences in pain sensitivity and tolerance. Several studies reported that a woman's phase in the menstrual cycle or her reproductive status (i.e., pregnant or not pregnant) can affect pain intensity ratings. However, with regard to changes in pain perception associated with the menstrual cycle, the pattern of responses differs considerably across the different studies. Some studies reported that women have greater pain during the premenstrual phase of the cycle (Procacci, Zoppi, Meresca, & Romano, 1974), others at ovulation (Goolkasian, 1980, 1983), and others following menses (Hapidou & De Catanzaro, 1988; Kuczmierczyk & Adams, 1986); however, others reported no changes in pain sensitivity during the various phases of the menstrual cycle (Amodie & Nelson Gray, 1989; Veith, Anderson, & Slade, 1987).

An additional psychosocial factor that may influence the responses of men and women to experimentally induced pain is the gender of the individual performing the experiments. In one study (Levine & De Simone, 1991), the researchers found that men reported less pain in front of a female experimenter than a male experimenter. However, the gender of the experimenter did not influence the responses of the female participants. In contrast, in at least two studies (Feine, Bushnell, Miron, & Duncan, 1991; Otto & Dougher, 1985), the investigators found that gender differences in pain sensitivity were not affected by the gender of the experimenter.

The data on gender differences in experimentally induced pain in humans are somewhat inconclusive. As noted by Berkley (in press), the findings from experimental pain studies suggest that gender differences in pain thresholds and tolerance

do exist, with females generally reporting lower pain thresholds and less tolerance to noxious stimuli. However, the gender differences are small and inconsistently observed, being most prominent for pressure or electrical stimuli. Furthermore, even under rigorously controlled experimental conditions, the presence and direction of the gender differences in pain perceptions appear to be influenced by the gender of the experimenter, the type of noxious stimulus, and the hormonal status of the participant.

It should be noted that most of the experimental studies that have evaluated gender differences in pain perception have focused on an evaluation of the sensory dimension of the human experience of pain. Additional research is warranted to determine if there are gender differences in the multiple dimensions of the human experience of pain (e.g., affective dimension, cognitive dimension, sociocultural dimension).

PERCEPTIONS OF MEN AND WOMEN ON THE HUMAN EXPERIENCE OF PAIN

One qualitative study (Bendelow, 1993) explored the relationships between perceptions of pain and various social characteristics of the individual, with a special emphasis on the influence of gender on the perception of pain. An emphasis was placed on trying to understand the meaning of the "lay" person's understanding of the phenomenon of pain as opposed to that of patients or health care professionals. This study was conducted in two phases. In phase 1, participants were asked to complete a questionnaire that was aimed at examining their beliefs about health, illness, and pain and to discover themes that would be investigated in more detail in phase 2 during in-depth interviews with a subsample of the study participants.

One of the major findings from the questionnaire data was that significantly more women than men thought that anxiety, fear, and depression affected their perception of pain. In fact, twice as many men as women did *not* complete the items on the questionnaire that evaluated the impact of emotions on the individual's perception of pain. This finding suggests that men may dwell more on the physiological dimension of the pain experience and tend to ignore the psychological dimension of the pain experience.

An additional finding from this study is that 66% of the females and 33% of the males believed that women were better able to cope with pain than men. As one woman explained, "Women are made to suffer pain because we have periods and childbirth. Whatever the social climate, women end up child rearing. Therefore they don't have the 'privilege' of giving in to pain and sickness" (Bendelow, 1993, p. 286). Both men and women expressed the view that the combination of female biology and the reproductive role serve to equip women with a "natural" capacity to endure pain both physically and emotionally. In essence, both men and women believed that women were better able to cope with pain because they were somehow equipped by nature to cope with the pain of childbirth.

Another finding from Bendelow's study (1993) that may contribute to the gender differences in pain perceptions is that children are socialized from a very young age to think about pain and react to painful events in certain ways. Boys are actively discouraged from expressing emotions, and male participants reported that they felt an obligation to display stoicism in response to pain. The role that socialization concerning pain may have on the ways women and men behave when they are in pain requires additional investigation.

Gender Differences in Reports of Acute Pain

In one large-scale study of young adults who were undergoing surgery for removal of third molars, Faucett, Gordon, and Levine (1994) evaluated gender differences in reports of postoperative pain following recovery from anesthesia but immediately prior to the administration of an analgesic medication. Pain intensity ratings were obtained using a visual analogue scale from 543 patients. Women reported significantly higher pain intensity scores (mean = 44.3 mm on a 0–100 visual analogue scale) than men (34.6 mm) regardless of ethnic group (i.e., Asian, African American, European, or Latino), age, education, or difficulty of the surgical extraction procedure. The findings from this study appear to support the findings from the animal literature, as well as the findings from experimental pain studies in humans, that females may be more sensitive to painful stimuli than males. However, when evaluating the results of this study, clinicians need to consider whether a difference of 0.7 mm on a visual analogue scale, although statistically significant, is clinically significant and warrants a different level of intervention.

Several studies have evaluated gender differences in reports of acute pain in critically ill patients or patients in the emergency room setting (Caldwell, Pelter, & Drew, 1996; Cunningham et al., 1989; Gregor et al., 1994; Herlitz, Karlson, Wiklund, & Bengtson, 1995; Puntillo & Weiss, 1994). Most of these studies have evaluated gender differences in reports of chest pain.

In one study, Cunningham and colleagues (1989) assessed the relationship between gender and the clinical manifestations of coronary artery disease by evaluating the common clinical problem of acute chest pain. A total of 7,734 patients (50% of the sample was female) who were admitted to an emergency room with acute chest pain were evaluated, and the incidence of myocardial infarction (MI) in each gender group was determined. The results of the study indicate that the clinical features that predict MI in men (i.e., an electrocardiogram strongly suggestive of MI with new Q waves, ST elevation or depression in ≥ 2 leads, diaphoresis, substernal pain, pressure-type chest pain, pain like prior MI or worse than previous angina, past history of MI) predict MI in women to a similar extent. However, female gender was associated with a 40% lower rate of MI except when classic electrocardiographic evidence was present on the electrocardiogram done in the emergency department. An additional finding from this study that is worth noting is that men without MI and without ischemic heart disease were admitted to the hospital at a significantly higher rate than women, suggesting that men with chest pain may be treated somewhat more conservatively than women with chest pain.

Garber, Carleton, and Heller (1992) conducted a study to determine the validity of the Rose Questionnaire (Rose, 1965) as a measure of myocardial ischemia by comparing it with results obtained using exercise thallium-201 myocardial scintigraphy. Geoffrey Rose developed the Rose Questionnaire as a standardized measure for angina pectoris. In this study, 47 male and 97 female patients with chest pain who were referred for clinical exercise testing were evaluated. The sensitivity of the Rose Questionnaire was similar in women (41%) and men (44%). However, the specificity of the questionnaire was 77% for men, whereas for women it was significantly lower (56%). The accuracy of the Rose Questionnaire in predicting myocardial ischemia was 0.19 in women and 0.48 in men. The authors speculate that the lower specificity of the Rose Questionnaire for women might be due to differences in the etiology of chest pain in women. In addition, they pointed out that, particularly for women, the Rose Questionnaire did not differentiate well between patients with and without myocardial ischemia as demonstrated by thallium-201 myocardial imaging.

In another study (Gregor et al., 1994), the Halifax County MONICA database was used to estimate the gender bias in presentation, pre-hospital, and in-hospital treatment and the 28-day mortality of patients with an episode of acute chest pain. During the 6-year study period, 9,737 patients were evaluated (32.6% were women). In this study, men were more likely to undergo coronary angiography (24% in men, 18% in women) and to have an exercise stress test (23% for men, 18% for women). Although the data from this study were obtained through chart review, the authors concluded that although mortality associated with treatment of chest pain appears to be gender-independent, the disease pattern appears to be different in men and women. Women appear to experience the "typical symptoms" of acute myocardial infarction less frequently than men do.

In another study of emergency department patients, Herlitz and colleagues (1995) studied whether there were gender differences in mortality and frequency of various symptoms 1 year after patients were sent home from the emergency department following an evaluation for chest pain. A total of 2,175 patients (54% male, 46% female) were sent a 1-year follow-up questionnaire that asked about the occurrence of cardiac symptoms (e.g., chest pain at rest, dyspnea at rest). In addition, patients were asked to rate the frequency of psychosomatic symptoms (e.g., headache, dizziness, gastritis) and psychological symptoms (e.g., anxiety, depression, indecision) using a 6-point scale that ranged from *not at all* to *all the time*. No gender differences were found in the overall mortality rate at 1 year (i.e., 3% for both men and women). However, compared to men, women more frequently reported chest pain at rest, chest pain at night, and dyspnea with both severe and light physical exertion. In addition, female patients with and without cardiac disease reported more psychosomatic and psychological complaints than male patients with and without cardiac disease. These findings are consistent with previous studies that showed that women report more symptoms than men do (Hunt, McEwen, & McKenna, 1984) and that women are more likely to seek health care than men (Verbrugge & Wingard, 1987).

Puntillo and Weiss (1994) evaluated 60 patients who underwent coronary artery bypass surgery (44 male, 16 female) and 14 patients who underwent vascular surgery (13 male, 1 female) to determine the extent to which age, gender, personality adjustment, and amount of analgesics predicted the magnitude of pain (i.e., pain intensity, pain affect, pain sensation) during the person's stay in a critical care unit. Pain intensity was measured using a 10-cm horizontal numeric rating scale. Pain affect and pain sensation were measured using the word descriptor list of the McGill Pain Questionnaire—Short Form. A hierarchical regression analysis demonstrated that women reported a greater magnitude of pain sensation than men did. However, no gender differences were found in patients' ratings of pain intensity or pain affect. The authors suggest that women are better able to fully describe their pain sensations than men are or are more willing to describe them, especially to female nurses.

Another study of acute pain (Caldwell et al., 1996) evaluated patients who were undergoing percutaneous transluminal coronary angioplasty (PTCA). The purposes of this study were to determine if there were gender differences in ischemia-induced pain intensity and to examine the relationship between the amount of ischemia and the intensity of ischemic pain in both men and women. The results of the study indicate that men and women reported similar pain intensity scores (i.e., 5.4 and 6.0, respectively) during the period of myocardial ischemia induced by balloon inflation during PTCA. In addition, there was no relationship between pain intensity and the amount of myocardial ischemia in either men or women.

The findings from these studies of acute pain suggest that men and women may express themselves differently when describing the sensations of pain associated with a specific clinical problem. For example, the "typical" descriptions of chest pain or postoperative pain may be biased to one gender group. This bias may not allow clinicians to accurately diagnose a specific clinical problem if their expectations are that the same "typical" words will be used by both men and women to describe the pain associated with a specific clinical condition. Additional research is needed to determine how our "typical" descriptions of common pain problems may need to be revised if there are specific differences in how men and women describe these pain problems.

EPIDEMIOLOGICAL STUDIES OF GENDER DIFFERENCES IN CLINICAL PAIN PROBLEMS

Undoubtedly, experimental pain studies are important in helping us to elucidate some of the basic physiological principles and mechanisms that may underlie across-gender and within-gender group differences in responses to painful stimuli. However, perhaps a more relevant area for consideration and further investigation is the apparent gender differences observed in a variety of clinically painful conditions. Additional investigations of these "real" pain problems may help us to discern how men and women differ on many of the multiple dimensions of the human experience of pain. In addition, by evaluating how men and women cope with clinical pain problems, we may be able to design gender-specific interventions for acute and chronic pain problems.

In an excellent review article, Unruh (1996) suggests that several chronic pain problems have a specific gender distribution (see Table 25.1). Findings from several epidemiological studies of common clinical pain problems suggest that women compared to men report greater pain with the same pathology (Berkanovic, Telesky, & Reider, 1981; Moulin, Foley, & Ebers, 1988), greater pain with a similar degree of tissue injury (Puntillo & Weiss, 1994; Savedra, Holzemer, Tesler, & Wilkie, 1993), and a greater number of painful sites (Andersson, Ejlertsson, Leden, & Rosenberg, 1993; Lester, Lefebvre, & Keefe, 1994); they are also more likely to develop a chronic pain syndrome after equivalent trauma (Von Korff, Dworkin, & LeResche, 1990). In addition, women are reported to use analgesics more frequently than men do (Eggen, 1993).

Data from three epidemiological studies suggest that women in the general population report a higher rate of abdominal pain (Adelman, Revicki, Magaziner, & Hebel, 1995), migraine headaches (Honkasalo, Kaprio, Heikkila, Sillanpaa, & Kos-

kenvuo, 1993), and a variety of chronic pain problems (Andersson et al., 1993). The findings from the large-scale epidemiological studies on gender differences in the prevalence of certain painful conditions are often interpreted to mean that women are more sensitive to painful stimuli than men and that women report pain problems more frequently than men do. However, both Berkley (in press) and Unruh (1996) cautioned against interpreting the findings from large-scale epidemiological studies so simplistically.

Numerous factors may influence the data reported in large-scale epidemiological studies. First of all, when women and men are surveyed and asked to recall how frequently they access a health care system for a variety of health problems, women report more visits (Dawson & Adams, 1986; Henderson et al., 1994; Otto & Dougher, 1985; Veith, Anderson, & Slade, 1987; Verbrugge, 1980, 1985) and more return visits (Brit et al., 1993) than men. However, when a prospective design was used to evaluate for gender differences in health care utilization, both Berkanovic and colleagues (1981) and Rakowski, Julius, Hickey, Verbrugge, and Halter (1988) found no differences in the number of health care visits made by men and women. Therefore, one needs to consider that gender differences in the memory of health care visits and the willingness to report health care visits may have some bearing on the outcomes of the retrospective epidemiological studies of clinical pain problems.

EFFECTS OF GENDER DIFFERENCES IN PAIN RESPONSES ON CLINICAL MANAGEMENT

One important consideration in the studies on the gender biology of pain is whether gender differences in pain perception and responses to acute and chronic pain problems affect the clinical management of pain. In other words, do health care professionals respond differently to men's and women's reports of pain and pain behaviors and provide analgesics based on their perceptions rather than on the men's and women's self-reports of pain? In other words, do stereotypes and preconceived notions of gender roles and pain behaviors influence clinicians' management of acute and chronic pain?

Several lines of evidence support the idea that health care professionals are influenced to manage pain differently in men and women. Some of these studies were reviewed earlier in this chapter. Addi-

TABLE 25.1. Gender Distribution of Some Common Pain Problems

Migraine headache (F, 3:1)
Cluster headache (M, 8:1)
Trigeminal neuralgia (F, 2:1)
Rheumatoid arthritis (F, 3:1)
Carpal tunnel syndrome (F, 2:1)
Temporomandibular joint disorder (F, 2:1 to 8:1)

Note. F, female; M, male.

tional studies suggest that although neither men nor women appear to receive adequate amounts of analgesics for the management of acute or chronic pain, the disadvantage may be greater for women.

Faherty and Grier (1984) reported that physicians prescribed significantly less pain medication for women who were 55 years of age or older than for men in the same age group following abdominal surgery. In addition, the researchers found that nurses administered significantly less pain medication to women between the ages of 25 and 54. In another postoperative pain study, Calderone (1990) evaluated whether the frequency of pain and sedative medications administered to postoperative coronary artery bypass graft (CABG) patients differed according to the patient's gender. The author hypothesized that women are perceived as being more emotionally labile than men and therefore may be more apt to exaggerate complaints of pain than men. Therefore, women may be taken less seriously than men and may, in fact, receive more sedative medication to inhibit their expressive behavior. Based on a review of the CABG patients' medical records (30 men and 30 women), it was determined that male patients received pain medication significantly more frequently than female patients and that female patients received sedative medications significantly more frequently than male patients.

Only one study could be found that evaluated differences in clinicians' responses to postoperative pain management in children (Beyer, De Good, Ashley, & Russell, 1983). Although the major purpose of this study was to examine differences in postoperative prescription and administration of analgesics following cardiac surgery in children (n = 50) and adults (n = 50), the investigators noted that significantly more codeine was prescribed for boys following open heart surgery, whereas more acetaminophen was prescribed for girls. It should be noted that all of the acute postoperative pain studies cited here possess one significant limitation. None of the studies evaluated whether men and women received adequate analgesia based on the dose of analgesics administered.

Recently, biases in pain management affecting women were reported by Cleeland and colleagues (1994) in a multisite study of 1308 outpatients with metastatic cancer who were being treated at one of 54 sites affiliated with the Eastern Cooperative Oncology Group. The adequacy of prescribed analgesics was assessed using guidelines developed by the World Health Organization. An index of pain management was constructed based on the most potent analgesic prescribed by the physician for the patient's reported level of pain. Forty-two percent of the patients who were experiencing pain were not given adequate analgesic therapy. However, women were given significantly less pain medication (odds ratio 1.5) than men.

One additional study (Brietbart et al., 1996) suggests a similar gender bias on the part of health care professionals who were treating patients with AIDS. In this study, the adequacy of analgesic management was evaluated in 366 ambulatory AIDS patients. Adequacy of analgesic therapy was assessed using the methodology reported by Cleeland and colleagues (1994). Results indicated that nearly 85% of the patients were classified as receiving inadequate analgesic therapy. Again, women with HIV disease were significantly more likely than men to receive inadequate analgesic therapy.

Taken together, these findings suggest that there might be a gender bias in how health care professionals respond to men's and women's reports of acute and chronic pain. Additional research is warranted to determine which factors on the part of the patient (e.g., pain behaviors, descriptions of pain problems), as well as of the health care professional (e.g., gender of the physician or the nurse), influence the clinical management of pain.

GENDER DIFFERENCES IN ANALGESIC RESPONSES

Recently a series of studies was published that reported gender differences in analgesic responses in patients who were undergoing standardized surgery for removal of third molars (Gear, Gordon, et al., 1996; Gear, Miaskowski, et al., 1996; Gordon et al., 1995). All of the surgical procedures were performed by the same oral surgeon. Patients received intravenous diazepam, nitrous oxide, and a local anesthetic without vasoconstrictor to achieve a nerve block of short duration.

The duration of any one experiment is 5 hours. Pain intensity is measured using a visual analogue scale. Following administration of the study drug, pain ratings are taken every 20 minutes for a total of 2.5 hours.

In the first study (Gordon et al., 1995), the effects of preoperative administration of baclofen on the analgesia produced by the postoperative administration of morphine (i.e., a predominantly mu-opioid agonist) or pentazocine (i.e., a predominantly kappa-opioid agonist) were evaluated. Baclofen is a

GABA-B agonist that is commonly used to treat spasticity associated with multiple sclerosis or spinal cord injury. Studies in animals have shown that baclofen, administered intrathecally or supraspinally, produces analgesic effects (Wilson & Yaksh, 1978; Yaksh & Reddy, 1981; Zieglgansberger, 1988).

The results of the experiment demonstrate that the analgesic efficacy of morphine was enhanced by the preoperative administration of baclofen. However, no gender differences were found in the analgesic responses to either morphine alone or morphine given in combination with baclofen. In contrast, in the pentazocine experiments, regardless of drug group (i.e., pentazocine alone or pentazocine and pretreatment with baclofen), women reported consistently better analgesic effects than men (Gordon et al., 1995).

In a subsequent study using the same postoperative paradigm, Gear, Gordon, and colleagues (1996) evaluated gender differences in the analgesic effects of pentazocine administered intravenously. Again, the analgesic efficacy of pentazocine was found to be greater in women than in men.

With the positive results obtained with the mixed agonist–antagonist, pentazocine, these researchers decided to investigate further the hypothesis that gender differences in responses to analgesics is a characteristic of the kappa-opioid receptor. In order to determine if there were gender differences associated with kappa-opioid activity, the analgesic efficacy of two other predominantly kappa-opioid agonists (i.e., nalbuphine and butorphanol) was compared in men and women who underwent surgery for removal of third molar teeth (Gear, Miaskowski, et al., 1996). Consistent with the findings with pentazocine, 2 mg of intravenously administered butorphanol significantly prolonged the duration of analgesia in female compared to male patients. In addition, similar effects were observed with 10 mg of nalbuphine. Taken together, the results of these studies demonstrate that women reported either better analgesic effects or a significantly prolonged duration of analgesia using kappa-opioid analgesics (i.e., pentazocine, butorphanol, nalbuphine) than men did. The findings from these studies suggest that women respond better to kappa-opioid analgesics than do men and that this class of analgesics is more efficacious in women.

The physiological basis for these sex differences in analgesic responses to kappa-opioid analgesics is not known at the present time. It is possible that a male-related hormone, such as testosterone, interacts negatively with kappa-opioid agonists. Another possibility is that a female hormone, such as estrogen or progesterone, may potentiate the action of kappa opioids. A third possibility that might explain the gender differences in analgesic responses is that some other factors unrelated to sex steroid hormones may account for these differences. Additional research with other clinical models of pain is warranted to determine the mechanisms underlying the gender differences in analgesic responses.

SUMMARY

The major findings from the various studies on gender differences in pain perception and responses to treatment are summarized in Table 25.2. Taken together, the findings from research studies done to date on gender differences in responses to painful stimuli and analgesic medications suggest that men

TABLE 25.2. Summary of the Findings from Research Studies on the Role of Gender in Pain Perception and Responses to Treatment

Pain perception

1. Animal studies that have examined sex differences in responses to painful stimuli have produced variable results.
2. The findings from experimental pain studies in humans suggest that gender differences in pain thresholds and tolerance do exist, with women generally reporting lower pain thresholds and less tolerance to painful stimuli.
3. Men and women believe that the combination of female biology and the reproductive role serve to equip women with a "natural" capacity to endure pain, both physically and emotionally.
4. Findings from acute pain studies in humans suggest that men and women may express themselves differently when describing the sensations of pain associated with a specific clinical problem.
5. Several chronic pain problems appear to have a specific gender distribution.
6. Findings from several research studies suggest that there may be a gender bias in how health care professionals respond to men's and women's reports of acute and chronic pain.

Responses to treatment

The results of several studies suggest that women reported either better analgesic effects or a significantly prolonged duration of analgesia using kappa-opioid analgesics (i.e., pentazocine, butorphanol, nalbuphine) than did men.

and women do respond differently to both painful stimuli and pain medication. Clinicians need to be mindful of these gender differences as they plan the care of an individual man or woman who is experiencing pain. Pain assessments and management strategies must be focused on the individual experiencing the pain. However, determining the mechanisms that underlie the gender differences found in the studies summarized in this chapter may provide insight for the use of different assessment tools and pain management strategies for men and women.

ACKNOWLEDGMENT

This work was partially supported by Grant No. RO1-NR03923 from the National Institute of Nursing Research.

REFERENCES

Adelman, A. M., Revicki, D. A., Magaziner, J., & Hebel, R. (1995). Abdominal pain in an HMO. *Family Medicine, 27,* 321–325.

Amodie N., & Nelson Gray, R. O. (1989). Reactions of dysmenorrheic and nondysmenorrheic women to experimentally induced pain throughout the menstrual cycle. *Journal of Behavioral Medicine, 12,* 373–385.

Andersson, H. I., Ejlertsson, G., Leden, I., & Rosenberg, C. (1993). Chronic pain in a geographically defined general population: Studies of differences in age, gender, social class, and pain localization. *Clinical Journal of Pain, 9,* 174–182.

Beatty, W. W., & Beatty, P. A. (1970). Hormonal determinants of sex differences in avoidance behavior and reactivity to electric shock in the rat. *Journal of Comparative and Physiological Psychology, 73*(3), 445–455.

Beatty, W. W., & Fessler, R. G. (1977). Gonadectomy and sensitivity to electrical shock in the rat. *Physiology and Behavior, 19,* 1–6.

Bendelow, G. (1993). Pain perceptions, emotions, and gender. *Sociology of Health and Illness, 15*(3), 273–294.

Berkanovic, E., Telesky, C., & Reider, S. (1981). Structural and social psychological factors in the decision to seek medical care for symptoms. *Medical Care, 19,* 693–709.

Berkley, K. J. (in press). Sex differences in pain. *Behavioral and Brain Sciences.*

Beyer, J. E., De Good, D. E., Ashley, L. C., & Russell, G. A. (1983). Patterns of postoperative analgesic use with adults and children following cardiac surgery. *Pain, 17*(1), 71–81.

Breitbart, W., Rosenfeld, B. D., Passik, S. D., McDonald, M. V., Thaler, H., & Portenoy, R. K. (1996). The undertreatment of pain in ambulatory AIDS patients. *Pain, 65*(2–3), 243–249.

Brennum, J., Kjeldsen, M., Jensen, K., & Jensen, T. S. (1989). Measurements of human pressure-pain thresholds on fingers and toes. *Pain, 38,* 211–217.

Brit, H., Miles, D. A., Bridges-Webb, C., Neary, S., Charles, J., & Traynor, V. (1993). A comparison of country and metropolitan general practice. *Medical Journal of Australia, 159,* 514–557.

Buchanan, H. M., & Midgley, J. A. (1987). Evaluation of pain threshold using a simple pressure algometer. *Clinical Rheumatology, 6,* 510–517.

Calderone, K. (1990). The influence of gender on the frequency of pain and sedative medication administered to postoperative patients. *Sex Roles, 23,* 11–12.

Caldwell, M. A., Pelter, M. M., & Drew, B. J. (1996). Chest pain is an unreliable measure of ischemia in men and women during PTCA. *Heart and Lung, 26,* 423–429.

Cleeland, C. S., Gonin, R., Hatfield, A. K., Edmonson, J. H., Blum, R. H., Stewart, J. A., & Pandya, K. J. (1994). Pain and its treatment in outpatients with metastatic cancer. *New England Journal of Medicine, 33*(9), 592–596.

Cunningham, M. A., Lee, T. H., Cook, E. F., Brand, D. A., Rouan, G. W., Weisberg, M. C., & Goldman, L. (1989). The effect of gender on the probability of myocardial infarction among emergency department patients with acute chest pain: A report from the multicenter chest pain study group. *Journal of General Internal Medicine, 4,* 392–398.

D'Amour, F. E., & Smith, D. L. (1941). A method for determining loss of pain sensation. *Journal of Pharmacology and Experimental Therapeutics, 72,* 74–79.

Dawson, D. A., & Adams, P. F. (1986). *Current estimates from the National Health Interview Survey: United States.* Hyattsville, MD: National Center for Health Statistics.

Drury, R. A., & Gold, R. M. (1978). Differential effects of ovarian hormones on reactivity to electric footshock in the rat. *Physiology and Behavior, 20,* 187–191.

Eggen, A. E. (1993). The Tromsø study: Frequency and predicting factors of analgesic drug use in a free-living population (12–56 years). *Journal of Clinical Epidemiology, 46,* 1297–1304.

Evans, E. D. (1961). A new technique for the investigation of some analgesic drugs on reflexive behavior in the rat. *Psychopharmacologia, 2,* 318–325.

Faherty, B. S., & Grier, M. R. (1984). Analgesic medication for elderly people post-surgery. *Nursing Research, 33*(6), 369–372.

Faucett, J., Gordon, N., & Levine, J. D. (1994). Differences in postoperative pain severity among four different ethnic groups. *Journal of Pain and Symptom Management, 9*(6), 383–389.

Federal Register. (1994). *NIH guidelines on the inclusion of women and minorities as subjects in clinical research* (Federal Register 59, No. 59, 14508). Bethesda, MD: National Institutes of Health.

Feine, J. S., Bushnell, M. C., Miron, D., & Duncan, G. H. (1991). Sex differences in the perception of noxious heat stimuli. *Pain, 44,* 255–262.

Fillingim, R. B., & Maixner, W. (1995). Gender differences in the responses to noxious stimuli. *Pain Forum, 44,* 209–221.

Fisher, A. A. (1987). Pressure algometry over muscles. Standard values, validity, and reproducibility of pressure threshold. *Pain, 30,* 115–126.

Garber, C. E., Carleton, R. A., & Heller, G. V. (1992).

Comparison of the "Rose Questionnaire Angina" to exercise thallium scintigraphy: Different findings in males and females. *Journal of Clinical Epidemiology, 45*(7), 715–720.

Gear, R. W., Gordon, N. C., Heller, P. H., Paul, S., Miaskowski, C., & Levine, J. D. (1996). Gender differences in analgesic response to the kappa-opioid pentazocine. *Neuroscience Letters, 205,* 207–209.

Gear, R. W., Miaskowski, C., Gordon, N. C., Paul, S. M., Heller, P. H., & Levine, J. D. (1996). Significantly greater analgesia in females compared to males after kappa-opioids. *Nature Medicine, 2,* 1248–1250.

Goolkasian, P. (1980). Cyclic changes in pain perception: An ROC analysis. *Perception and Psychophysiology, 27,* 499–504.

Goolkasian, P. (1983). An ROC analysis of pain reactions in dysmenorrheic and nondysmenorrheic women. *Perception and Psychophysiology, 34,* 381–386.

Gordon, N. C., Gear, R. W., Heller, P. H., Paul, S., Miaskowski, C., & Levine, J. D. (1995). Enhancement of morphine analgesia by the GABA-B agonist baclofen. *Neuroscience, 69,* 345–349.

Gregor, R. D., Bata, I. R., Eastwood, B. J., Garner, J. B., Guernsey, J. R., Mackenzie, B. R., Rautaharju, P. M., & Wolf, H. K. (1994). Gender differences in the presentation, treatment, and short-term mortality of acute chest pain. *Clinical and Investigative Medicine, 17,* 551–562.

Hall, E. G., & Davies, S. (1991). Gender differences in perceived intensity and affect of pain between athletes and nonathletes. *Perceptual and Motor Skills, 73,* 779–786.

Hapidou, E. G., & De Catanzaro, D. (1988). Sensitivity to cold pressor pain in dysmenorrheic and nondysmenorrheic women as a function of menstrual cycle phase. *Pain, 34,* 277–283.

Henderson, G., Akin, J., Zhiming, H., Shuiago, J., Haijiang, M., & Keyou, G. (1994). Equity and the utilization of health services: Report of an eight-province survey in China. *Social Science and Medicine, 39,* 687–699.

Herlitz, J., Karlson, B. W., Wiklund, I., & Bengtson, A. (1995). Prognosis and gender differences in chest pain patients discharged from an ED. *American Journal of Emergency Medicine, 13,* 127–132.

Honkasalo, M. L., Kaprio, J., Heikkila, K., Sillanpaa, M., & Koskenvuo, M. (1993). A population-based study of headache and migraine in 22,809 adults. *Headache, 33,* 403–412.

Hunt, S. M., McEwen, J., & McKenna, S. P. (1984). Perceived health: Age and sex comparisons in a community. *Journal of Epidemiology and Community Health, 38*(2), 156–160.

Jensen, R., Rasmussen, B. K., Pedersen, B., Louis, I., & Olesen, J. (1992). Cephalic muscle tenderness and pressure pain threshold in a general population. *Pain, 48,* 197–203.

Kepler, K. L., Kest, B., Kiefel, J. M., Cooper, M. L., & Bodnar, R. J. (1989). Roles of gender, gonadectomy, and estrous phase in the analgesic effects of intracerebroventricular morphine in rats. *Pharmacology, Biochemistry, and Behavior, 34*(1), 119–127.

Kuczmierczyk, A. R., & Adams, H. E. (1986). Autonomic arousal and pain sensitivity in women with premenstrual syndrome at different phases of the menstrual cycle. *Journal of Psychosomatic Research, 30,* 421–428.

Lester, N., Lefebvre, J. C., & Keefe, F. J. (1994). Pain in young adults: I. Relationship to gender and family history. *Clinical Journal of Pain, 10,* 282–289.

Levine, F. M., & De Simone, L. L. (1991). The effects of experimenter gender on pain report in male and female patients. *Pain, 44,* 69–72.

Marks, H. E., Fargason, B. D., & Hobbs, S. H. (1972). Reactivity to aversive stimuli as a function of alterations in body weight in normal and gonadectomized female rats. *Physiology and Behavior, 9,* 539–544.

Marks, H. E., & Hobbs, S. H. (1972). Changes in stimulus reactivity following gonadectomy in male and female rats of different ages. *Physiology and Behavior, 8*(6), 1113–1119.

McCaul, K. D., & Haugtvedt, C. (1982). Attention, distraction, and cold pressor pain. *Journal of Personality and Social Psychology, 43,* 154–162.

Miaskowski, C. (1996). Pain management in women. In B. J. McElmurry & R. S. Parker (Eds.), *Annual review of women's health* (Vol. 3, pp. 245–255). New York: National League for Nursing Press.

Miaskowski, C. (1997). Women and pain. *Critical Care Nursing Clinics of North America, 9*(4), 453–458.

Moulin, D. E., Foley, K. M., & Ebers, G.C. (1988). Pain syndromes in multiple sclerosis. *Neurology, 38,* 1830–1834.

Otto, M. W., & Dougher, M. J. (1985). Sex differences and personality factors in responsibility to pain. *Perceptual and Motor Skills, 61,* 383–390.

Pare, W. P. (1969). Age, sex, and strain differences in the aversive threshold to grid shock in the rat. *Journal of Comparative Physiology and Psychology, 69,* 214–218.

Procacci, P., Zoppi, M., Meresca, M., & Romano, S. (1974). Studies of pain threshold in men. In J. J. Bonica (Ed.), *Advances in neurology* (Vol. 4, pp. 107–113). New York: Raven Press.

Puntillo, K., & Weiss, S. J. (1994). Pain: Its mediators and associated morbidity in critically ill cardiovascular surgical patients. *Nursing Research, 43,* 31–36.

Rakowski, W., Julius, M., Hickey, T., Verbrugge, L., & Halter, J. B. (1988). Daily symptoms and behavioral responses: Results of a health diary with older adults. *Medical Care, 26,* 278–295.

Romero, M. T., Cooper, M. L., Komisaruk, B. R., & Bodnar, R. J. (1988). Gender-specific and gonadectomy specific effects upon swim analgesia: Role of steroid replacement therapy. *Physiology and Behavior, 44,* 257–265.

Romero, M. T., Kepler, K. L., Cooper, M. L., Komisaruk, B. R., & Bodnar, R. J. (1987). Modulation of genetic-specific effects upon swim analgesia in gonadectomized rats. *Physiology and Behavior, 40,* 39–45.

Rose, G. A. (1965). Chest pain questionnaire. *Milbank Memorial Fund Quarterly, 43,* 32–36.

Savedra, M. C., Holzemer, W. L., Tesler, M. D., & Wilkie, D. (1993). Assessment of postoperation pain in children and adolescents using the adolescent pediatric pain tool. *Nursing Research, 42,* 5–9.

Unruh, A. M. (1996). Gender variations in clinical pain experience. *Pain, 65,* 123–167.

Veith, J., Anderson, J., & Slade, S. (1987). Plasma ß-endorphin, pain thresholds, and anxiety levels across the human menstrual cycle. *Physiology and Behavior, 32,* 31–34.

Verbrugge, L. (1980). Sex differences in complaints and diagnoses. *Journal of Behavioral Medicine, 3,* 327–355.

✳ Verbrugge, L. (1985). Gender and health: An update on hypotheses and evidence. *Journal of Health, Sociology and Behavior, 26,* 156-182.

Verbrugge, L. M., & Wingard, D. L. (1987). Sex differentials in health and mortality. *Health Matrix, 5*(2), 3-19.

Von Korff, M., Dworkin, S. F., & LeResche, L. (1990). Graded chronic pain status: An epidemiological evaluation. *Pain, 40,* 279-291.

Wilson, P. R., & Yaksh, T. L. (1978). Baclofen is anti-nociceptive in the spinal intr... *European Journal of Pharmacol...*

Yaksh, T. L., & Reddy, S. V. (1981). S... on the analgetic effects associated w... tions of opiates, alpha-adrenergic agonist... *Anesthesiology, 54,* 451-467.

Zieglgansberger, W. (1988). Dorsal horn neur... cology: Baclofen and morphine. *Annals of ... York Academy of Sciences, 531,* 150-156.

s of Chronic Pain

αιια Response to Treatment

ROBERT J. GATCHEL
JAKE EPKER

As Gatchel and Turk (1996) have pointed out, perhaps one of the most universal forms of stress encountered is pain. Indeed, pain accounts for over 80% of all physician visits. The treatment of chronic pain patients accounts for the bulk of the $70 billion in annual health care costs and lost productivity in the United States. With this background of great economic costs and traditionally poor outcomes among chronic pain patients, it has become increasingly more important for researchers to develop effective and efficient ways of managing this patient population. This has stimulated two approaches to attacking this problem, both of which are reviewed in this chapter.

The first approach aims at developing reliable methods for predicting which acute pain patients are at greater risk for developing more chronic problems. If one can prevent chronicity, huge cost savings can be realized. For example, Linton and Bradley (1996) have noted that, although there is still a paucity of cost-effectiveness studies in the scientific literature pertaining to pain management, the ones that have been reported highlight the significant cost-savings associated with early intervention programs for pain-related disorders. Thus, if we can identify reliable predictors for these patients who are at greater risk for developing chronic pain, then early interventions may be a powerful means of reducing costs. The first section of this chapter

addresses the current status of such risk assessment attempts.

With the advent of the biopsychosocial perspective of pain, which has been comprehensively reviewed by Turk and Flor (Chapter 2, this volume), more effective treatment programs for pain are beginning to emerge. An important concurrent emerging interest is to develop a method for predicting which patients respond best to such treatments. As Turk and Gatchel (in press) have recently noted, there is currently little data available to determine "what set of patients with what characteristics are most likely to benefit from what set of treatment modalities." Research is greatly needed to address these issues because of the obvious cost-savings and treatment-outcome implications. The second part of this chapter addresses the issue of what individual psychosocial variables may help predict response to treatment.

PSYCHOSOCIAL PREDICTORS OF CHRONIC PAIN

Chronic Pain

As is discussed throughout this volume, chronic pain is a demoralizing condition that affects hundreds of thousands of people in the United States every year. On an individual level, one must confront not only the stress induced by the pain itself but also the ongoing stress of seeking relief that often remains unattained. Such unsuccessful attempts to achieve relief can result in feelings of helplessness, hopelessness, and depression. In addition, chronic pain also levies a heavy toll on those who try to support such an individual, as they become frustrated after efforts to alleviate the pain are unsuccessful.

Chronic pain also results in significant societal costs, manifested in lost productivity, increased health care, and soaring disability benefits. It is a significant problem because of the frequent ineffectiveness of traditional medical approaches. This ineffectiveness is demonstrated, in part, by the many patients who repeatedly seek treatment, regardless of the success rate in treating various chronic pain conditions. In turn, individuals disabled by chronic pain conditions, such as chronic low back pain (CLBP) and temporomandibular joint disorder (TMD), account for substantial costs to society. For example, with CLBP patients, Mayer and Gatchel (1988) concluded that when work measures, such as social security and loss of productivity, were considered in addition to treatment costs, the annual cost ranged from 20 to 60 billion dollars. More recently, Leigh, Markowitz, Fahs, Shin, and Landigran (1997) reported that, based on adjusted 1992 estimate costs, occupational injuries and disabilities account for $145 billion annually in the United States. To date, there is no treatment available that consistently and permanently alleviates pain for all patients. A better understanding of the psychosocial factors that contribute to the onset and maintenance of chronic pain, as well as the implication of such factors on treatment, should assist clinicians in developing more effective treatments for individuals with chronic pain.

Acute versus Chronic Pain

It is important to make a distinction between acute and chronic pain, for many people experience acute episodes of pain but are not disabled by chronic pain conditions. According to Grzesiak (1991), acute pain serves as a biological signal. It points to the underlying somatic problem and, by definition, tells the clinician what is necessary to effect a cure. The key to acute pain is that the location, pattern, and description of the pain usually lead the diagnostician to the underlying cause. However, with chronic pain, this is not the case. Chronic

pain lacks biological utility and tells the clinician only that something is wrong somewhere in the patient's life. The problem may have its origin in biological, psychological, or social difficulties or in a combination of these factors. As the chronicity of the pain increases, these factors play an increasingly important role in the maintenance of the pain behavior. As discussed by Turk and Flor (Chapter 2, this volume), a biopsychosocial model of pain best incorporates these interactive factors.

This differentiation is similar to that made between "disease" and "illness." S. Dworkin (1990) explains that "disease" is most usefully defined as a biological event representing a disruption of a body structure or organ system as a result of anatomical and/or physiological change. The disease process may involve single or multiple organs and organ systems, may advance, regress, or remain dormant, and may or may not be clinically apparent. "Illness," however, is defined as encompassing the subjective experience of physical discomforts, emotional perturbation, behavioral limitations, and psychosocial disruption of usual or expected activities and relationships. Mechanic (1985) defined "illness behavior" as the manner in which persons monitor their bodies, define and interpret symptoms, take remedial action, and utilize various sources of help in response to their illness concerns. Therefore, one's pain experience is a complex combination of physiological, psychological, and social factors that are interrelated. However, efforts to understand chronic pain conditions have not always incorporated such a biopsychosocial approach.

Pain and the Biopsychosocial Model

Efforts to study chronic pain conditions have broadened from antiquated, unidimensional models to complex, multidimensional models of pain that take into account physiological, psychological, and social variables. Evidence suggests that with medical patients in general and with chronic pain patients in particular there is a high comorbidity between psychological disturbances and physical disorders (e.g., Gatchel, 1996; Kinney, Gatchel, Polatin, Fogarty, & Mayer, 1993; Polatin, Kinney, Gatchel, Lillo, & Mayer, 1993; Kinney, Gatchel, Ellis, & Holt, 1992; Katon & Sullivan, 1990). Models have been proposed that identify the various factors that contribute to and maintain these comorbid conditions (Cohen & Rodriguez, 1995). Current efforts to utilize a multidimensional approach to the understanding of chronic pain disorders depend on physical measurements, psychological variables, and social/cultural factors. However, this was not always the case.

Traditional medical models have tended to view chronic pain as being a unidimensional phenomenon. Medicine has tended to dichotomize pain complaints as being either "organic" or "psychogenic" in nature, with those chronic pain patients who continue to seek treatment tending to be categorized as having a "psychogenic" problem. The conceptualization of pain has evolved from a simplistic, biomedical model to a multidimensional model that takes into account biological, psychological, and social factors in attempts to explain the occurrence and report of pain.

The biomedical model's inability to account for psychological factors that contribute to the pain experience led to inquiries into the role of such factors. Concepts such as "psychogenic pain" (Engel, 1959) and the associated "pain-prone disorder" evolved from this movement. Melzack and Wall (1965) attempted to take into account many of the diverse psychophysiological aspects that appear to be involved in the pain perception process with their "gate control" theory of pain. In this model, central nervous system mechanisms provide the physiological basis for psychological involvement in pain perception; it is the interplay between these mechanisms that is critical in determining if and to what extent a specific stimulus leads to pain. Specifically, a neurophysiological mechanism in the dorsal horns of the spinal cord serves a gate-like function, controlling the flow and transmission of nerve impulses from peripheral fibers to the central nervous system (CNS). Although this model underwent criticism, it represented a significant advance in our conceptualization of pain by being comprehensive enough to account for specific physiological and psychological mechanisms.

Other scientists pointed to the importance of factors other than the physiological and psychological in the pain experience. Mechanic (1966, 1972) pointed out that, in addition to psychological factors, social components should be considered in the study of the pain experience. As such, he recognized that one's response to symptoms may be seen as a function of the social implications of that behavior (e.g., attention from significant others, escape from unwanted responsibilities, financial compensation, etc.). Turk and Rudy (1988) synthesized these various aspects of the chronic pain experience and developed a biopsychosocial model of pain that stresses the necessity to incorporate

cognitive, affective, social, behavioral, and physiological data. In a review of the concepts of illness behavior, Dworkin (1990) indicates that the diversity in expression of any illness, including its severity, duration, and consequences for the individual, is accounted for by the interrelationship among biological changes, psychological status, and the social and cultural contexts that shape the patient's perceptions and responses to illness.

It is widely accepted in the various arenas of chronic pain research that psychological, social, and physical factors all have a significant role in the maintenance of pain behaviors. The common acceptance of such an approach has become the norm as opposed to the exception. In fact, a recent study (Glaros, Glass, & McLaughlin, 1994) assessed practicing dentists' knowledge of and beliefs about TMD and chronic pain in regard to four domains: psychophysiological, psychiatric disorders, chronic pain, and pathophysiology. The investigators found that dentists generally agreed with experts in the psychophysiological and psychiatric disorders domains. The findings suggest that the role of psychophysiological factors and psychiatric disorders in the etiology and/or maintenance of TMD is generally accepted among practitioners in the field. In addition, a factor analytic study (Rudy, Turk, Zaki, & Curtin, 1989) investigated functional and psychological impairment across subgroups of TMD patients and found that psychological factors played a major role in symptom presentation regardless of biological factors.

The search for psychosocial factors that aid in the prediction of identifying who becomes chronic and who does not has a long history. Early attempts often utilized specific psychological measures in efforts to identify a "pain personality." Although most such efforts failed to identify such a personality type, the evolution and results of these investigations provides insight into characteristics that are commonly seen in chronic pain populations.

Use of the Minnesota Multiphasic Personality Inventory as a Predictor Variable

Investigation of psychological factors in chronic pain has frequently been explored with the Minnesota Multiphasic Personality Inventory (MMPI), a psychological instrument designed to identify both acute areas of difficulty and more stable personality traits and styles. One of the earliest such studies was conducted by Hanvick (1951) in an evaluation of patients who were then considered either as having chronic pain with "organic" causes or else as having "functional disorders." This study conceptualized chronic pain according to the earlier models as being either "organic" or "psychogenic" in nature, although he referred to them as "organic" and "functionally disordered," respectively. Even though such a distinction has, fortunately, been replaced with the more comprehensive biopsychosocial model, this study provided the basis of subsequent studies on the interaction of psychological profiles and chronic pain disorders.

Hanvick found 25 items on the MMPI that differentiated the "organic" and "functionally disordered" groups. He noted that the latter group had elevations on scales 1, 2, 3, 4, 7, and 8 (Hypochondriasis, Depression, Hysteria, Psychopathic deviate, Psychasthenia, and Schizophrenia, respectively), with the "conversion-V" pattern (1, 2, 3 elevated with 2 lower than 1 and 3) present. The former group displayed this conversion-V pattern as well, but to a lesser degree. Further research has shown inconsistency in replicating these findings, with a majority of studies unable to support Hanvick's conclusions (McCreary, Turner, & Dawson, 1977; Sternbach, Wolf, Murphy, & Akeson, 1973).

Studies investigating the use of the MMPI in predicting chronicity in pain populations have some similarities. Several studies have demonstrated that patients with chronic pain tend to show certain patterns of elevations versus healthy controls and versus acute pain patients. For example, Schumann, Zweiner, and Nebrich (1988) found elevations on the neurotic triad (i.e., Hypochondriasis [scale 1], Depression [scale 2], and Hysteria [scale 3]) in TMD patients versus healthy controls. However, in a discriminant function analysis, 19.4% of the participants were not correctly separated into the groups of patients and controls. Thus the level of elevation on scales 1, 2, and 3 of the MMPI demonstrated poor discrimination in this study. Nevertheless, other researchers have noted the high incidence of elevations on the neurotic triad as well. Etscheidt and Steiger (1995) reported that elevations within the neurotic triad accounted for 56% of all two-point code types in their study of chronic pain patients.

In the TMD population, McCreary, Clark, Merril, and Oakley (1991) examined the MMPI profiles of three groups of patients: those with myalgia, those with temporomandibular joint problems, and those with pain arising from both muscle and joint problems. The myalgia group displayed elevated scales 1, 2, 3, and 6 (Hypochondriasis,

Depression, Hysteria, and Paranoia, respectively), with these scores being higher than the elevations of the other two groups. The myalgia group also demonstrated higher scores on the Beck Depression Inventory (BDI) and measures of anxiety when compared to the other two groups.

In the CLBP population, high scale 3 (Hysteria) scores have been associated with individuals reporting acute pain (Bigos et al., 1991; Fordyce, Bigos, Battie, & Fisher, 1992; Gatchel, Polatin, & Kinney, 1995; Gatchel, Polatin, & Mayer, 1995). In one longitudinal study, Bigos and colleagues (1991) found elevations on scale 3 of the MMPI to be predictive of development of low back pain in workers. Bombardier, Divine, Jordan, Brooks, and Neelon (1993) demonstrated that as the MMPI profile appears more distressed, the individual is facing more psychosocial difficulties. Other researchers have demonstrated that the scales of the MMPI become increasingly elevated as the length of disability increases (Garron & Leavitt, 1983; Sternbach, Wolf, Murphy, & Akeson, 1973). In yet another similar study, Barnes, Gatchel, Mayer, and Barnett (1990) found that patients undergoing successful functional restoration rehabilitation for CLBP evidenced significant decreases in scales 1, 2, and 3 between the time of admission and 6 months following discharge. They concluded that the elevations are sensitive to situational stressors and may be a reaction to the illness and resultant life changes.

Although there have been several efforts to identify "pain profiles" with the use of the MMPI, such studies have been strongly criticized (e.g., Main & Spanswick, 1995). Findings from studies utilizing the MMPI for this purpose provide variable and inconsistent results. One of the controversies surrounding the use of the MMPI with chronic pain populations is the overlap of symptoms of a particular disorder and items on the MMPI. Thus positive responses to symptoms of a chronic pain disorder might lead to erroneous estimates of psychopathology. For example, Pincus, Callahan, Bradley, Vaughn, and Wolfe (1987) identified five items on the MMPI that reflect both the presence and the severity of rheumatoid arthritis (RA). Each of these items code on both scales 1 and 3 (Hypochondriasis and Hysteria, respectively), and three items also code on scale 2 (Depression). If positive responses to these five items are not counted, the T scores for these three scales declines 4–10 points. Such findings in the RA population suggest that similar confounds may exist in other chronic pain populations.

In the field of psychosomatic medicine, the search for specific personality and psychosocial factors predisposing individuals to develop chronic pain problems has always been a major focus. For example, investigators have attempted to identify specific disorder-personality types (such as "migraine personality"), as well as a more general "pain-prone personality" (Blumer & Heilbrom, 1982). By and large, though, these efforts have received little empirical support and have been greatly challenged (e.g., Mayer & Gatchel, 1988; Turk & Salovey, 1984).

Part of the problem in attempts to uncover a "pain personality" is that people present with a variety of problems that differs depending on the period of time that they have perceived themselves to be in pain. For example, one study (Sternbach et al., 1973) compared the personality profiles of acute versus chronic pain patients with the use of the MMPI. They found that chronic pain patients reported significantly more psychological distress as evidenced by their higher elevations on scales 1, 2, and 3. These results indicate that early reports of pain are not associated with reports of major psychological distress. On the other hand, an increase in the length of the pain experience results in an increase in the report of psychological disturbance. These changes are likely due to the sustained physical discomfort, emotional despair, and preoccupation with the pain that become a focus in the lives of these patients. The occurrence of changes along the developmental course of chronic pain has been proposed by Gatchel (1991).

Progression of Pain

These psychological changes, which occur concomitantly with a shift toward chronicity, have been referred to as the result of a layering of behavioral/psychological problems over the original nociception of pain experience itself (Gatchel, 1996). This idea of "layering" was best explained by Gatchel's (1991) model of the progression of pain. This model consists of three successive stages (acute, subacute, and chronic disability, respectively) that follow from the experience of an identifiable injury. Stage 1 begins with a perceived pain and includes the resulting emotional reactions, such as fear, anxiety, and worry, that arise as a consequence of that perception. When this proceeds past a reasonably acute, normal healing time period (2–4 months), the progression into Stage 2 occurs. During this stage, the development and/or exacer-bation of psychological and behavioral problems occurs, such as learned helplessness/depression, distress/anger, and somatization. Gatchel (1991) suggests that the manifestation of these difficulties is dependent on the individual's premorbid psychological characteristics, as well as current socioeconomic and other environmental conditions. Therefore, if an individual has preexisting depression and suffers economically after losing his or her job due to pain and disability, the depressive symptoms will show a significant increase in intensity during this stage. Likewise, an individual with premorbid hypochondriacal characteristics who receives a great deal of secondary gain for being disabled will likely display significant somatization and symptom magnification.

In this model, the individual has certain pre-existing characteristics that are exacerbated by the stress of attempting to cope with the chronic pain. This complex interaction of physical, psychological, and social elements leads to Stage 3. At this point, as the patient's life begins to become consumed by the pain and the concomitant psychological and behavioral difficulties, the patient begins to accept a "sick role." In doing so, the patient may be excused from regular responsibilities and social obligations and receive compensation and therefore be reinforced to maintain the sick role. Indeed, Fordyce et al. (1984) originally noted that pain behavior initially elicited by tissue damage can persist in some patients long after normal healing time because these behavioral responses lead to positive consequences, such as solicitous attention from a spouse, financial compensation, and/or avoidance of unwanted responsibilities. If patients having persistent pain continue to use maladaptive cognitive and behavioral coping strategies, then the degree of suffering and functional disability associated with the pain may be significantly increased.

In Gatchel's model (1991), an additional factor that serves as another "layer" of behavioral and psychological difficulties is "physical deconditioning," which generally occurs when patients progress toward chronic disability. This refers to the incremental lack of use of the body, which leads to muscle atrophy, decreased endurance, and so forth. Research has shown that this can, in turn, lead to "mental deconditioning." Therefore, physical deconditioning has a negative impact on one's psychological health and self-esteem (Gatchel, Baum, & Krantz, 1989). However, this is not the end of it, for a vicious cycle can develop. These negative psychological reactions can reinforce the physical deconditioning by promoting decreased motivation to participate in work and recreational activities. Finally, this combination may also have a negative impact on the initial perception of pain by the patient. For example, when a patient engages in an activity that produces an acute pain, he or she tends to associate that pain with the initial hurt and resultant progressive chronic course suffered in the past. This causes the patient to avoid not only pain but also potentially pain-inducing situations because of a fear that there will be a recurrence of the harm from the past. Therefore, it is important that patients be taught the difference between hurt and harm (Fordyce, 1988). In fact, for some chronic pain conditions (e.g., CLBP), there is often pain associated with the physical reconditioning, rehabilitation, and additional steps needed in order to resume regular responsibilities and social obligations.

The implication of the view that chronic pain conditions are psychophysiological disorders is that their expression may include psychological distress and psychosocial impairment. Numerous studies have therefore attempted to identify psychiatric conditions that are implicated in the onset and/or exacerbation of chronic pain. These efforts have often utilized psychiatric diagnosis as an indicator of psychopathology in chronic pain populations. The assumption is that there is not one primary preexisting "pain personality" or psychological disorder. Rather, there is a general nonspecificity in the relationship between personality/psychosocial problems and pain (Gatchel, 1996). Pain is viewed as a stressor that exacerbates or produces psychosocial distress problems.

Psychological Disturbance and Chronic Pain

Studies have demonstrated that the presence of character pathology leads to poorer prognosis in the course of both physical and psychological illness (Peselow, Fieve, & DiFiglia, 1992; Clark, Watson, & Mineka, 1994). Also, as noted earlier, evidence suggests that with medical patients in general and with chronic pain patients in particular there is a high comorbidity between psychological disturbances and physical disorders. There remains debate as to which is the primary cause, the physical illness or the psychological disturbance. For example, in patients with irritable bowel syndrome (IBS), research indicates that individuals who seek treatment are more psychologically dis-

tressed than non-help-seeking IBS sufferers (Drossman et al.,1988). Blanchard (1993) notes that it is unknown whether this co-occurrence is causal. It may be that the IBS sufferer who becomes a patient has premorbid psychological distress and develops IBS symptoms or else that the severity and duration of IBS symptoms lead to both psychological disturbance and the seeking of medical attention. This is the age-old "chicken or egg" question.

A similar situation exists with individuals who suffer from headache, with depression reported to be the most common psychological disturbance encountered in this population (Adler, Alder, & Packard, 1987; Breslau, Davis, & Andreski, 1991; Nappi, Bono, Sandrini, Martignoni, & Micieli, 1991). Some depression in headache patients is likely a result of living with pain, since chronic pain can cause sleep disturbance, disruption of occupational and psychosocial activities, and severe strain on social support mechanisms (Hatch, 1993). However, the picture becomes less clear as the complex interaction of various aspects of this pain condition become more apparent: Depression can alter one's perception of pain, as depression has been associated with a lowering of pain threshold and pain tolerance level (Rome, Harness, & Kaplan, 1990). In this population, therefore, it appears that the interaction of variables results in the phenomenon of the pain experience.

Some evidence indicates that those who are unable to obtain effective alleviation of their pain through conventional medical procedures may develop psychopathology as a result. Dworkin, Von Korff, and LeResche (1990) assessed multiple pain conditions and their association with affective disturbance, somatization, and psychological distress based on questionnaire data from a sample of 1016 enrollees of a large health maintenance organization. Among other findings, they reported that individuals with two or more pain conditions were at an elevated risk of an algorithm diagnosis of major depression. Number of pain conditions was a better predictor of major depression than were important measures of pain experience, including pain severity and pain persistence. In this study, the findings point to a relationship between multiple pain conditions and increased risk of depression in individuals. It is reasonable, therefore, that individuals with chronic pain who tend to be somatic (i.e., have many physical complaints) may also tend to have an increased risk of affective disturbance, such as depression. Essentially, both depression and somatization have been heavily implicated in chronic pain (Dworkin, Von Korff, & LeResche, 1990; Romano & Turner, 1985).

Another study (Polatin et al., 1988) suggests that a large proportion of the chronic pain population has endured substantial psychological problems prior to the experience of their pain condition. Studies investigating such psychological problems have typically utilized the SCID, or Structured Clinical Interview for DSM (*Diagnostic and Statistical Manual of Mental Disorders*), to determine Axis I clinical disorders and Axis II personality disorders. Studies of both the CLBP population and the TMD population have found that the incidence of Axis I and Axis II disorders far exceeds the base rates for the general population (Gatchel, 1996). For example, Gatchel, Polatin, Mayer, and Garcy (1994) evaluated 152 CLBP patients undergoing treatment in a functional restoration program. They found that on entering the program almost all patients met criteria for at least one Axis I disorder (with somatoform pain disorder, substance abuse, and major depression being most common) and that over 50% met criteria of at least one Axis II disorder (with paranoid personality disorder being most common).

Kinney, Gatchel, Ellis, and Holt (1992) also used the SCID to assess psychological disorders in 50 chronic TMD patients. They found that 86% of the chronic TMD patients received at least one Axis I diagnosis, whereas 46% met criteria for two or more diagnoses. Not surprisingly, somatoform pain disorder (i.e., a preoccupation with pain without adequate physical findings to account for the pain) was diagnosed in a large percentage (40%) of the chronic TMD population. Even when somatoform disorders were excluded from the analyses, 84% of the chronic TMD patients still met lifetime diagnostic criteria for other Axis I disorders. Excluding somatoform pain disorder, the most frequently diagnosed Axis I disorders were major depression (74%), substance abuse disorders (30%), and anxiety disorders (24%). These rates also exceed the base rates in the general population. In addition, 40% of the TMD patients met criteria for at least one personality disorder. Again, this rate exceeds the prevalence of personality disorders in the general population.

Studies such as these point to the high incidence of comorbid psychological disorders in pain populations such as CLBP and TMD. Psychosocial predictors of chronic pain, by definition, must include social parameters, as well as the more specifically psychological factors previously discussed. Several researchers have also pointed to the impor-

tance of coping strategies in the development and/or maintenance of chronic pain (Fordyce, Roberts, & Sternbach, 1985; Lazarus & Folkman, 1984; Turk & Flor, 1987).

Coping Skills/Strategies

Turk and Kerns (1983) have noted that pain assessment should consist of a number of components, including the individual's coping strategies. For example, among RA patients, those who respond with negative, exaggerated, and/or catastrophizing thoughts and those who perceive themselves as unable to reduce or control their pain report much more severe and disabling pain (Keefe, Brown, Wallston, & Caldwell, 1989). RA patients who use coping self-statements and perceptions of resourcefulness tend to report less pain (Flor & Turk, 1988). In addition, active coping strategies (i.e., staying busy, ignoring pain, distraction) are associated with less pain, whereas passive coping strategies (i.e., restricting activities due to pain, engaging in wishful thinking, depending on others to relieve pain) are associated with more severe pain (Brown & Nicassio, 1987). Finally, Zautra and Manne (1992) note that patients who rely on passive, avoidant, or emotion-focused mechanisms for coping with RA usually report lower self-esteem, poorer adjustment, and greater negative affect as opposed to patients who utilize active, problem-solving strategies. Boothby, Thorn, Stroud, and Jensen (Chapter 21, this volume) provide a more thorough review of the importance of coping styles and pain.

Kerns, Turk, and Rudy (1985) set out to develop a multidimensional instrument that was psychometrically sound, theoretically linked to a cognitive-behavioral perspective, and specifically for use with chronic pain patients. The result of their research efforts was the West Haven–Yale Multidimensional Pain Inventory, or Multidimensional Pain Inventory (MPI), as it is currently known. It provides a brief but comprehensive assessment of the subjective experience of pain that can be included as part of an extended assessment protocol in conjunction with other procedures (Kerns et al., 1985). The instrument's strength is its taxonomy, which was empirically derived and makes no assumption about the classification of chronic pain patients other than to acknowledge the relevance of cognitive, affective, and behavioral data for establishing group membership.

In a subsequent study (Turk & Rudy, 1988), a cluster analysis was performed on the MPI scales to group heterogeneous samples of chronic pain patients according to similarities between their profile patterns. This analysis revealed three clusters of patient profiles, and the three-cluster solution was replicated on a second sample of subjects. The three profiles identified reflect coping styles and were labeled "dysfunctional" (43% of the sample), "interpersonally distressed" (28% of the sample), and "adaptive copers" (29.5% of the sample). The first cluster included patients who indicated the severity of their pain to be higher and said that it interfered to a greater extent in their lives. The second cluster consisted of patients who held the common perception that their families and significant others were not very supportive of them. The third cluster, adaptive copers, appeared to have in common: (1) lower levels of pain severity, perceived interference, and affective distress and (2) higher levels of daily activity and life control. Cluster analysis of MPI data in other pain populations have provided similar results (Walter & Brannon, 1991). However, few studies demonstrating this measure's potential usefulness in predicting chronicity have been published. We are currently conducting such an investigation with individuals who suffer from TMD .

The "Psychosocial Disability Factor"

The results of the studies presented above reiterate that chronic pain disability reflects more than just the presence of some physical symptom or a single psychosocial characteristic, such as an elevation of a specific scale of the MMPI or the diagnosis of a psychological disorder. Chronic pain disability is a complex psychosocioeconomic phenomenon. In fact, some researchers have argued that only approximately half of the total disability phenomenon in someone complaining of chronic back pain can be attributed to physical impairment (e.g., Waddell, Main, Morris, DiPaola, & Gray, 1984). For example, physical findings, such as radiographic results, have not been found to be reliable indices of low back pain (Mayer & Gatchel, 1988). Most cases of low back pain are classified as "soft-tissue injuries" because they are ill-defined and unverified on physical examination. In addition, in a study of magnetic resonance imaging by Jenson and colleagues (1994), significant spinal abnormalities were found in patients who were not experiencing back pain. Similar results have been found in other chronic pain conditions, such as TMD, where there is a dissociation between reports of

pain and actual physical abnormalities (Moss & Garrett, 1984).

It is apparent that psychological and/or emotional factors contribute significantly to determining who develops chronic pain disability. In RA patients, greater disability is reported by individuals with: greater hypochondriasis, depression, and denial of affective problems (McFarlane & Brooks, 1988); state and trait anxiety and arthritis helplessness (Hagglund, Haley, Reveille, & Alarcón, 1989); catastrophization (Keefe et al., 1989); and the utilization of passive coping strategies (Brown & Nicassio, 1987). However, this does not necessarily mean that such patients are "malingerers" who are "faking" their level of disability. As indicated earlier, chronic pain is a complex phenomenon, one in which psychosocial factors can interact with physical symptoms to contribute to disability. For instance, Lehmann, Spratt, and Lehmann (1993) evaluated 55 CLBP patients referred by occupational physicians and followed them for 6 months. Disabling CLBP, as defined by not returning to work after 6-months, was found to be correlated only with marital status, as married patients returned to work more quickly than single patients.

In a large-scale prospective study, a total of 504 acute low back pain patients were evaluated with a standardized battery of psychosocial assessment tests (Gatchel, Polatin, & Mayer, 1995). They were then tracked over the year after the initial evaluation in order to assess return-to-work status, as well as any recurrence of back pain or a new back injury. In addition, complete information about workers' compensation or personal injury insurance status was collected at this point in time. Logistic regression analyses were applied to these data in order to differentiate between those patients who were back at work after this 1-year period versus those who were not because of the original back injury. Results revealed the importance of two psychosocial variables: (1) level of self-reported pain and disability and (2) scores on scale 3 (Hysteria) of the MMPI. In addition, two other variables were found to be significant: gender of the patient and workers' compensation/personal injury insurance status at 1 year. Thus the model isolated the following characteristics of patients who were more likely not to be at work after 1 year: they were female, they had workers' compensation or personal injury insurance-related injuries, and they scored high on self-reported pain and disability, as well as on scale 3 of the MMPI, during the initial evaluation. The model correctly identified 90.7% of the cases. There were no differences between the two groups for the physician-rated severity of the initial back injury or the physical demands of the job to which patients had to return. Thus these results demonstrate that there is a robust "psychosocial disability factor" among injured workers that is important not only in pain perception but also in subsequent development of chronic pain-related disability. As in the other areas of the growing field of behavioral medicine, medical personnel will need to be concerned with the psychosocial characteristics of their acute-care patients in order to prevent costly effects (both economic and human productivity losses) of prolonged bouts of disability due to back pain injury. Indeed, Melamed (1995) has reviewed studies clearly demonstrating how psychological and physical disorders are "intertwined in a complex way" (p. 371). Early intervention that directly "flags" these psychosocial variables is essential in order to prevent such chronic disability.

Such psychosocial factors will therefore need to be attended to carefully in primary care settings. A medical evaluation of a chronic pain condition, such as low back pain or temporomandibular disorder, requires attention to more than the biomechanical and physical factors for a complete assessment that potentiates effective pain management. An understanding of the specific factors thus far demonstrated to be predictive of chronicity in various chronic pain domains should assist clinicians in their efforts to effectively treat pain patients.

We now discuss the importance of psychosocial factors that predict chronicity in specific pain disorders. Those pain disorders that have received the most scientific investigation in this area are presented.

Chronic Low Back Pain

Besides the just-reviewed study by Gatchel, Polatin, and Mayer (1995), other studies have recognized the report of high severity of pain and disability as potentially important in predicting those with an acute episode who subsequently develop chronic problems and those with chronic problems who do not respond to treatment (Biering-Sorenson, 1983; Mooney, Cairns, & Robertson, 1975; Lancourt & Kettelhut, 1992). In two studies of individuals with a first episode of acute back pain, chronic back pain at a 6-month follow-up was predicted by greater intensity of acute pain (Phillips, Grant, & Berkowitz, 1991; Williams & Slater,

1995). Studies such as these provide considerable evidence that severity of acute pain is a factor that tends to differentiate which patients with acute pain become chronic. Moreover, in terms of the other psychosocial factors found to be important, scale 3 of the MMPI has been found to be predictive of the development of low back pain in uninjured workers in a large-scale study of Boeing employees (Bigos et al., 1991).

Von Korff, Deyo, Cherkin, and Barlow (1993) evaluated 1,128 primary care back pain patients 1 year after they sought care. Outcome was determined by using an index of chronic pain grade, which was based on a rating of characteristic pain intensity, a disability score, and the number of disability days. Poor outcome (i.e., high disability and moderately limiting back pain or high disability and severely limiting back pain) was best predicted by pain-related disability, days in pain, lower educational level, and gender (female). The authors note that recency of onset was not a predictor of outcome, and thus it may be more appropriate and clinically meaningful to differentiate patients with chronic low back pain on the basis of levels of pain intensity, pain-related disability, and pain persistence rather than by a classification of acute versus chronic pain.

Dionne and colleagues (1997) interviewed 1,213 adult enrollees of a large health maintenance organization approximately 1 month after a consultation for back pain, and then followed these subjects each year thereafter. Outcome in this study was assessed with a modified version of the Roland–Morris scale, which measures limitations in behavior for the previous 2 weeks due to back pain. Of the various factors acquired at the 1-month assessment, measures of depression (SCL-90-R), somatization (SCL-90-R), functional limitations, and pain were the strongest predictors of 2-year outcome among a random sample of 569 subjects. Stepwise linear regression analyses retained initial depression and somatization scores, 1-month modified Roland–Morris score, and number of pain days in the past 6-months. When the 2-year Roland–Morris score was dichotomized at 50%, recursive partitioning identified two variables—SCL-90-R Depression and Somatization scores—that correctly classified 85.2% of the participants. The authors note that (1) the distinction made between participants with and without functional limitations at 1-month did not appear to be very useful in predicting return-to-work status and (2) the robustness of the association between psychological variables and back pain outcome suggests that psychological factors may represent the best criteria on which to base clinical decision rules.

Fenerstein, Berkowitz, and Peck (1997) conducted a large-scale study of musculoskeletal-related disability in United States Army personnel. In addition to finding that back-related disorders were the most prevalent sources of disability in the Army, these investigators also isolated a number of risk factors for developing such chronic low back pain disability. Besides isolating certain high-risk jobs, they found that gender (females) and psychosocial stressors (e.g., interpersonal stressors, role conflict, repetitive/boring work) are contributing risk factors. Thus, again, psychosocial factors appear to be closely related to chronicity development. Sanders (1995) has also independently demonstrated the significance of psychosocial variables as risk factors for chronic low back pain and disability. In a comprehensive review of epidemiological studies, he delineated various risk factors as barriers to recovery that were found to be consistently associated with an increased likelihood of an acute low back pain episode developing into a more chronic disability. In terms of psychosocial factors, MMPI scale 3 elevations, depression, low activity–high pain behavior, and negative beliefs for pain and activity were found to be important risk factors for developing chronic disability. In addition, Volinn (1996) has pointed out that psychosocial variables are more likely to have a greater influence on chronic back pain disability than the back pain itself! Jayson (1997) has also highlighted the strong association between psychosocial morbidity and back pain.

Finally, as a guide to assessing psychosocial risk factors for long-term low back pain disability and work loss, the National Advisory Committee on Health and Disability of New Zealand (1997) developed a method of screening for such risk factors in acute low back pain patients who were at risk for developing or perpetuating long-term disability. These comprehensive guidelines, based on findings from the scientific literature, are meant to help health care professionals better manage acute low back pain patients who have these risk "flags" in order to avoid chronicity problems. Table 26.1 summarizes these psychosocial risk variables. As can be seen, many are similar to those delineated in studies we have previously reviewed in this chapter.

Headache

Headache results in over 11 million people in the United States suffering various degrees of disability

TABLE 26.1. Summary of Psychosocial Risk Factors Delineated by the National Advisory Committee on Health and Disability of New Zealand (1997)

- Maladaptive attitudes and beliefs about back pain
- Display of frequent pain behaviors
- Reinforcement of pain behaviors by family members
- Lack of social support
- Compensation issues
- Heightened emotional reactivity
- Job dissatisfaction

every year (Stewart, Lipton, Celentano, & Reed, 1992). As with other chronic pain conditions, headache is a pain phenomenon with a large psychosocial component, and much psychological research has been conducted in attempts to identify a "headache personality." Although different types of headache patients have been described in terms of personality characteristics, research using standardized psychological measures has revealed little evidence for the existence of a "headache personality" (Kohler & Kosanic, 1992; Pfaffenrath, Hummelsberger, Pollman, Kaube, & Rath, 1991). Nevertheless, certain psychological characteristics, such as depression and anxiety, are found to be more common in headache patients versus normal controls. In fact, depression is the most frequently encountered psychological disturbance in patients with headache (Adler et al., 1987; Breslau et al., 1991; Nappi et al., 1991).

Studies of personality characteristics that contribute to the headache experience have typically been performed using such measures as the MMPI, the BDI, and the State–Trait Anxiety Inventory (STAI). Blanchard and Andrasik (1985) used the MMPI and determined that cluster headache patients and normal controls are not significantly different in terms of psychological functioning, whereas patients with migraine headache demonstrated elevated scores (T scores > 60) only on scale 3 (Hysteria). The greatest amount of psychological disturbance, as measured by the MMPI, was found in patients with tension-type headache. These individuals had elevated scores on scales 1 (Hypochondriasis), 2 (Depression), 3 (Hysteria), 7 (Psychasthenia), and 8 (Schizophrenia). An earlier study by Cox, Freundlich, and Meyer (1975) found that type of headache was matched by an increase in degree of psychological disturbance, as measured by the BDI and STAI. Such a pattern led Blanchard and Andrasik (1985) to conclude that severity of psychological disturbance is a function of "headache density," or number of days per week of headache suffering.

An early thorough review of the literature (Bakal, 1975) on tension-type and migraine headaches led the author to conclude that headache appears to be a psychological reaction to stressful stimulation. Kohler and Haimerl (1990) demonstrated that migraine headache is associated with psychological stress the day of or the day before the attack. Although it is difficult to define "stress" clinically, it has been argued that headache patients appraise stressful events, especially daily hassles, more negatively and cope with them less effectively than pain-free individuals (DeBenedittis & Lorenzetti, 1992; Holm, Holroyd, Hursey, & Penzien, 1986). Unfortunately, few prospective studies have been conducted with the purpose of determining which psychosocial factors predict the development of chronicity. A preliminary study by Blanchard, Kirsch, Applebaum, and Jaccard (1989) did, though, provide some initial support for an association between psychological factors and chronic headache pain. The authors appropriately noted that a direct answer to the question of whether the psychological disturbances often seen in chronic headache are the consequence of years of living with chronic pain or are predisposing factors in the initial development of the pain awaits a prospective longitudinal study. However, they took an initial step in attempting to indirectly answer this question through a series of statistical analyses of cross-sectional data on a large number of headache patients of various ages and at different points in their lifetime course of headache. Although the investigators pointed out that such analyses must be viewed as quite tentative, some modest support was found for the hypothesis that preexisting psychopathology may be one significant factor in "helping to cause" chronic headache. Such results are quite intriguing, but await validation from a prospective study.

Irritable Bowel Syndrome

Drossman and colleagues (1988) found that 20–30% of IBS patients demonstrated significant elevations (T score > 70) on various scales of the MMPI versus 5–17% of non-treatment-seeking IBS patients and 0–4% of normal subjects. This suggests that, as a group, IBS sufferers who seek medical attention are significantly more psycho-

logically disturbed than the other two groups. In fact, in a comparison of IBS patients to chronic headache patients, Blanchard and colleagues (1986) found the former to be more psychologically distressed.

Identification of potential psychological characteristics that contribute to the development and maintenance of pain conditions such as IBS remains a goal of many researchers. Evidence for chronic pain conditions resulting from the interaction of various psychological and physiological characteristics continues to mount. Blanchard, Radnitz, Schwartz, Neff, and Gerardi (1987) assessed depression and anxiety before and after a brief (approximately 4 months) behavioral treatment. Those IBS sufferers whose gastrointestinal symptoms were substantially relieved also showed a decrease in levels of anxiety and depression, as measured by the BDI and STAI, with posttreatment scores in the normal range. For those with no change in GI symptoms, there was also no change in levels of anxiety and depression. Thus it appears that sufficient severity and duration of IBS symptoms lead to, at least, greater psychological distress and eventual seeking of treatment. Nevertheless, many IBS sufferers who seek treatment show no notable elevations on such standardized tests as the BDI and STAI (Blanchard, 1993).

Finally, Walker, Gelfand, and Gelfand (1996) reported that IBS patients who had current depressive and anxiety disorders, relative to IBS patients with no such current psychiatric disorders, suffered significantly more gastrointestinal symptoms, unexplained symptoms such as headache and dizziness, and perceived themselves as being more disabled by their emotional symptoms. These results again demonstrate a comorbidity of IBS pain/disability and psychological factors.

Rheumatoid Arthritis

Research implicating the role of psychological factors in RA has appeared in the literature for a number of years. More recent efforts have continued to find specific psychosocial associations, especially between depression and the pain experience of RA. Brown (1990) utilized causal modeling with data from a longitudinal research design in an effort to prospectively study the relationship between pain and depression. The results support the notion that pain contributes to subsequent increases in depression, even after controlling for prior levels of depression. It has been suggested that the use of passive coping strategies may moderate this relationship (Brown, Nicassio, & Wallston, 1989).

A well-controlled study by Hagglund et al. (1989) found that the most robust predictors of pain intensity were measures of anxiety and depression, as assessed by the STAI and BDI, respectively. In a similar prospective study, researchers found that depression was associated with more intense pain, independent of pain activity (Affleck, Tennon, Urrows, & Higgins, 1991). Lorish, Abraham, Austin, Bradley, and Alarcón (1991) demonstrated that arthritis helplessness, as measured by the Arthritis Helplessness Index (AHI), significantly predicted impairment 12 months later, again independent of disease activity.

Other psychosocial variables have been implicated in the pain experience of RA. Goodenow, Reisine, and Grady (1990) demonstrated that, even after physical factors were controlled for, social support was a significant predictor of level of physical functioning and that the perceived quality of that support was more relevant than social integration. Higher support levels were associated with fewer declines in performance of activities. In a similar study, Zautra and Manne (1992) demonstrated that patients who describe their spouses as supportive engage in more adaptive coping behaviors. Similarly, the quality of social support and one's satisfaction with the level of support received have been shown to be positively related to psychological adjustment (Smith & Wallston, 1992).

Temporomandibular Joint Disorder

Vassend, Krogstad, and Dahl (1995) examined trait anxiety, subjective somatic symptoms, and pain associated with TMD in a combined cross-sectional and prospective study, with one of their primary intents being to examine the magnitude of the effect of these predictors on self-report of TMD-related pain and discomfort at a 2-year follow-up. Following correlational analyses, regression analyses were used to determine the effects of the initial anxiety and somatic complaints on later TMD-related pain. The authors concluded that the best predictors of later TMD pain (i.e., chronic TMD pain) were general somatic complaints, followed by initial pain and trait anxiety. Unfortunately, in this study chronic TMD pain was limited to a combination of self-report of (1) present pain/discomfort in the face and jaw, (2) jaw function, and (3) frequency of headache. Another limitation was that a relatively low number of subjects required that

the analyses be limited to models with few (two–four) independent variables. Nevertheless, this investigation demonstrated that psychological factors, such as trait anxiety and somatization, were predictive of maintenance of self-reported TMD pain after 2 years.

More recently, Garofalo, Gatchel, Wesley, and Ellis (1998) utilized the Research Diagnostic Criteria for TMD (RDC) as one of the psychosocial measures assessed in an effort to predict which patients presenting with acute TMD symptoms subsequently became chronic. The RDC (Dworkin & LeResche, 1992) is a dual-axis approach to classifying TMD. Prior to its development, there were numerous diagnostic systems for classifying TMD; this led to inconsistencies across studies because these various classification systems defined TMD differently. The RDC was developed with the intent of establishing a system of classification that would be universal, thus lending itself to comparisons across studies, as well as providing a "common language" for clinicians and researchers who investigate TMD. Axis I of the RDC is devoted to clinical diagnosis reflecting physical status, whereas Axis II pertains specifically to psychosocial classification. Garofalo and colleagues found that both RDC Axis I and Axis II data were able to predict chronicity. Specifically, Characteristic Pain Intensity, Graded Chronic Pain Severity, nonspecific physical symptoms (i.e., somatization), Group I disorders (i.e., myofacial pain with or without limited opening), and gender emerged as significant risk factors. Predictive models using these variables correctly classified 77% of the patients into chronic versus nonchronic groups.

Additional studies such as this, which utilize sound biopsychosocial measures that are empirically based and validated, will undoubtedly provide a greater understanding of the factors that predict chronicity in TMD. Ultimately, the goal of future investigations should be to arrive at a model for prediction of chronicity in TMD that accounts for a majority of the variance and thus most accurately predicts which patients are most likely to become chronic.

Other Pain Disorders

Dworkin (1997) has recently provided a comprehensive review of prospective studies that have evaluated risk factors for the development of pain chronicity in patients with acute pain. He primarily focused on three chronic pain syndromes: phantom pain, postherpetic neuralgia, and back pain.

For these three pain syndromes, it has been found that biomedical (greater physical pathology) and psychosocial (more severe self-reported acute pain and greater psychosocial distress) factors appear to increase the risk for developing chronic pain. Although he appropriately notes that replication is needed because several of the findings that led to this conclusion were based on single studies, the findings nevertheless again highlight the importance of psychosocial factors involved in the development of chronic pain.

In a study evaluating potential predictors of chronicity in 102 patients complaining of acute chest pain at their first admission, Kisely, Guthrie, Creed, and Tew (1997) measured outcome at 3 months and at 5 years. Outcome measures involved chest pain, change in physical activity, return to work, smoking, psychiatric disorder, and mortality. A major finding of this study was that a previous history of psychiatric disorder was associated with a fivefold increase in the risk of chronic chest pain at the 5-year follow-up evaluation. Thus these results again demonstrate a close link between psychosocial factors (in this case, a psychiatric disorder) and the development of chronic pain.

Other pain conditions that have increased at an alarming rate during the past decade—upper extremity disorders, such as carpal tunnel syndrome—have received attention as well. Feuerstein and Huang (1998) summarized factors that have been found to be associated with delayed recovery in patients with such occupationally related pain disorders. In addition to a number of medical and ergonomic variables, they isolated the significance of the following array of psychosocial factors found in various studies: high perceived work load, lack of social support, high perceived level of occupational stress, monotonous work, anxiety, and depression. Burton, Polatin, and Gatchel (1997) have also highlighted the important role of such factors, especially anxiety, in upper extremity disorders. Moreover, in terms of chronic musculoskeletal pain in general, Linton, Larden, and Gillow (1996) have found that a past history of sexual abuse was associated with higher levels of emotional distress and chronic pain.

Finally, Linton and Bradley (1996) have recently provided a comprehensive review of risk factors that are important to consider for the prevention of chronic pain. These include medical factors and demographic variables, as well as psychosocial factors such as work stressors, family involvement, sexual/physical abuse history, psychopathology, beliefs, and coping skills.

Treatment Implications

There is little doubt that psychosocial factors significantly contribute to pain perception and the subsequent pain-related disability seen in chronic pain patients. However, due to frequent inconsistencies in psychosocial measures utilized in the research, there remains debate as to specifically which factors contribute most significantly to the chronic pain experience. Nevertheless, such factors must be an area of focus if health care professionals hope to prevent the costly effects, both emotional and economical, that result from chronic pain disability. Early intervention is a key ingredient to preventing chronicity, since many patients possess premorbid psychological and personality characteristics (a diathesis) that become magnified when the individual is "stressed" and when attempting to cope with pain. This diathesis–stress model of pain, however, does not "paint" the complete picture. Other important socioeconomic and environmental variables, such as the secondary gain afforded by workers' compensation, can greatly impact the development of chronicity. However, it is those individuals with an array of predisposing factors who are the most likely to subsequently become chronic. Table 26.2 summarizes those psychosocioeconomic risk factors that appear to significantly predict the development of chronic pain disability, based on all the studies just reviewed. Of course, the exact algorithm or combination of these factors will obviously vary depending on the specific pain disorder.

TABLE 26.2. Summary of Psychosocioeconomic Risk Factors That May Predict the Development of Chronic Pain Disability

- High self-reported pain and disability
- Elevation of MMPI scale 3 (Hysteria)
- Depression
- Somatization
- Poor coping skills/strategies
- Poor quality of social support
- Unresolved workers' compensation/personal injury cases
- Gender
- Reinforcement of pain behaviors
- Job dissatisfaction
- Maladaptive attitudes and beliefs about pain
- History of childhood sexual abuse

This does not mean that these predisposing characteristics make chronic pain cases "functional" disorders or that chronic pain is "all in the patient's head." Chronic pain and disability represent a complex interaction of physical, psychological, and socioeconomic variables. Figure 26.1 illustrates the sequence of variables that may lead to chronicity. Efforts to treat such complex illnesses often benefit from multimodal treatment approaches. Moreover, treatment of the specific psychosocial issues involved usually falls into the broad category of cognitive-behavioral approaches (e.g., Gatchel & Turk, 1996). Specifically, modalities such as biofeedback and relaxation training, in addition to multidisciplinary treatment, have all been shown to be effective in controlled clinical trials (Gatchel & Blanchard, 1993; Flor, Haag, & Turk, 1986; Härkäpää, Mellin, Järvikoski, & Hurri, 1990; Mellin, Härkäpää, Hurri, & Järvikoski, 1990; Phillips, 1988; Sargent, Solbach, Coyne, Spohn, & Segerson, 1986).

We now review research addressing an issue that has traditionally been a major focus of attention in medical and psychological treatment research: Are there any psychosocial variables that can be used to predict a patient's response to treatment?

PSYCHOSOCIAL PREDICTORS OF RESPONSE TO TREATMENT

Chronic Low Back Pain

A study by Elkayam et al. (1996) assessed 67 patients before and after a comprehensive 4-week

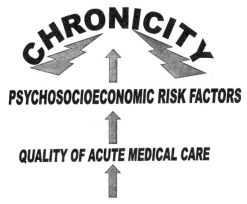

FIGURE 26.1. Sequence of variables that may lead to chronicity after the onset of a physical disease or injury.

multidisciplinary program. The results demonstrated that the presence of personality disorders was highly correlated with poor outcome, as were psychosocial stressors such as divorced marital status and unemployment. In a recent study evaluating treatment outcomes for CLBP patients, McMahon, Gatchel, Polatin, and Mayer (1997) assessed 473 consecutive graduates of a functional restoration program for the presence of childhood abuse via a structured interview. In this study, a history of childhood abuse was neither related to poorer outcome in any physical capacity measure nor a factor in successful completion of the actual program. However, such a history was found to be related to higher levels of psychological distress and poorer socioeconomic outcomes (i.e., lower work retention rates and higher postrehabilitative operations to the same area of injury) when compared to those without a history of childhood abuse. The authors note that a history of childhood abuse does not interfere with an initial positive response to an effective tertiary rehabilitation program but may cause a later resumption of other self-defeating disability behaviors.

There have also been a number of other studies linking psychosocial factors to treatment outcome. For example, Hildebrandt, Pfingsten, Saur, and Jansen (1997) evaluated 90 chronically disabled low back pain patients who were admitted to an 8-week program of functional restoration and behavioral support. They found that the most important variable in predicting a successful treatment outcome was a reduction in the patients' subjective feelings of disability. In another study, Härkäpää, Järvikoski, and Estlander (1996) reported that a patient's optimistic expectations and locus of control beliefs significantly predicted increased functional capacity in a group of 175 chronic low back pain patients who underwent an intensive multimodal treatment program. In addition, Rainville, Sobel, Hartigan, and Wright (1997) found that compensation involvement had an adverse effect on self-reported pain, depression, and disability, both before and after a spine rehabilitation program in a group of 192 chronic low back pain patients. Vaccaro, Ring, Scuderi, Cohen, and Garfin (1997) also reported that active workers' compensation and litigation issues negatively affected results of operative management of chronic low back pain patients with low-grade spindylolisthesis. Finally, in patients undergoing lumbar surgery, de Groot, Boeke, van den Berge, Duivenvoorden, Bonke, and Passchier (1997) found that preoperative anxiety predicted more postoperative anxiety and physical complaints.

Although studies such as the above indicate that certain psychosocial variables are associated with outcome, few studies have been performed with the specific intent of developing predictive models of treatment outcome. Burton, Tillotson, Main, and Hollis (1995), though, conducted a prospective study of 250 low back pain patients undergoing standard osteopathic treatment. Patients were classified as acute if their presenting symptoms lasted less than 3 weeks, subchronic if they lasted between 3 and 52 weeks, and chronic if they lasted more than 1 year. Psychosocial variables were assessed on presentation to a primary care facility, and outcome was measured at 1 year and determined by a back pain disability questionnaire. Stepwise discriminant function analysis was used to determine the best discrimination of good versus poor outcome. The model for all patients retained five variables (depressive symptoms, coping strategies of praying/hoping, somatic perception, leg pain, and duration of current spell) and correctly allocated 75.4% of the cases into recovered versus not recovered groups. The authors note that despite the many clinical variables included in the initial assessment, psychological status at presentation has a much stronger influence on outcome than does conventional clinical information.

A recent study of patient response to spinal cord stimulation (SCS) was conducted on 40 patients with chronic low back and/or leg pain, 85% of whom were diagnosed with failed back surgery syndrome (Burchiel et al., 1995). Treatment outcomes were found to improve significantly after 3 months of stimulation. Regression analysis revealed that patient age, MMPI scale 2 (Depression), and the evaluative subscale of the McGill Pain Questionnaire (MPQ) were important predictors of posttreatment pain status. Specifically, higher age and scale 2 scores were associated with worse pain status, whereas higher MPQ score correlated with improved pain status. Using a definition of success as a 50% decrease in visual analogue pain rating scale (VAS) level, the equation derived using these three variables correctly predicted success or failure in 88% of the study sample.

In a similar study, Hasenbring, Marienfeld, Kuhlendahl, and Soyka (1994) examined various physiological, psychological, and social variables for predictive value of short-term and long-term follow-up of 111 consecutively selected patients with acute radicular pain and a lumbar disc prolapse or protrusion. Outcome was measured by the intensity of persistent pain at the time of discharge from the hospital and 6 months later, as well as the application for early retirement at the 6-month follow-up. The results indicated that persistent pain was best predicted by a combination of physiological (degree of disc displacement), psychological (depression and pain coping strategies of avoidance behavior, endurance strategies, nonverbal pain behavior, and search for social support), and social parameters (social status and sitting position). These factors provided a correct prediction in 88% of the patient population. With regard to the application for early retirement at 6 month follow-up, depression and stress at work were the best predictors.

Headache

Gatchel, Deckel, Weinberg, and Smith (1985) found the Millon Behavioral Health Inventory (MBHI) to significantly predict response to treatment for chronic headache patients. They administered the MBHI to individuals with chronic headache ($n = 23$), chronic pain without headache ($n = 24$), and normal controls ($n = 21$). Response to treatment was measured by (1) number of daily headaches, (2) duration of headaches, (3) intensity of headaches, and (4) all medications taken. With regard to the headache group, comparison of pre- and postassessments revealed that those who scored highest on 11 of the 20 scales (Inhibited Style, Sensitive Style, Recent Stress, Premorbid Pessimism, Future Despair, Somatic Anxiety, Allergic Inclination, Gastrointestinal Susceptibility, Pain Treatment Responsivity, Life Threat Reactivity, and Emotional Vulnerability) subsequently demonstrated the greatest number of headaches following treatment (i.e., less treatment improvement). Those who scored lower on these scales responded best to treatment. Only four scales (Sensitive Style, Somatic Anxiety, Pain Treatment Responsivity, and Emotional Vulnerability) were correlated with duration of headaches, and only the Emotional Vulnerability scale was associated with the medications variable. Therefore, for all four of the outcome measures, only the Emotional Vulnerability scale was found to be consistently related to them all. Individuals who scored high on this scale responded the least to treatment in this study.

Osterhaus et al. (1993) evaluated the outcome of a combined behavioral treatment (which included relaxation training and temperature biofeedback) and cognitive training for 41 schoolchildren (32 in an experimental group, 9 in a wait-list control group) with migraine headache. Results indicated that 45% of the children in the experimental group were clinically improved at the posttreatment assessment, with improvements maintained at 7-month follow-up. Predictors of outcome were gender, headache history, age, and psychosomatic complaints before training.

Irritable Bowel Syndrome

As with other chronic pain conditions, IBS is the result of complex interactions between psychological, social, and physiological factors. As we have discussed, research has not verified that there is a "pain personality" for the development of IBS. However, studies have determined that certain characteristics have significant impact on outcome of treatment. For example, Guthrie, Creed, Dawson, and Tomeson (1991) present data on 51 patients who completed treatment versus 47 treatment controls. Variables associated with a good outcome were found to be the following: (1) initial presence of anxiety or depression (65% of improved versus 25% of unimproved); (2) abdominal pain exacerbated by stress (65% vs. 17%); (3) shorter duration of illness; and (4) absence of constant abdominal pain (67% vs. 23%). However, it is unclear as to why these authors did not report data on their entire sample of treatment completers, which they reported to number 79.

Blanchard, Schwarz, and Neff (1988) report data collected from 45 treated IBS patients. They found three potential predictors of treatment outcome: (1) trait anxiety from the STAI, (2) frequency of symptom-free days at baseline, and (3) gender. Specifically, having lower initial levels of trait anxiety, being male, and having more episodic symptoms (i.e., more symptom-free days) were associated with successful outcomes. Harvey, Hinton, Gunary, and Barry (1989) found that patients with psychological disturbance, as indicated by a score of 5 or greater on the General Health Questionnaire (GHQ), responded poorly to hypnotherapy (38% improved vs. 68% improved with lower GHQ score). Age was not a significant predictor in this study.

More recently, Blanchard et al. (1992) analyzed data from 90 patients treated previously and found that neither trait anxiety, gender, nor baseline symptom-free days predicted outcome. The only variable that significantly predicted outcome was the presence or absence of an Axis I disorder as measured by the Anxiety Disorders Interview

Schedule–Revised (ADIS-R; DiNardo & Barlow, 1988). They found that the absence of an Axis I disorder predicted more than twice the likelihood of successful outcome from treatment.

Rheumatoid Arthritis

Although Young (1993) notes that, in nine group outcome studies of cognitive-behavioral treatment of RA patients, there was no clear delineation of patient demographic characteristics that were associated with better outcomes, Radojevic, Nicassio, and Weisman (1992) reported that spousal participation in treatment tends to enhance outcome. Nevertheless, there are few studies that provide predictive models of those factors that can accurately predict which RA patients are most likely to have positive versus negative responses to treatment. Obviously, additional clinical research in this area is greatly needed.

Temporomandibular Joint Disorder

Much research has been conducted in the last two decades investigating the role of psychosocial factors in the development and maintenance of TMD. However, few studies have evaluated those psychosocial variables that serve to predict response to treatment. Schwartz, Greene, and Laskin (1979) evaluated 42 TMD patients who underwent conservative treatments (i.e., splints, physical therapy, and exercise). Those patients who did not respond to the treatment differed from those who did by having greater elevations on several scales of the MMPI: scales 1, 2, 3, 4, 7, and 8 (Hypochondriasis, Depression, Hysteria, Psychopathic Deviant, Psychasthenia, and Schizophrenia). Similar findings were reported by Milstein-Prentsky and Olsen (1979) with 74 TMD patients undergoing treatment. These elevations have been interpreted to indicate a tendency toward excessive pain sensitivity and agitated depression in TMD patients unresponsive to treatment (Block, 1996).

Rudy, Turk, Kubinski, and Zaki (1995) conducted a study in which they utilized a psychosocial measure–the MPI–to classify TMD patients within three psychosocial-behavior-based subgroups and then evaluated their differential responses to treatment. In this study, 133 TMD patients were assessed and then treated with a combination of intraoral appliance, biofeedback, and stress management. Six months after termination of treatment, patients were assessed. Although, as a group overall, patients improved significantly, comparisons across the aforementioned subgroups revealed differential patterns of response to treatment. The most notable changes occurred with the subgroup characterized by the greatest amount of psychological distress (Dysfunctional), as they demonstrated significantly greater improvements on measures of pain intensity, perceived impact of TMD symptoms on their lives, depression, and negative thoughts, compared with subgroups characterized by greater interpersonal problems (Interpersonally Distressed) and those patients who appeared to be less disabled by TMD (Adaptive Copers). The authors note that these data provide support for such a classification system and that future research utilizing such an approach to individualized treatments and outcome measures could improve treatment efficacy and outcome evaluation.

Subsequently, Kight (1996) analyzed multiple psychosocial variables in an effort to show which predicted response to treatment in a group of TMD patients treated with either cognitive therapy, biofeedback, or a combination of the two. The most robust predictor of poor response to treatment was coping ability as measured by the MPI. Those subjects who were categorized as either "dysfunctional" or "interpersonally distressed" displayed significantly poorer response to treatment. These results were somewhat different from those reported above by Rudy and colleagues (1995). The most likely reason was the different treatment protocols used in the two studies. This highlights the fact that there may be different predictors of outcome success for the same disorder, depending on the treatment program administered.

A study by Fricton and Olsen (1996) evaluated 94 participants with chronic TMD prior to entering a multidisciplinary treatment program to determine factors most predictive of outcome. Treatment outcome was determined by significant decreases in the Craniomandibular Index and the Symptom Severity Index from pre- to posttreatment. Variables were regressed on a random sample of half of the subjects (n = 47; criterion group), with the predictive model subsequently applied to the other half of the subjects. Low self-esteem, feeling worried, low energy, and sleep activity were identified as useful predictors of treatment outcomes in the criterion group (it is noteworthy that all these measures are symptoms of depression). The discriminant analysis using these four variables accounted for 49% of the variance in treatment response, was statistically significant, and correctly predicted treatment outcome for 87% of the par-

ticipants in the criterion group. The discriminant function correctly predicted treatment outcome for 79% of the cross-validation group and explained 28% of the variance in treatment response. The authors note that these findings indicate that symptoms of depression mediate treatment response for chronic TMD patients.

Finally, Suvinen, Hanes, and Reade (1997) evaluated factors that predicted treatment outcome in the conservative physical therapy management of TMD. They reported that "rapid" responders to conservative physical therapy evidenced greater psychosocial coping strategies relative to "slow" responders. These investigators conclude that such psychosocial factors cannot be ignored in managing TMD patients.

Response to Implantable Spinal Cord Stimulators

As Neban, Kennington, Novy, and Squitieri (1996) have noted, there has been an expanding role of spinal cord stimulation (SCS) as a treatment option for chronic pain in recent years. Along with this expansion, there has also been a concomitant increase in attempts to develop more effective patient selection criteria in order to increase SCS treatment outcome. These authors have delineated the following screening criteria that should be used to exclude patients from consideration for SCS implantation: (1) active psychosis, (2) active suicidality, (3) active homicidality, (4) untreated or poorly treated major mood disorders such as major depression, (5) an unusually high level of somatization or other somatoform disorders, (6) substance abuse disorders, (7) unresolved workers' compensation or litigation cases, (8) lack of appropriate social support, and (9) cognitive defects that compromise adequate reasoning and memory.

Neban and colleagues (1996) also discuss a host of other psychosocial parameters that need to be considered. Moreover, they emphasize that, although patient screening for SCS treatment is still a somewhat imprecise service, there can be no doubt that such parameters, when more refined, will make an important contribution to reliable prediction of response to treatment.

Treatment Outcome Implications

Taken as a whole across the various pain disorders that we have discussed, Table 26.3 summarizes

TABLE 26.3. Summary of Potential Psychosocioeconomic Predictors of Response to Treatment

- Depression
- Somatization
- History of childhood abuse
- Psychiatric disturbance (presence of Axis I clinical disorders)
- MPI subgroup categories
- Elevation of the Emotional Vulnerability scale of the MBHI
- Poor coping skills/strategies
- Unresolved workers' compensation/personal injury cases
- Positive attitudes and expectations about pain and disability

those variables that appear to hold promise for differentiating between those patients who respond and those who do not respond to a particular treatment program (as will be noted, some of these variables are similar to those presented in Table 26.2 that were associated with predicting the development of chronicity). It should be kept in mind, however, that even for the same pain condition there may be a different array of predictor variables, depending on the specific type of treatment program administered. Such *response specificity* should always be kept in mind.

Finally, one predictor variable, which is actually a component of a treatment method for pain reduction, is hypnotic susceptibility. By way of a historical overview, even before ether was discovered in the mid-1800s, there were dramatic reports of some physicians who performed major surgery on patients using hypnosis as the only method of analgesia (Bakal, 1979). Since that time, medical hypnosis has been used as a method to reduce pain. However, as Hilgard and Hilgard (1975) noted, only about 1 out of 10 individuals are hypnotizable to the extent that they can experience pain anesthesia. For these "high" hypnotizable patients, some studies have shown that hypnosis can achieve greater pain relief than medications, such as morphine and certain anxiolytics (Stern, Brown, Ulett, & Sleten, 1977). The reasons why and how hypnosis reduces pain, what types of pain it is most suitable for, and the effects of individual differences on response to the method remain questions for future research.

SUMMARY AND CONCLUSIONS

Several pain conditions have been presented that have received the attention of researchers in the field of behavioral medicine. Our conceptualization of pain and the progression of pain has evolved from unidimensional models to integrative, biopsychosocial models that take into account the many disparate factors that may contribute to the pain experience in any given individual. Those interested in achieving a better understanding of such chronic pain conditions have abandoned traditional medical models of explanation and have turned their attention to the multitude of physiological, psychological, social, and economic variables that are intertwined or interact to produce the pain experience.

Studies have been cited that demonstrate our growing understanding of these complex, interactive processes in a variety of chronic pain conditions. Some conditions, such as CLBP, have been more extensively investigated than others. Nevertheless, there remains this multidimensional approach that has become commonly accepted among researchers in the field. Through continued efforts to incorporate biological, psychological, and social aspects of pain, our understanding of these pain conditions can continue to flourish. Such strides in our understanding will not only help clinicians in their efforts to effectively treat patients in pain but will potentially help save billions of dollars through efficient application of available resources and effective avoidance of continued pain behavior in patients.

ACKNOWLEDGMENT

The writing of this chapter was supported in part by National Institutes of Health Grant Nos. R01 DE10713 and K02 MH01107.

REFERENCES

Adler, C. S., Alder, S. M., & Packard, R. C. (1987). *Psychiatric aspects of headache*. Baltimore: Williams & Wilkins.

Affleck, G., Tennon, H., Urrows, S., & Higgins, P. (1991). Individual differences in the day-to-day experience of chronic pain: A prospective daily study of rheumatoid arthritis patients. *Health Psychology, 10,* 419–426.

Bakal, D. A. (1975). A biopsychological perspective. *Psychological Bulletin, 82,* 369–382.

Bakal, D. A. (1979). *Psychology and medicine: Psychobiological dimensions of health and illness.* New York: Springer.

Barnes, D., Gatchel, R. J., Mayer, T. G., & Barnett, J. (1990). Changes in MMPI profiles of chronic low back pain patients following successful treatment. *Journal of Spinal Disorders, 3,* 353–355.

Biering-Sorenson, F. (1983). A prospective study of LBP in a general population: II. Location, character, aggravating and relieving factors. *Scandinavian Journal of Rehabilitation Medicine, 15,* 75–81.

Bigos, S. J., Battie, M. C., Spengler, D. M., Fisher, L. D., Fordyce, W. E., Hansson, T. H., Nachemson, A. L., & Wortley, M. D. (1991). A prospective study of work perceptions and psychosocial factors affecting the report of back injury. *Spine, 16,* 1–6.

Blanchard, E. B. (1993). Irritable bowel syndrome. In R. J. Gatchel & E. B. Blanchard (Eds.), *Psychophysiological disorders: Research and clinical applications.* Washington, DC: American Psychological Association

Blanchard, E. B., & Andrasik, F. (1985). *Management of chronic headache: A psychological approach.* Elmsford, NY: Pergamon Press.

Blanchard, E. B., Kirsch, C. A., Applebaum, K. A., & Jaccard, J. (1989). Role of psychopathology in chronic headache: Cause or effect? *Headache, 29,* 295–301.

Blanchard, E. B., Radnitz, C., Evans, D. D., Schwarz, S. P., Neff, D. F., & Gerardi, M. A. (1986). Psychological comparison of irritable bowel syndrome to chronic tension and migraine headache and nonpatient controls. *Biofeedback and Self-Regulation, 11,* 221–230.

Blanchard, E. B., Radnitz, C., Schwarz, S. P., Neff, D. F., & Gerardi, M. A. (1987). Psychological changes associated with self-regulatory treatments of irritable bowel syndrome. *Biofeedback and Self-Regulation, 12,* 31–38.

Blanchard, E. B., Scharff, L., Payne, A., Schwarz, S. P., Suls, J. M., & Malamood, H. (1992). Prediction of outcome from cognitive-behavioral treatment of irritable bowel syndrome. *Behavior Therapy, 30,* 647–650.

Blanchard, E. B., Schwarz, S. P., & Neff, D. F. (1988). Two-year follow-up of behavioral treatment of irritable bowel syndrome. *Behavior Therapy, 19,* 67–73.

Block, A. R. (1996). *Presurgical psychological screening in chronic pain syndromes.* Hillsdale, NJ: Erlbaum.

Blumer, J. P., & Heilbrom, T. (1982). Chronic pain as a variant of depressive disease: The pain-prone disorder. *Journal of Nervous and Mental Disease, 170,* 381–406.

Bombardier, C. H., Divine, G. W., Jordan, J. S., Brooks, W. B., & Neelon, F. A. (1993). Minnesota Multiphasic Personality Inventory (MMPI) cluster among chronically ill patients: Relationship to illness adjustment and treatment outcome. *Journal of Behavioral Medicine, 16,* 467–484.

Breslau, N., Davis, G. C., & Andreski, P. (1991). Migraine, psychiatric disorders, and suicide attempts: An epidemiologic study of young adults. *Psychiatry Research, 37,* 11–23.

Brown, G. K. (1990). A causal analysis of chronic pain and depression. *Journal of Abnormal Psychology, 99,* 127–137.

Brown, G. K., & Nicassio, P. M. (1987). Development of a questionnaire for the assessment of active and passive coping strategies in chronic pain patients. *Pain, 31,* 53–64.

Brown, G. K., Nicassio, P. M., & Wallston, K. A. (1989). Pain coping strategies and depression in rheumatoid arthritis. *Journal of Consulting and Clinical Psychology, 57,* 652–657.

Burchiel, K. J., Anderson, V. C., Wilson, B. J., Denison, D. B., Olson, K. A., & Shatin, D. (1995). Prognostic factors of spinal cord stimulation for chronic back and leg pain. *Neurosurgery, 36,* 1101–1110.

Burton, A. K., Tillotson, K. M., Main, C. J., & Hollis, S. (1995). Psychosocial predictors of outcome in acute and subchronic low back trouble. *Spine, 20,* 722–728.

Burton, K., Polatin, P. B., & Gatchel, R. J. (1997). Psychosocial factors and the rehabilitation of patients with chronic work-related upper extremity disorders. *Journal of Occupational Rehabilitation, 7,* 139–147.

Clark, L. A., Watson, D., & Mineka, S. (1994). Temperament, personality, and the mood and anxiety disorders. *Journal of Abnormal Psychology, 103,* 103–116.

Cohen, S., & Rodriguez, M. S. (1995). Pathways linking affective disturbances and physical disorders. *Health Psychology, 14*(5), 371–373.

Cox, D. J., Freundlich, A., & Meyer, R. G. (1975). Differential effectiveness of electromyographic feedback, verbal relaxation, and medication placebo with tension headaches. *Journal of Consulting and Clinical Psychology, 43,* 892–898.

de Benedittis, G., & Lorenzetti, A. (1992). The role of stressful life events in the persistence of primary headache: Major events vs. daily hassles. *Pain, 51,* 35–42.

de Groot, K. I., Boeke, S., van den Berge, H. J., Duivenvoorden, H. J., Bonke, B., & Passchier, J. (1997). The influence of psychological variables on postoperative anxiety and physical complaints in patients undergoing lumbar surgery. *Pain, 69,* 19–25.

DiNardo, P. A., & Barlow, D. H. (1988). *Anxiety Disorders Interview Schedule-Revised (ADIS-R).* Albany, NY: State University of New York, Center for Stress and Anxiety Disorders.

Dionne, C. E., Koepsell, T. D., Von Korff, M., Deyo, R. A., Barlow, W. E., & Checkoway, H. (1997). Predicting long-term functional limitations among back pain patients in primary care settings. *Journal of Clinical Epidemiology, 50,* 31–43.

Drossman, D. A., McKee, D. C., Sandler, R. S., Mitchell, C. M., Cramer, E. M., Lowman, B. C., & Burger, A. L. (1988). Psychosocial factors in the irritable bowel syndrome: A multivariate study of patients and nonpatients with irritable bowel syndrome. *Gastroenterology, 95,* 701–708.

Dworkin, R. H. (1997). Which individuals with acute pain are most likely to develop a chronic pain syndrome? *Pain Forum, 6,* 127–136.

Dworkin, S. F. (1990). Illness behavior and dysfunction: Review of concepts and application to chronic pain. *Canadian Journal of Physiological Pharmacology, 69,* 662–667.

Dworkin, S. F., & LeResche, L. (1992). Research diagnostic criteria for temperomandibular disorders: Review, criteria, examinations and specifications, critique. *Journal of Craniomandibular Disorders: Facial and Oral Pain, 6*(4), 302–355.

Dworkin, S. F., Von Korff, M. R., & LeResche, L. (1990). Multiple pains and psychiatric disturbance: An epidemiologic investigation. *Archives of General Psychiatry, 47,* 239–244.

Elkayam, O., Ben Itzhak, S., Avrahami, E., Meidan, Y., Doron, N., Eldar, I., Keidar, I., Liram, N., & Yaron,

M. (1996). Multidisciplinary approach to chronic back pain: Prognostic elements of the outcome. *Clinical and Experimental Rheumatology, 14,* 281–288.

Engel, G. L. (1959). "Psychogenic" pain and the pain-prone patient. *American Journal of Medicine, 26,* 900–918.

Etscheidt, M. A., & Steiger, H. G. (1995). Multidimensional Pain Inventory profile classifications and psychopathology. *Journal of Consulting and Clinical Psychology, 51*(1), 29–36.

Fenerstein, M., Berkowitz, S. M., & Peck, C. A. (1997). Musculoskeletal-related disability in U. S. Army personnel: Prevalence, gender, and military occupational specialties. *Journal of Occupational and Environmental Medicine, 39,* 68–78.

Feuerstein, M., & Huang, G. D. (1998). Preventing disability in patients with occupational musculoskeletal disorders. *American Pain Society Bulletin, 8,* 9–11.

Flor, H., Haag, G., & Turk, D. C. (1986). Long-term efficacy of EMG biofeedback for chronic rheumatic back pain. *Pain, 27,* 195–202.

Flor, H., & Turk, D. C. (1988). Chronic back pain and rheumatoid arthritis: Predicting pain and disability from cognitive variables. *Journal of Behavioral Medicine, 11,* 251–265.

Fordyce, W. E. (1988). Pain and suffering: A reappraisal. *American Psychologist, 43,* 276–283.

Fordyce, W. E., Bigos, S., Battie, M., & Fisher, L. (1992). MMPI Scale 3 as a predictor of back injury report: What does it tell? *Clinical Journal of Pain, 8,* 222–226.

Fordyce, W. E., Lansky, D., Calsyn, D. A., Shelton, J. L., Stolov, W. C., & Rocket, D. C. (1984). Pain measurement and pain behavior. *Pain, 18,* 53–65.

Fordyce, W. E., Roberts, A. H., & Sternbach, R. A. (1985). The behavioral management of chronic pain: A response to critics. *Pain, 22,* 113–125.

Fricton, J. R., & Olsen, T. (1996). Predictors of outcome for treatment of temporomandibular disorders. *Journal of Orofacial Pain, 10,* 54–65.

Garofalo, J. P., Gatchel, R. J., Wesley, L., & Ellis, E. (1998). Predicting chronicity with the Research Diagnostic Criteria in acute temporomandibular disorders. *Journal of the American Dental Association, 129,* 438–447.

Garron, D., & Leavitt, F. (1983). Chronic low back pain and depression. *Journal of Clinical Psychology, 39,* 486–493.

Gatchel, R. J. (1991). Early development of physical and mental deconditioning in painful spinal disorders. In T. G. Mayer, V. Mooney, & R. J. Gatchel (Eds.), *Contemporary conservative care for painful spinal disorders.* Philadelphia: Lea & Febiger.

Gatchel, R. J. (1996). Psychological disorders and chronic pain: Cause-and-effect relationships (pp. 33–52). In R. J. Gatchel & D. C. Turk (Eds.), *Psychological approaches to pain management: A practitioner's handbook.* New York: Guilford Press.

Gatchel, R. J., Baum, A., & Krantz, D. (1989). *An introduction to health psychology* (2nd ed.). New York: McGraw-Hill.

Gatchel, R. J., & Blanchard, E. B. (1993). *Psychophysiological disorders: Research and clinical applications.* Washington, DC: American Psychological Association.

Gatchel, R. J., Deckel, A. W., Weinberg, N., & Smith, J. E. (1985). The utility of the Millon Behavioral Health Inventory in the study of chronic headaches. *Headache, 25,* 49–54.

Gatchel, R. J., Polatin, P. B., & Kinney, R. K. (1995).

Predicting outcome of chronic back pain using clinical predictors of psychopathology: A prospective analysis. *Health Psychology, 14,* 415–420.

Gatchel, R. J., Polatin, P. B., & Mayer, T. G. (1995). The dominant role of psychosocial risk factors in the development of chronic low back pain disability. *Spine, 20*(24), 2702–2709.

Gatchel, R. J., Polatin, P. B., Mayer, T. G., & Garcy, P. (1994). Psychopathology and the rehabilitation of patients with chronic low back pain disability. *Archives of Physical Medicine and Rehabilitation, 75,* 666–670.

Gatchel, R. J., & Turk, D. C. (Eds.). (1996). *Psychological approaches to pain management: A practitioner's handbook.* New York: Guilford Press.

Glaros, A. G., Glass, E. G., & McLaughlin, L. (1994). Knowledge and beliefs of dentists regarding temporomandibular disorders and chronic pain. *Journal of Orofacial Pain, 8*(2), 216–222.

Goodenow, C., Reisine, S. T., & Grady, K. E. (1990). Quality of social support and associated social and psychological functioning in women with rheumatoid arthritis. *Health Psychology, 9,* 266–284.

Grzesiak, R. C. (1991). Psychologic considerations in temporo-mandibular dysfunction: A biopsychosocial view of symptom formation. *Temporomandibular Disorders and Orofacial Pain, 35*(1), 209–226.

Guthrie, E., Creed, F., Dawson, D., & Tomeson, B. (1991). A controlled trial of psychological treatment for the irritable bowel syndrome. *Gastroenterology, 100,* 450–457.

Hagglund, K. J., Haley, W. E., Reveille, J. D., & Alarcón, G. S. (1989). Predicting individual differences in pain and functional impairment among patients with rheumatoid arthritis. *Arthritis and Rheumatism, 32,* 851–858.

Hanvick, L. J. (1951). MMPI profiles in patients with low-back pain. *Journal of Consulting Psychology, 15,* 350–353.

Härkäpää, K., Järvikoski, A., & Estlander, A. M. (1996). Health optimism and control beliefs as predictors for treatment outcome of a multimodal back treatment program. *Psychology and Health, 12,* 123–134.

Härkäpää, K., Mellin, G., Järvikoski, A., & Hurri, H. (1990). A controlled study of the outcome of inpatient and outpatient treatment of low back pain: III. Long term follow-up of pain, disability, and compliance. *Scandinavian Journal of Rehabilitation Medicine, 22,* 181–188.

Harvey, R. F., Hinton, R. A., Gunary, R. N., & Barry, R. E. (1989). Individual and group hypnotherapy in treatment of refractory irritable bowel syndrome. *Lancet,* 424–425.

Hasenbring, M., Marienfeld, G., Kuhlendahl, D., & Soyka, D. (1994). Risk factors of chronicity in lumbar disc patients: A prospective investigation of biologic, psychologic, and social predictors of therapy outcome. *Spine, 19,* 2759–2765.

Hatch, J. P. (1993). Headache. In R. J. Gatchel, A. Baum, & D. Krantz, (Eds.), *An introduction to health psychology* (2nd ed.). New York: McGraw-Hill.

Hildebrandt, J., Pfingsten, M., Saur, P., & Jansen, J. (1997). Predictors of success from a multidisciplinary treatment program for chronic low back pain. *Spine, 22,* 990–1001.

Hilgard, E. R., & Hilgard, J. R. (1975). *Hypnosis in the relief of pain.* Los Altos, CA: Kaufman.

Holm, J. E., Holroyd, K. A., Hursey, K. G., & Penzien, D. B. (1986). The role of stress in recurrent tension headache. *Headache, 26,* 160–167.

Jayson, M. I. J. (1997). Why does acute pain become chronic? *Spine, 22,* 1053–1056.

Jenson, M. C., Brant-Zawadzki, M. N., Obuchowski, N., Modic, M. T., Malkasian, D., & Ross, J. S. (1994). Magnetic resonance imaging of the lumber spine in people without back pain. *New England Journal of Medicine, 331,* 69–73.

Katon, W., & Sullivan, M. D. (1990). Depression and chronic medical illness. *Journal of Clinical Psychiatry, 51,* 3–11.

Keefe, F. J., Brown, G. K., Wallston, K. A., & Caldwell, D. S. (1989). Coping with rheumatoid arthritis pain: Catastrophizing as a maladaptive strategy. *Pain, 37,* 51–56.

Kerns, R. D., Turk, D. C., & Rudy, T. E. (1985). The West Haven-Yale Multidimensional Pain Inventory (WHYMPI). *Pain, 23,* 345–356.

Kight, M. K. (1996). Differential treatment of temporomandibular disorders: Biofeedback and cognitive-behavioral skills training. Unpublished doctoral dissertation, University of Texas Southwestern Medical Center, Dallas.

Kinney, R. K., Gatchel, R. J., Ellis, E., & Holt, C. (1992). Major psychological disorders in chronic TMD patients: Implications for successful management. *Journal of the American Dental Association, 123,* 49–54.

Kinney, R. K., Gatchel, R. J., Polatin, P. B., Fogarty, W. T., & Mayer, T. G. (1993). Prevalence of psychopathology in acute and chronic low back pain patients. *Journal of Occupational Rehabilitation, 3,* 95–103.

Kisely, S., Guthrie, E., Creed, F., & Tew, R. (1997). Predictors of mortality and morbidity following admission with chest pain. *Journal of the Royal College of Physicians of London, 31*(2), 177–183.

Kohler, T., & Haimerl, C. (1990). Daily stress as a trigger of migraine attacks: Results of thirteen single-subject studies. *Journal of Consulting and Clinical Psychology, 58,* 870–872.

Kohler, T., & Kosanic, S. (1992). Are persons with migraine characterized by a high degree of ambition, orderliness, and rigidity? *Pain, 48,* 321–323.

Lancourt, J., & Kettlehut, M. (1992). Predicting return to work for lower back pain patients receiving workers' compensation. *Spine, 17,* 629–640.

Lazarus, R. S., & Folkman, S. (1984). *Stress, appraisal, and coping.* New York: Springer.

Lehmann, T. R., Spratt, K. F., & Lehmann, K. K. (1993). Predicting long-term disability in low back injured workers presenting to a spine consultant. *Spine, 18,* 1103–1112.

Leigh, J. P., Markowitz, S. B., Fahs, M., Shin, C., & Landrigan, P. J. (1997). Occupational injury and illness in the United States: Estimates of costs, morbidity, and mortality. *Archives of Internal Medicine, 157,* 1557–1567.

Linton, S. J., & Bradley, L. A. (1996). Strategies for the prevention of chronic pain. In R. J. Gatchel & D. C. Turk (Eds.), *Psychological approaches to pain management: A practitioner's handbook* (pp. 438–457). New York: Guilford Press.

Linton, S. J., Larden, M., & Gillow, A. M. (1996). Sexual abuse and chronic musculoskeletal pain: Prevalence and psychological factors. *Clinical Journal of Pain, 12,* 215–221.

Lorish, C. D., Abraham, N., Austin, J., Bradley, L. A., & Alarcón, G. S. (1991). Disease and psychosocial factors related to physical functioning in rheumatoid arthritis. *Journal of Rheumatology, 18,* 1150–1157.

Main, C. J., & Spanswick, C. C. (1995). Personality assessment and the Minnesota Multiphasic Personality Inventory: 50 years on: Do we still need our security blanket? *Pain Forum, 4,* 90–96.

Mayer, T. G., & Gatchel, R. J. (1988). *Functional restoration for spinal disorders: The sports medicine approach.* Philadelphia: Lea & Febiger.

McCreary, C. P., Clark, G. T., Merril, V., & Oakley, M. A. (1991). Psychological distress and diagnostic subgroups of temporomandibular patients. *Pain, 44,* 29–34.

McCreary, C. P., Turner, J., & Dawson, E. (1977). Differences between functional versus organic low-back pain patients. *Pain, 4,* 73–78.

McFarlane, A. C., & Brooks, P. M. (1988). An analysis of the relationship between psychological morbidity and disease activity in rheumatoid arthritis. *Journal of Rheumatology, 15,* 926–931.

McMahon, M. J., Gatchel, R. J., Polatin, P. B., & Mayer, T. G. (1997). Early childhood abuse in chronic spinal disorder patients: A major barrier to treatment success. *Spine, 22,* 2408–2415.

Mechanic, D. (1966). Response factors in illness: The study of illness behavior. *Social Psychiatry, 1*(1), 11–20.

Mechanic, D. (1972). Social psychological factors affecting the presentation of bodily complaints. *The New England Journal of Medicine, 286*(21), 1132–1139.

Mechanic, D. (1985). Illness behavior: An overview. In S. McHugh & T. Vallis (Eds.), *Illness behavior: A multidisciplinary model.* New York: Plenum.

Melamed, B. G. (1995). Introduction to the special section: The neglected psychological-physical interface. *Health Psychology, 14,* 371–373.

Mellin, G., Härkäpää, K., Hurri, H., & Järvikoski, A. (1990). A controlled study of the outcome of inpatient and outpatient treatment of low back pain: IV. Long term effects on physical measurements. *Scandinavian Journal of Rehabilitation Medicine, 22,* 181–188.

Melzack, R., & Wall, P. D. (1965). Pain mechanisms: A new theory. *Science, 150,* 971–979.

Milstein-Prentsky, S., & Olsen, R. E. (1979). Predictability of treatment outcome in patients with myofascial pain-dysfunction (MPD) syndrome. *Journal of Dental Research, 58,* 1341–1346.

Mooney, V., Cairns, D., & Robertson, J. (1975). The psychological evaluation and treatment of the chronic low back pain patient: II. A new approach. *Orthopedic Nurses Association Journal, 2,* 187–189.

Moss, R. A., & Garrett, J. C. (1984). Temporomandibular joint dysfunction syndrome and myofacial pain dysfunction syndrome: A critical review. *Journal of Oral Rehabilitation, 11,* 3–28.

Nappi, G., Bono, G., Sandrini, G., Martignoni, E., & Micieli, G. (Eds.). (1991). *Headache and depression: Serotonin pathways as a common clue.* New York: Raven Press.

National Advisory Committee on Health and Disability. (1997). *Guide to assessing yellow flags in acute low back pain.* Wellington, New Zealand: Ministry of Health.

Neban, D. V., Kennington, M., Novy, D. M., & Squitieri, P. (1996). Psychological selection criteria for implantable spinal cord stimulators. *Pain Forum, 5,* 93–103.

Osterhaus, S. O., Passchier, J., Van Der Helm-Hylkema, H., De Jong, K. T., Orlebeke, J. F., De Grauw, A. J., & Dekker, P. H. (1993). Effects of behavioral psychophysiological treatment on schoolchildren with migraine in a nonclinical setting: Predictors and process variables. *Journal of Pediatric Psychology, 18,* 697–715.

Peselow, E. D., Fieve, R. R., & DiFiglia, C. (1992). Personality traits and response to desipramine. *Journal of Affective Disorders, 24,* 209–216.

Pfaffenrath, V., Hummelsberger, J., Pollmann, W., Kaube, H., & Rath, M. (1991). MMPI personality profiles of inpatients with primary headache syndromes. *Cephalagia, 11,* 263–268.

Phillips, H. C. (1988). Changing chronic pain experience. *Pain, 32,* 165–172.

Phillips, H. C., Grant, L., & Berkowitz, J. (1991). The prevention of chronic pain and disability: A preliminary investigation. *Behaviour Research and Therapy, 29,* 443–450.

Pincus, T., Callahan, L. F., Bradley, L. A., Vaughn, W. K., & Wolfe, F. (1987). Elevated MMPI scores for hypochondriasis, depression, and hysteria in patients with rheumatoid arthritis reflect disease rather than psychological status. *Arthritis and Rheumatism, 29,* 1456–1466.

Polatin, P. B., Kinney, R. K., Gatchel, R. J., Lillo, E., & Mayer, T. G. (1993). Psychiatric illness and chronic low back pain. *Spine, 18,* 66–71.

Radojevik, V., Nicassio, P. M., & Weisman, M. H. (1992). Behavioral intervention with and without family support for rheumatoid arthritis. *Behavior Therapy, 23,* 13–30.

Rainville, J., Sobel, J. B., Hartigan, C., & Wright, A. (1997). The effect of compensation involvement on the reporting of pain and disability by patients referred for rehabilitation of chronic low back pain. *Spine, 22,* 2016–2024.

Romano, J. M., & Turner, J. A. (1985). Chronic pain and depression: Does the evidence support a relationship? *Psychological Bulletin, 97,* 18–26.

Rome, H. P., Jr., Harness, D. M., & Kaplan, H. J. (1990). Psychologic and behavioral aspects of chronic facial pain. In A. L. Jacobson & W. C. Donlon (Eds.), *Headache and facial pain.* New York: Raven Press.

Rudy, T. E., Turk, D. C., Kubinski, J. A., & Zaki, H. S. (1995). Differential treatment responses of TMD patients as a function of psychological characteristics. *Pain, 61,* 103–112.

Rudy, T. E., Turk, D. C., Zaki, H. S., & Curtin, H. D. (1989). An empirical taxometric alternative to traditional classification of temporomandibular disorders. *Pain, 36,* 311–320.

Sanders, S. H. (1995). Risk factors for the occurrence of low back pain and chronic disability. *American Pain Society Bulletin, 5,* 1–5.

Sargent, J., Solbach, P., Coyne, L., Spohn, H., & Segerson, J. (1986). Results of a controlled, experimental, outcome study of nondrug treatments for the control of migraine headaches. *Journal of Behavioral Medicine, 9,* 291–323.

Schumann, N. P., Zweiner, U., & Nebrich, A. (1988). Personality and quantified neuromuscular activity of the masticatory system in patients with temperomandibular joint dysfunction. *Journal of Oral Rehabilitation, 15,* 35–47.

Schwartz, R. A., Greene, C. S., & Laskin, D. M. (1979). Personality characteristics of patients with myofacial pain-dysfunction (MPD) syndrome unresponsive to conventional therapy. *Journal of Dental Research, 58,* 1435–1439.

Smith, C. A., & Wallston, K. A. (1992). Adaption in patients with chronic rheumatoid arthritis: Application of a general model. *Health Psychology, 11,* 151–162.

Stern, J. A., Brown, M., Ulett, G. A., & Sleten, I. (1977). A comparison of hypnosis, acupuncture, morphine, valium, aspirin, and placebo in the management of experimentally induced pain. *Annals of the New York Academy of Sciences, 296,* 175–193.

Sternbach, R. A., Wolf, S. R., Murphy, R. W., & Akeson, W. H. (1973). Chronic low-back pain: The low-back pain "loser." *Postgraduate Medicine, 53,* 135–138.

Stewart, W. F., Lipton, R. B., Celentano, D. D., & Reed, M. L. (1992). Prevalence of migraine headache in the United States: Relation to age, income, race, and other sociodemographic factors. *Journal of the American Medical Association, 267,* 84–89.

Suvinen, T. I., Hanes, K. R., & Reade, P. C. (1997). Outcome of therapy in the conservative management of temporomandibular pain dysfunction disorder. *Journal of Oral Rehabilitation, 24,* 718–724.

Turk, D. C., & Flor, H. (1987). Pain and pain behaviors. The utility of the pain behavior construct. *Pain, 31,* 277–295.

Turk, D. C., & Gatchel, R. J. (in press). Multidisciplinary programs for rehabilitation of chronic low back pain patients. In W. H. Kirkaldy-Willis & T. N. Bernanerd (Eds.), *Managing low back pain* (4th ed.). New York: Churchill-Livingstone.

Turk, D. C., & Kerns, R. D. (1983). Conceptual issues in the assessment of clinical pain. *International Journal of Psychiatric Medicine, 13,* 15–26.

Turk, D. C., & Rudy, T. E. (1988). Toward an empirically derived taxonomy of chronic pain patients: Integration of psychological assessment data. *Journal of Consulting and Clinical Psychology, 56,* 233–238.

Turk, D. C., & Salovey, P. (1984). Chronic pain as a variant of depressive disease: A critical reappraisal. *Journal of Nervous and Mental Disease, 172,* 398–404.

Vaccaro, A. R., Ring, D., Scuderi, G., Cohen, D. S., & Garfin, S. R. (1997). Predictors of outcome in patients with chronic back pain in low-grade spondylolisthesis. *Spine, 17,* 2030–2035.

Vassend, O., Krogstad, B. S., & Dahl, B. J. (1995). Negative affectivity, somatic complaints, and symptoms of temporomandibular disorders. *Journal of Psychosomatic Research, 39*(7), 889–899.

Volinn, E. (1996). Back pain and associated disability in the United States. *American Pain Society Bulletin, 6*(6), 8.

Von Korff, M., Deyo, R. A., Cherkin, D., & Barlow, W. (1993). Back pain in primary care: Outcomes at one year. *Spine, 18,* 855–862.

Waddell, G., Main, C. J., Morris, E. W., DiPaola, M., & Gray, I. C. (1984). Chronic low back pain, psychologic distress, and illness behavior. *Spine, 9,* 209–213.

Walker, E. A., Gelfand, M. D., & Gelfand, A. N. (1996). The relationship of current psychiatric disorder to functional disability and distress in patients with inflammatory bowel disease. *General Hospital Psychiatry, 18,* 220-229.

Walter, L., & Brannon, L. (1991). A cluster analysis of the Multidimensional Pain Inventory. *Headache, 31,* 476-479.

Williams, R. A., Atkinson, J. H., & Slater, M. A. (1995). Psychosocial risk factors predict acute low back pain

patients' progression to chronicity. Los Angeles: American Pain Society.

Young, L. D. (1992). Psychological factors in rheumatoid arthritis. *Journal of Consulting and Clinical Psychology, 60,* 619-627.

Zautra, A. J., & Manne, S. L. (1992). Coping with rheumatoid arthritis: A review of a decade of research. *Annals of Behavioral Medicine, 14,* 31-39.

Chapter 27

Interdisciplinary Treatment of Chronic Pain Patients

ROBERT J. GATCHEL
DENNIS C. TURK

As has been noted in other chapters of this book, pain is a complex subjective phenomenon that comprises an array of factors, each of which contributes to the interpretation of nociception as pain. The complexity of pain becomes especially noteworthy when it persists over extended periods of time during which a range of psychosocioeconomic factors can significantly interact with physical pathology to modulate a patient's self-report of pain and concomitant disability and response to treatment. Chronic pain disability is now appropriately viewed as a complex and interactive psychophysiological behavior pattern that cannot be broken down into distinct, independent psychological and physical components. The intention of this chapter is to review the critical elements of an interdisciplinary treatment approach that has been demonstrated to be efficacious when patients have progressed to the chronic pain disability stage, at which point their management becomes much more complex because of the interactive psychosocioeconomic factors involved.

At the outset, one should be aware of differences among primary, secondary, and tertiary care. As Mayer et al. (1995) have clearly delineated, the care of acute pain problems is considered primary care, usually consisting of control of the pain symptom. Primary care usually lasts between 0–12 weeks following the occurrence of a painful episode and includes (but is not restricted to) "passive treatment modalities" such as electrical stimulation, manipulation, temperature modulation methods, and analgesic medications. Moreover, as these investigators note, on the basis of the natural history of many pain disorders, especially musculoskeletal disorders, most patients recover spontaneously or with relatively limited primary care. Secondary care refers to the first stage of reactivation during the transition from primary care to return to work or normal activities of daily living. This secondary care phase usually occurs 2–6 months after the initial pain occurrence and is designed for patients who do not respond to initial primary treatment in order to facilitate a return to productivity before progressive physical deconditioning and psychosocioeconomic barriers become firmly entrenched. Secondary care is meant to avoid the occurrence of chronic disability by preventing physical deconditioning and potential negative psychosocial reactions, as well as social habituation to disability. As Mayer and colleagues (1995) point out, the rationale for secondary care rehabilitation is to recognize and manage early risk factors or signs of the development of disability, thus preventing chronic or permanent disability. Thus, reactivation is often the most common need at this point in time.

Finally, tertiary care refers to rehabilitation directed at preventing or ameliorating permanent disability for the patient who already suffers the effects of disability and physical deconditioning. It is this tertiary care or rehabilitation that requires an interdisciplinary team in order to accurately assess the various interrelated factors of chronic disability and pain, which then must be linked to the careful administration of a multifaceted pain management program in order to effect recovery and reduce permanent disability. This is not to say that the interdisciplinary approach is not of potential value for secondary care. However, this form of tertiary care is quite different from secondary care because of the intensity of services required, duration of disability, treatment program protocol, more specificity of physical and psychosocial assessment, and the greater level of coordination among health care professionals. In this chapter, we will discuss this interdisciplinary approach, especially as applied to tertiary care.

We distinguish between interdisciplinary and multidisciplinary treatment. Multidisciplinary connotes the involvement of several health care providers. The integration of these services, as well as communication among providers, may be limited. Interdisciplinary, in our use of the concept, involves greater coordination of services in a comprehensive program and frequent communication among the health care professionals providing care. A key ingredient of interdisciplinary care is a common philosophy of rehabilitation and active patient involvement (Turk & Stieg, 1987). Before discussing the specific elements of an interdisciplinary treatment approach, we will provide a brief historical overview of the growth of such pain management approaches.

GROWTH OF PAIN CLINICS

As we have carefully delineated elsewhere (Turk & Gatchel, in press), a number of anesthesiologists developed pain clinics that used nerve block procedures as a primary model of diagnosis and therapy following World War II. This subsequently stimulated the rapid growth of such pain clinics, which resulted in the listing of 327 such clinics in a directory of pain clinics that was published in 1977 by the American Society of Anesthesiologists (ASA) Committee on Pain Therapy. Of these 327 pain clinics, 73% of them were within the United States. More recently, it has been estimated that there are more than 3,300 pain treatment facilities and solo pain practitioners in the United States, treating 2.9 million Americans each year (Market Data Enterprises, 1995). More than 176,000 patients are estimated to be treated in specialty pain treatment facilities each year. Melzack and Wall (1982) characterized this proliferation of pain clinics as one of the most important advances in patient care during the past 25 years.

The International Association for the Study of Pain (IASP) has delineated four levels of pain programs (see Loeser, 1990): multidisciplinary pain centers, multidisciplinary pain clinics, pain clinics, and modality-oriented clinics. The pain clinic is typically a health care facility that focuses on the diagnosis and management of patients with chronic pain. Such clinics may specialize in specific diagnoses or in pain related to a specific region of the body (e.g., headache). The modality-oriented clinic is a health care facility that provides a specific type of treatment but does not provide comprehensive assessment or pain management. Examples of such clinics include nerve block clinics and biofeedback clinics. In such clinics, there is no emphasis on an integrated or comprehensive interdisciplinary approach. A multidisciplinary pain (in our terms, interdisciplinary) center is composed of a group of health care professionals and basic scientists. Such centers include research, teaching, and patient care related to acute and chronic pain. These facilities include a wide array of health care professionals, including physicians, psychologists, nurses, physical therapists, occupational therapists, and other health care provider specialties. Multiple therapeutic modalities are available, and these centers are usually affiliated with major health science institutions and are able to provide evaluation and treatment. Finally, a multidisciplinary (interdisciplinary) pain clinic is a health care delivery facility staffed by physicians and other health care provider specialists. It differs from the multidisciplinary pain center in that it does not include research and teaching activities as regular features.

The prototypical pain clinic that most psychologists are familiar with is the one originally developed at the University of Washington by Fordyce and his colleagues (Fordyce, Fowler, Lehmann, & DeLateur, 1968). This clinic utilized "pure" operant or behavioral treatment programs in which reinforcement procedures for "well behavior" were the major components used for pain management. The program originally involved a 4- to 8-week inpatient-treatment protocol designed to increase gradually the general activity level and socialization of the patient and to decrease medication use.

As pain treatment specialists began to understand the complexity of evaluating and treating chronic pain problems, simple pain clinics and modality-oriented clinics soon were replaced by interdisciplinary pain centers or clinics (IPCs) in which it was conceived that patients would be best served by a team of specialists with different health care backgrounds. These IPCs were driven by the concept that a complaint of pain was not just the result of body damage but also had cognitive, affective, and environmental origins. Moreover, these IPCs treated not only the experience of pain but also associated patient distress, dysfunction, and disability. The major aim was to improve a patient's physical performance and coping skills and also to transfer the control of pain and management of its related problems back to the patient. The treatment plan was conceptualized to be rehabilitative rather than investigative or curative. It was designed to increase function so that the patient could make further changes in life quality, environmental stressors, and psychosocial factors (e.g., self-esteem and affect), all of which would assist in pain control and management. Such IPCs emphasized an integrated treatment plan that included comprehensive care, such as drug detoxification, cognitive-behavioral treatment methods, functional restoration, and total rehabilitation. These more comprehensive approaches do not ignore operant factors that influence the maintenance of pain and disability. Rather, they incorporate behavioral factors within a broader rehabilitative model.

In recent years, there has been an even greater emphasis on functional restoration as a driving force of these IPCs (Baum, Gatchel, & Krantz, 1997). The term "functional restoration," originally developed by Mayer and Gatchel (1988), refers not only to a treatment methodology for chronic pain patients but also to a broader conceptualization of the entire problem, its diagnosis, and its management. Rather than accepting current limits in history taking based solely on patients' self-report of pain and on diagnosis through imaging technology, this method involves more objective information. Objective assessment of physical capacity and effort, with comparison to a normative data base, adds a new dimension to diagnosis. In keeping with a "sports medicine" approach, this permits the development of treatment programs of varied intensity and duration aimed primarily at restoring physical functional capacity and social performance. Objectives are more ambitious than merely attempting to alter pain complaints and to decrease medications. It is assumed that improvements in quality of life will be greatly enlarged by focusing on increasing physical capacity and decreasing

social problems associated with pain. Attention is given to realistic goals such as returning to work, increasing activities of daily living, and reducing the use of the medical system. This functional restoration approach, which is discussed later in this chapter, has already helped to change the focus of traditional pain treatment programs, as well as the criteria for evaluation of effectiveness. With this brief historical overview in mind, we now turn to the major components of an interdisciplinary treatment program and the roles of each health care specialist in an interdisciplinary treatment program.

THE INTERDISCIPLINARY TREATMENT TEAM

Table 27.1 summarizes the makeup of the interdisciplinary treatment team. As we discussed earlier, the integration of these multiple disciplines for the treatment of pain has been one of the most significant advances in the modern care of chronic pain patients. It should also be clearly noted that this team of multidisciplinary specialists consists of more than a group of individuals from varying disciplines, each of whom is monitoring the patient. There *must* be constant communication among each of these group members and a common understanding of the overall goals of the assessment-treatment program offered to patients (Turk & Stieg, 1987)—hence, an interdisciplinary approach.

The regular evaluation of patients, during which all team members are present, is essential in order for team members to obtain the most valid perception of the patient, as well as to help one another to work more effectively with the patient. Awareness of what other team members are doing with the patient is essential. This also greatly aids in providing a consistent message to patients. Chronic pain patients are often quite adept at "splitting" health care professionals from one another by providing conflicting information: "Doctor, please increase my pain medication because I overdid it in physical therapy today." The constant review and monitoring of the patient by all treatment personnel will greatly aid in minimizing this potential "splitting" problem. Aligning goals and providing clear communication regarding direction and duration of treatment are vital from the beginning, and all treatment personnel must "buy into" the treatment program. Table 27.2 presents the important factors that can significantly contribute to the success of the program.

TABLE 27.1. Staff Composition of an Interdisciplinary Pain Management Center

Medical director/physician: Serves a leadership role; responsible for medical issues involved in the diagnoses and management of anatomical, pathological, and physiological processes associated with complaint of pain.

Nurse: Serves as a physician "extender," and plays a significant role in obtaining patient histories, monitoring medications, and evaluating lifestyle issues that may affect pain patients and their response to treatment.

Psychologist: Assesses the patient's psychosocial functioning, personality characteristics, social support, motivational status, and coping resources that will help treatment planning, provides treatments addressing these issues, and monitors therapeutic progress.

Physical therapist: Performs comprehensive musculoskeletal evaluation, including the examination of gait and postural abnormalities, range of motion, sensation, reflexes, and neurological indices. This information is then used to specifically tailor a therapeutic program to address any diagnosed defects.

Occupational therapist: Conducts pre- and posttreatment evaluations that focus on body mechanics and energy conservation needed for activities of daily living, work, and leisure. During treatment, supervises progressive increases in the performance of such functional activities so that patients can return to as normal a level of functioning as possible. Also often serves as the liaison between employers and injured workers and may aid in developing job modifications for accommodation of the injured worker.

Medical-disability case manager: An occupational therapist or vocational rehabilitation professional, often employed to promote vocational and social reactivation throughout the treatment program. Monitors progress compliance and performance, postprogram follow-up, and occupational planning and sequencing, with coordination of socioeconomic issues.

In the next section of this chapter, we describe the roles and responsibilities of the different members of the interdisciplinary team. In many instances, there is a blurring of the boundaries between the disciplines in the educational components of the treatment. This is intentional, as it serves to reinforce the common message of functional restoration and self-management.

The Physician's Role in Interdisciplinary Rehabilitation

The essential medical issues involved in the diagnosis and management of anatomical, pathologi-

TABLE 27.2. Important Factors That Determine the Success of an Interdisciplinary Pain Treatment Program

- Understanding and acceptance of the philosophy of the treatment program by all staff

- Systematic monitoring of treatment outcomes in order to maximize quality assurance

- Regular meetings in order to maximize frequent communication among team members and mutual reinforcement of the overall goals for each patient

- Mutual reinforcement among team members for each other's role and efforts; communication of respect for each other's skills with patients

cal, and physiological processes related to the complaint of pain make up the primary role for the physician in interdisciplinary treatment. A physician usually serves as the medical director of the treatment program and often comes from a background specializing in rehabilitation care, but he or she may also come from training in psychiatry, orthopedic or neurologic surgery, physiatry, occupational medicine, or internal medicine. In a sense, the physician is responsible for the medical direction of the treatment team, as well as for providing a leadership role for the entire interdisciplinary team. There may also be a number of other physicians who actually manage the patient and who are responsible for synthesizing, interpreting, and translating viewpoints of various past medical records and consultants, as well as monitoring all medications, comorbid medical conditions, and any changes in symptoms that may occur during the course of the treatment program. Together with nurses and/or physician assistants, who may provide backup as physician extenders, the physician plays a vital role in the different phases of the treatment program. It is the physician who needs to sanction the physical activation program that may be prescribed, as well as endorse the emphasis on patient assumption of responsibility and safe management that is communicated to patients by all the other members of the treatment team.

It should also be noted that an important component of interdisciplinary treatment involves the process of patient education. Many times, physicians lead educational sessions on topics related to the basic physiology and anatomy of the pain condition, pointing out the distinction between impairment, disability, cure, and rehabilitation, discussing doctor–patient relationship issues, and explaining the rationale for the self-management approach that is emphasized in the treatment philosophy (Turk & Stacey, 1997). Such education sessions are developed in order to provide information, as well as to be interactive, so that patients become actively involved in the process rather than merely being passive recipients of the information. This patient education process is also led by other members of the treatment team. During these education sessions, pain should always be discussed openly and honestly but also with instruction in pain-reduction or management techniques. Thus, patients will learn to expect certain patterns of pain and will begin to take responsibility for their own treatment. Patients learn that, although they may not be able to achieve a total pain-free state, they can indeed gain significant control over their pain.

The Role of the Nurse in Interdisciplinary Treatment

As a natural "physician extender," the nurse plays an important role in obtaining patient histories, assisting in the monitoring of medications (as well as medication tapering regimens when needed), and in evaluating lifestyle issues that may affect pain patients (e.g., compliance issues, smoking and dietary problems, etc.). The nurse is also invaluable in providing instruction to patients concerning possible medication side effects, medication interactions, and the use of over-the-counter medications. They also play an important role in the education of patients by discussing healthy lifestyle characteristics that include diet, weight, blood pressure, smoking, alcohol use, sexuality, and sleep. Moreover, whenever anesthesiology procedures such as nerve blocks are used as a treatment modality, the nurse will assist in patient preparation during the procedure and in monitoring patients during the recovery phase. Nurses are also very important in conducting follow-up contacts with patients when the patients return home. They support and advise during the essential period when patients are bridging the gap between the interdisciplinary program and self-care at home. Faucett (1994) has concisely presented the results of a survey that describes the many roles that nurses play at different interdisciplinary pain programs.

The Role of the Psychologist in Interdisciplinary Treatment

As health care professionals have become more aware of the important role that psychosocial variables play in the rehabilitation of patients with chronic disabilities, the role of the psychologist has become especially important in helping to manage chronic pain patients in an interdisciplinary program. In fact, a psychologist must be included for a pain treatment facility to be certified by the Committee on the Accreditation of Rehabilitation Facilities (CARF).

Many of these pain patients present to the treatment staff with diagnosable clinical syndromes such as major depressive disorders, anxiety disorders, substance abuse disorders, and somatoform pain disorders (e. g., Polatin, Kinney, Gatchel, Lillo, & Mayer, 1993). Moreover, as Gatchel (1996) has emphasized, chronic pain should be viewed as a major stressor that can exact a considerable toll on a person's mental health that, in turn, can interfere with the patient's return to a productive lifestyle. It is therefore important that the interdisciplinary treatment team be aware of many potential psychosocial barriers to recovery that can significantly affect the successful course of treatment. Thus, one role of the psychologist is to assess many important characteristics of the patient: psychosocial functioning, personality characteristics, mental status, social support resources, motivational state, beliefs and attitudes, and available coping resources, as well as any barriers to increasing behavioral activities. It is important that the psychologist determine whether any of these above variables can positively contribute to the patient's full participation in the rehabilitation program or act as potential barriers that the treatment team needs to be fully aware of in order to carry out their particular rehabilitation duties.

During the treatment program itself, another important role of the psychologist is to emphasize to patients that they have an ability to exert control over their responses to pain. Often, it is useful to have patients focus on the role of stress and cognitive appraisals on pain perception and exacerbation. Psychologists also provide significant support in helping patients deal with depressed mood and interpersonal or family problems, as well as helping with problem-solving skills and stress management. The psychologist helps the patients to reconceptualize their pain situation from one of hopelessness to one that is more manageable through self-control.

Finally, the major mode of psychological treatment in pain management programs is the use of cognitive and behavioral coping skills that include relaxation, distraction, and imagery methods, as well as cognitive restructuring methods. Patients are taught behavioral skills that include controlling pain through activity–rest cycling and pacing, the setting up of realistic activity goals, and interacting effectively with spouse, family members, and significant others. Self-control over their pain is consistently emphasized. Gatchel and Turk (1996) have recently edited a volume that provides a comprehensive review of various psychological approaches used in such pain management programs.

The Role of the Physical Therapist in Interdisciplinary Treatment

Physical therapists play an important role in reducing pain, controlling inflammation, and protecting the injured tissue involved in the pain syndrome. They perform comprehensive musculoskeletal evaluations, during which they can evaluate factors such as gait and postural abnormalities, range-of-motion limitations, and sensation and reflex deficits, and they also perform preliminary neurological testing. Not all physical therapists can work well in an interdisciplinary treatment team. Besides having a basic knowledge of orthopedics, neurology, and pathology, they must also understand nonphysiological signs of chronic pain symptomatology. Moreover, they must be aware of not only the pathology of the injury but also the various physical and psychosocial sequelae of such painful injuries. Many physical therapists, because of an educational background that emphasizes the role of a single therapist working with a patient in isolation from a team of other specialists, have to be reoriented to the perspective that constant input from various other disciplines is extremely important in order for their job to be done more effectively and efficiently.

In general, physical therapy involves a combination of instruction and exercises. The instructional component of therapy needs to focus on providing patients with the following: (1) information concerning basic anatomical and physiological bases of pain and physical activity; (2) the use of proper body mechanics; (3) the effects of inap-propriate posture and distorted gait on pain; (4) the value of active exercise regimens versus passive modalities; (5) physical activity distraction techniques to control pain flare-ups; and (6) self-management modalities for home use, such as ice, heat, massage, and other assistive devices. The physical therapist needs to carefully customize programs to address any loss of flexibility, strength, or endurance that is part of the "deconditioning syndrome" often present with chronic pain patients. A very active approach is emphasized whenever possible in which patients are instructed in progressive daily exercises that focus on stretching, flexibility, strength, endurance, and general conditioning. In contrast, passive modalities are de-emphasized. Again, in keeping with the general overall philosophy of the interdisciplinary treatment program, issues of self-control, self-responsibility, and self-management are emphasized to patients throughout the physical therapy regimen.

The Role of the Occupational Therapist in Interdisciplinary Treatment

For a majority of chronic pain patients in an interdisciplinary treatment program, a significant challenge is to get back to work after often having been away from a work situation for an extended period of time (months or years). Therefore, a major goal of an occupational therapist is to work with these difficult patients who have a number of significant barriers that hinder their return to a functional lifestyle. These patients often feel uncertain about future job plans and lack self-confidence with regard to physical functioning in any potential job situation or life situation in general that they encounter. Such patients may be difficult to motivate toward rehabilitation, and they require a cohesive team approach in order to be successful.

Occupational therapists play an important role in both assessment and treatment. They conduct pre- and posttreatment evaluations that focus on body mechanics and energy conservation in performing activities of daily living, work activities, and leisure activities. An occupational therapist will also conduct physical capacity evaluations and job evaluations. In unison with a physical therapist, the occupational therapist will provide information, as well as design and supervise specific exercise programs, directed at returning patients to reasonable levels of functional activities of daily living and job demands. However, in contrast to physical therapists, who focus on general conditioning, the occupational therapist focuses on information about, and training for, energy conservation and functional performance related to specific activities of daily living and work-related activities. They simulate these functional activities and supervise patients in progressively increasing performance so that the patient can return to as normal a level of functioning as possible.

The occupational therapist plays an important role within the interdisciplinary team. His or her major goals include gaining the patient's trust in developing long-term plans; motivating the patient to increase physical progression in order to accomplish a return to normal functioning in activities of daily living or employment situations; and modifying various aspects of pain, work, and social behavior. He or she often also serves as the liaison between the employers and the injured workers and may help develop job modifications that will better accommodate injured workers for return to work. From the occupational therapist's perspective, the motivation of the patient goes hand-in-hand with increasing his or her physical progression. Such physical progression in occupational therapy is usually based on functional "whole body" activities such as lifting, twisting, bending, reaching, pulling, pushing, climbing, walking, and carrying. Again, like other team members, the occupational therapist will need to be adept at dealing with pain symptoms while patients are working through physical progression. He or she must be aware of the fact that such symptoms are usually initially magnified but can be dealt with safely as progression increases. Again, like other team members, the occupational therapist needs to address such issues through education and information related to the body's healing process.

Finally, the occupational therapist can also serve as a medical case manager, since he or she often acts as the liaison between employers and injured workers. Nurses also often play this role. These case-managing duties often include resolving any issues concerning a return to work (such as developing job modifications to accommodate the injured worker), vocational retraining when full return to work cannot be accomplished, as well as postprogram support and tracking to make sure that the patient stays on target in achieving desired postprogram levels of activities of daily living or return to work. They can serve as the major arbitrator between doctor and patient, between the patient and such external "players" as insurance adjusters, referring physicians, and possible employers, and between the treatment team and the external community. Again, all of these duties are carried out within the context of the interdisciplinary treatment team. In this capacity, the occupational therapist also monitors program compliance and performance, as well as aligning goals and providing clear communication regarding direction and duration of treatment from the very beginning of the treatment program.

THE MAJOR GOALS OF AN INTERDISCIPLINARY TREATMENT PROGRAM

Table 27.3 presents the major goals that interdisciplinary treatment programs should strive to achieve. As can be seen, these are all goals that can be objectively monitored and quantified. Indeed, emphasizing such objective functional and socioeconomic outcomes has been discussed by numerous clinical investigators (e. g., Feuerstein & Zastowny, 1996; Hazard, 1995; Mayer & Gatchel, 1988).

An Example of an Interdisciplinary Treatment Program

Functional restoration, as originally developed by Mayer and Gatchel (1988), can be used to illustrate what has proven to be an effective interdisciplinary treatment approach for chronic musculoskeletal pain disability. There are, though, other types of IPC programs that have been shown to be effective (Turk & Gatchel, in press; Turk & Stacey, 1997).

As mentioned earlier in this chapter, functional restoration incorporates a sports-medicine approach that emphasizes active involvement by patients in a treatment program that is aimed primarily at restoring physical functional capacity and

TABLE 27.3. Major Goals of an Interdisciplinary Pain Treatment Program

- Return the patient to productivity
- Maximize function, thus minimizing pain
- Help patient assume responsibility for self-management and progress
- Reduce or eliminate future medical utilization
- Avoid recurrence of injury, maintain therapeutic gains
- Avoid medication dependence and abuse

social performance. By focusing on increasing physical capacity and decreasing social problems associated with chronic disability, improvements in quality of life are greatly expanded. These goals are viewed as just as important as attempting to alter pain complaints and decrease medications. Moreover, attention to realistic socioeconomic outcomes, such as return to work and reducing the use of the health care system, are used as criteria for evaluation of treatment effectiveness. Of course, attention to such realistic outcomes does not suggest that one ignore self-reported pain when treating pain in this manner. Rather, self-report of pain is interpreted only in the context of overall functioning. In fact, adaptive, positive functioning is sometimes associated with an initial increase in pain complaints. Thus the phrase "no pain, no gain" is often emphasized to patients who are undergoing functional restoration. Rather than halting or delaying further physical training because of such pain complaints, the patient may have to learn to "work through" the pain. Psychological pain coping strategies are taught to patients while they undergo this physical reconditioning. The success of this program is dependent on all of the previously mentioned psychology and other specialty staff members who are required for a true interdisciplinary treatment program (e.g., Gatchel, Mayer, Hazard, Rainville, & Mooney, 1992; Hazard, 1995).

The success of this interdisciplinary functional restoration approach to chronic pain management has been unequivocally documented in a number of different investigations (e.g., Bendix & Bendix, 1994; Bendix et al., 1996; Hazard et al., 1989; Hildebrandt, Pfingsten, Saur, & Jansen, 1997; Mayer, Gatchel, et al., 1985; Mayer et al., 1987). For example, in the study by Mayer et al. (1987), patients who had undergone the functional restoration program were followed up 2 years after completion of the program. Results clearly demonstrated significant changes in a number of important socioeconomic outcome measures: Nearly 90% of the treatment group were actively working, as compared with only about 41% of a nontreatment comparison group; about twice as many comparison group patients required additional spine surgery and had unsettled worker's compensation litigation relative to the treatment group; the comparison group also had approximately five times more patient visits to health care professionals and had higher rates of recurrence of injury relative to the functional restoration group. There were also significant improvements in self-report measures

and physical function measures such as back strength and range of motion in the functional restoration treatment group. Thus, these findings demonstrate the significant impact that an interdisciplinary program such as functional restoration can have on a range of important self-report, physical functioning, and socioeconomic outcome measures.

Finally, it should be noted that the original functional restoration program was independently replicated by Hazard et al. (1989) in the United States, by Bendix and Bendix (1994) and Bendix et al. (1996) in Denmark, by Hildebrandt et al. (1997) in Germany, and by Corey, Koepfler, Etlin, and Day (1996) in Canada. The fact that different clinical treatment teams, functioning in different states (Texas and Vermont) and different countries, with markedly different economic-social conditions and workers' compensation systems, produced comparable outcome results speaks highly for the robustness of the research findings and the utility, as well as the fidelity, of this functional restoration approach. In addition, Burke, Harms-Constas, and Aden (1994) have recently demonstrated its efficacy in 11 different rehabilitation centers across seven states. Hazard (1995) has also recently reviewed the overall effectiveness of functional restoration.

It should be noted that besides functional restoration, there are other forms of interdisciplinary treatment programs for chronic pain that have been shown to be efficacious with chronic pain sufferers (Turk & Gatchel, in press; Turk & Stacey, 1997). These other programs differ from functional restoration mainly in terms of a decreased emphasis on the direct quantification of function used to drive the "sports medicine" philosophy of that approach. Overall, Turk and Gatchel (in press) have pointed out that the cost savings of all IPCs can be quite significant. In addition, it was emphasized that more research is needed to examine what combinations of variables are most important in being able to prescribe the most efficient and effective therapeutic "package" in an interdisciplinary treatment program. Future investigation is needed to address this important issue so as to increase the efficiency in time, cost, and outcome of this promising interdisciplinary treatment approach to pain management.

SUMMARY AND CONCLUSIONS

In a review of the literature, Flor, Fydrich, and Turk (1992) concluded that the overall therapeutic results emanating from such IPCs were quite promising, with significant changes demonstrated not only in self-reported pain and mood but also in important socioeconomic variables such as the return to work and the use of the health care system. The cost of hospital and medical charges for chronic pain have been estimated to be in excess of $125 billion (Frymoyer & Durett, 1997). Based on the meta-analysis published by Flor et al. (1992) that included 3,089 patients, even when the cost of treatment of the IPC was included, Turk and Gatchel (in press) calculated a savings of over $1 billion over a period of 19 years. Recall that this estimate is based on 3,089 patients. The market data survey (Market Data Enterprises, 1995) estimated that over 176,000 patients were treated at IPCs each year. Extrapolating potential savings of IPCs would be in excess of $1.5 billion each year.

It was also emphasized that more research is needed to examine what combinations of variables are most important to the ability to prescribe the most efficient and effective therapeutic "package" in an interdisciplinary treatment program. As we conclude, to date "there are no data available to determine what set of patients with what characteristics are most likely to benefit from what set of treatment modalities, provided in what type of format" (Turk & Gatchel, in press). Future investigation is needed to address this important issue so as to increase the efficiency in time, cost, and outcome of this promising interdisciplinary treatment approach to pain management.

REFERENCES

American Society of Anesthesiologists Committee on Pain Therapy. (1977). *Directory of pain clinics*. Chicago: Author.

Baum, A., Gatchel, R. J., & Krantz, D. (1997). *Introduction to health psychology* (3rd ed.). New York: McGraw Hill.

Bendix, A. E., Bendix, T., Vaegter, K., Lund, C., Frolund, L., & Holm, L. (1996). Multidisciplinary intensive treatment for chronic low back pain: A randomized, prospective study. *Cleveland Clinic Journal of Medicine, 63*, 62–69.

Bendix, T., & Bendix, A. (1994, June). Different training programs for chronic low back pain—A randomized, blinded one-year follow-up study. Paper presented at the meeting of the International Society for the Study of the Lumbar Spine, Seattle, WA.

Burke, S. A., Harms-Constas, C. K., & Aden, P. S. (1994). Return to work/work retention outcomes of a functional restoration program: A multi-center, prospective study with a comparison group. *Spine, 19*, 1880–1886.

Corey, D. T., Koepfler, L. E., Etlin, D., & Day, H. I. (1996). A limited functional restoration program for injured workers: A randomized trial. *Journal of Occupational Rehabilitation, 6*, 239–249.

Faucett, J. (1994). What is the role of nursing in the Multidisciplinary pain treatment center? *American Pain Society Bulletin, 4*, 6–8.

Feuerstein, M., & Zastowny, T. R. (1996). Occupational rehabilitation: Multidisciplinary management of work-related musculoskeletal pain and disability. In R. J. Gatchel & D. C. Turk (Eds.), *Psychological approaches to pain management: A practitioner's guide* (pp. 458–485). New York: Guilford Press.

Flor, H., Fydrich, T., & Turk, D. C. (1992). Efficacy of multidisciplinary pain treatment centers: A meta-analytic review. *Pain, 49*, 221–230.

Fordyce, W. E., Fowler, R. S., Lehmann, J. F., & DeLateur, B. J. (1968). Some implications of learning in problems of chronic pain. *Journal of Chronic Diseases, 21*, 179–190.

Frymoyer, J. W., & Durett, C. L. (1997). The economics of spinal disorders. In J. W. Frymoyer et al. (Eds.), *The adult spine* (2nd ed., pp. 193–196). Philadelphia: Lippincott-Raven.

Gatchel, R. J. (1996). Psychological disorders and chronic pain: Cause-and-effect relationship. In R. J. Gatchel & D. C. Turk (Eds.), *Psychological approaches to pain management: A practitioner's handbook* (pp. 33–52). New York: Guilford Press.

Gatchel, R. J., Mayer, T. G., Hazard, R. B., Rainville, J., & Mooney, V. (1992). Functional restoration—Pitfalls in evaluating efficacy [Editorial]. *Spine, 17*, 988–994.

Gatchel, R. J., & Turk, D. C. (Eds.). (1996). *Psychological approaches to pain management: A practitioner's handbook*. New York: Guilford Press.

Hazard, R. G. (1995). Spine update: Functional restoration. *Spine, 20*, 2345–2348.

Hazard, R. G., Fenwick, J. W., Kalisch, S. M., Redmond, J., Reeves, V., Reid, S., & Frymoyer, J. W. (1989). Functional restoration with behavioral support: A one-year prospective study of patients with chronic low back pain. *Spine, 14*, 157–161.

Hildebrandt, J., Pfingsten, M., Saur, P., & Jansen, J. (1997). Prediction of success from a multidisciplinary treatment program for chronic low back pain. *Spine, 22*, 990–1001.

Loeser, J. D. (1990). *Desirable characteristics for pain treatment facilities*. Seattle, WA: IASP.

Market Data Enterprises (1995). *Chronic pain management programs: A market analysis*. Valley Stream, NY: Market Data Enterprises.

Mayer, T. G., & Gatchel, R. J. (1988). *Functional restoration for spinal disorders: The sports medicine approach*. Philadelphia: Lea & Febiger.

Mayer, T. G., Gatchel, R. J., Kishino, N., Keeley, J., Capra, P., Mayer, H., Barnett, J., & Mooney, V. (1985). Objective assessment of spine function following industrial injury: A prospective study with comparison group and one-year follow-up. *Spine, 10*, 482–492.

Mayer, T. G., Gatchel, R. J., Mayer, H., Kishino, N. D., Keeley, J., & Mooney, V. (1987). A prospective two-year study of functional restoration in industrial low back injury utilizing objective assessment. *Journal of the American Medical Association, 258*, 1763–1767.

Mayer, T. G., Polatin, P., Smith, B., Smith, C., Gatchel, R. J., Herring, H., Hall, H., Donelson, J., Dickey, J., & English, W. (1995). Contemporary concepts in spine care–spine rehabilitation: Secondary and tertiary nonoperative care. *Spine, 20,* 2060–2066.

Melzack, R., & Wall, P. D. (1982). *The challenge of pain.* New York: Basic Books.

Polatin, P. B., Kinney, R., Gatchel, R. J., Lillo, E., & Mayer, T. G. (1993). Psychiatric illness and chronic low back pain: The mind and the spine—Which goes first? *Spine, 18,* 66–71.

Turk, D. C., & Gatchel, R. J. (in press). Multidisciplinary programs for rehabilitation of chronic low back pain

patients. In W. H. Kirkaldy-Willis & T. N. Bernard, Jr. (Eds.), *Managing low back pain.* New York: Churchill Livingstone.

Turk, D. C., & Stacey, B. R. (1997). Multidisciplinary pain centers in the treatment of chronic back pain. In J. W. Frymoyer (Ed.), *The adult spine* (2nd ed.). New York: Lippincott-Raven.

Turk, D. C., & Stieg, R. L. (1987). Chronic pain: The necessity of interdisciplinary communication. *Clinical Journal of Pain, 3,* 163–167.

Chapter 28

Family Therapy for Adults with Chronic Pain

ROBERT D. KERNS

Attention to the role of the family in a broad array of health- and illness-related issues has a long history in sociology, psychology, and medicine. In most contexts, the family is viewed as a critical environment in which health-related beliefs and behaviors are learned and in which most health care is delivered (Litman, 1974; Litman & Venters, 1979; Ramsey, 1989). Across the lifespan, research and clinical observation support roles for the family in the development of children's conceptualizations of health and illness and the development of health behaviors in determining responses to acute illness and medical interventions among adults and in issues of aging and geriatric care (Turk & Kerns, 1985). Theory-driven research, as well as the consumerism movement in health care and a growing appreciation of positive relationships between involvement of the family in the delivery of care and patient outcomes and satisfaction, encourage increased attention to the role of the family in illness prevention, management, and treatment.

The management of chronic illness continues to dominate many discussions of health care research and health care delivery. Multiple explanatory models have been proposed for the family's role in determining the course of chronic illness and in the adaptation of the chronically ill family member (e.g., Kerns & Weiss, 1994; Olson, 1989; Patterson & Garwick, 1994). An expanding body

of empirical research documents important roles of the family in the etiology, care, and treatment of a range of chronic illnesses (Kerns, 1995). Associated with the proliferation and refinement of contemporary models of chronic illness adaptation that articulate roles of the family and supporting empirical research have been calls for inclusion of the family in clinical efforts to promote optimal management of the illness.

There has long been a call in the chronic pain literature to consider the role of the family, among other psychosocial variables, in the perpetuation of the problem (Flor, Turk, & Rudy, 1987a; Payne & Norfleet, 1986; Roy, 1992). This search for alternative explanations has been encouraged by the recognition that medical diagnoses of chronic pain conditions often have limited explanatory power and that traditional medical interventions are often ineffective and by a growing acceptance of multidimensional, as opposed to purely somatosensory, models of pain. Early psychosomatic models of illness, for example, frequently referred to chronic pain conditions as examples of the relevance of their models. These include Parson's "sick role" model (Parsons, 1951; Levine & Kozloff, 1978), Hill's "family stress" model (Hill, 1949), and Minuchin's family systems model (Minuchin, 1974). Refinements or extensions of these models of family functioning and family stress have proliferated (cf. Ramsey, 1989). However, none of these

445

models have had widespread influence in the field of chronic pain, in part because of the complexity of the models, difficulties in operationalizing key constructs, and the absence of empirical data supporting the effectiveness of interventions based on the models (Kerns & Weiss, 1994).

Informed by operant theory and clinical observation of chronic pain patients, Fordyce (1976) proposed an alternative to these family systems perspectives. According to the model, important social contingencies (e.g., positive attention from family members, disability compensation) for expressions of pain and disability are hypothesized to contribute to the maintenance of the experience of pain and disability. The dominance of behavioral and cognitive-behavioral models in the fields of health psychology and behavioral medicine over the past 20 years, early empirical support for Fordyce's model (Fordyce, 1988), and the development and demonstration of effective treatment programs based on the operant model (Keefe, Dunsmore, & Burnett, 1992; Keefe, Gil, & Rose, 1986) have encouraged widespread adoption of the model. Cognitive-behavioral refinements of this model (Turk, Meichenbaum, & Genest, 1983) and recently articulated multidimensional models of the development and perpetuation of the experience of chronic pain have continued to emphasize the role of the family (Flor, Birbaumer, & Turk, 1990; Kerns & Jacob, 1995).

The elaboration of these integrative theoretical models and a growing volume of supportive theory-driven research encourages development of clinical assessment and intervention strategies that include attention to family variables. Unfortunately, to date, clinical programs appear to largely maintain an individual focus. The few empirical studies of the effectiveness of chronic pain treatment that included a family member have not incorporated refinements that appear to be specifically theoretically informed. None of these studies have demonstrated enhanced outcome by inclusion of family members.

The primary goal of this chapter is to provide suggestions for refinements in available treatments for chronic pain that include attention to the family. To the extent possible, these suggestions will be consistent with contemporary theoretical models of the experience of chronic pain and supporting empirical data. The chapter begins with elaboration of a cognitive-behavioral transactional model of family functioning and its relevance for understanding the perpetuation of the chronic pain experience. This is followed by a review of the avail-

able data regarding families and chronic pain, as well as specific recommendations for theory-driven research. A clinical model for assessment, conceptualization, prescriptive treatment planning, and treatment delivery based on theory and data will be outlined. General and specific recommendations for family or couple interventions close the chapter.

THE COGNITIVE-BEHAVIORAL TRANSACTIONAL MODEL

Cognitive-behavioral perspectives have dominated the fields of health psychology and behavioral medicine since their emergence in the late 1970s. Consistent with their roots in social learning theory, these perspectives hypothesize a central role of social interactions in virtually all aspects of health promotion and illness prevention and management. Turk and Kerns have offered a specific elaboration of this perspective to explicate further the role of families relevant to health and illness issues (Kerns, 1995; Kerns & Payne, 1996; Kerns & Weiss, 1994; Turk & Kerns, 1985). Termed the cognitive-behavioral transactional model of family functioning, this model shares several key features with other models of family stress and coping (Patterson & Garwick, 1994), as well as other cognitive-behavioral models of couples and families (Fincham & Bradbury, 1990; Jacobson & Margolin, 1979).

Like all family systems models, the cognitive-behavioral transactional model encourages consideration of the family as the basic unit of analysis, although individual differences among family members continue to be important to assess as well. The model proposes that the family and its members actively interact with the environment, constantly seeking out and evaluating information about sources of stress (e.g., disease) and available resources to cope with the stress. The family, as a function of this appraisal process, considers alternative responses, acts, and evaluates the effectiveness of the response. The model, then, places emphasis on the family's and its members' cognition, particularly appraisals of threat and efforts to meet the challenges posed by the stress.

As has been hypothesized for individuals, families develop relatively stable beliefs or schemata about the world, the family and its members, and interactions between the family and its environment. Similarly, families develop a spectrum of coping resources. These beliefs and resources develop as a function of the family's history and sociocultural context. Many, but not necessarily all, of the family's idiosyncratic beliefs are shared among the family members. These family paradigms influence daily problem solving, as well as the family's response to challenges such as those posed by illness in a family member.

Paradigms or schemata hypothesized by other family theorists to guide family functioning may be relevant to refinements of the cognitive-behavioral transactional model. Reiss's (1989) family paradigm model of family functioning, for example, may prove useful in helping to identify patterns or dimensions underlying the structure of core beliefs common among subgroups of families. Reiss has articulated three primary dimensions of family functioning. "Configuration" refers to the family's worldview, "coordination" refers to its view of the degree of integration of the family itself, and "closure" refers to perceptions of the family that directly influence its flexibility and adaptability in facing new challenges. Olson (1989; Olson, Sprenkle, & Russell, 1979) has labeled two similar core dimensions of family functioning, namely "cohesion" and "adaptability." These constructs have important implications for describing if not explaining differences among families in their response to chronic illness. They may also be useful in understanding how families may appear to do well in adjusting to some aspects of the illness relative to others.

Although perceptions of stress occur within the family system, individual family members also experience them uniquely. Observation of symptoms of stress among one or more of its members triggers the family's appraisal process. The family's schemata and specific appraisals of the stress and available resources will interact to determine the family's experience of stress and its response. Central to the model is the hypothesis that the family's response influences the response of its members. The reciprocal and dynamic relationship of these interactions is a key feature of the family's response to stress. Finally, as is emphasized in Breunlin's (1989) oscillation theory, the family's own resources are enhanced through the growth of an individual member's coping capacities and their incorporation into the family's arsenal of resources.

Patterson's (1989; Patterson & Garwick, 1994) family adjustment and adaptation response (FAAR) model proposes a process of appraisal that appears to be quite similar and directly relevant to the cognitive-behavioral transactional perspective. According to this and other family stress theories, the degree of stress experienced by the family is a function of the interaction between challenges to the family and the family's resources to meet the challenges. Challenges may be experienced as specific problems or may be associated with the more global meanings or schemata associated with perceptions of the challenge. Resources may include physical, psychological, and social resources, as well as the coping behaviors of the family. The primary goal of the family is maintenance of homeostasis and overall adjustment to stress. Ultimately, the value of the FAAR model may be the fact that several psychometrically sound measures of key constructs have been developed. Unfortunately, overlap and ambiguity among several key constructs and the overall complexity of the model may limit its applicability.

THE ROLE OF THE FAMILY IN CHRONIC PAIN

Kerns and his colleagues have articulated an explanatory model of chronic pain that emphasizes the social and particularly the family context in which the multidimensional experience of chronic pain develops (Kerns & Jacob, 1995; Banks & Kerns, 1996). According to this model, the family is the central environment in which complex interactions occur between the challenges or problems commonly associated with the perception of pain and the individual's efforts to meet these challenges. Kerns and his colleagues have offered a further elaboration of this model that incorporates the cognitive-behavioral transactional model of family functioning (Kerns & Payne, 1996; Kerns & Weiss, 1994). It is hoped that greater attention to family process variables will aid in our developing understanding of the development and perpetuation of the chronic pain experience and lead to treatment refinements that improve pain management for a larger proportion of individuals.

The general model, described as a diathesis–stress model of chronic pain, identifies several key components. As a developmental model, prior strengths or vulnerabilities (i.e., diatheses) of the individual (and family) that may be relevant to efforts to meet the challenges or problems posed by pain are considered. These strengths or vulnerabilities are described as occurring in four primary domains, namely, biological (e.g., the integrity of brain systems relevant to the regulation of pain and affect), cognitive (e.g., problem-solving competence), affective (e.g., baseline levels of anxiety), and behavioral (e.g., instrumental skill) domains. Similar dimensions may be useful in categorizing the multiple common challenges or problems posed by the experience of pain. The experience of persistent and often constant aversive stimulation almost certainly challenges the individual's biological homeostasis. The intrusiveness of the experience may interfere with optimal cognitive functioning. Associated physical impairment, pain itself, and the fear of pain or further injury may contribute to behavioral inhibition and functional disability. Finally, failure to effect relief from pain may be associated with sadness, anger, anxiety, and more general challenges to affective regulation.

Also central to the model is the notion that the experience of pain is itself a multidimensional phenomenon. Again, four primary dimensions of the experience of chronic pain have been articulated, namely, the disease or pathology presumed to be related to nociception, the experience of pain, functional disability, and affective distress. Although these dimensions of the experience are likely to be significantly interrelated, the model acknowledges their relative independence, that is, the likelihood that an individual may experience varying degrees of dysfunction in each of these domains. This model, then, proposes that attention to each of these domains is critical in fully describing the complex and multidimensional experience of chronic pain (Kerns, 1996). It further explicitly acknowledges that perceptions of intense pain and/or substantial disability may be associated with minimal evidence of structural pathology (Deyo, 1986) or that symptoms of depression or anxiety disorder may develop at varying levels of pain (Banks & Kerns, 1996; Kerns & Haythornthwaite, 1988; Haythornthwaite, Seiber, & Kerns, 1991).

According to the model, the multidimensional experience of chronic pain develops and persists as a function of the interaction of specific diatheses and challenges, or stressors. According to the model, the experience of pain, disability, or distress may develop in situations in which available resources are outstripped by the specific challenges or problems posed in association with the experience of persistent pain. Conversely, negative outcomes of the experience of pain may be minimized to the extent that available resources or strengths of the individual and family are well matched and successful in meeting the specific challenges posed by the pain problem.

Consistent with its roots in social learning theory, the diathesis–stress model of chronic pain emphasizes that the entire developmental process occurs in its social context. As already noted, this context includes the family, as well as other important social systems. Resources to meet the challenges of pain, and, conversely, vulnerabilities, develop through interactions with these systems. At the individual level, adaptive cognitive and behavioral coping skills, for example, are hypothesized to be conditioned or learned as a function of the specific reinforcement contingencies manifested by the family and its members. Through a similar process, the family's resources develop and are refined as a function of its interactions with other relevant social systems. Appraisals of these resources and their availability, as well as appraisals of the pain problem itself, occur within these contexts as well. Family perspectives on these processes consistently emphasize the critical if not defining role of the family in determining these appraisals. Ultimately, the individual's and family's efforts to solve the problems posed, including the consideration of alternative responses, the selection of specific responses, and evaluations of the effectiveness of the responses, occurs within these social learning environments.

As a learning model, the response of the family and its members contingent on the behavioral manifestations of the individual's experience of pain is hypothesized to be critical in determining the future responses of the individual (Fordyce, 1976). However, as a complex, multidimensional, and dynamic model of the development of chronic pain, the family's response to one set of discrete observable behaviors (e.g., pain behaviors such as grimacing or complaining of pain) may have unexpected direct and indirect effects on another behavioral domain (e.g., the affective response). The model, therefore, may aid in understanding the observed positive effects of a family's response on one domain while adversely affecting another. For example, it has been observed that individuals' perceptions of support from family members are associated with a decreased frequency of depressive symptoms while simultaneously being associated with increased reports of pain and disability (e.g., Turk, Kerns, & Rosenberg, 1992). Thus theory and supporting empirical evidence encourages behavioral specificity when examining the impact of the family on the chronic pain experience.

As described in the preceding discussion, the cognitive-behavioral transactional model suggests that identifiable cognitive schemata and processes that are relatively characteristic of the family may predict the family's response to discrete behavioral manifestations of the experience of pain. Also consistent with the multidimensional model of chronic pain, however, it may be reasonable to predict that different beliefs and attitudes may underlie the family's responses to differing behaviors on the part of the individual with pain. For example, the family may respond in a relatively solicitous manner to expressions of suffering as a function of beliefs consistent with an acute model of pain and associated caregiving roles. At the same time, family members may encourage continued work functioning consistent with attitudes about family responsibility and fear of financial loss. This perspective encourages assessment of the family members' behavioral responses, as well as their underlying beliefs and attitudes. Attention to family members' appraisals of the meaning of the responses of others may be particularly important.

Unfortunately, to date, specific measures of family appraisals and beliefs informed by the cognitive-behavioral perspective have not been developed. Recent advances in the cognitive-behavioral marital literature, such as measures of causal attributions for spouse communication, may prove to be useful in assessing family cognition. Adaptation of measures informed by the family adjustment and adaptation model might also prove useful (e.g., the Family Environment Scale; Moos & Moos, 1981).

EMPIRICAL EVIDENCE

The models just described are clear in proposing that both the individual's experience of chronic pain, as well as the family's response, will be multiply and reciprocally determined. Theory and available data encourage a multidimensional analysis of the chronic pain experience and further reveal that, for example, the persistence of pain is not necessarily predictive of significant disability or affective distress. Similarly, the cognitive-behavioral transactional model predicts that the family's response will be a function of a complex array of appraisals of the individual's observable behavioral manifestations of the chronic pain experience. Thus predictions that chronic pain in a family member will inevitably be associated with family dysfunction and distress are not consistent with this model.

Investigation of the functioning of the family and its members in the presence of an individual member experiencing chronic pain are indeed inconclusive. Although some studies have offered evidence of marital and sexual dysfunction, increased prevalence of psychophysiological disorders, heightened emotional distress and depressive symptoms among the partners of individuals

with chronic pain (e.g., Ahern, Adams, & Follick, 1985; Feuerstein, Sult, & Houle, 1985; Flor, Turk, & Scholz, 1987; Maruta, Osborne, Swenson, & Holling, 1981; Mohamed, Weisz, & Waring, 1978), others have not found evidence of dysfunction or distress (e.g., Revenson & Majerovitz, 1990; Deyo, 1986). Methodological shortcomings of these studies (e.g., lack of adequate controls) and their generally descriptive nature compromise confidence in any conclusions that might be drawn. Research on the impact of chronic pain on the family informed explicitly by either family systems or cognitive-behavioral transactional family perspectives is in its infancy (e.g., Elliot, Trief, & Stein, 1986; Kopp et al., 1995; Thomas & Roy, 1989). Efforts to identify individual difference variables and/or theory-based and reliable variables related to family functioning that moderate or mediate the family's response may prove to be particularly fruitful avenues for future research.

The cognitive-behavioral transactional model predicts that the response of the individual to the challenges associated with the onset of pain will be significantly influenced by the family's appraisals of the behaviors exhibited by the individual and, ultimately, by the family's response. Also consistent with the multidimensional model of chronic pain just described, the family's appraisals and responses may differentially affect the varying dimensions of the individual's experience of chronic pain. Efforts to characterize the family's response as either adaptive or maladaptive in a global sense are inconsistent with this multidimensional perspective. Rather, judgments about the family's appraisals and responses, as well as the family's attitudes and beliefs that influence these processes, should be based on the observed relationships between the family's response and measures of the individual's cognition and behavioral manifestations of the chronic pain experience.

Empirical research investigating the influence of the family on the individual's adaptation to chronic pain has begun to proliferate over the past 15 years. The focus of this research has largely been restricted to the role of spouses, for both practical reasons and reasons of parsimony, and because of the presumed primary importance of this dyadic relationship. These studies have specifically been informed by operant formulations of chronic pain that hypothesize a key role of positive social reinforcement contingent on demonstrations of pain in the perpetuation of pain and disability (Fordyce, 1976). According to this model, families, and particularly spouses, are hypothesized to play a central role due to the presumed high frequency of interaction with the individual family member experiencing chronic pain and because of their high reinforcement potential. Specifically, expressions of pain, termed pain behaviors, such as complaints of pain and incapacity, withdrawal and inactivity, and paraverbal expressions such as moaning or sighing, are hypothesized to be maintained by attention and explicit positive responses of significant others contingent on their expression, even in the absence of continued nociception.

Results to date are highly consistent with this behavioral model. Numerous studies document significant positive relationships between perceived spouse solicitousness and reports of pain intensity (e.g., Block, Kremer, & Gaylor, 1980; Flor, Kerns, & Turk, 1987; Flor, Turk, & Rudy, 1989; Kerns, Haythornthwaite, Southwick, & Giller, 1990; Kerns & Turk, 1984; Lousberg, Schmidt, & Groenman, 1992; Turk et al., 1992), reports of pain behavior frequency (Kerns et al., 1991), observed pain behavior frequency (Lousberg et al., 1992; Paulsen & Altmaier, 1995; Romano et al., 1992), and reports of inactivity, behavioral interference, and disability (Flor, Kerns, & Turk, 1987; Kerns & Turk, 1984; Turk et al., 1992). Consistent with multidimensional models of pain, depressive symptom severity and reports of affective distress have been reported to be more reliably related to frequency of negative pain-relevant responding from the spouse (e.g., Kerns et al., 1990; Kerns et al., 1991) and inversely related to the presence of spousal support (Brown, Wallston, & Nicassio, 1989; Kerns & Turk, 1984).

Global marital satisfaction appears to have a strong and reliable moderating role on these relationships. On the one hand, studies have been consistent in failing to identify a relationship between global marital satisfaction and reports of pain and disability. However, the relationship between degree of perceived solicitousness and these variables appears to be magnified in the context of a more generally positive relationship. It may be that pain-relevant support is more reinforcing when it is delivered by a spouse who is generally positive and reinforcing (Kerns & Weiss, 1994). On the other hand, the relationship between negative responding to pain and depressive symptom severity appears to be manifested only in the context of a more generally distressing relationship. Alternatively, it may be that a globally satisfying relationship and the availability of alternative sources of positive reinforcement from the spouse serves to buffer the individual experiencing chronic pain

from the otherwise deleterious effects of pain-specific negative responding (Goldberg, Kerns, & Rosenberg, 1993; Kerns et al., 1990; Kerns & Turk, 1984; Kerns & Weiss, 1994).

Kerns and Weiss (1994) have articulated four specific avenues for future research in this area. First, these authors argue for the use of direct observation methods for assessing the role of family interactions in the perpetuation of pain such as those described by Romano and her colleagues (Romano et al., 1991). At the very least, reports of other family members should be used to supplement the reports of the individual experiencing chronic pain (Kerns & Rosenberg, 1995).

Second, complex patterns of pain-relevant interactions should be examined in addition to the main effects of more general categories of significant-other responding. In one study, Weiss and Kerns (1995) reported that, depending on the specific criterion measure examined (i.e., pain severity, disability, depression), regression models that incorporated all possible interaction terms among measures of solicitous, distracting, and negative pain-relevant responding, as well as a measure of global marital satisfaction, accounted for up to 33% of the variance. As one example, pain intensity was highest among individuals who reported a high frequency of both positive *and* negative pain-relevant responding. This pattern is possibly understood by considering the power of intermittent or variable schedules of reinforcement.

Theoretical and empirical advances in the cognitive-behavioral marital literature have encouraged attention to individuals' appraisals of the meaning and perceived intent of their spouses' responses (Bradbury & Fincham, 1990). Attention to similar cognitive appraisal processes in the chronic pain literature is a third specific recommendation. For example, it may be that an individual's appraisal of the positive nature of a spouse's response will vary depending on the perceived intent of the response. Conversely, the causal attributions of spouses for the behavior of their partners, their beliefs about the effectiveness of available responses, and appraisals of their roles in relation to their partners may all be expected to influence their responses. Development of reliable measures to assess these dimensions will be necessary prior to examination of these hypotheses.

Finally, research in this area must move away from its sole focus on dyadic relationships toward a more integrative examination of the role of family functioning. Again, operationalization and measurement of key constructs currently appears to remain a stumbling block to systematic investigation. Measures informed by family systems and family stress models, however, should be evaluated for their behavioral specificity, refined or modified, if necessary, and potentially utilized as a point for initiating this line of important research.

Additional areas of investigation can also be cited. One area of potential importance is the examination of the effects of perceived stress or conflict among family members and perceptions of pain and pain behaviors (Schwartz, Slater, & Birchler, 1994). A second is the examination of psychophysiological responding and its role in mediating the responses of significant others (e.g., Stampler, Wall, Cassisi, & Davis, 1997). Continued efforts to clarify the constructs of support and solicitousness in the context of the family and chronic pain may prove to be particularly important in accounting for apparent inconsistencies in this literature and advancing the field (e.g., Paulsen & Altmaier, 1995; Turk et al., 1992).

Perhaps most remarkable is the observation that, to date, there have been no published reports on controlled investigations of the efficacy of family therapy for chronic pain. Only a few have examined the effectiveness of couple treatment (Moore & Chaney, 1985; Radojevic, Nicassio, & Weisman, 1992; Saarijarvi, 1991), and, in these studies, the incremental value of couple treatment relative to individual treatment remained unclear. The most sophisticated of these studies is that published by Radojevic and her colleagues. In this controlled and otherwise well-designed study, a behavioral-oriented couple treatment was designed that incorporated education of spouses to cue and reinforce home practice of relaxation exercises, activities, and constructive reappraisals. Unfortunately, despite evidence of incremental effectiveness immediately posttreatment relative to individual treatment and nonspecific couple treatment, these advantages were not present at follow-up. Nevertheless, this study and the couple-treatment approach evaluated is encouraging and serves as a model for future research. Future efforts to develop and evaluate family, or at least couple, treatment of chronic pain that is informed by contemporary family theory is strongly encouraged.

COGNITIVE-BEHAVIORAL FAMILY THERAPY FOR CHRONIC PAIN

Family therapy based on the cognitive-behavioral transactional model of family functioning should follow guidelines similar to those that have been frequently articulated for individual cognitive-behavioral treatment. The key refinement is, of course, the characterization of the family system as the primary unit of analysis and focus. This focus is certainly not new either, having been encouraged as the appropriate perspective for health care problems in general (Litman, 1974; Turk & Kerns, 1985), as well as for chronic pain more specifically (Karoly, 1985). However, as noted by Kerns and Payne (1996), this family perspective on the management of chronic pain is clearly contrary to contemporary clinical practice.

Before proceeding, it is important to realize that involvement of the family commonly is limited to some subset of members, most often a single member such as the spouse or live-in partner or an adult child or parent. Close friends, particularly someone with whom the individual lives or shares frequent activities, may act as a surrogate for a more typical portrait of the family. Principles described below for "family" treatment are similarly indicated for any situation involving more persons than the individual experiencing chronic pain.

A family focus of pain treatment has several implications for the therapeutic goals and process. Goals of family treatment ultimately emphasize the family's overall adjustment and accommodation to the problems associated with a family member's experience of pain. Consistent with individual cognitive-behavioral treatment approaches, treatment is designed to (1) encourage reappraisal of the problems of chronic pain that reduce the experience of stress and challenge, (2) reinforce existing effective coping and problem solving, and (3) promote the development of additional resources. Adoption of a constructive and flexible approach to problem solving specific to each family is encouraged in order to achieve specified goals for treatment and to promote continued health, adaptive functioning, and affective well-being beyond the termination of active treatment. Adoption of a chronic-illness perspective to the problem of chronic pain is encouraged to promote long-term maintenance of treatment gains and incorporation of a self-management approach into the life of the family.

These family-oriented goals are, of course, in addition to goals related to the health of the individual family member experiencing chronic pain. The multidimensional model of chronic pain encourages simultaneous attention to several goals. These are to promote optimal (1) management of the illness or structural pathology presumed to be associated with nociception (e.g., adherence to medication and exercise prescriptions), (2) pain control, (3) functioning across multiple domains, and (4) emotional well-being. Finally, goals such as improved mood and productive functioning may be established for other individual family members.

The process of family therapy involves constant attention to the dynamic and reciprocal relationships among family members, as well as to interactions with social systems external to the family. At times the clinician may focus on one dyadic pair, for example, the marital relationship, while at the same time continuing to reframe these interactions within a family context. The clinician is challenged to attend to and frame feedback in terms of "chains" of reciprocal interactions. A unidirectional focus that stands the risk of inferring causality should be avoided. Also consistent with this perspective, the clinician works to encourage participation of each family member. Individual members' perspectives are valued and specifically acknowledged, while at the same time the clinician attempts to identify shared beliefs, attitudes, coping skills, problem-solving processes, and so forth.

A model that integrates the cognitive-behavioral transactional model of family functioning and a multidimensional model of chronic pain encourages a multidimensional and multimodal approach to assessment and the design of effective interventions. The model specifies several targets for assessment, such as the domains of the chronic pain experience, as well as appraisals of additional challenges or problems posed by this ongoing experience and resources available to meet these challenges. The family perspective emphasizes the importance of assessing the experience of the family and its members with regard to each of these variables in order to develop a more comprehensive and integrative conceptualization. As a dynamic and learning-based model, this perspective encourages attention to the transactions of the family over time, including direct observation of current general and pain-specific interactions. Finally, the model highlights the importance of assessing attitudes, beliefs, and attributions, as well as the behavioral and affective responses shared among family members.

The integrative model is also used to inform a hypothesis-generation and hypothesis-testing approach to clinical assessment, conceptualization, and treatment planning and treatment delivery. The clinician enters the clinical situation with prior hypotheses about the nature of the problems experienced by the individual and family (e.g., presence of significant disability on the part of the in-

dividual experiencing chronic pain) based on documented base rates of these problems. Numerous theory- and research-based hypotheses about possible contributors to these problems are also considered (e.g., disability is maintained by a high rate of solicitous responding by family members). These hypotheses are used to inform general methods and targets for assessment. As the assessment process proceeds, these hypotheses are either supported, discarded, or refined, leading to alterations in the subsequent assessment process. This process leads to the development of an integrative conceptualization of the problems experienced by the family and its members and the likely contributing or maintaining factors. A prescriptive approach to treatment planning based on this conceptualization and incorporating empirically supported interventions is then undertaken (Kerns, 1994). Evaluation of the effectiveness of specific treatment components ultimately provides support for the conceptualization or encourages further revision and alternative interventions.

Clinical assessment typically begins with a broad clinical interview designed to scan each of the relevant domains of the experience of chronic pain, relevant historical factors, and ongoing challenges or problems. As hypotheses emerge about potential contributing factors, the interview becomes increasingly narrow and focused in an effort to gather information relevant to the hypotheses. In addition to the family's views of the nature of the pain problem itself, emphasis is placed on other dimensions of members' experience, including their causal attributions, expectations for recovery, and perceived effects on the family. Care should be taken to involve each family member in the discussion and reflection when there appear to be a shared "family view" and when there appear to be individual differences in perspectives. Standardized questionnaires, inventories, diaries, and other self-monitoring procedures are commonly used to supplement the interviewing process.

Goals for treatment and strategies and processes to accomplish the goals are determined via a process of active collaborative discussion involving the family and clinician. The clinician initiates this process by offering specific feedback about the results of the evaluation. Feedback from the family is elicited in an effort to engage the family in a process leading to a shared conceptualization of the problem and likely contributing factors. Consistent with a multidimensional perspective on chronic pain and the added complexities associated with a family emphasis, a potentially large number of targets for intervention may be identified. It is important to emphasize that goals may target the individual experiencing chronic pain (e.g., improved sleep, medication reduction), other individual family members (e.g., increased frequency of activities away from home, otherwise labeled "respite"), and the family unit (e.g., increased frequency of family activities). Through an active process of problem identification, negotiation, and decision making, a hierarchical list of goals and treatment strategies can be developed. Most often this process leads to an identification of a few key processes that are hypothesized to play important roles in perpetuating several problems. Ultimately, success of this process is contingent on the ability of the clinician to help the family develop a consensus plan for intervention. Expectations about family members' participation, including expectations for attendance at treatment sessions and roles and responsibilities during and outside of therapy, should be specified before proceeding.

The overall process and therapeutic techniques employed are similar to those articulated for individual cognitive-behavior therapy for chronic pain (Turk et al., 1983). Several specific refinements of these strategies to take advantage of the involvement of the family can be articulated as well. More detailed elaboration of these strategies for couples and families is available elsewhere (e.g., Jacobson & Gurman, 1995).

Central to the therapeutic process and to the primary goals of individual and family adjustment and well-being are efforts to promote accurate appraisals of problems and available resources. Although initiated during the assessment and reconceptualization phases, this process continues early in treatment through more directed and explicit discussion. Examples of these discussions include the "meaning" of perceived changes and losses within the family, such as fears related to financial burden, anger associated with increased responsibilities of other family members, concern about the impact on children, and generally heightened distress. Perceptions of helplessness among family members and perceptions of burden experienced by the member with chronic pain are particularly common and are important to address. Discussions promoting more accurate and adaptive reframing of specific problems, consideration of alternative solutions to these problems, and specification of plans for action can then be promoted. These discussions usually are followed by a consensus to incorporate some of these specific plans and goals into the treatment process.

Woven throughout the discussions with the family members about their concerns and understanding of the problems of chronic pain is explicit patient and family education about alternative models for understanding the problems and about potentially effective strategies for intervention. A broad array of information may appropriately be provided. Specific information and discussion about any of the theoretical models outlined in this chapter, for example, may be indicated. Most often it is useful to at least offer information about models that encourage chronic-illness and multidimensional perspectives on chronic pain, to replace unidimensional (i.e., sensory, pain-focused) and acute illness (i.e., pain as an indication for medical attention) models. Theoretical and intuitively compelling links between the experience of pain and other frequent concomitants and sequelae can be described with specific reference to data elicited from the family members.

Three particularly common and potentially useful models can be described. One is the link between pain, decline in activity, and deconditioning and increased pain with activity. A second emphasizes understandable mediators between pain and depressive symptoms, including decline in pleasurable and constructive activity and developing perceptions of helplessness and hopelessness. A third is the role of stress and negative emotions in fostering exacerbations in the experience of pain. The process of education and collaborative discussion of these and other models often contributes to a rapid reduction in the family's distress, and concerns are "normalized." Development of perceptions of understanding and clarification of a credible plan for action encourage enhanced perceptions of self-efficacy and optimism for improved outcomes. Development of a common language for further discussions and further elaboration of goals within these explanatory frameworks are additional benefits of this process.

Central to the cognitive-behavioral transactional model is the focus on communication within the family. Theory and research reviewed in this chapter have led to the identification of several common "patterns" of family, or at least dyadic, communication that may contribute to or potentiate the experience of pain, disability, and distress, if not the underlying disease or pathology itself. These patterns can range from families who appear to be highly solicitous in responding to expressions of pain and incapacity to those who evidence an inconsistent pattern of responding to those that are pervasively negative. Explicit targeting of hypothesized maladaptive patterns of communication is, therefore, a critical component of effective family therapy for chronic pain. Ultimately, theory and research encourage efforts to reduce pain-specific communication, to reduce negative communication of a pain-specific or more general nature, and to promote positive, constructive communication, especially communication that encourages effective problem solving, active listening, and assertiveness. Application of cognitive and behavioral strategies for communication training to facilitate these efforts is encouraged (Flor, Turk, & Rudy, 1987b).

Family members may also be invited to play key roles in cuing and reinforcing adaptive coping behaviors and steps toward identified goals. To maximize these efforts, the family is explicitly taught the language and basic principles of behavior modification. Behavioral rehearsal of appropriate responses, negotiation of specific goals, and contingency contracting among family members are particularly relevant techniques. These same strategies can be used to promote acquisition and practice of recommended self-management skills such as home practice of relaxation, exercise and activity goals, and intersession tasks assigned by the clinician. It is important to note that these strategies are unlikely to be appropriate in the context of a highly distressed family lacking in strong reinforcement potential.

Use of similar strategies to those just reviewed are potentially important avenues for targeting symptoms of depressive and anxiety disorders, marital dysfunction, anger control problems, and other concomitant behavioral problems. The presence of other chronic illnesses and their impact should also be addressed. Finally, chronic pain and other medical and psychological problems experienced by other family members are equally important targets for intervention.

SUMMARY AND CONCLUSION

Contemporary theory of chronic pain and pain treatment and a growing body of empirical evidence encourage explicit attention to if not inclusion of the family in efforts to promote adaptation and adjustment to the experience of chronic pain. To date, however, despite the availability of relatively specific guidelines for such treatment, empirical tests of the efficacy of such approaches, especially compared to individual treatment approaches, have been few and inconclusive. A growing awareness of the limitations of individual treatment should

offer a further inducement to pursue the option of family treatment.

REFERENCES

Ahern, D., Adams, A., & Follick, M. (1985). Emotional and marital disturbance in spouses of chronic low back pain patients. *Clinical Journal of Pain, 1*, 69–74.

Banks, S. M., & Kerns, R. D. (1996). Explaining high rates of depression in chronic pain: A diathesis–stress framework. *Psychological Bulletin, 119*, 95–110.

Block, A., Kremer, E., & Gaylor, M. (1980). Behavioral treatment of chronic pain: The spouse as a discriminative cue for pain behavior. *Pain, 9*, 243–252.

Bradbury, T. N., & Fincham, F. D. (1990). Attribution in marriage: Review and critique. *Psychological Bulletin, 107*, 3–33.

Breunlin, D. C. (1989). Clinical implications of oscillation theory: Family development and the process of change. In C. N. Ramsey (Ed.), *Family systems in medicine*. New York: Guilford Press.

Brown, G. K., Wallston, K. A., & Nicassio, P. M. (1989). Social support and depression in rheumatoid arthritis. *Journal of Applied Social Psychology, 19*, 1164–1181.

Deyo, R. A. (1986). The early diagnostic evaluation of patients with low back pain. *Journal of General Internal Medicine, 1*, 328–338.

Elliot, D. J., Trief, P. M., & Stein, N. (1986). Mastery, stress, and coping in marriage among chronic pain patients. *Journal of Behavioral Medicine, 9*, 549–558.

Feuerstein, M., Sult, S., & Houle, M. (1985). Environmental stressors and chronic low back pain: Life events, family and work environment. *Pain, 22*, 295–307.

Fincham, F. D., & Bradbury, T. N. (Eds.). (1990). *The psychology of marriage: Basic issues and applications*. New York: Guilford Press.

Flor, H., Birbaumer, N., & Turk, D. C. (1990). The psychobiology of chronic pain. *Advances in Behavioral Research and Therapy, 12*, 47–84.

Flor, H., Kerns, R. D., & Turk, D. C. (1987). The role of spouse reinforcement, perceived pain and activity levels of chronic pain patients. *Journal of Psychosomatic Research, 31*, 251–259.

Flor, H., Turk, D. C., & Rudy, T. E. (1987a). Pain and families: I. Etiology, maintenance and psychosocial impact. *Pain, 30*, 3–27.

Flor, H., Turk, D. C., & Rudy, T. E. (1987b). Pain and families: II. Assessment and treatment. *Pain, 30*, 29–45.

Flor, H., Turk, D. C., & Rudy, T. E. (1989). Relationship of pain impact and significant other reinforcement of pain behaviors: The mediating role of gender, marital status and marital satisfaction. *Pain, 38*, 45–50.

Flor, H., Turk, D. C., & Scholz, O. B. (1987). Impact of chronic pain on the spouse: Marital, emotional, and physical consequences. *Journal of Psychosomatic Research, 31*, 63–71.

Fordyce, W. E. (1976). *Behavioral methods for chronic pain and illness*. St. Louis, MO: Mosby.

Fordyce, W. E. (1988). Pain and suffering: A reappraisal. *American Psychologist, 43*, 276–283.

Goldberg, G. M., Kerns, R. D., & Rosenberg, R. (1993). Pain relevant support as a buffer from depression among chronic pain patients low in instrumental activity. *Clinical Journal of Pain, 9,* 34–40.

Haythornthwaite, J., Seiber, W. J., & Kerns, R. D. (1991). Depression in the chronic pain experience. *Pain, 46,* 177–184.

Hill, R. (1949). *Families under stress.* New York: Harper & Row.

Jacobson, N. S., & Gurman, A. S. (Eds.). (1995). *Clinical handbook of couple therapy.* New York: Guilford Press.

Jacobson, N. S., & Margolin, G. (1979). *Marital therapy: Strategies based on social learning and behavior exchange principles.* New York: Brunner/Mazel.

Karoly, P. (1985). Assessment of pain: Concepts and procedures. In P. Karoly (Ed.), *Measurement strategies in health psychology.* New York: Wiley.

Keefe, F. J., Dunsmore, J., & Burnett, R. (1992). Behavioral and cognitive-behavioral approaches to chronic pain: Recent advances and future directions. *Journal of Consulting and Clinical Psychology, 60,* 528–536.

Keefe, F. J., Gil, K. M., & Rose, S. C. (1986). Behavioral approaches in the multidisciplinary management of chronic pain: Programs and issues. *Clinical Psychology Review, 6,* 87–113.

Kerns, R. D. (1994). Pain management. In M. Hersen & R. T. Ammerman (Eds.), *Handbook of prescriptive treatments for adults.* New York: Plenum Press.

Kerns, R. D. (1995). Family assessment in intervention in chronic illness. In P. Nicassio & T. Smith (Eds.), *Managing chronic illness: A biopsychosocial perspective.* Washington, DC: American Psychological Association.

Kerns, R. D. (1996). Psychosocial factors: Primary or secondary outcomes? In J. N. Campbell & M. J. Mitchell (Eds.), *Pain treatment centers at a crossroads: A conceptual reappraisal.* Seattle, WA: IASP Press.

Kerns, R. D., & Haythornthwaite, J. A. (1988). Depression among chronic pain patients: Cognitive-behavioral analysis and effect on rehabilitation outcome. *Journal of Consulting and Clinical Psychology, 56,* 870–876.

Kerns, R. D., Haythornthwaite, J., Southwick, S., & Giller, E. L. (1990). The role of marital interaction in chronic pain and depressive symptom severity. *Journal of Psychosomatic Research, 34,* 401–408.

Kerns, R. D., & Jacob, M. C. (1995). Toward an integrative diathesis–stress model of chronic pain. In A. J. Goreczny (Ed.), *Handbook of health and rehabilitation psychology.* New York: Plenum Press.

Kerns, R. D., & Payne, A. (1996). Treating families of chronic pain patients. In R. J. Gatchel & D. C. Turk (Eds.), *Psychological approaches to pain management: A practitioner's handbook.* New York: Guilford Press.

Kerns, R. D., & Rosenberg, R. (1995). Pain-relevant responses from significant others: Development of a significant-other version of the WHYMPI scales. *Pain, 61,* 245–249.

Kerns, R. D., Southwick, S., Giller, E. L., Haythornthwaite, J., Jacob, M. C., & Rosenberg, R. (1991). The relationship between reports of pain-related social interactions and expressions of pain and affective distress. *Behavior Therapy, 22,* 101–111.

Kerns, R. D., & Turk, D. C. (1984). Depression and chronic pain: The mediating role of the spouse. *Journal of Marriage and the Family, 46,* 845–852.

Kerns, R. D., & Weiss, L. H. (1994). Family influences on

the course of chronic illness: A cognitive-behavioral transactional model. *Annals of Behavioral Medicine, 16,* 116–130.

Kopp, M., Richter, R., Rainer, J., Kopp-Wilfling, P., Rumpold, G., & Walter, M. H. (1995). Differences in family functioning between patients with chronic headache and patients with chronic low back pain. *Pain, 63,* 219–224.

Levine, S., & Kozloff, M. A. (1978). The sick role: Assessment and overview. *Annual Review of Sociology, 4,* 317–343.

Litman, T. J. (1974). The family as basic unit in health and medical care: A social-behavioral overview. *Social Science and Medicine, 8,* 495–519.

Litman, T. J., & Venters, M. (1979). Research on health care and the family: A methodological review. *Social Science and Medicine 13,* 379–385.

Lousberg, R., Schmidt, A. J. M., & Groenman, N. H. (1992). The relationship between spouse solicitousness and pain behavior: Searching for more experimental evidence. *Pain, 51,* 75–79.

Maruta, T., Osborne, D., Swenson, D. W., & Holling, J. M. (1981). Chronic pain patients and spouses: Marital and sexual adjustment. *Mayo Clinic Procedures, 56,* 307–310.

Minuchin, S. (1974). *Families and family therapy.* Cambridge, MA: Harvard University Press.

Mohamed, S. N., Weisz, G. N., & Waring, E. M. (1978). The relationship of chronic pain to depression, marital adjustment, and family dynamics. *Pain, 5,* 285–292.

Moore, J. E., & Chaney, E. F. (1985). Outpatient group treatment of chronic pain. *Journal of Consulting and Clinical Psychology, 53,* 326–334.

Moos, R., & Moos, B. (1981). *Family Environment Scale Manual.* Palo Alto, CA: Consulting Psychologists Press.

Olson, D. H. (1989). Circumflex model and family health. In C. N. Ramsey (Ed.), *Family systems in medicine.* New York: Guilford Press.

Olson, D. H., Sprenkle, D., & Russell, C. (1979). Circumplex model of marital and family systems: I. Cohesion and adaptability dimensions, family types, and clinical applications. *Family Process 18,* 3–28.

Parsons, T. (1951). *The social system.* New York: Free Press.

Patterson, J. M. (1989). A family stress model: The family adjustment and adaptation response. In C. N. Ramsey (Ed.), *Family systems in medicine.* New York: Guilford Press.

Patterson, J. M., & Garwick, A. W. (1994). The impact of chronic illness on families: A family systems perspective. *Annals of Behavioral Medicine, 16,* 131–142.

Paulsen, J. S., & Altmaier, E. M. (1995). The effects of perceived versus enacted social support on the discriminative cue function of spouses for pain behaviors. *Pain, 60,* 103–110.

Payne, B., & Norfleet, M. A. (1986). Chronic pain and the family: A review. *Pain, 26,* 1–22.

Radojevic, V., Nicassio, P. M., & Weisman, M. H. (1992). Behavioral intervention with and without family support for rheumatoid arthritis. *Behavior Therapy, 23,* 13–30.

Ramsey, C. N., Jr. (Ed.). (1989). *Family systems in medicine.* New York: Guilford Press.

Reiss, D. (1989). Families and their paradigms: An ecologic approach to understanding the family in its social world. In C. N. Ramsey (Ed.), *Family systems in medicine*. New York: Guilford Press.

Revenson, T. A., & Majerovitz, S. D. (1990). Spouses' support provision to chronically ill patients. *Journal of Social and Personal Relationships, 7,* 575–586.

Romano, J. M., Turner, J. A., Friedman, L. S., Bulcroft, R. A., Jensen, M. P., & Hops, H. (1991). Observational assessment of chronic pain patient–spouse behavioral interactions. *Behavior Therapy, 22,* 549–567.

Romano, J. M., Turner, J. A., Friedman, L. S., Bulcroft, R. A., Jensen, M. P., Hops, H., & Wright, S. F. (1992). Sequential analysis of chronic pain behaviors and spouse responses. *Journal of Consulting and Clinical Psychology, 60,* 777–782.

Roy, R. (1992). *The social context of the chronic pain sufferer.* Toronto: University of Toronto Press.

Saarijarvi, S. (1991). A controlled study of couple therapy in chronic low back pain patients: Effects of marital satisfaction, psychological distress and health attitudes. *Journal of Psychosomatic Research, 35,* 265–272.

Schwartz, L., Slater, M. A., & Birchler, G. R. (1994). Interpersonal stress and pain behaviors in patients with chronic pain. *Journal of Consulting and Clinical Psychology, 62,* 861–864.

Stampler, D. B., Wall, J. R., Cassisi, J. E., & Davis, H. (1997). Marital satisfaction and psychophysiological responsiveness in spouses of patients with chronic pain. *International Journal of Rehabilitation and Health, 3,* 159–170.

Thomas, M., & Roy, R. (1989). Pain patients and marital relations. *Clinical Journal of Pain, 5,* 255–259.

Turk, D. C., & Kerns, R. D. (1985). *Health, illness and families: A life span perspective.* New York: Wiley.

Turk, D. C., Kerns, R. D., & Rosenberg, R. (1992). Effects of marital interaction on chronic pain and disability: Examining the down side of social support. *Rehabilitation Psychology, 37,* 259–274.

Turk, D. C., Meichenbaum, D., & Genest, M. (1983). *Pain and behavioral medicine: A cognitive–behavioral perspective.* New York: Guilford Press.

Weiss, L. H., & Kerns, R. D. (1995). Patterns of pain-relevant social interactions. *International Journal of Behavioral Medicine, 2,* 157–171.

Chapter 29

Evaluation of Treatment Effectiveness in Patients with Intractable Pain: Measures and Methods

RAYMOND C. TAIT

The evaluation of treatment effectiveness is a topic of increasing importance in applied pain research for a combination of financial, clinical, and theoretical reasons. Financial impetus comes from insurance carriers and employers who demand data regarding the benefits likely to accrue from dollars expended (Kulich & Lande, 1997; Webster & Snook, 1994). Clinical impetus comes from a growing need to identify components of treatment necessary for successful outcomes to occur (Bloch, 1987; North, Ewend, Lawton, & Piantadosi, 1991). Outcome assessment hinges on consideration of conceptual questions, such as what dimensions of the pain experience should be assessed (Turk & Rudy, 1992; Waddell, 1996), and methodologic questions, such as what level of change should be considered clinically meaningful (Slater, Doctor, Pruitt, & Atkinson, 1997). The latter questions cut across both surgical (Taylor, 1989) and nonsurgical treatments (Cutler et al., 1994).

This chapter focuses primarily on these conceptual and methodological questions, not on questions of treatment efficacy for nonsurgical treatment. The latter topic has been extensively and critically reviewed in a number of recent articles (Cutler et al., 1994; Flor, Fydrich, & Turk, 1992; Turk & Rudy, 1990, 1991; Turk, Rudy, & Sorkin, 1993). Obviously, it is impossible to address the area of program evaluation exhaustively in the pages of a single chapter, even when a reasonably narrow focus such as that described above is defined. Hence, readers will be referred throughout the chapter to reviews that more thoroughly summarize particular topics. Thus the overarching goal of this chapter is to summarize critical issues in program evaluation in a manner that can provide a template for the interested reader to use in further exploration of this complex topic.

DIMENSIONS FOR ASSESSMENT

Clinical pain research has occurred without a well-accepted taxonomy to facilitate classification of patients and comparisons among studies (Bonica, 1979; Turk & Rudy, 1992). Although the absence is recognized, attempts to bridge the gap with "framework" (e.g., Staats, Hekmat, & Staats, 1996) or structural (Novy, Nelson, Francis, & Turk, 1995) models have been largely unsuccessful. Thus there are a number of classification schemes that have been proposed, based on both empirical and theoretical strategies, none of which have been universally embraced.

Consequently, no matter how important, the choice of any heuristic to focus attention on particular outcome dimensions is somewhat arbitrary. That having been said, the heuristic used in this chapter is the Glasgow Illness Model (Waddell, 1996). As Figure 29.1 indicates, this model views pain as a biopsychosocial phenomenon involving pain, cognitive mediating events, psychological distress, and disability/illness behavior, all of which interact in the context of a sick role. Aside from its conceptual appeal, several factor analytic studies have demonstrated empirical support for its elements as consistently important elements of the pain experience (DeGagne, Mikail, & D'Eon, 1995; Tait, Chibnall, Duckro, & Deshields, 1989). Moreover, it has provided a useful organization in a previous review of assessment instruments of psychosocial contributors to disability (Tait, 1993).

Aside from its organizational value, the latter model also is interesting to consider in terms of its implications for "consumers" with potentially differing perspectives on program evaluation. For example, a patient is likely to be most interested in and/or satisfied with treatment that can provide reductions in pain and/or ways of coping more effectively with pain (Desbiens et al., 1996). A patient's family may be interested in programs that can provide the patient and family members with improved quality of life (Miaskowski, Zimmer, Barrett, Dibble, & Wallhagen, 1997). A referring physician may be most interested in reduction of health care utilization and/or opioid use (Deathe & Helmes, 1993). An employer is likely to be invested in return to work. An insurance carrier and/or case manager may be interested in cost effectiveness (Kulich & Lande, 1997). Because satisfaction with treatment is greatest when expectations are met (Shutty, DeGood, & Tuttle, 1990),

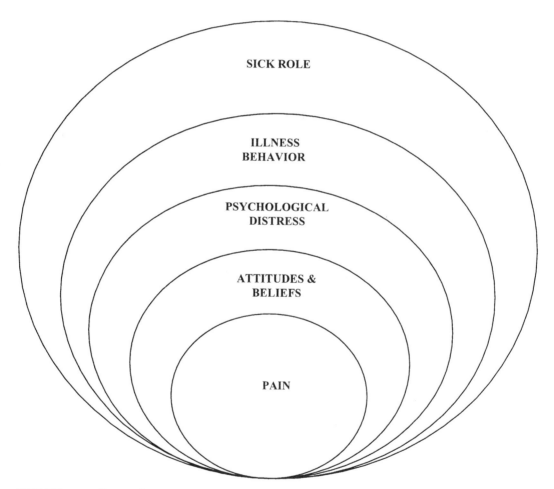

FIGURE 29.1. Glasgow illness model. Adapted from Waddell et al. (1993). Copyright 1993 by Elsevier Science. Adapted by permission.

outcomes that are satisfactory to one set of consumers may not satisfy other consumers with different expectations. To address the needs of each of the consumer groups, outcome assessment must be capable of speaking to each of these perspectives.

The following sections review measures that have been used to assess each of the latter dimensions in the evaluation of multidisciplinary pain treatment. The first section examines measures used to assess nociceptive aspects of pain, including intensity and distribution. The second section reviews instruments that have been used to evaluate attitudes, beliefs, and coping skills. The third section examines measures of psychological adjustment and/or distress. In the fourth section, a variety of self-report and performance measures are reviewed. Finally, measures relevant to the sick role are reviewed, including return to work and health care utilization.

PAIN

Because pain is a complex event, multiple approaches to its assessment have been developed (Turk & Melzack, 1992). In a review of the topic, Jensen and Karoly (1992) classified measures of pain as involving the categories of intensity, affect, and distribution. This section reviews only the measures concerning intensity and distribution, as measures of affect will be considered in a subsequent section. Because there is a vast literature concerning the psychometric properties of instruments used to measure the latter constructs (well beyond the scope of this chapter), the chapter focuses only on the elements of each construct that have implications for outcome assessment. The interested reader is referred to Jensen and Karoly (1992) for a more thorough review of the psychometric literature.

Pain Intensity

Although the clinical significance of self-reported pain intensity has come under fire in recent years (Mayer et al., 1987), measurement of pain intensity was part of every outcome study that I could find, probably because of its clinical salience and relative ease of assessment. Pain intensity has been assessed primarily through self-report measures, although psychophysiological parameters also have been examined (Flor, Miltner, & Birbaumer, 1992). Commonly used measures of pain inten-

sity have included verbal ratings scales, numerical rating scales, and visual analogue scales (Jensen & Karoly, 1992).

Verbal rating scales (VRS) are composed of lists of adjectives ranked in order of the level of pain intensity that they represent. Generally, these measures have demonstrated validity (Jensen, Karoly, & Braver, 1986) and sensitivity to change (Rybstein-Blinchik, 1979). Disadvantages include the ordinal nature of the data that these scales provide and the need for patients to understand the words that compose the lists (Jensen & Karoly, 1992).

The most common, but certainly not the only (e.g., Tursky, Jamner, & Friedman, 1982), VRS measure is the McGill Pain Questionnaire (MPQ; Melzack, 1975). The MPQ is composed of 20 lists of verbal descriptors of sensory, affective, and evaluative dimensions of pain; patients circle a descriptor in each list that best describes their pain. A Pain Rating Index (PRI) has been used to score the sensory subscale: Ranks are assigned to descriptors on lists relevant to that dimension, and the ranks of endorsed descriptors are summed to yield a total score. In addition to the PRI score, the total number of words chosen also can be calculated in order to gauge the general intensity of the patient's pain experience.

The MPQ has been used in numerous studies of pain that have documented its reliability, validity, and sensitivity to change (Melzack & Katz, 1992). While research has shown that the three dimensions it was designed to measure are correlated (Holroyd et al., 1992), its value as a classification tool is well documented, as it has been used to classify patients with different pain syndromes (Melzack, Terrence, Fromm, & Amsel, 1986). Because standard scoring protocols yield ordinal level data, however, it has been recommended that measures such as the PRI be supplemented with measures yielding interval or ratio level data in outcome research (Jensen & Karoly, 1992).

Unlike VRS measures, numerical rating scales (NRS) and visual analogue scales (VAS) yield ratio level data, although the data are generated in different ways. With NRS measures, patients choose a number that reflects level of pain intensity, usually with 0 representing no pain and numbers that range from 10 to 100 representing worst possible or excruciating levels of pain (Jensen, Turner, & Romano, 1994). VAS measures require patients to indicate a point on a line to indicate level of pain, with the line usually anchored with descriptors similar to those described for an NRS measure.

With ratio level data, a reduction in pain from 80/100 at pretreatment to 40/100 at posttreatment can be viewed as a change of 50%, allowing more robust statistical analysis than is available with ordinal level data. VRS and VAS measures have been shown to be valid and sensitive to change (Jensen & Karoly, 1992). Because of their ease of administration and conceptual simplicity, NRS and VAS measures now are commonly used in outcome research.

One question involving NRS measures involves the optimum number of gradations needed to adequately assess intensity. Pain intensity has been measured with scales ranging from as few as four to as many as 101 points (e.g., Jensen, Romano, & Turner, 1994). The latter study examined the comparability of scales of differing ranges in a sample of 124 patients seen in multidisciplinary treatment who rated their worst, least, usual, and current pain levels. High scale correlations ($r > .98$) were found for 11-, 21-, and 101-point scales, whereas scales with lower ranges correlated less well (as low as $r = .59$) with the 101-point measure. More important, the scales with lower ranges were found to be less sensitive to changes in pain severity, a result consistent with previous research (Machin, Lewith, & Wylson, 1988). The authors concluded that patients generally are able to use only 21 points on a scale, and there is little to choose among scales with at least 11 levels of pain intensity.

Because all measures of pain intensity require memory, a matter of more conceptual and methodological concern involves the impact of memory on reported levels of pain intensity. It has been shown that ratings of pain are biased by the patient's pain status at the time that he is asked to recall previous pain intensities (Eich, Rachman, & Lopatka, 1990; Salovey, Smith, Turk, Jobe, & Willis, 1993). Obviously, these memory effects are most pernicious in retrospective treatment designs in which patients are asked to compare their current with their pretreatment status (e.g., Duckro, Margolis, Tait, & Korytnyk, 1985). Even in more sophisticated research designs, however, patients often are asked to estimate usual levels of pain intensity (e.g., Ralphs, Williams, Richardson, Pither, & Nicholas, 1994), a methodology that is susceptible to memory pitfalls.

Several approaches have been suggested to increase the accuracy of pain intensity measurement. Jensen, Turner, Turner, and Romano (1996) compared weekly average ratings of worst, least, and usual pain with data collected through daily pain diaries, a methodology with documented validity for evaluating daily levels of pain and activity (Cruise, Broderick, Porter, Kaell, & Stone, 1996; Follick, Ahern, & Laser-Wolston, 1984). They found that the best single predictor of actual average level of pain over a 2-week period was patient rating of least pain ($r = .81$) and that the best composite predictor was the average of least and usual pain ($r = .87$). Although the correlation was somewhat lower than that for least pain, it is interesting that patient ratings of usual level of pain also correlated reasonably well with actual average level of pain ($r = .78$).

Another approach to developing an accurate measure of actual average level of pain also has been proposed (Jensen & McFarland, 1993). They investigated the frequency and time period over which diary recordings were needed to provide valid indicators of actual average pain. With three daily ratings over a 4-day period, they computed a composite score that had stable, high correlations with actual average pain.

Finally, daily diary ratings of pain have been examined (e.g., Keefe et al., 1997). Patients in the latter study completed daily ratings of pain intensity and a variety of other measures (e.g., measures of coping) over extended periods of time (e.g., 30 days). Rather than decompose the ratings into average numbers, data were examined in a sophisticated, within-subject design that enabled the investigators to identify lagged relations between day-to-day changes in pain and coping. Clearly, this methodology offers the most powerful approach yet to the study of pain intensity.

Although the latter approach is powerful, it is also costly (in terms of finance and labor), so it may not be applicable to many clinical operations interested in collecting outcome data regarding pain intensity. Obviously, other approaches to program evaluation that involve composite scores derived from pain diaries also can provide valid information (Jensen & McFarland, 1993). In fact, reasonably valid data can be derived on a weekly or twice-weekly basis as well (Salovey, Smith, Turk, Jobe, & Willis, 1993). Thus there are a range of options open to clinicians and researchers that can provide useful information on pain intensity as part of program evaluation.

Pain Distribution

Relative to the vast attention given to measurement of pain intensity, that given to pain distribution is markedly less, despite its common use in assessment batteries (e.g., Melzack, 1975). Nonetheless, a number of scoring systems have been developed for measurement of pain distribution. Ransford, Cairns, and Mooney (1976) developed a scoring system in which penalty points were assigned to elements of pain drawings that reflected "psychological involvement" with the pain condition, such as markings outside the body outline or distributed in nondermatomal patterns. Although the penalty point methodology has high interrater reliability (Ransford, Cairns, & Mooney, 1976; Margolis, Tait, & Krause, 1986), it has been criticized on two grounds: (1) the information that it yields overlaps with straightforward measures of pain extent, suggesting that penalty points may be contaminated by the extent of pain (Margolis, Tait, & Krause, 1986); (2) the link between psychological involvement and pain may be complex, such that psychological distress may be a consequence rather than a cause of pain (Wallis, Lord, & Bogduk, 1997).

Other measures of pain distribution have assigned numerical values to pain distributions by measuring the percentage of painful body surface (Margolis, Tait, & Krause, 1986) or by dividing the body into distinct regions and summing the number of regions that patients shade as painful (Toomey, Gover, & Jones, 1983). Such methods have been shown to have high interrater (Margolis, Tait, & Krause, 1986) and test–retest reliability (Margolis, Chibnall, & Tait, 1988) and to correlate with other important dimensions of the pain experience (Tait, Chibnall, & Margolis, 1990; Toomey, Gover, & Jones, 1983).

North, Nigrin, Fowler, Szymanski, and Piantadosi (1992) describe an interesting application of an automated pain drawing procedure to implantable dorsal column stimulation. Using an interactive, computerized technology, patients undergoing electrode placement can indicate areas where they experience stimulation paresthesias relative to their sites of pain. This approach has facilitated optimal placement of electrodes for pain relief. Despite novel applications such as the latter and widespread use of pain drawings, each of which indicates that pain distribution assesses a dimension of pain not tapped by measures of pain intensity, pain drawings have not been assessed systematically in outcome studies. This is certainly an area for further research, especially in anesthesiological, medical, and/or physical therapy-based treatments in which changes in pain are the most frequently assessed barometers of improvement (Feine & Lund, 1997; White & Harth, 1996).

ATTITUDES, BELIEFS, AND COPING RESPONSES

Recent studies have identified attitudes and beliefs as important elements of the pain experience (DeGood & Shutty, 1992; Fernandez & Turk, 1989). Attitudes have been defined as affective responses to a topic, whereas beliefs reflect a person's understanding of the topic (Ajzen & Fishbein, 1977). Each has been distinguished from coping responses, which refer to "purposeful efforts to manage . . . the negative impact of stress" (Jensen, Turner, & Romano, 1991, p. 250). All of the above have been linked to adjustment to pain (Jensen, Turner, Romano, & Lawler, 1994; Strong, Ashton, & Chant, 1992) and to response to treatment (Schwartz, DeGood, & Shutty, 1985; Carosella, Lackner, & Feuerstein, 1994).

Attitudes

The Survey of Pain Attitudes (SOPA; Jensen, Turner, Romano, & Lawler, 1994) has emerged as the major measure of pain-related attitudes. It has been modified several times since it was initially developed (Jensen, Karoly, & Huger, 1987), and it presently includes subscales that assess attitudes toward solicitude, emotionality and pain, likelihood of a medical cure, control over pain, pain as an indicator of bodily harm, pain as disabling, and medication as a preferred treatment for pain. The SOPA has been associated with psychosocial functioning (Jensen & Karoly, 1991; Jensen, Turner, Romano, & Lawler, 1994), levels of physical activity (Jensen & Karoly, 1991), utilization of medical services (Jensen & Karoly, 1992), and with measures of physical disability (Jensen, Turner, Romano, & Lawler, 1994). The major downside of the SOPA involves its length (57 items), although a 30-item version of the SOPA has been developed that may facilitate wider use of the instrument (Tait & Chibnall, 1997).

Beliefs

Beliefs and expectancies also have been linked to treatment outcomes (DeGood & Shutty, 1992). Several measures of beliefs have been developed. The Pain Information and Beliefs Questionnaire (PIBQ), a two-part questionnaire designed to measure knowledge about conservative pain management and a patient's agreement with a conservative treatment philosophy measure, is designed to be administered after exposure to an informational videotape (Schwartz, DeGood, & Shutty, 1985). Degree of agreement has been found to correlate with treatment satisfaction and with level of change in pain and function associated with treatment (Shutty, DeGood, & Tuttle, 1990). Due to its construction, the PIBQ is useful primarily to assess beliefs that mediate responsiveness to treatment.

By contrast, the Pain Beliefs and Perceptions Inventory (PBPI; D. Williams & Thorn, 1989; D. Williams, Robinson, & Geisser, 1994) is a 16-item self-report inventory that is more easily administered. Although the initial study described three subscales (D. Williams & Thorn, 1989), more recent research suggests that it contains four scales: pain as a mystery, self-blame, pain permanence, and pain constancy (Strong, Ashton, & Chant, 1992; D. Williams, Robinson, & Geisser, 1994). Each subscale appears associated with distinct elements of adjustment to pain, suggesting that interventions that change pain beliefs may have functional implications. Unfortunately, this hypothesis has yet to be tested, as beliefs have not yet been the focus of intervention studies.

Self-efficacy beliefs have been defined as the expectancies that a person can produce behaviors likely to yield desirable outcomes (Bandura, 1977). Hence self-efficacy is related to the levels of effort and/or persistence that individuals will demonstrate in executing such behavior. The self-efficacy construct has been investigated in several studies of patients with intractable pain. For example, Dolce, Crocker, Moletteire, and Doleys (1986) measured self-efficacy ratings of patients who were given progressive exercise quotas as part of treatment, finding that self-efficacy increased and ratings of concern about reinjury decreased among patients who completed their quotas. Council, Ahern, Follick, and Kline (1988) measured task-specific efficacy and pain expectations among low back pain patients asked to perform 10 specific movements, finding that both efficacy and pain expectations correlated with performance of exercise.

In light of the relation between performance and self-efficacy/pain expectations, it is not surprising that they have been the focus of outcome studies. Several studies have shown that self-efficacy scores improve with multidisciplinary treatment, with self-efficacy correlated with follow-up measures of work status, medication use, exercise, and self-ratings of improvement (Dolce, Crocker, & Doleys, 1986; Kores, Murphy, Rosenthal, Elias, & North, 1990). In a related line of research, several studies

have focused on pretreatment evaluation of patient expectations regarding their likelihood of returning to work following treatment. Hildebrandt, Pfingsten, Saur, and Jansen (1997) found that self-perceived disability and, especially, patient estimates of their likelihood of returning to work were more predictive of return to work than were measured changes in their functional capacity, a finding supported by other recent work (Carosella, Lackner, & Feuerstein, 1994; Pfingsten, Hildebrandt, Leibing, Franz, & Saur, 1997).

Although self-efficacy is a construct of obvious relevance to outcome assessment, research has been hindered by a relative lack of pain-specific measures of the construct (DeGood & Shutty, 1992). One instrument that has been used is the Arthritis Self-Efficacy scale (ASE), a 20-item self-report measure developed for use with arthritis patients that has shown construct and concurrent validity (Lorig, Chastain, Ung, Shoor, & Holman, 1989). The ASE has three subscales: (1) self-efficacy for physical functioning, (2) self-efficacy for pain control, and (3) self-efficacy for controlling other arthritis symptoms. In a recent study, all three ASE scales were shown to correlate with pain behavior, suggesting that it measures a construct with important implications for behavior (Buckelew et al., 1994). Of course, due to its construction, the ASE is best suited for arthritis patients.

Anderson, Dowds, Pelletz, Edwards, and Peeters-Asdourian (1995) recently developed a 22-item self-efficacy questionnaire designed for the broad pain population, the Chronic Pain Self-Efficacy Scale (CPSS). The scale has three subscales that parallel the ASE: (1) self-efficacy for pain management, (2) self-efficacy for coping with other symptoms, and (3) self-efficacy for physical function. Although the CPSS has shown good psychometric properties across two patient samples used in its development, it has not yet been used as part of an outcome assessment protocol.

It should be noted that there are several other instruments that have been developed for use in assessing pain-related beliefs, although their relations to outcomes have been less studied than the measures discussed here, including the Cognitive Error Questionnaire (Lefebvre, 1981) and the Pain and Impairment Relationship Scale (Riley, Ahern, & Follick, 1988; Slater, Itall, Atkinson, & Garfin, 1991). Similarly, the Multidimensional Health Locus of Control Scale (Wallston, Wallston, & DeVellis, 1978) has been used with chronic pain patients, and there is some evidence of its predictive validity for treatment outcomes with low back pain (Härkäpää, Järvikoski, Mellin, Hurri, & Luoma, 1991). With further research on their relations with outcome, these instruments may have value as part of a program evaluation protocol.

Coping Responses

A vast literature has accumulated regarding coping skills (Jensen, Romano, Turner, & Karoly, 1991), well beyond the scope of this chapter. In general, the literature supports the effectiveness of cognitive coping skills (e.g., imagery) in alleviating pain (Fernandez & Turk, 1989). Although several measures of coping strategies exist that are of potential use in studying coping relevant to pain (e.g., the Ways of Coping questionnaire; Folkman & Lazarus, 1980; the Vanderbilt Pain Management Inventory; Brown & Nicassio, 1987), the Coping Strategies Questionnaire (CSQ; Rosenstiel & Keefe, 1983) has been used in the vast majority of pain research. The CSQ is a 42-item self-report inventory that assesses seven coping strategies: diverting attention, reinterpreting pain sensation, use of coping self-statements, ignoring pain sensation, praying and hoping, catastrophizing, and increasing activity level. Two further items ask patients to rate their abilities to control and reduce pain. The CSQ appears to have three factors: cognitive coping (ignoring pain, coping self-statements), self-efficacy belief (ability to control pain, ability to reduce pain), and pain avoidance (diverting attention, praying and hoping). Catastrophizing and increasing activity seem not to load consistently on any factor (Lawson, Reesor, Keefe, & Turner, 1990).

Two trends are evident in studies of the CSQ. First, patients who catastrophize about pain and feel helpless in regard to its management appear to be more disabled and depressed (Keefe, Brown, Wallston, & Caldwell, 1989). It is likely that catastrophizing occasions higher levels of depression and, through depression, greater disability. Second, patients who cope with pain through attention diversion, reinterpretive strategies, and praying/hoping demonstrate high levels of pain and disability. Thus the latter coping tactics appear dysfunctional in dealing with pain of a chronic nature.

Although less studied, the Vanderbilt Pain Management Inventory (VPMI; Brown & Nicassio, 1987) is a brief, 19-item instrument with good psychometric properties that measures active and passive approaches to coping with pain. In addition, a longitudinal study showed that rheumatoid arthritis patients who used passive coping strategies over a 6-month period demonstrated increasingly severe levels of depression (Brown, Nicassio, & Wallston, 1989). A recent study, although supporting the validity of the active and passive coping dimensions of the VPMI, found it to be psychometrically weaker than the CSQ (Snow-Turek, Norris, & Tan, 1996).

Several questions have been raised about the CSQ in particular and about coping strategies more generally. Although the CSQ has been found to correlate with self-reports of disability and poor adjustment to pain (Martin et al., 1996), there is little research relevant to coping strategies and a healthy adjustment to pain. Thus the CSQ appears to identify only coping strategies that are dysfunctional. A more general criticism has been raised in recent research examining long-term (12-month) follow-up of multidisciplinary treatment (Pfingsten, Hildebrandt, Leibing, Franz, & Saur, 1997). Relative to beliefs about disability and/or self-efficacy, coping strategies accounted for very little variance in return-to-work. Thus, although coping strategies appear relevant to affective distress and to selected elements of disability, they may carry less weight than other cognitive variables with regard to outcome variables such as work status.

PSYCHOLOGICAL DISTRESS

Psychological distress is another vast domain that has received wide attention in outcome research. Two general domains relevant to psychological distress can be distinguished: (1) global measures of psychological adjustment, and (2) measures of affective distress. As was the case with measures of pain, the focus of this section is not to summarize all of the research that has been conducted on these dimensions but to highlight only research pertinent to outcome assessment. Thus instruments such as semistructured interviews (e.g., Psychosocial Pain Inventory; Heaton et al., 1982) may have value for purposes of psychological evaluation but lack characteristics necessary for outcome assessment.

Global Measures of Adjustment

Two measures of global adjustment will be reviewed: (1) the Minnesota Multiphasic Personality Inventory (MMPI), and (2) the Symptom Checklist 90—Revised (SCL-90-R). Although other general measures also have been used (e.g., the Millon Behavioral Health

Inventory; Millon, Green, & Meagher, 1983), the former measures have been used more heavily. Of these, the MMPI is the more psychiatrically based (Bradley, Haile, & Jaworsky, 1992), whereas the SCL-90-R is constructed to be applicable to both psychiatric and medical populations (Derogatis, 1983).

The MMPI is a 566-item questionnaire designed to assess psychological disturbance that employs a true/false format to generate a profile that includes 10 clinical scales and 3 validity scales. In 1989 the MMPI was revised to develop current norms for the inventory, to make it more representative of the U.S. population, and to update item content (Butcher, Dahlstrom, Graham, Tellegen, & Kaemmer, 1989). The MMPI-2 contains 567 items and is generally continuous with its predecessor. The MMPI has been widely used in psychological assessment of patients in pain (Love & Peck, 1987), despite its length and the well-documented problems with selected somatic items in its subscales that, with pain patients, can reflect disease rather than psychological processes (J. Moore, McFall, Kivlahan, & Capestany, 1988; Prokop, 1986).

These problems notwithstanding, the MMPI has seen considerable use in outcome assessment. One use has involved pre- and postcomparison of scale profiles. Studies have shown MMPI profiles following successful surgical (Dvorak, Valach, Fuhrimann, & Heim, 1988) and nonsurgical treatment (Barnes, Gatchel, Mayer, & Barnett, 1990; Gatchel, Mayer, Capra, Diamond, & Barnett, 1986; M. Moore, Berk, & Nypaver, 1984) to be less elevated than those prior to treatment. Thus the MMPI has demonstrated sensitivity to treatment changes, although its length and scoring protocol have been criticized relative to briefer, more symptom-specific inventories (Bernstein, Jaremko, & Hinkley, 1994).

Another outcome-related use of the MMPI has involved predicting response to treatment based on MMPI profile patterns (Bradley, Prokop, Margolis, & Gentry, 1978). Bradley and Van der Heide (1984) identified a number of behavioral correlates associated with empirically derived MMPI subgroups and proposed that the subgroups could be used to predict the outcome of treatment. Unfortunately, several studies that followed up on that proposal failed to identify relations between profile patterns and treatment outcome (Guck, Meilman, Skultety, & Poloni, 1988; J. Moore, Armentrout, Parker, & Kivlahan, 1988). Hence the MMPI appears to be of little value as an outcome predictor.

The SCL-90-R is a briefer (90-item), Likert-type instrument with several subscales that are more suited to medical patients, including somatization, depression, and a general measure of symptom severity (Global Severity Index; GSI). There is factor-analytic evidence that the SCL-90-R may be a one-factor measure of maladjustment among patients with low back pain (Bernstein et al., 1994; Kinney, Gatchel, & Mayer, 1991). In addition, the response patterns of pain patients have been shown to differ from those of patients with psychiatric diagnoses (Buckelew, DeGood, Schwartz, & Kerler, 1986). Nonetheless, because research has shown the SCL-90-R to be both sensitive to change in clinical status (e.g., Spinhoven & Linssen, 1991; Wallis, Lord, & Bogduk, 1997) and not objectionable to patients (Bernstein et al., 1994), it continues to be used as a general indicator of psychological adjustment.

Depression

Because depression is common among patients with intractable pain (Dworkin & Gitlin, 1991; Romano & Turner, 1985), it has been assessed frequently in outcome studies. A variety of treatments have been shown effective in treatment of depression among patients with intractable pain, including pharmacological treatment (Max et al., 1991; Ward, 1986; White & Harth, 1996), surgical treatment (Dvorak, Valach, Fuhrimann, & Heim, 1988), behaviorally oriented treatment (Spinhoven & Linssen, 1991; Turner & Clancy, 1986), functional restoration treatment (Alaranta et al., 1994; Mayer et al., 1987), and multidisciplinary pain management programs (Duckro, Margolis, Tait, & Korytnyk, 1985; Peters, Large, & Elkind, 1992; A. Williams et al., 1996). Depression has been measured both through administration of established psychometric instruments (e.g., Peters, Large, & Elkind, 1992; A. Williams et al., 1996) and through rating scales in which the patient is asked to report present mood state or changes in mood compared to pretreatment status (e.g., Duckro, Margolis, Tait, & Korytnyk, 1985; Max et al., 1991).

Not surprisingly, a number of self-report instruments have been used to measure depression among patients in pain, including the Beck Depression Inventory (BDI), the Center for Epidemiologic Studies–Depression scale (CES-D), and the Zung Self-Rating Depression Scale (Zung, 1965). This chapter focuses on the two most widely used instruments, the BDI and the CES-D. Of the two, the most used has been the BDI, a 21-item self-report inventory with good psychometric properties (Beck,

Ward, Mendelson, Mock, & Erlbaugh, 1961). The BDI has demonstrated good discrimination between pain patients with and without depression (Turner & Romano, 1984; Geisser, Roth, & Robinson, 1997). On the other hand, questions have been raised about the factor structure of the BDI (Chibnall & Tait, 1994a; Novy, Nelson, Berry, & Averill, 1995; Turk & Okifuji, 1994), suggesting that there is possible inflation of depression scores by somatic items. Several studies have shown patients in pain to differentially endorse somatic items over affective and cognitive items on the scale (Wesley, Gatchel, Polatin, Kinney, & Mayer, 1991; A. Williams & Richardson, 1993). Recent research suggests, however, that depression may modulate responses even to somatic items, so that the inclusion of these items actually improves the discriminative capacity of the instrument, although it also raises the level of the cutoff used to assess clinical significance (Geisser, Roth, & Robinson, 1997).

An instrument that has received increased use in pain research is the CES-D (Radloff, 1977), a measure normed on a population sample, not a psychiatric sample. Relative to the BDI, its validity appears less compromised by somatic items (Berkman et al., 1986; Turk & Okifuji, 1994). In addition, the CES-D appears somewhat more sensitive to changes in severity of depressive symptoms (Santor, Zuroff, Ramsey, Cervantes, & Palacios, 1995). Geisser, Roth, and Robinson (1997) found the CES-D and the BDI to be comparable in detecting depression among patients in pain.

Several caveats should be kept in mind when using any measure of depression. First, responses are influenced by a patient's emotional status at the time of assessment, a factor of considerable importance in retrospective designs in which patients indicate change in mood from pre- to posttreatment from the perspective of a single point in time (e.g., Duckro, Margolis, Tait, & Korytnyk, 1985). Second, as with any self-report instrument, measures of mood are vulnerable to response biases (Furnham, 1986), especially social desirability effects (Deshields, Tait, Gfeller, & Chibnall, 1995).

Anxiety

The role of anxiety in assessment is a topic of relatively recent interest. General levels of anxiety have been assessed primarily with the Spielberger State–Trait Anxiety Inventory (STAI). Although the STAI is a well-established measure (Spielberger, Gorsuch, & Lushene, 1970) that has shown sensitivity to

change in program evaluation of patients in pain (e.g., A. Williams et al., 1996), recent research has focused more specifically on pain-specific measures of anxiety/fear/avoidance of pain. Several self-report inventories have been used in research, as have task-specific assessments of pain expected with movement.

McCracken and associates (1992) developed the Pain Anxiety Symptom Scale (PASS) to assess cognitive, physiological, and motoric aspects of fear of pain, finding that PASS scores correlated with affective and functional measures. Subsequently, they found that PASS scores were associated with higher predictions of pain and lower range of motion on a straight leg raising task (McCracken, Gross, Sorg, & Edmands, 1993). PASS scores also have been found to correlate with dysfunctional responses to pain as measured with the Multidimensional Pain Inventory (Asmundson, Norton, & Allerdings, 1997). Research also has supported the validity of another measure of pain avoidance, the Tampa Scale for Kinesiophobia (TSK; Kori, Miller, & Todd, 1990). TSK scores reflecting fear of movement have been shown to correlate with self-limiting behavior when patients have been asked to perform simple movements (Vlaeyen, Kole-Snijders, Boeren, & van Eek, 1995).

Another paper-and-pencil measure that assesses beliefs is the Fear and Avoidance Beliefs Questionnaire (FABQ; Waddell, Newton, Henderson, Somerville, & Main, 1993). The FABQ has two components, one involving a general fear of activity and the other involving fear of work-related activities. The latter subscale was more strongly associated with lost work time than were several medical markers, suggesting that the scale has value in assessing psychological factors that interfere with return to work.

Several studies have examined fear of pain relative to specific movements. In a study previously discussed, Council, Ahern, Follick, and Kline (1988) found fear of pain to be associated with restriction of movement in a set of 10 specific exercises. Rainville, Ahern, Phalen, Childs, and Sutherland (1992) also examined pain anticipated with activity among patients being treated through a functionally oriented restoration program. Although there were significant improvements in performance associated with treatment, ratings of pain anticipated with activity did not decrease from pre- to posttreatment. They concluded that fear of pain should not be considered a deterrent to progress in rehabilitation. On the other hand, pain management approaches to treatment have been shown to reduce pain anticipated with movement while also increasing tolerance for activity (A. Williams et al., 1996). Further study of relations between fear of movement and performance is needed as part of assessment of program evaluation to establish more clearly its relations with function, especially over the long term.

DISABILITY

Disability assessment has seen tremendous growth in outcome research with the development of a host of self-report and behavioral measures (Flores, Gatchel, & Polatin, 1997). As noted earlier, the growth is partly attributable to input from insurance carriers, especially worker's compensation carriers, who are interested in outcomes relevant to return to work and cost containment (Webster & Snook, 1994), criteria that guide decisions regarding the use of expensive, multidisciplinary treatment protocols. Additionally, attention to disability related to pain has been boosted by research that has shown that pain-related interference with function is predictive of long-term adjustment (Von Korff, Dworkin, & Le Resche, 1990). Finally, there has been considerable evolution in instrumentation used to measure function and/or disability (Flores, Gatchel, & Polatin, 1997). Because of the wealth of information regarding assessment of disability in outcome research, that research will be divided into two sections. The first will examine self-report measures that are commonly used. The second will examine behavioral measurement, including both measures of pain behavior and measures of performance.

Self-Report

Two measures of general health status have been used with patients in pain, the Sickness Impact Profile (SIP) and the Medical Outcomes Study Short Form–36 (SF-36). Because of its careful scale development and psychometric properties (Bergner, Bobbit, Carter, & Gilson, 1981), the SIP has probably been the most heavily used measure in pain outcome research (Brooks, Jordan, Divine, Smith, & Neelon, 1990; Bruin, Witte, Stevens, & Diederiks, 1992; Romano et al., 1988; Slater, Doctor, Pruitt, & Atkinson, 1997). The SIP is composed of 136 items in a yes/no format in which patients indicate the impact of health problems on 12 areas of function that can be summed to form

three scales: physical (involving problems in ambulation, body care, and mobility); psychosocial (representing problems in alertness, emotionality, communication, and social interactions); total (including physical and psychosocial subscores and additional problems in sleep, eating, work, home management, and recreation). Although widely used and having well-documented reliability and validity with pain patients, the SIP has drawbacks that include its length, the inclusion of items not relevant to patients in pain, problems associated with scoring (it is common to have unequal numbers of items on pre/post assessment due to its yes/no format), and questions about its sensitivity to change (Deyo & Centor, 1986).

The SF-36, another self-report measure of general health status, consists of 36 Likert-type items and also has well-established data regarding reliability, validity, and sensitivity to change (Ware & Sherbourne, 1992). There are eight subscales that are clustered into three health dimensions: functional status (including physical functioning, social functioning, role limitations attributed to physical problems, and role limitations attributed to emotional problems); well-being (mental health, energy and fatigue, pain); and overall health (general health perception). Aside from its brevity, advantages of the SF-36 include its successful use in treatment research involving patients in pain (Lansky, Butler, & Waller, 1992; Osterhaus, Townsend, Gandek, & Ware, 1994), as well as the volume of research across settings that promote comparisons with established norms, making it possible to draw population-based conclusions in addition to sample-specific conclusions (Ware, 1995). Its primary limitation involves its lack of specificity relative to pain. Because the instrument was developed to assess the general impact of illness, patient responses to items can be affected by health problems other than pain. Hence it has been suggested that disease-specific instruments be administered in conjunction with the SF-36 in order to assess both specific and general changes in health status (Ruta, Garratt, Wardlaw, & Russell, 1994).

The Multidimensional Pain Inventory (MPI) is a 52-item questionnaire developed exclusively for use with patients in pain. It has 12 subscales that cut across topics that include pain severity, pain-related interference with activity, affective distress, and support/concern from significant others. There is support for subscale reliability and validity (Kerns, Turk, & Rudy, 1985), especially the pain and activity subscales (Holmes & Stevenson, 1990; Rudy, Turk, Kubinski, & Zaki, 1995). Although there is evidence of its sensitivity to change as an outcome measure (Kerns & Haythornthwaite, 1988; Kerns, Turk, Holzman, & Rudy, 1986), the MPI subscales have less empirical support than do measures of more specific constructs (e.g., affective distress, disability). Hence, some studies have used the MPI for purposes of clustering/describing patients prior to treatment, while using other measures to assess treatment-related change (e.g., Rudy, Turk, Kubinski, & Zaki, 1995; A. Williams et al., 1996).

Aside from these comprehensive inventories, a number of brief, disability-specific inventories also have been developed. Of these, three are discussed in this chapter that have seen considerable use among pain patients: the Oswestry Low Back Pain Questionnaire (OLBPQ), the SIP Roland scale (SIP-R), and the Pain Disability Index (PDI). Readers who are interested in discussions of other brief, pain-specific instruments are referred to several recent reviews (Deyo, 1986; Kerns & Jacob, 1992; Tait, 1993).

The OLBPQ is a 10-item inventory that was developed to assess pain-related interference in everyday activities among patients with low back pain (Fairbank, Couper, Davies, & O'Brien, 1980) using a percentage score as a marker of general levels of pain-related disability. Since its inception, it has been found to be a reliable and valid measure of disability (Deyo, 1986; Gronblad et al., 1993; Strong, Ashton, & Large, 1994), making it useful in studies examining treatment outcomes (e.g., Meade, Dyer, Browne, Townsend, & Frank, 1990). Relative to other instruments, however, it may be a less sensitive indicator of change in functional status (Beurskens, de Vet, & Koke, 1996; Little & MacDonald, 1994; Strong, Ashton, & Large, 1994).

The SIP-Roland is a 24-item inventory derived from the SIP that was designed to assess low back pain (Roland & Morris, 1983a). It has been shown to have adequate test-retest reliability (Roland & Morris, 1983b; Deyo, 1986) and validity (Deyo, 1986), although the latter study showed it to correlate more highly with the SIP Physical scale than with the SIP Psychosocial scale. It also has been shown to be sensitive to treatment-related change (Hadler, Curtis, Gillings, & Stinnett, 1987; Klein & Eek, 1990). Finally, a recent revision found it to be suitable for assessment of patients with a variety of pain conditions, not just low back pain (Jensen, Strom, Turner, & Romano, 1992). The sensitivity to change of the modified instrument has yet to be examined.

The final brief measure to be discussed is the PDI, a 7-item inventory developed to assess interference in role functioning associated with pain (Pollard, 1984). There is considerable evidence supporting its validity and reliability with a broad population of patients in pain (Gronblad et al., 1993; Jerome & Gross, 1991; Tait, Chibnall, & Krause, 1990). Research on large samples has shown it to measure a single disability factor, and norms have been reported for patients referred to comprehensive pain centers (Chibnall & Tait, 1994b). There is evidence that it is more sensitive to change than other brief measures of pain-related disability (Strong, Ashton, & Large, 1994) and that it taps a set of patient self-perceptions that are predictive of return-to-work outcomes for patients treated in multidisciplinary programs (Hildebrandt, Pfingsten, Saur, & Jansen, 1997). Its main disadvantage, in common with other self-report measures (Robinson et al., 1997), involves its face validity, which makes it vulnerable to manipulation by patients who may want to magnify their levels of disability.

Behavioral Measures

This section reviews two observational measures of pain behavior that have been used in outcomes research, a pain behavior observation protocol developed by Keefe and Block (1982) and the University of Alabama Pain Behavior Scale (Richards, Nepomuceno, Riles, & Suer, 1982). As with other sections in this chapter, these represent only a portion of the observational systems that have been developed for patients in pain. The reader interested in a more thorough discussion of these instruments is referred to a recent review of that research (Keefe & Williams, 1992).

The Pain Behavior Observation System (PBOS) involves a standardized set of activities performed by patients who are videotaped for subsequent scoring. With the initial protocol, a series of discrete time intervals were selected from the videotape, and viewers rated the occurrence of a target behavior within a time interval, a rating process that yielded high interrater reliability. Pain behaviors assessed through the PBOS have been shown to correlate with a variety of constructs that support the validity of the measure in a variety of populations (Keefe et al., 1987; Keefe, Brantley, Manuel, & Crisson, 1985; Keefe & Williams, 1992) and to be sensitive to treatment-related change (e.g., Romano et al., 1988). Although a major drawback of the original protocol was its inflexibility and cost of administration, time sampling protocols have been developed that make the PBOS sufficiently flexible to be employed in more naturalistic settings (Keefe, Crisson, & Trainor, 1987).

The UAB Pain Behavior Scale (PBS) is a rating system designed expressly for use in more naturalistic settings, using a time sampling design in which raters indicate the frequency with which patients demonstrate pain behaviors such as limping and grimacing. It has demonstrated good interrater reliability across a range of settings, as well as correlations with self-reported disability (Tait, Chibnall, & Krause, 1990), duration of sick leave following work-related low back injury (Ohlund et al., 1994), and residual functional capacity (Fishbain et al., 1994). Although both the PBS and PBOS have shown utility as predictors of treatment outcome (Connally & Sanders, 1991), further work remains to establish relations between observed pain behaviors and other measures of function and/or risk of relapse over time.

Performance Measures

Performance measures of disability, including range of motion, strength, and endurance, have proliferated as a result of their use in goal-oriented programs designed for workers with compensable low back injuries that focus on restoration of function (e.g., Hazard, 1994; Mayer et al., 1987). A recent article provides an extensive review of these measures, and the interested reader is referred to that article for more detail on the topic (Flores, Gatchel, & Polatin, 1997). This section reviews four types of measures that have been used to assess physical changes related to treatment in patients with low back pain: (1) range of motion, (2) spine strength, (3) lifting capacity, and (4) other functional assessment techniques. In addition, there is some discussion of measurement of effort, always an important consideration when assessing physical performance.

Range of Motion

Range of motion of the lumbar spine has long been considered a marker for musculoskeletal dysfunction (Loebl, 1967). A number of measures have been used to evaluate range of motion in the lumbar spine, including measurement of the distance from fingertips to the floor at maximum flexion,

change in distance between spinous processes and straight leg raising (SLR), all of which demonstrate significant reliability problems (Robinson, Greene, O'Connor, Graves, & MacMillan, 1992). Inclinometry, a technique that has been accepted by the American Medical Association (1993), involves placement of instruments on the sacrum and at the first lumbar vertebra and yields reliable information regarding both sagittal and axial movement (Keeley et al., 1986). There is recent evidence that range increases with functionally oriented treatment (Mayer et al., 1987) and that functional gains are associated with more confident patterns of movement (Mayer, Tabor, Bovasso, & Gatchel, 1994).

Strength

Deconditioning is recognized as a significant component of pain-related disability (Spektor, 1990). Accordingly, there are multiple machines commercially available to measure lumbar strength (Flores, Gatchel, & Polatin, 1997). Although there is increasing evidence that isokinetic and/or isoinertial testing is preferable to isometric testing as a gauge of strength and effort in patients with low back pain, problems remain with test-retest reliability and with the validity of these devices as predictors of work performance (Hazard, Reeves, & Fenwick, 1992). Despite these difficulties, there is evidence that pain patients can improve back strength with functional treatment (Kohles, Barnes, Gatchel, & Mayer, 1990), although not to levels demonstrated by pain-free subjects (Brady, Mayer, & Gatchel, 1994).

Lifting Capacity

Lifting capacity is another physical measure that has been used to assess function in low back pain patients. Although computer technologies have allowed more accurate assessment of lifting capacity, it has proved difficult to develop computer technologies that adequately assess this parameter because lifting is a complicated biomechanical task (Flores, Gatchel, & Polatin, 1997). Hence progressive isoinertial lifting tasks have been used to simulate workplace lifting. Although these measures appear to have validity, they are less amenable to computerized scoring protocols (Mayer et al., 1988). As with other measures of physical function, lifting capacity has been shown to improve with functionally oriented treatment, even to levels comparable to those of pain-free subjects (Curtis, Mayer, & Gatchel, 1994).

Other Performance Measures

Aside from the rather specific measures described here, more global approaches also have been used to measure general functional capacity evaluation (FCE). FCEs also can be modified to assess specific job requirements. Standardization of FCEs is problematic, however, as they can vary according to treatment philosophy, leaving questions about reliability/validity of measurement. Isernhagen (1994) has provided an excellent review of this methodology.

Harding and colleagues (1994) recently developed a battery of physical performance measures for use with pain patients designed to assess speed/endurance in walking, stair climbing, sit-to-stand movements, balance, sit-ups, arm endurance, grip strength, and peak respiratory flow. Aside from balance, the measures demonstrated good test-retest reliability at a 12-week time interval (all r's > .70). In addition, they have been shown to be sensitive to multidisciplinary treatment and to correlate with other measures of function such as the SIP and return to work (A. Williams et al., 1996). Obviously, because of its relative ease of administration and measurement properties, this performance protocol deserves further study.

Effort

Although the above sections give reason to believe that objective measures of function can be applied with reliability and validity to patients in pain, actual performance is affected by multiple factors, including subjective phenomena such as the effort a patient is willing to expend (Hazard, Reid, Fenwick, & Reeves, 1988). Multiple physiological indices of effort have been proposed, including variation in peak force between repeated isometric (Harber & SooHoo, 1984) and isokinetic tasks (Hazard, Reeves, Weisman, Fleming, & Pope, 1991). Unfortunately, test-retest reliability for these instruments is sufficiently poor that they cannot be considered good barometers of effort (Robinson, Greene, O'Connor, Graves, & MacMillan, 1992; Robinson, MacMillan, O'Connor, Fuller, & Cassisi, 1991). Hazard, Reeves, and Fenwick (1992) have observed that isokinetic and isoinertial tasks are preferable to isometric tasks in assess-

ing variability in effort; they classified normal volunteers into maximal and submaximal effort categories with these measures with better than 60% accuracy. Although this classification percentage is better than chance, it is sufficiently low that its application to single cases is problematic.

A recent study by Hildebrandt, Pfingsten, Saur, and Jansen (1997) sheds an interesting light on functional measures as predictors of return to work. Of 90 patients with chronic low back pain, 82 were treated through functional restoration with behavioral support and followed for 12 months, the primary criterion variable being return to work. Patients demonstrated progress on a number of pain, performance, medical, and psychological parameters, and discriminant functions were computed using the parameters as predictors. Analyses showed that reduction in self-perceived disability was a much more powerful predictor of return to work than was performance change, leading the authors to conclude that "modification of beliefs is more important for the rehabilitation of patients . . . than changes in the patients' objective physical status" (p. 999). Given that beliefs are associated with persistence of effort, the role of these subjective phenomena as mediators of functional gain clearly requires further investigation.

SICK ROLE

The sick role (Parsons, 1951) is a socially prescribed phenomenon in which expectations are suspended for functioning in a productive role and replaced with expectations relevant to sickness, making it a concept with clear socioeconomic implications. Several socioeconomic indices relevant to the sick role have been considered in recent treatment studies. In fact, along with functional capacity, the socioeconomic implications of intractable pain have been a major focus of attention in recent years (Webster & Snook, 1994). This section focuses on two socioeconomic issues, return to work and health care utilization.

Return to Work

Assessment of return to work has become a standard for functional restoration programs (Alaranta et al., 1994; Burke, Harms-Constas, & Aden, 1994; Mayer et al., 1987; Polatin, Cox, Gatchel, & Mayer, 1997) and for multidisciplinary pain services(Altmaier, Lehmann, Russell, Weinstein, &

Kao, 1992; Deardorff, Rubin, & Scott, 1991; Hubbard, Tracy, Morgan, & McKinney, 1996; Peters, Large, & Elkind, 1992; A. Williams et al., 1996). In a meta-analysis of the literature, Cutler et al. (1994) concluded that these nonsurgical treatments are effective in returning patients to work.

Although these data are encouraging, several problems with return-to-work data should be noted. First, these data are generally based on patient self-report, and most studies do not indicate how data are screened for accuracy (Flores, Gatchel, & Polatin, 1997). Second, some studies fail to specify pretreatment work status, making it difficult to gauge change in work status (Cutler et al., 1994). Third, there is great disparity between return-to-work results among programs. It is difficult to determine whether the differential results are a function of differences in treatment protocols, differences in patients selected for treatment, or differences in the social environment in which treatment occurs (Alaranta et al., 1994; Turk, Rudy, & Sorkin, 1993). Thus, although return to work is a crucial concept, treatment and nontreatment factors that influence it require further investigation.

Health Care Utilization

Several parameters of health care utilization have been examined and found to be effectively treated through nonsurgical treatment in a recent meta-analytic review (Flor, Fydrich, & Turk, 1992): medication use (Deardorff, Rubin, & Scott, 1991; Gottlieb, Alperson, Schwartz, Beck, & Kee, 1988; Hubbard, Tracy, Morgan, & McKinney, 1996; Peters, Large, & Elkind, 1992; A. Williams et al., 1996), further health care visits (Deardorff, Rubin, & Scott, 1991; Mayer et al., 1987; Polatin, Cox, Gatchel, & Mayer, 1997; A. Williams et al., 1996), and further surgeries (Mayer et al., 1987; Polatin, Cox, Gatchel, & Mayer, 1997). All of the above are derived from patient self-reports, so there are unanswered questions regarding reliability and validity of much of the health care utilization data. In fact, it is rare for reports to describe explicit techniques used to assess the quality of data collected (Flores, Gatchel, & Polatin, 1997).

Efforts have also been made to address the question of socioeconomic outcome from a financial perspective (i.e., cost/benefit). Using data regarding average costs of disability payments, Peters, Large, and Elkind (1992) computed average savings associated with successful treatment of a small sample of patients, finding that costs associated

even with inpatient treatment more than offset costs attributable to disability. Strax, Turk, Rosomoff, and Jafri (1997) used a similar approach to compute savings offsets that insurance carriers would realize from multidisciplinary treatment relative to surgical treatment of intractable low back pain, again finding advantages to multidisciplinary treatment. In a study of management of acute work injuries, Matheson, Brophy, Vaughan, Nunez, and Saccoman (1995) took this approach one step further, comparing data regarding actual mean costs per case with average costs per case on a statewide basis. Obviously, these computations, while moving the field in an important direction, lack methodologic rigor compared to studies that provide direct comparisons of the cost effectiveness of different approaches to treatment.

One study has compared costs of functional restoration versus standard treatment of patients with work-related musculoskeletal pain (Mitchell & Carmen, 1994). The study found that 79% of functionally treated patients and 78% of control patients were working 12 months after treatment was completed. Treatment costs of the functionally treated patients were greater than those of the other group, although total costs (including duration of absence from work and disability award costs) were equivalent across groups. Although these data provide less than compelling support of multidisciplinary treatment, patient selection may have biased the results. Frank et al. (1996) have done computations indicating that cost effectiveness improves with (expensive) multidisciplinary treatment after 3 months, largely because many patients recover with little or no treatment prior to that time, whereas relatively few do so thereafter. Obviously, further study of cost effectiveness is needed, potentially through accessing large databases, such as those maintained by large insurers (Flores, Gatchel, & Polatin, 1997).

METHODOLOGICAL ISSUES

No discussion of program evaluation would be complete without some discussion of the difficult methodological issues that complicate such research. Several of these issues will be addressed: (1) the clinical significance of outcomes, (2) patient selection, (3) study architecture, and (4) follow-up evaluation. As with other topics considered here, detailed discussion of these methodological issues is well beyond the scope of the chapter, so the reader is referred to several recent reviews of these topics (Turk & Rudy, 1990, 1991; Turk, Rudy, & Sorkin, 1993).

Clinical Significance

Outcome research in behaviorally oriented treatment has been criticized because results can be reported that are statistically significant but of little clinical and/or practical consequence (Jacobson, Follette, & Revenstorf, 1984). Obviously, part of the benefit of socioeconomic indicators such as return to work and health care utilization involves their direct application to such issues. Other approaches have also been applied to program evaluation research, however, to obtain results that are both clinically and statistically meaningful.

For example, Roberts and Reinhardt (1980) developed strict criteria for treatment success that were subsequently adopted by others (e.g., Guck, Skultety, Meilman, & Dowdy, 1985): (1) patients had to be employed or, if not employed, unemployed for reasons other than pain; (2) they had to be active 8 hours per day; (3) they could not be receiving compensation for pain; (4) they reported no further surgeries or hospitalizations for pain; and (5) they were taking no prescription medication for pain. Malec, Cayner, Harvey, and Timming (1981) developed similar criteria, also adopted by others (Peters, Large, & Elkind, 1992): (1) patients were taking no opioid analgesics, tranquilizers, or muscle relaxants; (2) they were employed, active around the house, and continuing 50–100% of exercises; and (3) they reported ongoing control over pain.

Recently, Slater, Doctor, Pruitt, and Atkinson (1997) adopted a different approach. They defined "clinically significant change" as a level of performance following treatment that is "representative" of subjects who are functional. To identify criterion levels of representative function, data relevant to disability and depression were obtained from a sample of 17 orthopedic patients. Other procedures were used to identify "functional" levels of pain. These data were compared to those provided by 17 patients with intractable pain who underwent behavioral treatment. Compared to pain, disability, and depression data from the "functional" group, 40% (7 of 17) of the treated patients demonstrated clinically significant change on one of the outcome variables, whereas only one demonstrated change on all three instruments. Obviously, these data are sobering compared to data bearing only on statistical significance.

One other approach to the issue of clinical significance has been reported by Härkäpää, Järvikoski, Mellin, and Hurri (1990). They computed a reliability-of-change (RC) score, using pretreatment and 2½-year follow-up data derived from a low back disability index. The RC index reflected the difference score between pre- and posttreatment assessments divided by the standard error of the difference. Using these computations, they determined that patients needed to demonstrate at least a 5-point difference from pre- to posttreatment, a criterion met by 25% of the treated patients.

Patient Selection

A persistent and perplexing problem in evaluating studies of treatment outcome involves questions about the comparability of patients entered into treatment across settings (Turk & Rudy, 1990). A number of potentially important demographic characteristics have been identified that vary across settings (Holzman et al., 1985): gender, age, prior treatments, and pain duration. Not included in this list are a number of clinical variables that have been identified as predictive of outcome, including self-perceived disability (Hildebrandt, Pfingsten, Saur, & Jansen, 1997), congruence of patient expectations with actual treatment (Shutty, DeGood, & Tuttle, 1990), employment status (Dworkin, Handlin, Richlin, Brand, & Vannucci, 1985), litigation status (Talo, Hendler, & Brodie, 1989), level of pretreatment pain behavior (Connally & Sanders, 1991), level of dysfunction prior to treatment (Tait, Duckro, Margolis, & Wiener, 1988), and the social context within which treatment occurs (Alaranta et al., 1994). Depending on patient selection, comparable treatments can have widely discrepant results. In fact, some studies have reported return-to-work results for untreated patients in a comparison group (e.g., Mayer et al., 1987) that are better than results for treated patients in other studies (e.g., McArthur, Cohen, Gottlieb, Naliboff, & Schandler, 1987).

Although it is clear that these and other patient selection differences profoundly affect program outcomes, there are no clear solutions to the problem. As noted by Turk and Rudy (1990), statistical adjustments (e.g., covariance analyses) may be inappropriate due to heterogeneity of variance across samples, violating assumptions necessary to use these statistical techniques. Although program evaluations that address multiple levels of the pain experience (as outlined in this chapter) are likely to control at least some of these influences, the only way to address the matter adequately is through randomized controlled trials, difficult to perform with clinical populations.

Study Architecture

Bloch (1987) has described four designs of increasing power that are used in treatment studies of low back pain: (1) case studies, (2) case series without comparison groups, (3) cohort studies with comparison groups, and (4) randomized controlled trials with random assignment to treatment and comparison groups. Whereas early outcome research in pain treatment used case series designs in order to demonstrate that clinical improvement could be found with behavioral treatment (e.g., Fordyce et al., 1973), most recent studies have used cohort designs in which outcomes are compared for patients who are assigned (nonrandomly) to groups that receive different treatments (Flor, Fydrich, & Turk, 1992). Although these studies have shown that nonsurgical treatment can be effective, they have been critiqued on several grounds, most importantly for the use of problematic comparison groups.

A variety of comparison groups has been used: (1) patients denied treatment by reason of insurance (e.g., Mayer et al., 1987; Sturgis, Schaefer, & Sikora, 1984), (2) patients who dropped out of treatment (e.g., Cassisi, Sypert, Salamon, & Kapel, 1989), (3) waiting-list controls (A. Williams et al., 1996), (4) patients assigned to a different (medical/physical therapy) treatment (e.g., Burke, Harms-Constas, & Aden, 1994), and (5) patients assigned to a different intensity (e.g., inpatient vs. outpatient) treatment (Tait, Duckro, Margolis, & Wiener, 1988). Studies using all of the above designs have demonstrated treatment effectiveness, although they lack some methodological rigor because of their lack of randomization (Wen, Hernandez, & Naylor, 1995).

Several recent studies, however, have employed randomized methodologies. Two compared patients assigned either to inpatient or outpatient multidisciplinary pain treatment or to a control condition (Peters, Large, & Elkind, 1992; A. Williams et al., 1996), with each study finding highly significant effects associated with treatment. Interestingly, the last study also found long-term (12-month) benefits associated with inpatient treatment relative to outpatient treatment in terms of several clinical variables, including employment status. Less compelling findings emerged from a Finnish study (Alaranta et al., 1994) in which patients were assigned randomly to multidisciplinary functional restoration or to standard inpatient rehabilitation. Although multidisciplinary treatment was associated with greater reduction of self-reported pain and disability, it was no more effective than standard rehabilitation in reducing psychological distress or employment variables, a result at variance with results reported by Mayer and associates (e.g., Mayer et al., 1986) and which the authors attributed to differences in social climate between the United States and Finland.

Follow-Up Evaluation

It is well recognized that effective treatment should be characterized by durable clinical change, that is, change that is stable over time. Accordingly, many outcome studies have examined data collected not only immediately posttreatment but also at varying time intervals following treatment (up to 8 years; Roberts & Reinhardt, 1980). With the passage of time, research has shown a tendency among many patients to relapse (Turk & Rudy, 1991). Similarly, patients become increasingly difficult to reach, such that the response rate for some follow-up studies can be distressingly low (e.g., 24% at one year; Gottlieb, Alperson, Schwartz, Beck, & Kee, 1988).

A poor rate of response greatly complicates evaluation of long-term effects. Most studies address the issue by assuming that the rate of relapse is equivalent between responders and nonresponders, an assumption that probably is not tenable (Kerns & Haythornthwaite, 1988). At the other end of the spectrum, it could be assumed that all nonresponders have relapsed, an assumption that would greatly deflate the success rates of most studies of treatment outcome (Turk & Rudy, 1991). Although it is obvious that the truth regarding relapse and rate of response falls between the poles represented by the above assumptions, it also is obvious that a poor response rate leaves much room for error.

Recent research has paid more attention to response rates in follow-up. Bloch (1987) has suggested that high quality follow-up studies collect data on 80% of treated patients in order to minimize error associated with response rate. Many recent studies have collected follow-up data at or near that rate (e.g., Burke, Harms-Constas, & Aden, 1994; Hildebrandt, Pfingsten, Saur, & Jansen, 1997; Mayer et al., 1987). Collection of such data is time-consuming and costly, but there appears to be no other recourse.

CONCLUDING COMMENTS

There has been a tremendous growth in information available regarding outcomes of treatment for patients with intractable pain. Much of the information supports the effectiveness of nonsurgical treatments presently available (Cutler et al., 1994; Flor, Fydrich, & Turk, 1992). On the other hand, a number of important topics are highlighted by the research that has been done.

One topic involves comparability among studies, a problem partly due to patient selection and partly to proliferation of research instruments. In a recent review, Flor, Fydrich, and Turk (1992) counted 704 dependent variables among the 65 studies that they included in a meta-analysis. Since the publication of that article, additional instruments have been developed, some of which are presented in this chapter. Although it is unrealistic to expect that further instrument development will cease as investigators agree on measures to be used across studies, it may be possible to reach agreement on conceptually meaningful dimensions of the pain experience to be assessed in any comprehensive program evaluation without specifying the specific measures used to assess those dimensions. Obviously, this chapter has used dimensions suggested by the Glasgow Illness Model (Waddell, 1996) as a basis for organization, a model that has conceptual and empirical support. Other organizational schemas could have been used (Turk & Rudy, 1992). Whatever the schema, it is important that some agreement is reached for both conceptual and practical reasons.

Agreement on an evaluative conceptual schema could benefit program evaluation for surgical, medical, and physical therapy treatments of patients in pain as well. Several recent reviews of outcome research in those areas found that many studies lacked measures of disability and distress, and none included measures of attitudes and beliefs (Feine & Lund, 1997; White & Harth, 1996). With a broader range of variables, such studies could address both clinical and theoretical questions. For example, in a recent study of a radio-frequency neurotomy technique, Wallis, Lord, and

Bogduk (1997) included a measure of psychological adjustment (the SCL-90-R). Patients who obtained pain relief from the procedure reported significant reduction in distress, whereas patients who did not obtain relief reported no reduction in distress. The authors note that these findings support a somatopsychic rather than psychosomatic model of pain, a finding of obvious theoretical importance.

Although there is no doubt that a range of outcome data is needed if treatment programs are to remain viable and to continue to contribute to knowledge of pain, there are practical issues associated with the administration of research instruments. Some of the more robust data are generated by the most expensive and time-consuming techniques (e.g., FCEs, daily diary recordings), techniques not accessible for many pain services. Further research that focuses on brief assessment protocols and that establishes relations between such protocols and more sophisticated objective measures could improve the general quality of data available for program evaluation, while encouraging smaller clinics to engage in scientifically sound program evaluation. Continued progress in program evaluation is likely to be necessary if the field of multidisciplinary pain treatment is to be theoretically and fiscally viable.

REFERENCES

Ajzen, I., & Fishbein, M. (1977). Attitude-behavior relations: A theoretical analysis and review of empirical research. *Psychological Bulletin, 84*, 888–918.
Alaranta, H., Rytokoski, U., Rissanen, A., Talo, S., Ronnemaa, T., Puukka, P., Karppi, S.-L., Videman, T., Kallio, V., & Slatis, P. (1994). Intensive physical and psychosocial training program for pain with chronic low back pain: A controlled clinical trial. *Spine, 19,* 1339–1349.
Altmaier, E. M., Lehmann, T. R., Russell, D. W., Weinstein, J. N., & Kao, C. F. (1992). The effectiveness of psychological interventions for the rehabilitation of low back pain: A randomized controlled trial evaluation. *Pain, 49,* 329–335.
American Medical Association. (1993). *Guides to the Evaluation of Permanent Impairment* (4th ed.). Chicago: Author.
Anderson, K. O., Dowds, B. N., Pelletz, R. E., Edwards, W. T., & Peeters-Asdourian, C. (1995). Development and initial validation of a scale to measure self-efficacy beliefs in patients with chronic pain. *Pain, 63,* 77–84.
Asmundson, G. J. G., Norton, G. R., & Allerdings, M. D. (1997). Fear and avoidance in dysfunctional chronic back pain patients. *Pain, 69,* 231–236.
Bandura, A. (1977). Self-efficacy: Toward a unifying theory of behavioral change. *Psychology Review, 84,* 191–215.

Barnes, D., Gatchel, R. J., Mayer, T. G., & Barnett, J. (1990). Changes in MMPI profiles of chronic low back pain patients following successful treatment. *Journal of Spinal Disorders, 3,* 353–355.

Beck, A. T., Ward, C. H., Mendelson, M., Mock, J., & Erlbaugh, J. (1961). An inventory for measuring depression. *Archives of General Psychiatry, 4,* 53–63.

Bergner, M., Bobbitt, R. A., Carter, W. B., & Gilson, B. S. (1981). The Sickness Impact Profile: Development and final revision of a health status measure. *Medical Care, 19,* 787–805.

Berkman, L. F., Berkman, C. S., Kasl, S., Freeman, D. H., Jr., Ostfeld, A. M., Cornoni-Huntley, J., & Brody, J. A. (1986). Depressive symptoms in relation to physical health and functioning in the elderly. *American Journal of Epidemiology, 124,* 372–388.

Bernstein, I. H., Jaremko, M. E., & Hinkley, B. S. (1994). On the utility of the SCL-90-R with low-back pain patients. *Spine, 19,* 42–48.

Beurskens, A. J. H. M., de Vet, H. C. W., & Koke, A. J. A. (1996). Responsiveness of functional status in low back pain: A comparison of different instruments. *Pain, 65,* 71–76.

Bloch, R. (1987). Methodology in clinical back pain trials. *Spine, 12,* 430–432.

Bonica, J. J. (1979). The need of a taxonomy. *Pain, 6,* 247–252.

Bradley, L. A., Haile, J. M., & Jaworski, T. M. (1992). Assessment of psychological status using interviews and self-report instruments. In D. C. Turk & R. Melzack (Eds.), *Handbook of pain assessment* (pp. 193–213). New York: Guilford Press.

Bradley, L. A., Prokop, C. K., Margolis, R., & Gentry, W. D. (1978). Multivariate analyses of the MMPI profiles of low back pain patients. *Journal of Behavioral Medicine, 1,* 253–272.

Bradley, L. A., & Van der Heide, L. H. (1984). Pain-related correlates of MMPI profile subgroups among back pain patients. *Health Psychology, 3,* 157–174.

Brady, S., Mayer, T., & Gatchel, R. (1994). Physical progress and residual impairment quantification after functional restoration: II. Isokinetic trunk strength. *Spine, 19,* 395–400.

Brooks, W. B., Jordan, J. S., Divine, G. W., Smith, K. S., & Neelon, F. A. (1990). The impact of psychologic factors on measurement of functional status: Assessment of the Sickness Impact Profile. *Medical Care, 28,* 793–804.

Brown, G. K., & Nicassio, P. M. (1987). The development of a questionnaire for the assessment of active and passive coping strategies in chronic pain patients. *Pain, 31,* 53–65.

Brown, G. K., Nicassio, P. M., & Wallston, K. A. (1989). Pain coping strategies and depression in rheumatoid arthritis. *Journal of Consulting and Clinical Psychology, 57,* 652–657.

Bruin, A. F., Witte, L. P., Stevens, F., & Diederiks, J. P. M. (1992). Sickness Impact Profile: The state of the art of a generic functional status measure. *Social Science and Medicine, 35,* 1003–1014.

Buckelew, S. P., DeGood, D. E., Schwartz, D. P., & Kerler, R. M. (1986). Cognitive and somatic item response patterns of pain patients, psychiatric patients, and hospital employees. *Journal of Consulting and Clinical Psychology, 42,* 852–860.

Buckelew, S. P, Parker, J. C., Keefe, F. J., Deuser, W. E.,

Crews, T. M., Conway, R., Kay, D. R., & Hewett, J. E. (1994). Self-efficacy and pain behavior among subjects with fibromyalgia. *Pain, 59,* 377–384.

Burke, S. A., Harms-Constas, C. K., & Aden, P. S. (1994). Return to work/retention outcomes of a functional restoration program: A multi-center prospective study with a comparison group. *Spine, 19,* 1880–1885.

Butcher, J. N., Dahlstrom, W. G., Graham, J. R., Tellegen, A. M., & Kaemmer, B. (1989). *MMPI-2: Manual for Administration and Scoring.* Minneapolis: University of Minnesota Press.

Carosella, A. M., Lackner, J. M., & Feuerstein, M. (1994). Factors associated with early discharge from a multidisciplinary work rehabilitation program for chronic low back pain. *Pain, 57,* 69–76.

Cassisi, J. E., Sypert, G. W., Salamon, A., & Kapel, L. (1989). Independent evaluation of a multidisciplinary rehabilitation program for chronic low back pain. *Neurosurgery, 25,* 877–883.

Chibnall, J. T., & Tait, R. C. (1994a). The short form of the Beck Depression Inventory: Validity issues with chronic pain patients. *Clinical Journal of Pain, 10,* 261–266.

Chibnall, J. T., & Tait, R. C. (1994b). The Pain Disability Index: Factor structure and normative data. *Archives of Physical Medicine and Rehabilitation, 75,* 1082–1086.

Connally, G. H., & Sanders, S. H. (1991). Predicting low back pain patients' response to lumbar sympathetic nerve blocks and interdisciplinary rehabilitation: The role of pretreatment overt pain behavior and cognitive coping strategies. *Pain, 44,* 139–146.

Council, J. R., Ahern, D. K., Follick, M. J., & Kline, C. L. (1988). Expectancies and functional impairment in chronic low back pain. *Pain, 33,* 323–331.

Cruise, C. E., Broderick, J., Porter, L., Kaell, A., & Stone, A. A. (1996). Reactive effects of diary self-assessment in chronic pain patients. *Pain, 67,* 253–258.

Curtis, L., Mayer, T. G., & Gatchel, R. J. (1994). Physical progress and residual impairment quantification after functional restoration: III. Isokinetic and isoinertial lifting capacity. *Spine, 19,* 401–405.

Cutler, R. B., Fishbain, D. A., Rosomoff, H. L., Andel-Moty, E., Khalil, T. M., & Rosomoff, R. S. (1994). Does nonsurgical pain center treatment of chronic pain return patients to work?: A review and meta-analysis of the literature. *Spine, 19,* 643–652.

Deardorff, W. W., Rubin, H. S., & Scott, D. W. (1991). Comprehensive multidisciplinary treatment of chronic pain: A follow-up study of treated and non-treated groups. *Pain, 45,* 35–43.

Deathe, A. B., & Helmes, E. (1993). Evaluation of a chronic pain programme by referring physicians. *Pain, 52,* 113–121.

DeGagne, T. A., Mikail, S. F., & D'Eon, J. L. (1995). Confirmatory factor analysis of a 4-factor model of chronic pain evaluation. *Pain, 60,* 195–202.

DeGood, D. E., & Shutty, M. S., Jr. (1992). Assessment of pain beliefs, coping, and self-efficacy. In D. C. Turk & R. Melzack (Eds.), *Handbook of pain assessment* (pp. 214–234). New York: Guilford Press.

Derogatis, L. R. (1983). *SCL-90-R: Administration, scoring and procedures manual* (2nd ed.). Towson, MD: Clinical Psychometric Research.

Desbiens, N. A., Wu, A. W., Broste, S. K., Wenger, N. S., Connors, Jr., A. F., Lynn, J., Yasui, Y., Phillips, R. S., & Fulkerson, W. (1996). Pain and satisfaction with pain control in seriously ill hospitalized adults: Findings from the SUPPORT research investigations. *Critical Care Medicine, 24,* 1953-1961.

Deshields, T. L., Tait, R. C., Gfeller, J. D., & Chibnall, J. T. (1995). Relationship between social desirability and self-report in chronic pain patients. *Clinical Journal of Pain, 11,* 189-193.

Deyo, R. A. (1986). Comparative validity of the Sickness Impact Profile and shorter scales for functional assessment in low-back pain. *Spine, 11,* 561-565.

Deyo, R. A., & Centor, R. M. (1986). Assessing the responsiveness of functional scales to clinical change: An analogy to diagnostic test performance. *Journal of Chronic Disease, 39,* 897-906.

Dolce, J. J., Crocker, M. F., & Doleys, D. M. (1986). Prediction of outcome among chronic pain patients. *Behavior Research and Therapy, 14,* 313-319.

Dolce, J. J., Crocker, M. F., Molleteire, C., & Doleys, D. M. (1986). Exercise quotas, anticipatory concern and self-efficacy expectancies in chronic pain: A preliminary report. *Pain, 24,* 365-372.

Duckro, P. N., Margolis, R. B., Tait, R. C., & Korytnyk, N. (1985). Long-term follow-up of chronic pain patients: A preliminary study. *International Journal of Psychiatry in Medicine, 15,* 283-292.

Dvorak, J., Valach, L., Fuhrimann, P., & Heim, E. (1988). The outcome of surgery for lumbar disc herniation: II. A 4-17 years' follow-up with emphasis on psychosocial aspects. *Spine, 13,* 1423-1427.

Dworkin, R. H., & Gitlin, M. J. (1991). Clinical aspects of depression in chronic pain patients. *Clinical Journal of Pain, 7,* 79-94.

Dworkin, R. H., Handlin, D. S., Richlin, D. M., Brand, L., & Vannucci, C. (1985). Unraveling the effects of compensation, litigation, and employment on treatment response in chronic pain. *Pain, 23,* 49-59.

Eich, E., Rachman, S., & Lopatka, C. (1990). Affect, pain and autobiographical memory. *Journal of Abnormal Psychology, 99,* 174-178.

Fairbank, J. C. T., Couper, J., Davies, J., & O'Brien, J. P. (1980). The Oswestry low back pain disability questionnaire. *Physiotherapy, 66,* 271-273.

Feine, J. S., & Lund, J. P. (1997). An assessment of the efficacy of physical therapy and physical modalities for the control of chronic musculoskeletal pain. *Pain, 71,* 5-23.

Fernandez, E., & Turk, D. C. (1989). The utility of cognitive coping strategies for altering pain perception: A meta-analysis. *Pain, 38,* 123-135.

Fishbain, D. A., Abdel-Moty, E., Cutler, R., Khalil, T. M., Sadek, S., Rosomoff, R. S., & Rosomoff, H. L. (1994). Measuring residual functional capacity in chronic low back pain patients based on the Dictionary of Occupational Titles. *Spine, 19,* 872-880.

Flor, H., Fydrich, T., & Turk, D. C. (1992). Efficacy of multidisciplinary pain treatment centers: A meta-analytic review. *Pain, 49,* 221-230.

Flor, H., Miltner, W., & Birbaumer, N. (1992). Psychophysiological recording methods. In D. C. Turk & R. Melzack (Eds.), *Handbook of pain assessment* (pp. 169-190). New York: Guilford Press.

Flores, L., Gatchel, R. J., & Polatin, P. B. (1997). Objectification of functional improvement after non-operative care. *Spine, 22,* 1622-1633.

Folkman, S., & Lazarus, R. S. (1980). An analysis of coping in a middle-aged community sample. *Journal of Health and Social Behavior, 21,* 219-239.

Follick, M. J., Ahern, D. K., & Laser-Wolston, N. (1984). Evaluation of a daily activity diary for chronic pain patients. *Pain, 19,* 373-382.

Fordyce, W. E., Fowler, R. S., Jr., Lehmann, J. F., DeLateur, B. J., Sand, P. L., & Trieschmann, R. B. (1973). Operant conditioning in the treatment of chronic pain. *Archives of Physical Medicine and Rehabilitation, 54,* 399-408.

Frank, J. W., Brooker, A.-S., DeMaio, S. E., Kerr, M. S., Maetzel, A., Shannon, H. S., Sullivan, T. J., Norman, R. W., & Wells, R. P. (1996). Disability resulting from occupational low back pain: II. What do we know about secondary prevention? A review of the scientific evidence on prevention after disability begins. *Spine, 21,* 2918-2929.

Furnham, A. (1986). Response bias, social desirability, and dissimulation. *Personality and Individual Differences, 7,* 385-400.

Gatchel, R. J., Mayer, T. G., Capra, P., Diamond P., & Barnett, J. (1986). Quantification of lumbar function: VI. The use of psychological measure in guiding physical functional restoration. *Spine, 11,* 36-42.

Geisser, M. E., Roth, R. S., & Robinson, M. E. (1997). Assessing depression among persons with chronic pain using the Center for Epidemiological Studies-Depression Scale and the Beck Depression Inventory: A comparative analysis. *Clinical Journal of Pain, 13,* 163-170.

Gottlieb, H., Alperson, B. L., Schwartz, A. H., Beck, C., & Kee, S. (1988). Self-management for medication reduction in chronic low back pain. *Archives of Physical Medicine and Rehabilitation, 69,* 442-448.

Gronblad, M., Hupli, M., Wennerstrand, P., Jarvinen, E., Lukinmaa, A., Kouri, J.-P., & Karaharju, E. O. (1993). Intercorrelation and test-retest reliability of the Pain Disability Index (PDI) and the Oswestry Disability Questionnaire (ODQ) and their correlation with pain intensity in low back pain patients. *Clinical Journal of Pain, 9,* 189-195.

Guck, T. P., Meilman, P. W., Skultety, M., & Poloni, L. D. (1988). Pain-patient Minnesota Multiphasic Personality Inventory (MMPI) subgroups: Evaluation of long-term treatment outcome. *Journal of Behavioral Medicine, 11,* 159-169.

Guck, T. P., Skultety, F. M., Meilman, P. W., & Dowdy, E. T. (1985). Multidisciplinary follow-up study: Evaluation with a no-treatment control group. *Pain, 21,* 295-306.

Hadler, N. M., Curtis, P., Gillings, D. B., & Stinnett, S. (1987). A benefit of spinal manipulation as adjunctive therapy for acute low-back pain: A stratified controlled trial. *Spine, 12,* 703-706.

Harber, P., & SooHoo, K. (1984). Static ergonomic strength testing in evaluating occupational back pain. *Journal of Occupational Medicine, 26,* 877-884.

Harding, V. R., Williams, A. C. de C., Richardson, P. H., Nicholas, M. K., Jackson, J. L., Richardson, I. H., & Pither, C. E. (1994). The development of a battery of measures for assessing physical functioning of chronic pain patients. *Pain, 58,* 367-375.

Härkäpää, K., Järvikoski, A., Mellin, G., & Hurri, H. (1990). A controlled study on the outcome of inpatient and outpatient treatment of low back pain: III. Long-term follow-up of pain, disability and compliance. *Scandinavian Journal of Rehabilitation Medicine, 22,* 181-188.

Härkäpää, K., Järvikoski, A., Mellin, G., Hurri, H., & Luoma, J. (1991). Health locus of control beliefs and psychological distress as predictors for treatment outcome in low-back pain patients: Results of a 3-month follow-up of a controlled intervention study. *Pain, 46,* 35–41.

Hazard, R. G. (1994). Occupational low back pain: The critical role of functional goal setting. *APS Journal, 3,* 101–106.

Hazard, R. G., Reeves, V., & Fenwick, J. W. (1992). Lifting capacity: Indices of subject effort. *Spine, 17,* 1065–1070.

Hazard, R. G., Reeves, V., Weisman, G., Fleming, B. C., & Pope, M. H. (1991). Dynamic lifting capacity: The relationship between peak force and weight as an indicator of effort. *Journal of Spinal Disorders, 4,* 63–67.

Hazard, R. G., Reid, S., Fenwick, J. W., & Reeves, V. (1988). Isokinetic trunk and lifting strength measurements: Variability as an indicator of effort. *Spine, 13,* 54–57.

Heaton, R. K., Getto, C. J., Lehman, R. A. W., Fordyce, W. E., Brauer, E., & Groban, S. E. (1982). A standardized evaluation of psychosocial factors in chronic pain. *Pain, 12,* 165–174.

Hildebrandt, J., Pfingsten, M., Saur, P., & Jansen, J. (1997). Prediction of success from a multidisciplinary treatment program for chronic low back. *Spine, 22,* 990–1001.

Holmes, J. A., & Stevenson, C. A. Z. (1990). Differential effects of avoidant and intentional coping strategies on adaptation to chronic and recent-onset pain. *Health Psychology, 9,* 577–584.

Holroyd, K. A., Holm, J. E., Keefe, F. J., Turner, J. A., Bradley, L. A., Murphy, W. D., Johnson, P., Anderson, K., Hinkle, A. L., & O'Malley, W. B. (1992). A multi-center evaluation of the McGill Pain Questionnaire: Results from more than 1700 chronic pain patients. *Pain, 48,* 301–311.

Holzman, A. D., Rudy, T. E., Turk, D. C., Gerber, K. E., Sanders, S. H., Zimmerman, J., & Kerns, R. D. (1985). Chronic pain: A multi-setting comparison of patient characteristics. *Journal of Behavioral Medicine, 8,* 411–422.

Hubbard, J. E., Tracy, J., Morgan, S. F., & McKinney, R. E. (1996). Outcome measures of a chronic pain program: A prospective statistical study. *Clinical Journal of Pain, 12,* 330–337.

Isernhagen, S. (1994). Contemporary issues in functional capacity evaluation. In S. Isernhagen (Ed.), *The comprehensive guide to work injury management* (pp. 410–429). Gaithersburg, MD: Aspen.

Jacobson, R. S., Follette, W. C., & Revenstorf, D. (1984). Psychotherapy outcome research: Methods for reporting variability and evaluating clinical significance. *Behavior Therapy, 15,* 336–352.

Jensen, M. P., & Karoly, P. (1991). Control beliefs, coping efforts, and adjustment to chronic pain. *Journal of Consulting and Clinical Psychology, 59,* 431–438.

Jensen, M. P., & Karoly, P. (1992). Pain-specific beliefs, perceived symptom severity, and adjustment to chronic pain. *Clinical Journal of Pain, 8,* 123–130.

Jensen, M. P., Karoly, P., & Braver, S. (1986). The measurement of clinical pain intensity: A comparison of six methods. *Pain, 27,* 117–126.

Jensen, M. P., Karoly, P., & Huger, R. (1987). The development and preliminary validation of an instrument

to assess patients' attitudes toward pain. *Journal of Psychosomatic Research, 31,* 393–400.

Jensen, M. P., & McFarland, C. A. (1993). Increasing the reliability and validity of pain intensity measurement in chronic pain patients. *Pain, 55,* 195–203.

Jensen, M. P., Strom, S. E., Turner, J. A., & Romano, J. M. (1992). Validity of the Sickness Impact Profile Roland scale as a measure of dysfunction in chronic pain patients. *Pain, 50,* 157–162.

Jensen, M. P., Turner, J. A., & Romano, J. M. (1991). Self-efficacy and outcome expectancies: Relationship to chronic pain coping strategies and adjustment. *Pain, 44,* 263–269.

Jensen, M. P., Turner, J. A., & Romano, J. M. (1994). Correlates of improvement in multidisciplinary treatment of chronic pain. *Journal of Consulting and Clinical Psychology, 62,* 172–179.

Jensen, M. P., Turner, J. A., Romano, J. M., & Karoly, P. (1991). Coping with chronic pain: A critical review of the literature. *Pain, 47,* 249–283.

Jensen, M. P., Turner, J. A., Romano, J. M., & Lawler, B. K. (1994). Relationship of pain-specific beliefs to chronic pain adjustment. *Pain, 57,* 301–309.

Jensen, M. P., Turner, L. R., Turner, J. A., & Romano, J. M. (1996). The use of multiple-item scales for pain intensity measurement in chronic pain patients. *Pain, 67,* 35–40.

Jerome, A., & Gross, R. T. (1991). Pain Disability Index: Construct and discriminant validity. *Archives of Physical Medicine and Rehabilitation, 72,* 920–922.

Keefe, F. J., Affleck, G., Lefebvre, J. C., Starr, K., Caldwell, D. S., & Tennen, H. (1997). Pain coping strategies and coping efficacy in rheumatoid arthritis: A daily process analysis. *Pain, 69,* 35–42.

Keefe, F. J., & Block, A. R. (1982). Development of an observation method for assessing pain behavior in chronic low back pain patients. *Behavior Therapy, 13,* 363–375.

Keefe, F. J., Brantley, A., Manuel, G., & Crisson, J. E. (1985). Behavioral assessment of head and neck cancer pain. *Pain, 23,* 327–336.

Keefe, F. J., Brown, G. K., Wallston, K. A., & Caldwell, D. S. (1989). Coping with rheumatoid arthritis pain: Catastrophizing as a maladaptive strategy. *Pain, 37,* 51–57.

Keefe, F. J., Caldwell, D. S., Queen, K. T., Gil, K. M., Martinez, S., Crisson, J. E., Ogden, W., & Nunley, J. (1987). Osteoarthritic knee pain: A behavioral analysis. *Pain, 28,* 309–321.

Keefe, F. J., Crisson, J. E., & Trainor, J. J. (1987). Observational methods for assessing pain: A practical guide. In J. A. Blumenthal & D. C. McKee (Eds.), *Applications in behavioral medicine and health psychology: A clinician's source book* (pp. 67–94). Sarasota, FL: Professional Resource Exchange.

Keefe, F. J., & Williams, D. A. (1992). Assessment of pain behaviors. In D. C. Turk & R. Melzack (Eds.), *Handbook of pain assessment* (pp. 277–292). New York: Guilford Press.

Keeley, J., Mayer, T., Cox, R., Gatchel, R., Smith, J., & Mooney, V. (1986). Quantification of lumbar function: 5. Reliability of range of motion measures in the sagittal plane and an in vivo torso rotation measurement technique. *Spine, 11,* 31–35.

Kerns, R. D., & Haythornthwaite, J. A. (1988). Depression among chronic pain patients: Cognitive-behav ioral analysis and effect on rehabilitation outcome. *Journal of Clinical and Consulting Psychology, 56,* 870–876.

Kerns, R. D., & Jacob, M. C. (1992). Assessment of the psychosocial context of the experience of chronic pain. In D. C. Turk & R. Melzack (Eds.), *Handbook of pain assessment* (pp. 235–253). New York: Guilford Press.

Kerns, R. D., Turk, D. C., Holzman, A. D., & Rudy, T. E. (1986). Comparison of cognitive-behavioral and behavioral approaches to the outpatient treatment of chronic pain. *Clinical Journal of Pain, 1,* 195–203.

Kerns, R. D., Turk, D. C., & Rudy, T. E. (1985). The West Haven-Yale Multidimensional Pain Inventory (WHYMPI). *Pain, 21,* 345–356.

Kinney, R. K., Gatchel, R. J., & Mayer, T. G. (1991). The SCL-90-R evaluated as an alternative to the MMPI for psychological screening of chronic low-back pain patients. *Spine, 16,* 940–942.

Klein, R. G., & Eek, B. C. (1990). Low-energy laser treatment and exercise for chronic low back pain: Double-blind controlled trial. *Archives of Physical Medicine and Rehabilitation, 71,* 34–37.

Kohles, S., Barnes, D., Gatchel, R., & Mayer, T. (1990). Improved physical performance outcomes after functional restoration treatment in patients with chronic low-back pain: Early versus recent training results. *Spine, 15,* 1321–1324.

Kores, R. C., Murphy, W. D., Rosenthal, T. L., Elias, D. B., & North, W. C. (1990). Predicting outcome of chronic pain treatment via a modified self-efficacy scale. *Behavior Research and Therapy, 28,* 165–169.

Kori, S. H., Miller, R. P., & Todd, D. D. (1990, January/February). Kinesiophobia: A new view of chronic pain behavior. *Pain Management,* pp. 35–43.

Kulich, R., & Lande, S. D. (1997). Managed care: The past and future of pain treatment. *APS Bulletin, 7,* 1, 4–5.

Lansky, D., Butler, J. B. V., & Waller, F. T. (1992). Using health status measures in the hospital setting: From acute care to "outcomes management." *Medical Care, 30,* 57–73.

Lawson, K., Reesor, K. A., Keefe, J. J., & Turner, J. A. (1990). Dimensions of pain-related cognitive coping: Cross validation of the factor structure of the Coping Strategy Questionnaire. *Pain, 43,* 195–204.

Lefebvre, M. F. (1981). Cognitive distortion in depressed psychiatric and low back pain patients. *Journal of Consulting and Clinical Psychology, 49,* 517–525.

Little, D. G., & MacDonald, D. (1994). The use of the percentage change in Oswestry Disability Index score as an outcome measure in lumbar spinal surgery. *Spine, 19,* 2139–2143.

Loebl, W. Y. (1967). Measurement of spinal posture and range in spinal movements. *Annals of Physical Medicine, 9,* 103.

Lorig, K., Chastain, R. L., Ung, E., Shoor, S., & Holman, H. (1989). Development and evaluation of a scale to measure perceived self-efficacy in people with arthritis. *Arthritis and Rheumatology, 32,* 37–44.

Love, A. W., & Peck, C. L. (1987). The MMPI and psychosocial factors in chronic low back pain: A review. *Pain, 28,* 1–28.

Machin, D., Lewith, G. T., & Wylson, S. (1988). Pain measurement in randomized clinical trials: A comparison of two pain scales. *Clinical Journal of Pain, 4,* 161–168.

Malec, J., Cayner, J. J., Harvey, R. F., & Timming, R. C. (1981). Pain management: Long-term follow-up of an inpatient program. *Archives of Physical Medicine and Rehabilitation, 62,* 369–372.

Margolis, R. B., Chibnall, J. T., & Tait, R. C. (1988). Test-retest reliability of the pain drawing instrument. *Pain, 33,* 49–53.

Margolis, R. B., Tait, R. C., & Krause, S. J. (1986). A rating system for use with patient pain drawings. *Pain, 24,* 57–65.

Martin, M. Y., Bradley, L. A., Alexander, R. W., Alarcon, G. S., Triana-Alexander, M., Aaron, L. A., & Alberts, K. R. (1996). Coping strategies predict disability in patients with primary fibromyalgia. *Pain, 68,* 45–53.

Matheson, L. N., Brophy, R. G., Vaughan, K. D., Nunez, C., & Saccoman, K. A. (1995). Workers' compensation managed care: Preliminary findings. *Journal of Occupational Medicine, 5,* 27–36.

Max, M. B., Kishore-Kumar, R., Schafer, S. C., Meister, B., Gracely, R. H., Smoller, B., & Dubner, R. (1991). Efficacy of desipramine in painful diabetic neuropathy: A placebo-controlled trial. *Pain, 45,* 3–9.

Mayer, T. G., Barnes, D., Nichols, G., Kishino, N. D., Coval, K., Piel, B., Hoshino, D., & Gatchel, R. J. (1988). Progressive isoinertial lifting evaluation: II. A comparison with isokinetic lifting in a disabled chronic low-back pain industrial population. *Spine, 13,* 998–1002.

Mayer, T. G., Gatchel, R. J., Kishino, N., Keeley, J., Mayer, H., Capra, P., & Mooney, V. (1986). A prospective short-term study of chronic low back pain patients utilizing novel objective functional measurement. *Pain, 25,* 53–68.

Mayer, T. G., Gatchel, R. J., Mayer, H., Kishino, N. D., Keeley, J., & Mooney, V. (1987). A prospective two-year study of functional restoration in industrial low back injury. *Journal of the American Medical Association, 258,* 1763–1767.

Mayer, T. G., Tabor, J., Bovasso, E., & Gatchel, R. J. (1994). Physical progress and residual impairment quantification after functional restoration: Part I. Lumbar mobility. *Spine, 19,* 389–394.

McArthur, D. L., Cohen, M. J., Gottlieb, H. J., Naliboff, B. D., & Schandler, S. L. (1987). Treating chronic low back pain: II. Long-term follow-up. *Pain, 29,* 23–38.

McCracken, L. M., Gross, R. T., Sorg, P. J., & Edmands, T. A. (1993). Prediction of pain in patients with chronic low back pain: Effects of inaccurate prediction and pain-related anxiety. *Behaviour Research and Therapy, 31,* 647–652.

McCracken, L. M., Zayfert, C., & Gross, R. T. (1992). The Pain Anxiety Symptoms Scale: Development and validation of a scale to measure fear of pain. *Pain, 50,* 67–73.

Meade, T. W., Dyer, S., Browne, W., Townsend, J., & Frank, A. O. (1990). Low back pain of mechanical origin: Randomised comparison of chiropractic and hospital outpatient treatment. *British Medical Journal, 300,* 1431–1437.

Melzack, R. (1975). The McGill Pain Questionnaire: Major properties and scoring methods. *Pain, 1,* 277–299.

Melzack, R., & Katz, J. (1992). The McGill Pain Questionnaire: Appraisal and current status. In D. C. Turk & R. Melzack (Eds.), *Handbook of pain assessment* (pp. 152–168). New York: Guilford Press.

Melzack, R., Terrence, C., Fromm, G., & Amsel, R. (1986). Trigeminal neuralgia and atypical facial pain: Use of the McGill Pain Questionnaire for discrimination and diagnosis. *Pain, 27,* 297–302.

Miaskowski, C., Zimmer, E. F., Barrett, K. M., Dibble, S. L., & Wallhagen, M. (1997). Differences in patients' and family caregivers' perceptions of the pain experience influence patient and caregiver outcomes. *Pain, 72,* 217–226.

Millon, T., Green, C., & Meagher, R. (1983). *Millon Behavioral Health Inventory Manual* (3rd ed.). Minneapolis, MN: National Computer Systems.

Mitchell, R. I., & Carmen, G. M. (1994). The functional restoration approach to the treatment of chronic pain in patients with soft tissue and back injuries. *Spine, 19,* 633–642.

Moore, J. E., Armentrout, D. P., Parker, J. C., & Kivlahan, D. R. (1986). Empirically-derived pain-patient MMPI subgroups: Prediction of treatment outcome. *Journal of Behavioral Medicine, 9,* 51–63.

Moore, J. E., McFall, M. E., Kivlahan, D. R., & Capestany, F. (1988). Risk of misinterpretation of MMPI Schizophrenia scale elevations in chronic pain patients. *Pain, 32,* 207–213.

Moore, M. E., Berk, S. N., & Nypaver, A. (1984). Chronic pain: Inpatient treatment with small group effects. *Archives of Physical Medicine and Rehabilitation, 65,* 356–361.

North, R. B., Ewend, M. G., Lawton, M. T., & Piantadosi, S. (1991). Spinal cord stimulation for chronic, intractable pain: Superiority of "multi-channel" devices. *Pain, 44,* 119–130.

North, R. B., Nigrin, D. J., Fowler, K. R., Szymanski, R. E., & Piantadosi, S. (1992). Automated "pain drawing" analysis by computer-controlled patient-interactive neurological stimulation system. *Pain, 50,* 51–57.

Novy, D. M., Nelson, D. V., Berry, L. A., & Averill, P. M. (1995). What does the Beck Depression Inventory measure in chronic pain?: A reappraisal. *Pain, 61,* 261–270.

Novy, D. M., Nelson, D. V., Francis, D. J., & Turk, D. C. (1995). Selected theoretical perspectives of chronic pain: Specifying structural models. *Pain Forum, 4,* 265–272.

Ohlund, C., Lindstrom, I., Areskoug, B., Eek, C., Peterson, L.-E., & Nachemson, A. (1994). Pain behavior in industrial subacute low back pain: I. Reliability: Concurrent and predictive validity of pain behavior assessments. *Pain, 58,* 201–209.

Osterhaus, J. T., Townsend, J. F., Gandek, B., & Ware, J. E. (1994). Measuring the functional status and well-being of patients with migraine headaches. *Headache, 34,* 337–343.

Parsons, T. (1951). *The social system.* New York: Free Press.

Peters, J., Large, R. G., & Elkind, G. (1992). Follow-up results from a randomized controlled trial evaluating in- and outpatient pain management program. *Pain, 50,* 41–50.

Pfingsten, M., Hildebrandt, J., Leibing, E., Franz, C., & Saur, R. (1997). Effectiveness of a multimodal treatment program for chronic low-back pain. *Pain, 73,* 77–86.

Polatin, P. B., Cox, B., Gatchel, R. J., & Mayer, T. G. (1997). A prospective study of Waddell signs in patients with chronic low back pain: When they may not be predictive. *Spine, 22,* 1618–1621.

Pollard, C. A. (1984). Preliminary validity study of the Pain Disability Index. *Perceptual and Motor Skills, 59,* 974.

Prokop, C. K. (1986). Hysteria scale elevations in low back pain patients: A risk factor for misdiagnosis? *Journal of Consulting and Clinical Psychology, 54,* 558–562.

Radloff, L. (1977). The CES-D scale: A self-report depression scale for research in the general population. *Journal of Applied Psychological Measurement, 1,* 385–401.

Rainville, J., Ahern, D. K., Phalen, L., Childs, L. A., & Sutherland, R. (1992). The association of pain with physical activities in chronic low back pain. *Spine, 17,* 1060–1064.

Ralphs, J. A., Williams, A. C. de C., Richardson, P. H., Pither, C. E., & Nicholas, M. K. (1994). Opiate reduction in chronic pain patients: A comparison of patient-controlled reduction and staff controlled cocktail methods. *Pain, 56,* 279–288.

Ransford, A. O., Cairns, D. C., & Mooney, V. (1976). The pain drawing as an aid to the psychologic evaluation of patients with low-back pain. *Spine, 1,* 127–134.

Richards, J. S., Nepomuceno, C., Riles, M., & Suer, A. (1982). Assessing pain behavior: The UAB Pain Behavior Scale. *Pain, 14,* 393–398.

Riley, J. F., Ahern, D. K., & Follick, M. J. (1988). Chronic pain and functional impairment: Assessing beliefs about their relationship. *Archives of Physical Medicine and Rehabilitation, 59,* 579–582.

Roberts, A. H., & Reinhardt, L. (1980). The behavioral management of chronic pain: Long-term follow-up with comparison group. *Pain, 8,* 151–162.

Robinson, M. E., Greene, A. F., O'Connor, P., Graves, J. E., & MacMillan, M. (1992). Reliability of lumbar isometric torque in patients with chronic low back pain. *Physical Therapy, 72,* 186–190.

Robinson, M. E., MacMillan, M., O'Connor, P., Fuller, A., & Cassisi, J. (1991). Reproducibility of maximal versus submaximal efforts in an isometric lumbar extension task. *Journal of Spinal Disorders, 4,* 444–448.

Robinson, M. E., Myers, C. D., Sadler, I. J., Riley, J. L., Kvaal, S. A., & Geisser, M. E. (1997). Bias effects in three common self-report pain assessment measures. *Clinical Journal of Pain, 13,* 74–81.

Roland, M., & Morris, R. (1983a). A study of the natural history of back pain: I. Development of a reliable and sensitive measure of disability in low-back pain. *Spine, 8,* 141–144.

Roland, M., & Morris, R. (1983b). A study of the natural history of back pain: II. Development of guidelines for trials of treatment in primary care. *Spine, 8,* 145–150.

Romano, J. M., Syrjala, K. L., Levy, R. L., Turner, J. A., Evans, P., & Keefe, F. J. (1988). Observational assessment of pain behaviors: Relationship to patient functioning and treatment outcome. *Behavior Therapy, 19,* 191–201.

Romano, J. M., & Turner, J. A. (1985). Chronic pain and depression: Does the evidence support a relationship? *Psychological Bulletin, 97,* 18–34.

Rosenstiel, A. K., & Keefe, F. J. (1983). The use of coping strategies in chronic low back pain patients: Relationship to patient characteristics and current adjustment. *Pain, 17,* 33–44.

Rudy, T. E., Turk, D. C., Kubinski, J. A., & Zaki, H. S. (1995). Differential treatment responses of TMD patients as a function of psychological characteristics. *Pain, 61,* 103–112.

Ruta, D. A., Garratt, A. M., Wardlaw, D., & Russell, I. T. (1994). Developing a valid and reliable measure of health outcome for patients with low back pain. *Spine, 19,* 1887–1896.

Rybstein-Blinchik, E. (1979). Effects of different cognitive strategies on chronic pain experience. *Journal of Behavioral Medicine, 2,* 93–101.

Salovey, P., Smith, A. F., Turk, D. C., Jobe, J. B., & Willis, G. B. (1993). The accuracy of memory for pain: Not so bad most of the time. *American Pain Society Journal, 2,* 184–191.

Santor, D. A., Zuroff, D. C., Ramsey, J. O., Cervantes, P., & Palacios, J. (1995). Examining scale discriminability in the BDI and CES-D as a function of depressive severity. *Psychological Assessment, 7,* 131–139.

Schwartz, D. P. M, DeGood, D. E., & Shutty, M. S. (1985). Direct assessment of beliefs and attitudes of chronic pain patients. *Archives of Physical Medicine and Rehabilitation, 66,* 806–809.

Shutty, M. S., DeGood, D. E., & Tuttle, D. H. (1990). Chronic pain patients' beliefs about their pain and treatment outcomes. *Archives of Physical Medicine and Rehabilitation, 71,* 128–132.

Slater, M. A., Doctor, J. N., Pruitt, S. D., & Atkinson, J. H. (1997). The clinical significance of behavioral treatment for chronic low back pain: An evaluation of effectiveness. *Pain, 71,* 257–263.

Slater, M. A., Itall, H. F., Atkinson, J. H., & Garfin, S. R. (1991). Pain and impairment beliefs in chronic low back pain: Validations of the Pain and Impairment Relationship Scale (PAIRS). *Pain, 44,* 51–56.

Snow-Turek, A. L., Norris, M. P., & Tan, G. (1996). Active and passive coping strategies in chronic pain patients. *Pain, 64,* 455–462.

Spektor, S. (1990). Chronic pain and pain related disabilities. *Journal of Disability, 1,* 98–102.

Spielberger, C. D., Gorsuch, R. L., & Lushene, R. N. (1970). *Manual for the State–Trait Anxiety Inventory.* Palo Alto, CA: Consulting Psychologists Press.

Spinhoven, P., & Linssen, A. C. G. (1991). Behavioral treatment of chronic low back pain: I. Relation of coping strategy use to outcome. *Pain, 45,* 29–34.

Staats, P. S., Hekmat, H., & Staats, A. W. (1996). The psychological behaviorism theory of pain: A basis for unity. *Pain Forum, 5,* 194–207.

Strax, D. E., Turk, D. C., Rosomoff, H., & Jafri, I. (1997, Oct.). Outcome data collection and cost assessment utilizing different approaches. Symposium conducted at the 16th Annual Scientific Meeting of the American Pain Society, New Orleans.

Strong, J., Ashton, R., & Chant, D. (1992). The measurement of attitudes towards and beliefs about pain. *Pain, 48,* 227–236.

Strong, J., Ashton, R., & Large, R. G. (1994). Function and the patient with chronic low back pain. *Clinical Journal of Pain, 10,* 191–196.

Sturgis, E. T., Schaefer, C. A., & Sikora, T. L. (1984). Pain center follow-up study of treated and untreated patients. *Archives of Physical Medicine and Rehabilitation, 65,* 301–303.

Tait, R. C. (1993). Psychological factors in the assessment of disability among patients with chronic pain. *Journal of Back and Musculoskeletal Rehabilitation, 3,* 20–47.

Tait, R. C., & Chibnall, J. T. (1997). Development of a brief version of the Survey of Pain Attitudes. *Pain, 70,* 229–235.

Tait, R. C., Chibnall, J. T., Duckro, P. N., & Deshields, T. L. (1989). Stable factors in chronic pain. *Clinical Journal of Pain, 5,* 323–328.

Tait, R. C., Chibnall, J. T., & Krause, S. (1990). The Pain Disability Index: Psychometric properties. *Pain, 40,* 171–182.

Tait, R. C., Chibnall, J. T., & Margolis, R. B. (1990). Pain extent: Relations with psychological state, pain severity, pain history, and disability. *Pain, 41,* 295–301.

Tait, R. C., Duckro, P. N., Margolis, R. B., & Wiener, R. (1988). Quality of life following treatment: A preliminary study of in- and outpatients with chronic pain. *International Journal of Psychiatry in Medicine, 18,* 271–282.

Talo, S., Hendler, N., & Brodie, J. (1989). Effects of active and completed litigation on treatment results: Workers' compensation patients compared with other litigation patients. *Journal of Occupational Medicine, 31,* 265–269.

Taylor, M. E. (1989). Return to work following back surgery: A review. *American Journal of Industrial Medicine, 16,* 79–88.

Toomey, T. C., Gover, V. F., & Jones, B. N. (1983). Site of pain: Relationship to measures of pain description, behavior and personality. *Pain, 17,* 289–300.

Turk, D. C., & Melzack, R. (Eds.). (1992). *Handbook of pain assessment.* New York: Guilford Press.

Turk, D. C., & Okifuji, A. (1994). Detecting depression in chronic pain patients: Adequacy of self-reports. *Behaviour Research and Therapy, 32,* 9–16.

Turk, D. C., & Rudy, T. E. (1990). Neglected factors in chronic pain treatment outcome studies: Referral patterns, failure to enter treatment, and attrition. *Pain, 43,* 7–25.

Turk, D. C., & Rudy, T. E. (1991). Neglected topics in the treatment of chronic pain patients—relapse, noncompliance, and adherence enhancement. *Pain, 44,* 5–28.

Turk, D. C., & Rudy, T. E. (1992). Classification logic and strategies in chronic pain. In D. C. Turk & R. Melzack (Eds.), *Handbook of pain assessment* (pp. 409–428). New York: Guilford Press.

Turk, D. C., Rudy, T. E., & Sorkin, B. A. (1993). Neglected topics in chronic pain treatment outcome studies: Determination of success. *Pain, 53,* 3–16.

Turner, J. A., & Romano, J. M. (1984). Self-report screening measures for depression in chronic pain patients. *Journal of Clinical Psychology, 40,* 909–913.

Tursky, B., Jamner, I. D., & Friedman, R. (1982). The pain perception profile: A psychophysical approach to the assessment of pain report. *Behavior Therapy, 13,* 376–394.

Vlaeyen, J. W. S., Kole-Snijders, A. M. J., Boeren, R. G. B., & van Eek, H. (1995). Fear of movement/(re)injury in chronic low back pain and its relation to behavioral performance. *Pain, 62,* 363–372.

Von Korff, M., Dworkin, S., & Le Resche, L. (1990). Graded chronic pain status: An epidemiologic evaluation. *Pain, 40,* 279–291.

Waddell, G. (1996). Low back pain: A twentieth century health care enigma. *Spine, 21,* 2820–2825.

Waddell, G., Newton, M., Henderson, I., Somerville, D., & Main, C. (1993). A Fear-Avoidance Beliefs Questionnaire (FABQ) and the role of fear-avoidance beliefs in chronic low back pain and disability. *Pain, 52,* 157–168.

Wallis, B. J., Lord, S. M., & Bogduk, N. (1997). Resolution of psychological distress of whiplash patients following treatment by radiofrequency neurotomy: A randomised, double-blind, placebo-controlled trial. *Pain, 73,* 15–22.

Wallston, K. A., Wallston, B. S., & DeVellis, R. (1978). Development of the Multidimensional Health Locus of Control (MHLC) Scales. *Health Education Monographs, 6,* 160–170.

Ward, N. G. (1986). Tricyclic antidepressants for chronic low back pain: Mechanism of action and predictors of response. *Spine, 11,* 661–665.

Ware, J. E. (1995). The status of health assessment 1994. *Annual Review of Public Health, 16,* 327–354.

Ware, J. E., & Sherbourne, C. D. (1992). The SF-36 health status survey: I. Conceptual framework and item selection. *Medical Care, 30,* 473–483.

Webster, B. S., & Snook, S. H. (1994). The cost of 1989 workers' compensation low back pain claims. *Spine, 19,* 1111–1116.

Wen, S. W., Hernandez, R., & Naylor, C. D. (1995). Pitfalls in nonrandomized outcomes studies. *Journal of the American Medical Association, 274,* 1687–1691.

Wesley, A. L., Gatchel, R. J., Polatin, P. B., Kinney, R. A.,

& Mayer, T. G. (1991). Differentiation between somatic and cognitive/affective components components in commonly used measurements of depression in patients with chronic low-back pain: Let's not mix apples and oranges. *Spine, 16,* 5213–5215.

White, K. P., & Harth, M. (1996). An analytical review of 24 controlled clinical trials for fibromyalgia syndrome (FMS). *Pain, 64,* 211–219.

Williams, A. C., & Richardson, P. H. (1993). What does the BDI measure in chronic pain? *Pain, 55,* 259–266.

Williams, A. C., Richardson, P. H., Nicholas, M. K., Pither, C. E., Harding, V. R., Ridout, K. L., Ralphs, J. A., Richardson, I. H., Justins, D. M., & Chamberlain, J. H. (1996). Inpatient vs. outpatient pain management: Results of a randomised controlled trial. *Pain, 66,* 13–22.

Williams, D. A., Robinson, M. E., & Geisser, M. E. (1994). Pain beliefs: Assessment and utility. *Pain, 59,* 71–78.

Williams, D. A., & Thorn, B. E. (1989). An empirical assessment of pain beliefs. *Pain, 36,* 351–358.

Zung, W. W. K. (1965). A self-rating scale depression scale. *Archives of General Psychiatry, 12,* 63–70.

Chapter 30

Psychosocial Factors and Pain: Revolution and Evolution

DENNIS C. TURK
ROBERT J. GATCHEL

Over the past 3 decades, there has been a growing awareness that pain is more than a sensory phenomenon; rather, it is a complex perceptual experience comprised of the integration of psychosocial and behavioral–functional factors, as well as somatic ones. The shift away from the perception of pain as a purely sensory phenomenon to pain as a perceptual experience has been given the greatest impetus by the work of several psychologists and their collaborators from other disciplines. Some of the most notable contributions include the following:

> The formulation of the gate control theory of pain by Ronald Melzack and Patrick Wall (Melzack & Casey, 1968; Melzack & Wall, 1965).
> The application and extension of the principles of operant conditioning to pain by Wilbert Fordyce (1976).
> Demonstration of the conscious control of the autonomic nervous system by Neal Miller (1969) and John Basmajian (1963).
> Demonstration of the role of cognitive processes (e.g., beliefs, appraisals, and expectations) in disability and response to treatment (e.g., Sternbach, 1974; Gottlieb et al., 1977; Turk, Meichenbaum, & Genest, 1983).

Each of these areas has had a major impact in contributing to the understanding of pain, has

resulted in the development of assessment methods, and has converged to serve as the basis for innovative treatment methods. In a sense, by their efforts, these pioneering psychologists created a revolution in the field of pain. The preceding chapters in this volume have illustrated the tremendous advances that have been made. Before considering the future, it is worth spending some time reviewing the major impetuses that served as the basis for our current understanding and that will instigate continued evolution.

GATE CONTROL THEORY

Melzack and his collaborators (Melzack & Casey, 1968; Melzack & Wall, 1965) postulated that the experience of pain resulted from the neurophysiological integration of motivational–affective, cognitive–evaluative, and sensory–discriminative contributions. The gate control theory did not give priority to sensory input, nor did it treat sensory phenomena as isomorphic to pain. Rather, pain was postulated to result from the integration and interpretation of sensory and psychological processes and was, therefore, a perceptual process.

Melzack (1975) developed an assessment instrument, the McGill Pain Questionnaire (MPQ), designed to assess the three central components of the conceptual features of the gate control theory.

The MPQ provides a quantitative measurement of patients' ratings of pain intensity, as well as separate indexes of sensory, affective, and evaluative aspects of pain. Since its publication, the MPQ has served a variety of clinical and experimental purposes. Some of the uses include (1) characterization of the pain experienced by patients with diverse medical diagnoses, (2) use as a diagnostic tool to identify specific disease categories, and (3) use as an outcome measure to evaluate the impact of different treatment modalities on the components of pain proposed by the gate control theory.

In addition to increased understanding of the mechanisms underlying pain perception, the gate control theory has had an important impact on treatment. Melzack and Casey (1968) suggested: "The surgical and pharmacological attacks on pain might well profit by redirecting thinking toward the neglected and almost forgotten contributions of motivation and cognitive processes. Pain can be treated not only by trying to cut down sensory input by anesthetic blocks, surgical interventions and the like but by influencing the motivational and cognitive factors as well" (p. 435).

The gate control theory can be credited as a source of inspiration for diverse clinical applications to control or manage pain, including neurophysically based procedures, pharmacological advances, behavioral treatments, and those interventions targeting modification of attentional and perceptual processes in the pain experience (Abram, 1993; Turk et al., 1983). Treatment conceptualizations based on the gate control theory have led to increased emphasis on cognitive and affective contributors to the experience of pain, suffering, and disability. Thus, the gate control theory served as one of the conceptual bases, along with operant conditioning, for the cognitive-behavioral perspective and approach to pain management and functional restoration that, as is evident throughout this volume, has become a dominant paradigm for current treatment and rehabilitative approaches in chronic pain.

OPERANT CONDITIONING

The operant conditioning model, as originally described by Fordyce (1976), noted that when an individual is exposed to a stimulus that causes tissue damage, the immediate response is withdrawal and attempts to escape from the noxious sensations. This may be accomplished by avoidance of activity believed to cause or exacerbate pain, help-seeking to reduce symptoms, and so forth. These behaviors are observable and, consequently, subject to the principles of operant conditioning. The operant conditioning model does not concern itself with the initial cause or report of pain. Rather, it treats pain as an internal subjective experience that may be maintained after an initial physical cause of the symptom has resolved. The operant model draws attention to overt manifestations of pain, distress, and suffering—"pain behaviors"—such as limping, moaning, and avoiding activity.

According to the operant conditioning model, positive reinforcement, such as attention and avoidance of undesirable or feared activities, may serve to maintain the pain behaviors even in the absence of ongoing noxious sensory input. In this way, reflexive behaviors that occur following an acute injury may be maintained by reinforcement even after any tissue damage has resolved.

A particularly important feature of conditioning models of pain noted by Fordyce is pain avoidance. Fordyce and his associates (Fordyce, Shelton, & Dundore, 1982) hypothesized that avoidance behavior does not necessarily require intermittent sensory stimulation from the site of bodily damage, environmental reinforcement, or successful avoidance of aversive social activity to account for the maintenance of protective movements. They suggested that protective behaviors could be maintained by anticipation of aversive consequences based on prior learning, since nonoccurrence of pain is a potent reinforcer.

In addition to the direct effects of positive reinforcement on pain behaviors, operant factors can have an indirect effect on pain. This can be observed when an individual is negatively reinforced for an abnormal pain pattern (e.g., limping)—avoidance of nociception by means of an alteration of ambulatory pattern. Eventually, the maladaptive response patterns that develop may lead to nociception arising from myofascial syndromes that are a consequence of the compensatory activities of muscles associated with the distorted gait.

The learning principle of stimulus generalization is also important, as patients may come to avoid more and more activities that they believe share features in common with those that previously produced pain. Reduction of activity leads to greater physical deconditioning, more activities that elicit pain, and, consequently, even greater disability. Moreover, it is quite probable that the deconditioning following from reinforced inactivity can result directly in increased noxious sensory input. Muscles that were involved in the original injury generally heal rapidly but, due to underuse of these muscle, they are weakened and become subject to noxious stimulation when summoned into action.

The emphasis of Fordyce's operant formulation on pain behaviors has resulted in a number of efforts to develop assessment methods that can evaluate the presence and frequency of performance of these behaviors. Keefe and Block (1982) developed a systematic strategy in which patients are asked to engaged in a set of activities and the presence of different pain behaviors emitted during the performance of these activities is recorded. This method can lead to the identification of the prevalence of specific behaviors that may be targeted during treatment. Moreover, change in pain behaviors has been used as an outcome measure in treatment studies.

Treatments based on operant learning attempt to extinguish pain behaviors (e.g., "downtime") and reinforce well behaviors (e.g., exercise), irrespective of pain. Attention from significant others (e.g., health care professionals, family members) is withdrawn from pain behaviors and redeployed to well behaviors. A major tactic for increasing well behaviors is physical activity that promotes muscle strength, endurance, and flexibility. A shaping procedure is employed by which activity is gradually increased through progressive quotas and reinforced with rest, positive feedback, and verbal reinforcement (e.g., praise). Engagement in activity should lead to corrective feedback or reassurance that pain based on movement need not signal injury. Failure to perform an activity eliminates the learning opportunity. The reinforcing property of analgesic medications is diminished by switching medication schedules from an "as needed" basis to an interval basis (therefore, medication is time-contingent, not pain-contingent). The amount of medication is then reduced on a specific schedule.

Several studies have provided evidence that supports the underlying assumptions of the operant model. For example, Cairns and Pasino (1977) and Doleys, Crocker, and Patton (1982) demonstrated that pain behaviors and "well behaviors" (e.g., activity) could be decreased by verbal reinforcement. Block, Kremer, and Gaylor (1980) demonstrated that pain patients reported differential levels of pain in an experimental situation depending on whether they knew they were being observed by their spouses or ward clerks. The operant model has also generated what has proven to be an effective treatment for select samples of chronic pain patients (for a review, see Keefe & Williams, 1989) and, more recently, has been incorporated within the cognitive-behavioral model already mentioned, and which will be described later.

Besides operant conditioning mechanisms involved in the development of pain behaviors, classical conditioning is also another form of learning that is related to such behaviors. In an early dramatic indication of how pain perception and the resultant response can be modified through learning, Pavlov (1927) demonstrated what could happen when a slight change was made in a classical conditioning procedure. In a basic classical conditioning paradigm, instead of being preceded by a bell (the conditioned stimulus), the food (an unconditioned stimulus) was preceded by an aversive stimulus such as electric shock or a skin prick. Normally, such conditioned stimuli, when presented alone, would produce a variety of negative emotional responses. What Pavlov reported was that after this conditioning, the dogs failed to demonstrate any negative emotional response to the aversive stimuli. Rather, the dogs began to perceive these aversive stimuli as signals that food was imminent. These aversive stimuli actually elicited salivation and approach rather than avoidance behaviors. Yet another example of how pain can be learned and modified through basic learning principles. Operant conditioning can increase pain behaviors, just as such procedures can be used to modify pain behaviors. Similarly, classical conditioning procedures can be effectively used to decrease pain behavior and avoidance.

VOLUNTARY CONTROL OF AUTONOMIC NERVOUS SYSTEM

The demonstration by Basmajian (1963) and Miller (1969) that people could voluntarily control the somatic and autonomic nervous systems inspired a number of investigations relevant to pain. In particular, there has been some suggestion that physiological parameters such as electrical activity in muscles and skin temperature might be related to specific symptoms such as musculoskeletal pain (e.g., back pain, temporomandibular disorders, tension-type headaches) and vascular headache (migraine). The reasoning was that if maladaptive electrical activity in muscles and vascular activity were associated with specific pain syndromes, then teaching patients to control these maladaptive activities should reduce or eliminate the symptoms.

Electrophysiological methods have been devised to evaluate autonomic activity associated with different pain states (Flor, Miltner, & Birbaumer, 1992). Once maladaptive patterns are identified, these can become the targets of intervention. However, research on the association between autonomic activity and pain and the role of actual alteration of autonomic activity on symptoms are equivocal (Flor & Turk, 1989).

Treatments, most notably biofeedback and diverse relaxation methods, have been developed with the intent of teaching patients how to control maladaptive physiological activity believed to be associated with nociception. Biofeedback involves the use of instrumentation to monitor ongoing physiological signals, objectify these signals (into digital measures, for instance), and then present this information back to the subject with a view to changing it. Recordings of ongoing muscle activity (electromyographic [EMG]) can be detected by electrodes at the site of pain and then filtered and amplified into meaningful output such as a graph or digital display on a screen facing the subject; concurrent recordings of various physiological functions (e.g., EMG, peripheral finger temperature, skin conductance) can be obtained from multiple sites, and the feedback can be delivered in one or more modalities, including auditory, visual, and tactile.

The central idea of biofeedback is promotion of the patient's awareness of otherwise undetected physiological events that may be systematically related to pain. As the patient learns to discriminate changes in physiological events of interest, it becomes more feasible to voluntarily alter these events through cognitive strategies, such as self-talk and imagery, or through musculoskeletal mediation. Any alteration of the physiological process in the desired direction is instantly reinforced by knowledge of success conveyed through biofeedback. This is even more reinforcing if the new information and its corresponding physiological change is followed by a reduction in pain.

After gaining control over physiological responding in the clinic, patients are encouraged to practice and apply the techniques outside of the clinic setting and with proficiency in situations in which they are most relevant. It has been repeatedly demonstrated that, with practice, most people can learn to voluntarily control important physiological functions that may be associated directly with pain and stress.

Biofeedback and relaxation have become treatments for diverse chronic pain syndromes (e.g., headache, temporomandibular disorders, chronic back pain), either as self-contained treatments or as part of more comprehensive interventions. The actual mechanisms underlying the effectiveness of biofeedback is unclear, as several studies have shown minimal association between alterations of autonomic activity and reported pain (e.g., Holroyd et al., 1984; Nouwen & Solinger, 1979). Some have suggested that the efficacy of biofeedback is related more to the sense of control that patients achieve than to any actual control over autonomic activity (Blanchard, 1987; Holroyd et al., 1984).

Indeed, because there is limited evidence that the etiological variables and pathophysiology of the pain are known and can be voluntarily controlled, there is an inherent problem with using biofeedback as the sole treatment for pain patients. As we have seen, pain is a complex phenomenon and not merely a sensory experience. One cannot, therefore, expect that dealing solely with a physiological component of the pain process will completely eliminate the problem. At best, biofeedback should be used as an adjunctive treatment in a more comprehensive, therapeutic regimen.

APPRAISAL, BELIEFS, AND EXPECTATIONS

If one accepts that chronic pain is a complex, subjective phenomenon that is uniquely experienced by each individual, then knowledge about idiosyncratic beliefs, appraisals, and coping repertoires become critical for optimal treatment planning and for accurately evaluating treatment outcome. The cognitive activity of chronic pain patients may contribute to the exacerbation, attenuation, or maintenance of pain, pain behavior, affective distress, and dysfunctional adjustment to chronic pain (Turk, 1996; Turk et al., 1983).

Biological factors that may have initiated the original report of pain play less of a role in disability over time, although secondary problems associated with deconditioning may exacerbate and serve to maintain the problem. Inactivity leads to increased focus on and preoccupation with the body and pain, and these cognitive-attentional changes increase the likelihood of misinterpreting symptoms, preoccupation with symptoms, and the perception of oneself as being disabled. Reduction of activity, fear of reinjury, pain, loss of compensation, and an environment that, perhaps unwittingly, supports the "pain-patient role" can impede alleviation of pain, successful rehabilitation, reduction of disability, and improvement in adjustment.

Cognitive factors may not only affect the patient's behavior and, indirectly, his or her pain but also may actually have a direct effect on physiological factors believed to be associated with the experience of pain (Bandura, Taylor, Williams, Meffort, & Barchas, 1985; Bandura, O'Leary, Taylor, Gauthier, & Gossard, 1987; Flor, Turk, & Birbaumer, 1985).

The cognitive-behavioral formulation posed by Turk and his colleagues (Turk & Meichenbaum, 1984; Turk et al., 1983) was developed to integrate the cognitive factors with somatic factors into a broader understanding of pain and also as a flexible basis for treatment. As Turk and Meichenbaum (1984) suggested, the cognitive-behavioral perspective attempted to create a new way of thinking about individuals who experienced pain. The treatment based on this perspective made use of a whole range of cognitive and behavioral techniques designed to bring about change in how people came to view their situation and their ability to exert control over problems associated with pain.

The most important focus of the cognitive-behavioral model, similar to the operant model, is on the patient, rather than on symptoms and pathophysiology. Unlike the operant model, however, the cognitive-behavioral model places a great deal of emphasis on the patient's thoughts and feelings, as these will influence behavior. Conversely, the cognitive-behavioral model acknowledges that environmental factors can also influence behavior and that behavior can affect the patient's thoughts and feelings. Bandura (1977) refers to this as a process of reciprocal determinism.

As is obvious, the emphasis on the role of a diverse set of psychological factors in pain has resulted in the development of a range of assessment instruments too numerous to review here (see DeGood & Shutty, 1992, and Kerns & Jacob, 1992). Research is needed to systematically evaluate the similarities and overlap among these measures.

From the cognitive-behavioral perspective, assessment and, consequently, treatment of the patient with persistent pain requires a broader strategy than those based on the previous dichotomous models described, one that examines and addresses the entire range of psychosocial and behavioral factors in addition to biomedical ones. Similarly, a number of psychological factors have been demonstrated to be associated with the evolution from acute to chronic pain (e.g., Bigos et al., 1991; Gatchel, Polatin, & Kinney, 1995; see also Linton, Chapter 23, this volume) and response to surgical treatments (Love & Peck, 1987; see

also Block, Chapter 24, this volume). Thus attention to important psychological variables is important in assessing and possibly intervening with these individuals, as well as with chronic pain patients being considered for functional restoration and rehabilitation.

The cognitive-behavioral approach to therapy is implemented within the broad framework of learning theory for the extinction of maladaptive thoughts, feelings, and behaviors and the acquisition of alternatives. After a fundamental reeducation about the nature of pain (in particular, the links among thoughts, emotions, behavior, and physiological processes), the patient is taught a set of specific skills.

More than 250 treatment studies evaluating the efficacy of cognitive-behavioral therapies have been reported in the literature. To date, studies have demonstrated the benefits of this perspective and the approach that follows from it with diverse chronic pain syndromes, including osteoarthritis (e.g., Calfas, Kaplan, & Ingram, 1992), rheumatoid arthritis (e.g., O'Leary, Shoor, Lorig, & Holman, 1988), low back pain (Alaranta et al., 1994), irritable bowel syndrome (Greene & Blanchard, 1994), upper limb pain (Spence, 1989), recurrent abdominal pain (Sanders, Shepherd, Cleghorn, & Woolford, 1994), noncardiac chest pain (Klimes, Mayou, Pearce, & Fagg, 1990), fibromyalgia (Goldenberg et al., 1994; Turk, Okifuji, Sinclair, & Starz, 1998), pelvic pain (Gambone & Reiter, 1990), and temporomandibular disorders (Turk, Zaki, & Rudy, 1993).

People all come to treatment with diverse prior learning histories, sociocultural values, and sets of attitudes, beliefs, expectancies, and coping resources. What the four general areas of contribution by psychologists briefly described here suggest is the importance of addressing psychological and behavioral factors as they are likely to influence how patients adjust to nociceptive input, present themselves, and respond to treatments offered. Viewing all patients with the same medical diagnosis as being similar is likely to prove inadequate. It would seem more prudent to follow these guidelines:

> Attempt to identify patients' idiosyncratic beliefs and relevant reinforcement contingencies that may explain their behavior.
> Address those beliefs, the accompanying emotional state, behaviors, and physiological activity that may be subject to control.
> Increase patients' sense of control.

Match treatments to the individual characteristics of the patients.

Understanding and successfully treating chronic pain patients and, thereby, reducing pain and disability will require attention not only to the organic basis of their symptoms but also to the range of factors that modulate nociception, the pain experience, and disability. It is this realization that is the major contribution of psychology to the field of pain.

As stated by the godfather of the modern field of pain and an anesthesiologist, John Bonica (1953/1990):

> The crucial role of psychologic and environmental factors in causing chronic pain behavior in a significant number of patients only recently received attention. As a consequence, there has emerged a sketch plan of pain apparatus with its receptors, conducting fibers, its centers of elaboration, and its standard function, which is supposed to be applicable to all circumstances. But . . . in so doing, medicine has overlooked the fact that the activity of this apparatus is subject to a constantly changing influence of the mind. (p. 12)

The studies reviewed throughout this volume provide a great deal of support for the role of a range of psychological and behavioral factors in the maintenance and exacerbation of pain and disability. Assessment instruments and procedures have been developed that permit better understanding of the mediating and moderating role and impact of these factors. Treatment strategies have been developed that are designed to address the maladaptive thoughts, feelings, behaviors, and physiological activity associated with pain. Psychologists have become important clinical investigators increasing understanding of pain and have assumed essential roles in the clinical management of pain as parts of multidisciplinary teams and as consultants. We now look to the future and the ongoing evolution of the field of pain.

MAPPING OUT THE FUTURE

Psychologists have been accused of and venerated for their ability to read minds and predict the future. We know all too well how cloudy is the crystal ball that permits us to predict the future, although our hindsight appears to be 20/20. Thus it is with some trepidation that we turn now from reflecting on the psychological foundations of pain

to cast our gaze into the future and to be prescriptive, making some humble proposals for directions for research that will enable the continuing evolution of the field. We are fortunate that the previous chapters in this volume have provided some suggestions upon which we can build.

Integration of Physical, Psychosocial, and Behavioral Parameters

Examining the contributions of psychological research to pain as we did in the first part of this chapter revealed that major contributors to the evolution were based on the demonstrated relationship between psychological and physiological parameters. A number of the chapters in this book have described models attempting to integrate physiological, psychological, and behavioral factors to explain the perception of pain, disability, and response to treatment. The gate control model and conscious control of autonomic functioning were the forerunners of this movement. The biobehavioral model, the diathesis–stress conceptualization, and the emphasis on the physiological basis of consciousness have expanded thinking about pain, thus continuing the evolution.

Additional effort needs to be devoted toward more closely integrating physical and psychological factors. Sophisticated imaging methods, such as functional magnetic resonance imaging (fMRI) and positron emission tomography (PET), will permit us to examine the effects of psychological factors on brain structures. Greater understanding of the reciprocal interactions among hormonal, endocrine, and psychological factors should advance our understanding and ability to treat pain more effectively.

Research is needed to answer such questions as: How are the anatomy of the nervous system and physiological processes altered by psychological interventions? How do physiological processes and physical status affect mood, thoughts, and behavior? What is the role of genetic predispositions on pain perception and response? How are memories organized, stored, and retrieved so that they influence the pain experience?

Sociocultural and Demographic Influences

A good deal of attention has been given to the important role of significant others (e.g., spouses, partners, family) in influencing pain reports and overt communications of pain distress and suffering. Sociocultural factors are also likely to form a basis for how individuals respond to symptoms and seek and respond to treatment. With an increasingly pluralistic society, sociocultural factors and myths will affect the personal narratives of patients. Studies are needed to develop better understanding of the diverse sociocultural influences and to integrate this within the treatments offered.

Age and sex of individuals are a growing interest in the research community. Research is needed to go beyond the stereotypes and to understand the differential impact of symptoms throughout the life cycle. It is well known that there are significant differences in the prevalence of pain syndromes associated with the different sexes (Unruh, 1996). Some of these differences may be attributable to the meaning of symptoms, symptom presentations, and the stereotypes of health care providers (Weir, Growne, Tunks, Gafni, & Roberts, 1996). There is also a growing body of literature indicating that some of the sex differences may be associated with hormonal and neuroendocrine factors specific to males versus females. The psychological and physiological factors associated with sex are likely to be promising areas of research.

The Transition from Acute to Chronic Pain

The vast majority of individuals who are injured recover in a reasonable amount of time and do not go on to develop chronic disorders. Similarly, a significant number of people who develop chronic diseases associated with pain do not become physically and emotionally disabled. A number of efforts have been made to identify the predictors of disability among these groups (e.g., Gatchel et al., 1995; Turk, 1997). There are, however, few longitudinal studies, and replications are the exception rather than the rule.

Minimal attention has been given to those individuals who recover spontaneously or who make adequate and often exceptional accommodations to their conditions regardless of physical impairments and limitations. Much of what we know about chronic pain syndromes is based on patients who seek treatment. These may not be a representative group. It is most likely that people will seek treatment when they have exacerbations of their symptoms, when things are at their worst. Parenthetically, we can note that treatment seeking when symptoms are worse will likely result in almost any treatment appearing reasonably successful. There is likely to be some interaction between the treatment and statistical regression to the mean. We must be cautious about generalizing from groups seeking treatment to all who might have the same diagnosis. This may create a negative bias and lead to assumptions that may only be appropriate for treatment seekers and not for all people with the syndrome or disease. We must also be cautious about developing sophisticated models about people with a specific diagnosis based on what may be atypical clinical samples who are seen when they are most distressed by their symptoms. In other words, we often see rather biased samples. It is essential that research extend beyond the clinical population to community samples that are not seeking care.

We also need to be cautious about retrospective bias. People with different pain syndromes had prior learning histories that preceded symptom onset. Thus we need to consider the relevance of preceding factors and not focus exclusively on patients at one point in time, the point at which they are seeking treatment. On the flip side, however, we need to keep in mind that when patients who have had symptoms for many years are asked to recall features of their lives prior to symptom onset, they may produce invalid information. All people seek post hoc explanations and causal factors to explain their current situation. Thus the stories recalled and told may lack complete veracity, not because of conscious deception but because of the cognitive heuristics used (Tverskey & Kahneman, 1974; Turk & Salovey, 1986) and the influences of memory. We must resist the temptation to make inferences about causality from correlational data and retrospective interpretations.

A number of studies have begun to identify predictors of disability for injured workers with acute pain states and also predictors of response to treatment. But identifying predictors is insufficient. The next step is to determine whether knowledge of predictors can guide treatment design and the development of strategies for improving outcome. To paraphrase the old behavioral adage, "Insight without changing behavior is a waste of time."

Prevention of Disability

Prevention and earlier interventions hold promise for reduction in the extent of disability. Again, to paraphrase from the wisdom of others, this time the comment of the character Linus in the comic strip *Peanuts*, "There is nothing so anxiety-provoking as to be told one has great potential." The average individual treated at a multidisciplinary pain center averages over 85 months of pain (Flor, Fydrich, & Turk, 1992). By this time, patients have become so disabled that rehabilitation becomes a Herculean task, the outcomes, although reasonably good, could have been improved if implemented at an earlier stage. In Chapter 22 of this volume, Von Korff provided a detailed description of an early intervention program that was implemented in primary care. Linton and Bradley (1996) have reviewed a number of efforts that may be viewed as secondary preventions—that is, treatments used with those who have already had a first pain episode—designed to prevent long-term disability.

Given the natural history of many musculoskeletal pain disorders, it is important that early interventions be reasonably inexpensive. For example, the experience with back pain suggests that a significant percentage of individuals will recover in only a few weeks. Providing expensive interventions for groups with high rates of natural recovery is inefficient and costly. Von Korff reminds us that for a substantial minority of patients, pain will persist or recur even though they return to work in a short time. Efforts to prevent, or at least minimize, the consequences of exacerbations and relapse may be particularly cost-effective. The effects of early interventions are mixed, but the costs of chronicity are so extreme that research in this area is definitely warranted.

Prospective and Process Research

The majority of the research in the field of pain has been cross-sectional. We know little about the evolution and changes that accompany pain conditions over time, as well as throughout the process of treatment. Prospective studies with high-risk populations such as those preparing for amputation (see Katz & Gagliese, Chapter 18, this volume) and herpes zoster patients who are at risk for development of postherpetic neuralgia (Dworkin et al., 1992; see also Dworkin & Banks, Chapter 16, this volume) may be able to tell us a great deal about the changing pain experience, adaptation, and disability. These disorders offer the opportunity to study the evolution of the adaptive processes.

Process research is important not only for observing the evolution of chronic pain syndromes but also for learning about the co-occurrence of physical and psychological factors over time. That

is to say, rather than relying on retrospective reports, it will be useful to investigate the co-occurrences of thoughts, feelings, and behaviors over time. This process approach can also provide useful information about the manner in which changes occur during treatment. For example, what are the relationships between physical and psychological changes during the course of a treatment such as biofeedback? Do autonomic parameters change first, influencing symptoms, mood, thoughts, and behavior, or does mood change first, leading to a different interpretation of symptoms and a subsequent alteration in physiological responses?

Cost Effectiveness of Treatment

The issue of cost effectiveness has been alluded to previously. With changes in health care, cost effectiveness is assuming a role that is at least as important as clinical effectiveness. Chronic pain is expensive, with estimates as high as $125 billion annually for health care and indemnity costs. Specialized pain programs are expensive, averaging $8,1000 for comprehensive treatment programs (Marketdata Enterprises, 1995). If interdisciplinary pain programs are to survive, they will need to demonstrate that they are both clinically and cost effective (Turk & Okifuji, 1997; see also Gatchel & Turk, Chapter 27, this volume, and Cohen & Campbell, 1996).

Many treatments for chronic pain contain a host of components delivered in different ways (e.g., group vs. individual, inpatient vs. outpatient, daily vs. weekly) and include several health care providers. Little attempt has been made to isolate what features are necessary and sufficient to produce the optimal outcomes. Third-party payers are forcing us to consider cost effectiveness. The trend for evidence-based medicine requires that we demonstrate the clinical and cost effectiveness of the treatments that are provided. The research with headache patients demonstrating that "minimal therapist" contact can produce results comparable to those requiring more intensive effort by clinicians (Attanasio, Andrasik, & Blanchard, 1987; Griffiths & Martin, 1996) should encourage us to try to address the issue of what is both necessary and also sufficient to produce the best outcomes.

One size may fit all, but do all need the most extensive (read most expensive) treatment? If an individual has a vitamin A deficiency, he or she may benefit from a multivitamin (the shotgun approach), but it would be more cost efficient to treat him or her with vitamin A alone (the rifle approach). The efficiency of pain treatments will need to become a central focus of research.

Patient Differences and Treatment Matching

There seems no question that psychological and behavioral factors play an important role in pain perception, experience, and response. Many avenues of research still need to be pursued to understand the mechanisms by which these factors produce their effects on physiological processes and behavior. Research has demonstrated that groups of patients may differ in psychosocial and behavioral characteristics, even when the medical diagnosis is identical (Turk & Rudy, 1990; Turk & Okifuji, 1996; Turk, Sist, et al., 1998).

Conversely, people with the same medical diagnosis may vary significantly in their response to their symptoms. For example, Turk and his colleagues have shown that patients with disease and syndromes as diverse as metastatic cancer, back pain, and headaches show similar adaptation patterns, whereas patients with the same diagnosis may show marked variability in their degrees of disability (Turk & Rudy, 1990; Turk, Okifuji, et al., 1998). In one such study, Turk and Rudy (1990) demonstrated that the within-diagnosis variability in adaptation for patients with temporomandibular disorders, low back pain, and headaches was greater than between diagnosis variability. Although there are a number of studies that have identified subgroups of chronic pain patients based on psychological characteristics and psychosocial and behavioral responses, there are only a handful of studies that have actually begun to demonstrate that matching treatments to these characteristics is of any benefit (Rudy, Turk, Kubinski, & Zaki, 1995; Turk, Okifuji, et al., 1998; Turk, Okifuji, Sinclair, & Starz, 1996; Turk, Rudy, Kubinski, Zaki, & Greco, 1996).

The tradition has been to lump patients with the same medical diagnosis or set of symptoms together (e.g., chronic pain syndrome, back pain, fibromyalgia) and then to treat them the same way—again, as if one size fits all. But the differential response of these individuals with the same diagnosis to the same treatment should give us pause. Many common diagnoses for chronic pain syndromes such as low back pain, temporomandibular disorders, headache, and fibromyalgia syndrome are gross categories, and there may be unique features of patients given these generic diagnoses.

Averaging the results of standard treatments may mask the effects. That is, some patients may respond quite well to the treatment, whereas others might actually get worse or show no improvement. The strategy of aggregating these subsets together may mask important differences in outcome. Potentially useful treatments may be ignored because the group as a whole did not respond well.

In passing, it should also be noted that Blanchard (1979) cogently pointed out six important dimensions that one should consider in evaluating clinical applications of therapeutic modalities, using biofeedback as an example. These six dimensions would similarly hold true for the evaluation of pain management procedures and for the issues that we raised previously. The six dimensions that he listed were the following:

> The percentage or fraction of the treated patient sample that demonstrated significant therapeutic improvement.
>
> The degree of clinical meaningfulness of the therapeutic changes that were obtained.
>
> The degree of transfer of changes that were obtained in the clinical setting to the patient's natural environment.
>
> The degree of change in the biopsychosocial response for which the treatment was prescribed.
>
> The degree of replicability of the results by different clinicians and clinical sites.
>
> The extent and thoroughness of the follow-up date obtained.

Each of these are important factors that should be considered when evaluating the therapeutic efficacy of any pain management intervention.

As we noted, similar patterns of psychosocial disability are associated with common diseases and syndromes in which chronic pain is an important clinical feature. Careful reading of the chapters on specific disorders in this volume will reveal that all share features from the psychosocial domain in common—depression, limitations in activities, and increased health care utilization—while each retains those unique physical features from the biological or physical domain related to the specific body site (head, jaw, back) or pathophysiological processes (e.g., postherpetic neuralgia, cancer). Research that includes multiple pain disorders may be useful. We need to be less parochial in focusing our research on only one, our preferred, syndrome (irritable bowel disorder, back pain, cancer) with the assumption that it is uniquely different from others. Actually, those who suffer from different conditions may have more in common with each other than those with the same diagnosis do.

Studies are needed that will determine the benefits of matching interventions to specific patient characteristics (Turk, 1990). The important question is not whether a treatment is effective but rather what treatment components delivered in what way and when produce the most successful outcomes for individual pain sufferers with what set of characteristics.

Motivation for and Adherence to Treatment

The role of psychosocial, affective, cognitive, and behavioral factors in acceptance of treatment, motivation for self-management, and treatment adherence need to become targets of research (Turk & Rudy, 1991). Not all patients are equally ready for treatment (Kerns, Rosenberg, Jamison, Caudill, & Haythornthwaite, 1997). Assessment methods need to be developed to help identify impediments to treatment responsiveness. Intervention strategies that can be used to enhance motivation and receptiveness should be investigated (Jensen, 1996).

We know from many areas of behavior change that the risk of relapse is high. Treating people with recurrent pain and chronic pain often makes major demands for lifestyle changes—relaxing, pacing activities, communicating more effectively, performing exercises, and so forth. If we know that relapse is high for such behavior changes as reduction or elimination of substance use and weight reduction, why would we be surprised that relapse would be high for people with persistent and recurrent pain? Almost all psychological interventions for persistent pain have been shown to be effective, at least for some individuals, but the duration of the benefits varies. Strategies need to be investigated to enhance maintenance of therapeutic gains.

Indeed, a relapse-prevention model was originally developed by Marlatt and Gordon (1980, 1985) to address the problem of long-term maintenance of new health behaviors. It was developed as a means of aiding patients to acquire new coping skills that would reduce the risks of an initial relapse or recurrence, as well as preventing any minor lapses from escalating into a total relapse. The major element of the model, and how it differs from conventional treatment strategies, is that the problem of possible lapses and relapses is neither ignored nor attributed to failures of the treatment management program or the patient. Such lapses and relapses are viewed as an important part of the learning required for long-term successful behavioral change. Keefe and Van Horn (1993) have utilized this type of relapse-prevention model with chronic pain patients. They have outlined a number of relapse-prevention methods to use that can be integrated within a cognitive-behavioral treatment program.

We also need to go beyond the assumption that people who have problems coping with their pain and the problems associated with it simply suffer from a skills deficiency and that simply teaching them appropriate skills will alleviate their problems. Beyond consideration of the skills deficiency, we need to consider production deficiency. That is, what are the impediments to the use of the skills in the natural environment, and what can we do to help patients overcome these obstacles?

Closely aligned with maintenance is adherence. For a treatment to be effective, two things have to occur: The treatment must contain active ingredients, and the treatment must be carried out in an appropriate manner. All too often, we seem to be concerned about the details of the treatment but less about whether our patients adhere to the demands of the treatment. We make recommendations for significant changes in behaviors and expect that our patients will continue to engage in the behaviors that we prescribe. We have been somewhat naive in this expectation (hope, wish, prayer). Yet the long-term rates of adherence by chronic pain patients has been reported to be quite low in some studies (Lutz, Silbret, & Olshan, 1983). Greater attention needs to be given to adherence enhancement methods (Turk & Rudy, 1991). Importantly, we need to make sure that we assess adherence in our research.

We may view a treatment as ineffective when it may in fact have been very effective—but only for those who adhered to the prescriptive behaviors. This was illustrated in a study conducted by Basler and Rehfisch (1991). They evaluated the effectiveness of a cognitive-behavioral treatment for patients with ankylosing spondolitis. On the basis of the group outcome, the cognitive-behavioral treatment did not appear to lead to statistically significant benefits. This might lead to the conclusion that cognitive-behavioral treatment was not an effective treatment for this population. However, when Basler and Rehfisch compared the effects of the treatment for those who were adherent to the recommended behaviors to those who admitted they were nonadherent, it became apparent that the treatment was, indeed, effective but only for those who adhered to it. This is not very surprising—if people do not practice the exercises included within the treatment, why would we be surprised if they did not show positive outcomes? Here the poor results were not due to an inefficacious treatment but rather to the failure of a subset of patients to adhere to the treatment recommendations. Again, we see the importance of not just looking at the effectiveness of the treatment for a group; rather, we need to attend to the characteristics of patients who improved as opposed to the characteristics of those who do not.

Of course, there are many other research questions that are raised by the chapters in this volume. What we have attempted to do is to highlight some of what appear to us to be the most prominent. We have come a long way since the mechanistic, Cartesian dualistic model of pain that was so prominent prior to the 1960s. There have been major strides in understanding the complexity of pain and the important roles of psychosocial and behavioral, as well as physical, factors in the experience of pain. At the dawn of the new millennium, we can look ahead to new challenges and opportunities that await us. Research will assuredly help us to better understand pain, to prevent disability, and to treat the diverse conditions that come under the generic rubric, chronic pain. We expect that the revolution created and led largely by psychologists in the 1960s was only a beginning point that initiated an evolving process. The evolution will require continuing efforts if we hope to better understand pain, to prevent disability, and to provide optimal (clinical and cost effective) treatments.

REFERENCES

Abram, S. E. (1993). Advances in chronic pain management since gate control. *Regional Anesthesia, 18*, 66–81.

Alaranta, H., Rytokoski, U., Rissanen, A., Talo, S., Ronnemaa, T., Pukka, P., Karppi, S. -L., Videman, T., Kallio, V., & Slatis, P. (1994). Intensive physical and psychosocial training program for patients with chronic low back pain: A controlled clinical trial. *Spine, 19*, 1339–1349.

Attanasio, V., Andrasik, F., & Blanchard, E. B. (1987). Cognitive therapy and relaxation training in muscle contraction headaches: Efficacy and cost-effectiveness. *Headache, 27*, 254–260.

Bandura, A. (1977). *Social learning theory.* Englewood Cliffs, NJ: Prentice-Hall.

Bandura, A., O'Leary, A., Taylor, C. B., Gauthier, J., & Gossard, D. (1987). Perceived self-efficacy and pain control: Opioid and nonopioid mechanisms. *Journal of Personality and Social Psychology, 53*, 563–571.

Bandura, A., Taylor, C. B., Williams, S. L., Mefford, I. N., & Barchas, J. D. (1985). Catecholamine secretion as a function of perceived coping self-efficacy. *Journal of Consulting and Clinical Psychology, 53*, 406–414.

Basler, H. -D., & Rehfisch, H. P. (1991). Cognitive-behavioral therapy in patients with ankylosing spondolitis in a German self-help organization. *Journal of Psychosomatic Research, 35*, 345–354.

Basmajian, J. V. (1963). Control and training of individual motor units. *Science, 141*, 440–441.

Bigos, S., Battie, M., Spangler, D., Fisher, A., Fordyce, W., Hansson, T., Nachemson, A., & Wortley, J. (1991). A prospective study of work perceptions and psychosocial factors affecting the report of back injury. *Spine, 16*, 1–6.

Blanchard, E. B. (1979). Biofeedback and the modification of cardiovascular dysfunction. In R. J. Gatchel & K. P. Price (Eds.), *Clinical applications of biofeedback: Appraisal and status.* New York: Pergamon Press.

Blanchard, E. B. (1987). Long-term effects of behavioral treatment of chronic headache. *Behavior Therapy, 18*, 375–385.

Block, A. R., Kremer, A. F., & Gaylor, M. (1980). The spouse as a discriminative cue for pain behavior. *Pain, 9*, 245–252.

Bonica, J. J. (1990). *The management of pain* (2nd ed.). Philadelphia: Lea & Febiger. (Original work published 1953)

Cairns, D., & Pasino, J. A. (1977). Comparison of verbal reinforcement and feedback in the operant treatment of disability due to chronic low back pain. *Behavior Therapy, 8*, 621–630

Calfas, C. J., Kaplan, R. M., & Ingram, R. E. (1992). One year evaluation of cognitive-behavioral intervention in osteoarthritis. *Arthritis Care and Research, 5*, 202–209.

Cohen, M. J. M., & Campbell, J. N. (Eds.). (1996). *Progress in pain research and management: Vol. 7. Pain treatment centers at a crossroads: A practical and conceptual reappraisal.* Seattle, WA: IASP Press.

DeGood, D. E., & Shutty, M. S. (1992). Assessment of pain beliefs, coping and self-efficacy. In D. C. Turk & R. Melzack (Eds.), *Handbook of pain assessment* (pp. 214–234). New York: Guilford Press.

Doleys, D. M., Crocker, M., & Patton, O. (1982). Response of patients with chronic pain to exercise quotas. *Physical Therapy, 62*, 1111–1114.

Dworkin, R. H., Hartstein, G., Rosner, H. L., Walther, R. R., Sweney, E. W., & Brand, L. (1992). A high-risk method for studying psychosocial antecedents of chronic pain: The prospective investigation of herpes zoster. *Journal of Abnormal Psychology, 101*, 200–205.

Flor, H., Fydrich, T., & Turk, D. C. (1992). Efficacy of multidisciplinary pain treatment centers: A meta-analytic review. *Pain, 49*, 221–230.

Flor, H., Miltner, W., & Birbaumer, N. (1992). Psychophysiological recording methods. In D. C. Turk & R. Melzack (Eds.), *Handbook of pain assessment* (pp. 169–190). New York: Guilford Press.

Flor, H., & Turk, D. C. (1989). The psychophysiology of chronic pain: Do chronic pain patients exhibit symptom-specific psychophysiological responses? *Psychological Bulletin, 105*, 215–259.

Flor, H., Turk, D. C., & Birbaumer, N. (1985). Assessment of stress-related psychophysiological responses in chronic back pain patients. *Journal of Consulting and Clinical Psychology, 54*, 354–364.

Fordyce, W. E. (1976). *Behavioral methods for chronic pain and illness.* St. Louis: Mosby.

Fordyce, W. E., Shelton, J., & Dundore, D. (1982). The modification of avoidance learning pain behaviors. *Journal of Behavioral Medicine, 4,* 405–414.

Gambone, J. C., & Reiter, R. C. (1990). Nonsurgical management of chronic pelvic pain: A multidisciplinary approach. *Clinic Obstetrics and Gynecology, 33,* 205–211.

Gatchel, R. J., Polatin, P. B., & Kinney, R. K. (1995). Predicting outcome of chronic back pain using clinical predictors of psychopathology: A prospective analysis. *Health Psychology, 14,* 415–420.

Goldenberg, D. L., Kaplan, K. H., Nadeau, M. G., Broduer, C., Smith, S., & Schmid, C. H. (1994). A controlled study of a stress-reduction, cognitive-behavioral treatment program in fibromyalgia. *Journal of Musculoskeletal Pain, 2,* 53–66.

Gottlieb, H., Strite, L., Koller, R., Madorsky, A., Hockersmith, V., Kleeman, M., & Wagner J. (1977). Comprehensive rehabilitation of patients having chronic low back pain. *Archives of Physical Medicine and Rehabilitation, 58,* 101–108.

Greene, B., & Blanchard, E. B. (1994). Cognitive therapy for irritable bowel syndrome. *Journal of Consulting and Clinical Psychology, 62,* 576–582.

Griffiths, J. D., & Martin, P. R. (1996). Clinical- versus home-based treatment formats for children with chronic headache. *British Journal of Health Psychology, 1,* 151–166.

Holroyd, K. A., Penzien, D. B., Hursey, K. G., Tobin, D. L., Rogers, L., Holm, J. E., Marcille, P. J., Hall, J. R., & Chila, A. G. (1984). Change mechanisms in EMG biofeedback training: Cognitive change underlying improvements in tension headache. *Journal of Consulting and Clinical Psychology, 52,* 1039–1053.

Jensen, M. P. (1996). Enhancing motivation to change in pain treatment. In R. J. Gatchel & D. C. Turk (Eds.), *Psychological approaches to pain management: A practitioner's handbook* (pp. 78–111). New York: Guilford Press.

Keefe, F. J., & Block, A. R. (1982). Development of an observation method for assessing pain behavior in chronic low back pain patients. *Behavior Therapy, 13,* 165–173.

Keefe, F. J., & Van Horn, Y. V. (1993). Cognitive-behavioral treatment of rheumatoid arthritis pain: Maintaining treatment gains. *Arthritis Care and Research, 6,* 213–222.

Keefe, F. J., & Williams, D. A. (1989). New directions in pain assessment and treatment. *Clinical Psychology Review, 9,* 549–568.

Kerns, R. D., & Jacob, M. C. (1992). Assessment of the psychosocial context of the experience of chronic pain. In D. C. Turk & R. Melzack (Eds.), *Handbook of pain assessment* (pp. 235–253). New York: Guilford Press.

Kerns, R. D., Rosenberg, R., Jamison, R., Caudill, M. A., & Haythornthwaite, J. (1997). Readiness to adopt a self-management approach to chronic pain: The pain stages of change questionnaire (PSOCQ). *Pain, 72,* 227–234.

Klimes, I., Mayou, R. A., Pearce, M. J., & Fagg, J. R. (1990). Psychological treatment for atypical non-cardiac chest pain: A controlled evaluation. *Psychological Medicine, 20,* 605–611.

Linton, S. J., & Bradley, L. A. (1996). Strategies for the prevention of chronic pain. In R. J. Gatchel & D. C.

Turk (Eds.), *Psychological approaches to pain management: A practitioner's handbook* (pp. 438–457). New York: Guilford Press.

Love, A. W., & Peck, C. L. (1987). The MMPI and psychological factors in chronic low back pain: A review. *Pain, 28,* 1–12.

Lutz, R. W., Silbret, M., & Olshan, N. (1983). Treatment outcome and compliance with therapeutic regimens: Long-term follow-up of a multidisciplinary pain program. *Pain, 17,* 301–308.

Marketdata Enterprises (1995). *Chronic pain management programs: A market analysis.* Valley Stream, NY: Author.

Marlatt, G. A., & Gordon, J. R. (1980). Determinants of relapse: Implications for the maintenance of behavior change. In P. O. Davidson & S. M. Davidson (Eds.), *Behavioral medicine: Changing health lifestyles* (pp. 145–161). New York: Brunner/Mazel.

Marlatt, G. A., & Gordon, J. R. (Eds.). (1985). *Relapse prevention: Maintenance strategies in the treatment of addictive behaviors.* New York: Guilford Press.

Melzack, R. (1975). The McGill Pain Questionnaire: Major properties and scoring methods. *Pain, 1,* 277–299.

Melzack R., & Casey, K. L. (1968). Sensory, motivational and central control determinants of pain: A new conceptual model. In D. Kenshalo (Ed.), *The skin senses* (pp. 423–443). Springfield, IL: Thomas.

Melzack R., & Wall, P. D. (1965). Pain mechanisms: A new theory. *Science, 50,* 971–979.

Miller, N. E. (1969). Learning of visceral and glandular responses. *Science, 16,* 434–445.

Nouwen, A., & Solinger, J. W. (1979). The effectiveness of EMG biofeedback training in low back pain. *Biofeedback and Self-Regulation, 4,* 103–111.

O'Leary, A., Shoor, S., Lorig, K., & Holman, H. R. (1988). A cognitive-behavioral treatment for rheumatoid arthritis. *Health Psychology, 7,* 527–544.

Pavlov, I. P. (1927). *Conditioned reflexes.* New York: Dover.

Rudy, T. E., Turk, D. C., Kubinski, J. A., & Zaki, H. S. (1995). Differential treatment responses of TMD patients as a function of psychological characteristics. *Pain, 61,* 103–112.

Sanders, M. R., Shepherd, R. W., Cleghorn, G., & Woolford, H. (1994). The treatment of recurrent abdominal pain in children: A controlled comparison of cognitive-behavioral family intervention and standard pediatric care. *Journal of Consulting and Clinical Psychology, 62,* 306–314.

Spence, S. H. (1989). Cognitive behavior therapy in the management of chronic occupational pain of the upper limbs. *Behaviour Research and Therapy, 27,* 435–446.

Sternbach, R. A. (1974). *Pain patients: Traits and treatments.* New York: Academic Press.

Turk, D. C. (1990). Customizing treatment for chronic pain patients: Who, what, and why. *Clinical Journal of Pain, 6,* 255–270.

Turk, D. C. (1996). Biopsychosocial perspective on chronic pain. In R. J. Gatchel & D. C. Turk (Eds.), *Psychological approaches to pain management: A practitioner's handbook* (pp. 3–32). New York: Guilford Press.

Turk, D. C. (1997). The role of demographic and psychosocial factors in the transition from acute to chronic pain. In T. S. Jensen, J. A. Turner, & Z. Wisenfeld-Hallin (Eds.), *Proceedings of the Eighth World Congress on Pain* (pp. 185–214). Seattle, WA: IASP Press.

Turk, D. C., & Meichenbaum, D. (1984). A cognitive-behavioral approach to pain management. In P. D.

Wall & R. Melzack (Eds.), *Textbook of pain* (pp. 787–794). London: Churchill Livingstone.

Turk, D. C., Meichenbaum, D., & Genest, M. (1983). *Pain and behavioral medicine: A cognitive-behavioral perspective.* New York: Guilford Press.

Turk, D. C., & Okifuji, A. (1996). Perception of traumatic onset and compensation status: Impact on pain severity and emotional distress in chronic pain patients. *Journal of Behavioral Medicine, 19,* 435–455.

Turk, D. C., & Okifuji, A. (1997). Multidisciplinary pain centers: Boons or boondoggles? *Journal of Worker's Compensation, 6,* 9–26.

Turk, D. C., Okifuji, A., Sinclair, J. D., & Starz, T. W. (1996). Pain disability, and physical functioning in subgroups of fibromyalgia patients. *Journal of Rheumatology, 23,* 1255–1262.

Turk, D. C., Okifuji, A., Sinclair, J. D., & Starz, T. W. (1998). Differential responses by subgroups of fibromyalgia syndrome patients to an interdisciplinary treatment. *Arthritis Care and Research, 11,* 397–404.

Turk, D. C., & Rudy, T. E. (1990). Robustness of an empirically derived taxonomy of chronic pain patients. *Pain, 43,* 27–36.

Turk, D. C., & Rudy, T. E. (1991). Neglected topics in the treatment of chronic pain patients—relapse, noncompliance, and adherence enhancement. *Pain, 44,* 5–28.

Turk, D. C., Rudy, T. E., Kubinski, J. A., Zaki, H. S., &

Greco, C. M. (1996). Dysfunctional TMD patients: Evaluating the efficacy of a tailored treatment protocol. *Journal of Consulting and Clinical Psychology, 64,* 139–146.

Turk, D. C., & Salovey, P. (1986). Cognitive structures, cognitive processes, and cognitive-behavior modification: I. Client issues. *Cognitive Therapy and Research, 9,* 1–17.

Turk, D. C., Sist, T. C., Okifuji, A., Miner, M. F., Florio, G., Harrison, P., Massey. J., Lema, M. L., Zevon, M. A. (1998). Adaptation to metastatic cancer pain, regional/local cancer pain and non-cancer pain: Role of psychological and behavioral factors. *Pain, 74,* 247–256.

Turk, D. C., Zaki, H. S., & Rudy, T. E. (1993). Effects of intraoral appliance and biofeedback/stress management alone and in combination in treating pain and depression in TMD patients. *Journal of Prosthetic Dentistry, 70,* 158–164.

Tversky, A., & Kahneman, D. (1974). Judgment under uncertainty: Heuristics and biases. *Science, 185,* 1124–1131.

Unruh, A. M. (1996). Gender variations in clinical pain experience. *Pain, 65,* 123–167.

Weir, R., Growne, G., Tunks, E., Gafni, A., & Roberts, J. (1996). Gender differences in psychosocial adjustment to chronic pain and expenditures for health care services used. *Clinical Journal of Pain, 12,* 277–290.

Index

(*f* indicates a figure; *t* indicates a table)